Health and Wellness

Fifth Edition

Health and Wellness

Gordon Edlin
John A. Burns School of Medicine
University of Hawaii

Eric Golanty
Las Positas College

Kelli McCormack Brown
Department of Health Sciences
Illinois State University

Jones and Bartlett Publishers
Sudbury, Massachusetts
Boston   London   Singapore

Editorial, Sales, and Customer Service Offices
Jones and Bartlett Publishers
40 Tall Pine Drive
Sudbury, MA 01776
508-443-5000
800-832-0034

Jones and Bartlett Publishers International
Barb House, Barb Mews
London W6 7PA
England

Library of Congress Cataloging-in-Publication Data
Edlin, Gordon
     Health and wellness / Gordon Edlin, Eric Golanty, Kelli McCormack
  Brown.—5th ed.
        p.   cm.
     Includes bibliographical references and index.
     ISBN 0-86720-994-1
     1. Health.   2. Holistic medicine.   I. Golanty, Eric.   II. Brown, Kelli McCormack.   III. Title.
RA776.E24 1996
613--dc20   95-51780
                                                                  CIP

Chief Executive Officer: Clayton E. Jones
Chief Operating Officer: Donald W. Jones, Jr.
Vice President, Production and Manufacturing: Paula Carroll
Vice President and Editor-in-Chief: David P. Geggis
Director of Sales and Marketing: Rob McCarry
Marketing Manager: Anne T. King
Acquisitions Editor: Joseph E. Burns
Assistant Production Manager/Coordination: Judy Songdahl

Senior Manufacturing Buyer: Dana L. Cerrito
Design: Glenna Collett
Editorial Production: Books By Design, Inc.
Illustrations: JAK Graphics
Typesetting: The Clarinda Company
Color Separation: The Clarinda Company
Printing and Binding: Banta Company
Cover Printing: Henry N. Sawyer Company

Photo Credits:
Part One: p. 1, top left; p. 2, bachmann/Stock, Boston; p. 4, Frank Priegue/International Stock; p. 13, Lawrence Migdale/Photo Researchers, Inc.; p. 1, top right, p. 20, Bob Daemmrich/Stock, Boston; p. 30, Richard Hutchings/Photo Researchers, Inc.; p. 32, Asian Art Museum of San Francisco; p. 1, bottom left, p. 36, Bob Daemmrich/Stock, Boston; p. 49, Oliver Strewe/Tony Stone Images; p. 54, J. Gerard Smith/Photo Researchers, Inc.; p. 1, bottom right, p. 56, Joe Nettis/Photo Researchers, Inc.; p. 58, Richard Hutchings/Photo Researchers, Inc.; p. 67, Jeff Isaac Greenberg/Photo Researchers, Inc.; p. 70, Richard Hutchings/Photo Researchers, Inc. Part Two: p. 75, top right, p. 76, Anthony Blake/Tony Stone Worldwide; p. 79, Stanley Rowin/The Picture Cube; p. 94, Henryk T. Kaiser/The Picture Cube; p. 101, © Jen Morin; p. 103, © Jen Morin; p. 75, left, p. 108, Lori Adamski Peek/Tony Stone Images; p. 114, Frank Siteman/The Picture Cube; p. 117, Penny Tweedie/Tony Stone Images; p. 120, A. Perlstein/Jerrican/Photo Researchers, Inc.; p. 122, © Jen Morin; p. 75, bottom, p. 128, Lori Adamski Peek/Tony Stone Images; p. 131, Lawrence Migdale/Stock, Boston; p. 134, David Weintraub/Stock, Boston; p. 137, Porterfield Chickering/Photo Researchers, Inc.; p. 142, Will and Deni McIntyre/Photo Researchers, Inc. **Part Three:** p. 145, top left, p. 146, Richard Hutchings/Photo Researchers, Inc.; p. 149, Frank Siteman/Tony Stone Images; p. 150, Phyllis Picardi/The Picture Cube; p. 165, Bruce Ayres/Tony Stone Images; p. 169, Bruce Ayres/Tony Stone Images; p. 145, top right, p. 172, James Davis/International Stock; p. 178, Roger Tully/Tony Stone Images; p. 181, Barry Elz/International Stock; p. 184, David Young Wolff/Tony Stone Worldwide, Ltd.; p. 190, bottom left, Laurence Monneret/Tony Stone Images; p. 198, Charles Thatcher/Tony Stone Images; p. 210, Jeff Greenberg/Photo Researchers, Inc.; p. 216, Robert W. Ginn/The Picture Cube; p. 145, bottom right, p. 218, © Steven Ferry; p. 225, top, Biophoto Associates/Photo Researchers, Inc.; p. 225, bottom, CDC/Science Source/Photo Researchers, Inc.; p. 226, Dr. P. Marazzi/Science Photo Library/Photo Researchers, Inc. **Part Four:** p. 237, top left, p. 238, J. Griffin/The Image Works, Inc.; p. 240, left, NIBSC Science Photo Library/Photo Researchers, Inc.; p. 240, right, A. B. Dowsett/Science Photo Library/Photo Researchers, Inc.; p. 244, Roger Tully/Tony Stone Images; *Credits continued on p. 496 which constitutes a continuation of the copyright page.*

Printed in the United States of America
00 99 98 97 96   10 9 8 7 6 5 4 3 2 1

Brief Contents

Contents

part two

Eating and Exercising toward a Healthy Life-style   75

part three

Building Healthy Relationships 145

part four *Understanding and Preventing Disease* 237

part five

Explaining Drug Use and Abuse 325

part six

Making Healthy Choices 383

part
seven *Overcoming Obstacles*   *429*

Feature Contents

Managing Stress

Wellness Guide

Exploring Your Health

 Controversy in Health

Global Wellness

Health Update

Preface

When writing the first edition of *Health and Wellness,* we had no idea that our book would be received so warmly and enthusiastically by hundreds of instructors and thousands of students. We were particularly gratified by the many students who conveyed to us that *Health and Wellness* made a profound impact on their well-being. To all the students and instructors who chose our text, we say thank you very much. Your support prodded us to undertake a major revision of *Health and Wellness;* we hope it is a markedly improved view of personal health and self-responsibility that will be useful and practical for the turn-of-the-century college student of all ages.

Improvements and refinements have been made in each edition of *Health and Wellness,* but the underlying principles of the book have remained the same. We are committed to providing accurate information regarding health and wellness, focusing on self-responsibility. In this fifth edition of *Health and Wellness* we take a new look at health and wellness issues; we have incorporated eight new features, added two new chapters, and combined several chapters, resulting in 24 revised chapters. We are excited about this edition and hope you are, too!

We feel very fortunate that what began as a two-person collaboration 20 years ago has now evolved into a triad of authors. Kelli McCormack Brown is a Certified Health Education Specialist who has taught over 10 years at the university level. She has received numerous awards for excellence in teaching, research, and service. Her teaching and writing experience are a valuable addition to the team.

CONTENT AND ORGANIZATION OF *HEALTH AND WELLNESS*

For this edition several chapters were consolidated and two *new* chapters were developed, one on violence and one on preventing accidents. The theme of taking responsibility for your health is addressed early on and reinforced throughout the book. Each chapter has been carefully reviewed, revised, and updated. New pedagogical features provide information on newly emerging issues, and challenge the student to promote and maintain a healthy life-style.

Health and Wellness, Fifth Edition, is organized into seven parts with no more than four chapters per part, which we believe makes the book more learning-friendly.

- Part One, **Achieving Wellness,** provides the basic definitions and concepts of health and wellness that are the foundation of the book. This part emphasizes the importance of stress management and positive emotional health to one's overall health and well-being.
- Part Two, **Eating and Exercising toward a Healthy Life-style,** presents the basics of good health: good nutritional habits, weight control, and physical fitness as a way of life. All three chapters emphasize personal responsibility.
- Part Three, **Building Healthy Relationships,** addresses both the physical and social aspects of sexuality, including healthy intimate relationships, pregnancy and parenthood, fertility methods, abortion, sexually transmitted diseases, and AIDS.
- Part Four, **Understanding and Preventing Disease,** reinforces the importance of self-responsibility and knowledge, and how the two can help prevent infectious diseases, cancer, cardiovascular diseases, and AIDS. A unique chapter on birth defects and genetic diseases provides insight into increasingly diagnosable human genetic disorders.
- Part Five, **Explaining Drug Use and Abuse,** provides an understanding of three health habits that can be controlled by each of us. Self-responsibility includes wisely using over-the-counter drugs, prescription drugs, and alcohol, as well as eliminating cigarette and tobacco use.
- Part Six, **Making Healthy Choices,** facilitates making healthy decisions regarding health care. Under-

standing alternative choices to medical care will help guide you through sometimes difficult and confusing decisions. This part has a new chapter addressing accident prevention, including motor vehicle safety and workplace safety.

- Part Seven, **Overcoming Obstacles**, provides insight into how to age with health and vigor, and how environmental issues affect each of us personally. This part has a new chapter on violence, dealing with acquaintance rape, child abuse, and firearm violence.

NEW FEATURES OF THE FIFTH EDITION: A VISUAL WALK-THROUGH

This edition of *Health and Wellness* expands greatly on features of the previous editions. A popular feature has been the boxes, which provide interesting, up-to-date information on current topics in greater depth than in the text itself. In this edition, over 80 percent of the boxes are new.

Nine new features call attention to critical health-related issues and challenge students to reflect on their life-styles or health-related decisions they have made or will make.

Managing Stress: Written by Brian Luke Seaward, Managing Stress boxes facilitate coping with stressful situations, using a variety of relaxation methods and other mind-body techniques. Examples include:

- The Two-Minute Stress Reducer (page 54)
- Stress and Your Diet (page 93)
- Walking in Balance (page 132)

Wellness Guide: Provides "how to" health information. Many offer tips, techniques, or steps toward prevention and self-responsibility. Examples include:

- Ways to Prevent Skin Cancer (page 275)
- How to Interpret Blood Cholesterol and Lipid Measurements (page 302)

Managing Stress

Stress and Your Diet

Believe it or not, some see eating as a technique to reduce the symptoms of stress. The feeling of food in the stomach sends a message to the brain to calm down. Yet there are certain foods that can send your stress levels off the charts and most people are completely unaware of them. Moreover, repeated bouts of stress can deplete necessary nutrients, vitamins, and minerals creating a cycle of poor health. Here are some examples:

Sugar

An excess of simple sugars tends to deplete vitamin stores, particularly the vitamin B-complex (niacin, thiamine, riboflavin, and B₁₂). White sugar and even bleached flour flushed of its vitamin and mineral content require additional B-complex vitamins to be metabolized. These and other vitamins are crucial for optimal function of the central nervous system. A depletion of the B-complex vitamin may manifest in signs of fatigue, anxiety, and irritability. In addition, increased amounts of ingested simple sugars can cause major fluctuations in blood glucose levels resulting in pronounced fatigue, headaches, and general irritability.

Caffeine

Food sources that trigger the sympathetic nervous system are referred to as *sympathomimetic agents.* There is a powerful substance in caffeine called *methylated xanthine.* This chemical stimulant with amphetamine-like characteristics triggers in the sympathetic nervous system a heightened state of alertness and arousal; it can also stimulate the release of several stress hormones. The result is a intensified alertness which makes the individual more susceptible to perceived stress. Caffeine can be found in many foods, including chocolate, coffee, tea, and several other beverages. Current estimates suggest that the average American consumes three 6-ounce cups of coffee per day. A 6-ounce cup of caffinated coffee contains approximately 250 milligrams of caffeine, half the amount necessary to provoke adverse arousal of the central nervous system.

Salt

It seems that Americans have a love affair with salt. Many people add salt to their food without even tasting it. High sodium intake is associated with high blood pressure, as sodium acts to increase water retention. As water volume increases in a

closed system, blood p[...] increases. If this condi[...] may contribute to hype[...]

Vitamin and Mineral[...]

Chronic stress can dep[...] vitamins necessary for [...] metabolism and for the[...] response. The synthesi[...] requires vitamins. The [...] response activates seve[...] that mobilize and meta[...] and carbohydrates for [...] duction. The breakdow[...] carbohydrates requires [...] specifically vitamins C [...] B-complex. Inadequate [...] these vitamins may als[...] tal alertness, and prom[...] sion and insomnia. Str[...] associated with depleti[...] and the inability of bo[...] erly absorb calcium, se[...] stage for the developm[...] porosis, the demineral[...] bone tissue. The depletion is a controversial [...] anced diet usually pro[...] quate supply of vitami[...] nutrients for energy m[...] However, the majority [...] do not maintain a bala[...] Vitamin supplements [...] for individuals prone t[...] stress.

sugar **galactose.** When lactose is digested, the glucose and galactose are separated and the galactose is converted to glucose. Whereas almost all babies have the capacity to digest lactose (it is the major sugar in mother's milk), many older children and adults, particularly of black and Asian heritage, are not able to digest it because they lack a required enzyme **lactase,** which splits lactose into glucose and galactose. Lack of this enzyme causes gastrointestinal upset, diarrhea, and, occasionally, severe illness when lactase-deficient people consume dairy products. These individuals can supplement their diets with products containing lactase (e.g., Lactaid) or by eating yogurt, cheese, and other dairy products in which the lactose has been broken down by the fermentation process. Because dairy products are a

major source of calcium in the North[...] people who avoid dairy products shoul[...] cium-rich vegetables (e.g., broccoli and [...] bly take calcium supplements.

Complex Carbohydrates These [...] from grains (wheat, rice, corn, oats, b[...] (peas, beans); the leaves, stems, and root[...] some animal tissue. There are two mai[...] plex carbohydrates: **starch,** which is [...] **fiber,** which is not digestible.

Starch consists of many glucose m[...] together. It is a way organisms store gl[...] needed. In plants, starch is usually contai[...] within seeds, pods, or roots. Wheat flou[...]

Health Update

Radioactivity from Chernobyl Nuclear Power Plant Causes Cancer in People Living Nearby

On April 26, 1986, a Russian nuclear power plant in the Ukrainian city of Chernobyl broke down, releasing a large amount of radioactivity. The fallout from the radioactivity was greatest in the surrounding region, but was carried by winds across northern Europe where high levels of radioactivity were recorded.

One of the radioactive elements that was released was radioactive iodine, which is concentrated in the thyroid.

Children are particularly sensitive to radioactive iodine ingested in food and water. In 1986, only four cases of thyroid cancer were reported among thousands of children living in areas surrounding Chernobyl. By 1991, the number of thyroid cancer cases in children had risen to 55, and is expected to continue to rise. It is too early to detect increases in other forms of cancer among people who were exposed to this radioactive fallout, but increased cancer rates are anticipated.

have not been adequately tested. Of the thousands of chemical substances that have been tested, many have been found to be carcinogenic and should be avoided if at all possible. These carcinogens include cigarette smoke, pesticides, asbestos, heavy metals (lead, mercury, cadmium), benzene, and nitrosamines (Table 13.2).

I don't want to achieve immortality through my work; I want to achieve immortality by not dying.
Woody Allen

Despite the long list of carcinogenic substances, some scientists and public health officials argue that tobacco is the only substance of consequence with respect to the numbers of cancers caused. While the argument has some basis, it is of small consolation to those who acquire cancer from exposure, often without their knowledge, to other carcinogenic substances.

In some industries, workers suffer from cancers that

almost never arise in the general population. For example, **mesothelioma** is a rare form of lung cancer that only occurs among persons exposed to asbestos fibers. Long-term exposure to the heavy metals beryllium and cadmium increases workers' risk of prostate cancer. Workers exposed to vinyl chloride, the starting material for polyvinyl chloride (PVC) pipes and other products, develop a rare form of liver cancer not found in the general public. Fortunately, with current regulations we do not see high numbers of these types of cancer.

Although the total number of cancers attributable to industrial chemicals is relatively small compared to the risks of tobacco smoke and dietary factors, the fact remains that cancers caused by industrial hazards are

Wellness Guide

Ways to Prevent Skin Cancer

Sunscreen products contain chemicals that provide sun protective factors (SPFs) to varying degrees. The SPF value indicates how much additional time you can expose yourself to the sun without burning. For example, if someone usually burns after 15 minutes exposure to intense sun, a sunscreen product with an SPF of 10 should give protection for ten times as long or 150 minutes of exposure; 30 SPF means thirty times more protection. Generally, SPF values above 30 are not considered useful because the cream or lotion

wears off before its usefulness is exhausted. The effectiveness of a sunscreen product depends on the SPF number, how waterproof the product is, and how effectively it covers the skin.

The SPF number refers only to protection from UVB, so exposure to UVA still can harm the skin. The primary ingredients in sunscreen products are para-amino-benzoic acid (PABA) or Padimat-O, both of which absorb only UVB. Chemicals such as avobenzone or oxybenzone protect against UVA, so look for

sunscreen products that contain these substances or that claim to protect against both forms of UV.

Fear of skin cancer is driving many people to use chemical tanning products marketed in the form of lotions, creams, gels, and mousses. This tan-in-a-bottle industry has grown from sales of about $5 million in 1988 to more than $86 million in 1993. Clearly, looking tan is still a desirable goal for many people. These products may be safe, but they have not been in use long enough to know.

- Determining If You Are at Risk for Bearing a Genetically Disabled Child (page 320)

Exploring Your Health: Contains self-assessments that students can use to evaluate their health status in a particular area. Examples include:

- How Well Are You? (page 6)
- How Does Your Diet Rate for Variety? (page 82)
- How Intimate Are You? (page 166)
- Choosing the Best Contraceptive for You (page 210)

Controversy in Health: Introduces controversial issues in health where there are no clear-cut answers. This feature presents both sides of the issue, then asks the reader critical thinking questions requiring the student to choose and support a perspective. Examples include:

- Food Irradiation: Toxic to Bacteria, Safe for Humans (page 102)
- Lifting the Gay Ban in the Military (page 152)

- Should Students Be Tested for HIV? (page 231)
- Should People Be Tested for Inherited Cancer-Susceptibility Genes? (page 282)

Case Study: Presents scenarios ending with questions that help students understand how certain issues affect people in the world today. These questions present the issue and ask students "How would you react in a comparable situation?" Examples include:

- Beginning Your Fitness Routine (page 130)
- An HIV Ethical Dilemma (page 233)
- Driving under the Influence of Alcohol (DUI) (page 374)
- Contaminated Water in Milwaukee Sickens 400,000 Persons (page 473)

Global Wellness: Explores the multicultural aspects of health and wellness. Examples include:

- Yin and Yang: Finding Balance (page 22)

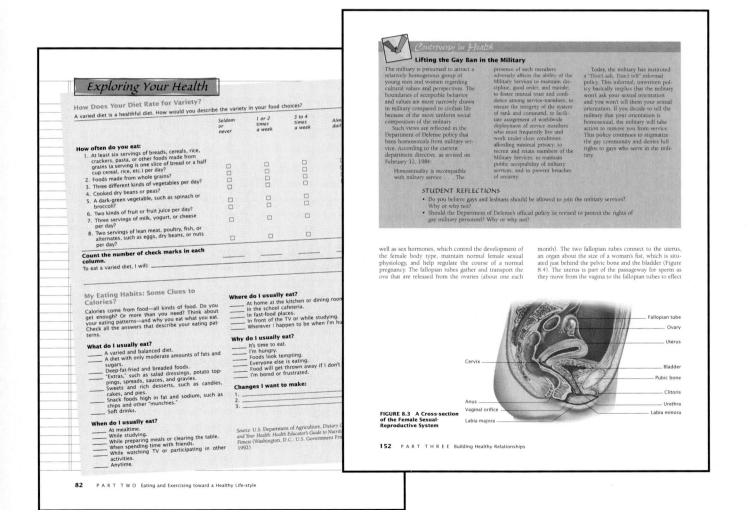

- Overwork Causes Death in Japan (page 49)
- HIV Cases Worldwide (page 228)
- Can Beliefs Influence Disease Susceptibility? (page 440)

Healthy People 2000: In 1991 the Surgeon General's office issued a report titled *Healthy People 2000,* which identified health promotion and disease prevention goals and objectives for all Americans for the year 2000. These objectives are annotated and included throughout the text. The annotations help put each objective in a relevant context for the student.

Health Update: Discusses current and relevant personal health trends and issues. Examples include:

- Youth and Tobacco Advertising (page 352)
- Take a Walk on the Safe Side (page 419)
- First Alzheimer's Drug Approved (page 438)
- "Fill You Full of Lead" Is No Joke (page 471)

Learning Objectives: The learning objectives, which begin each chapter, are a study guide for students, helping them focus on the most important concepts of each chapter.

Familiar Features

This edition of *Health and Wellness* has retained several features from previous editions with appropriate updates.

Health in Review is a brief review of the chapter's most important concepts. The reviews correspond closely with the chapter learning objectives.

Annotated Suggested Readings follow the References and provide students with resources for further study.

Epigrams, a favorite feature in past editions, continue to highlight each chapter with both humorous and serious quotes regarding specific health issues.

Key terms are defined on the page on which they are highlighted, as well as in the glossary at the end of the book.

References are found at the end of each chapter. As the chapters were updated, so were the References for continuity.

---

with stress, and fight off colds and other infections by boosting the immune system's defenses. Heart disease, obesity, and high blood pressure may not be an overriding concern today; however, your exercise and fitness behaviors today can affect your health in the future.

WHAT IS PHYSICAL ACTIVITY?

The health club and exercise equipment industries and the advertising and TV infomercials that support them can easily lead people to think that exercising for health requires considerable time, energy, money, and commitment. These investments can seem so overwhelming that some people forego exercising altogether.

Fortunately, physical activity does not require special equipment or spending a lot of money. Physical activity is anything you do when you are not sitting or lying down. Besides jogging, swimming, cycling, and aerobic dancing, physical activity includes yoga, tai chi ch'uan, martial arts training, gardening, and walking. For instance, regular walking strengthens muscles, increases aerobic capacity, clears and quiets the mind, reduces stress, expends calories, and is virtually injury-free. Other than appropriate shoes, walking requires no special clothing, equipment, or money, and it can be worked into a busy schedule. Instead of eating at breaks at work or between classes, you can walk to a job or class. Walk up stairs instead of using elevators. If you

need to drive, park and walk the last ten m... destination. Aerobic capacity can be incre... ing briskly enough to increase the heart ra... ing uphill or up stairs).

Once a commitment is made to an exer... other healthy behaviors often follow, such... eating habits and a reduction in heavy alco... tion. Such programs also may lessen stress... sirable stress-reducing behaviors such as ci... ing, overeating, or drug consumption are u...

If none of these points convinces you... benefits of exercise, think of it as setting a... attention for you. Many people feel overwh... demands of school, job, and family. Just... hours a week to exercise can give you t... relax, reflect, and indulge your imaginatio...

Physiological Benefits of Physical Activity

Research shows that only moderate, n... extensive exercise is sufficient for good heal... ple, for both women and men, the chance... heart disease, cancer, and several other dise... for individuals with sedentary life-styles th... engage in a daily brisk walk of 30 to 60 n... man, 1993). Moderate regular exercise, las... 30 minutes, five times a week also has b... improve health. In fact, high levels of exe... the risk of injuries.

CASE STUDY
Beginning Your Fitness Routine

Frank is a graduate student who took up jogging about a year ago because so many of his friends were runners, including his financée, Susan. Although he wasn't overweight, Frank nevertheless thought he could stand to have firmer muscles, especially in his thighs and abdomen. He began to run with Susan on the college track several times a week.

At first, Frank found running to be very hard. He had never before been physically active. In fact, he had always hated sports because of bad experiences in high school physical education classes. Also, he smoked about a pack of cigarettes a day, which severely limited his breathing ability. On the first day he could barely run one lap of the track—one-fourth of a mile—and without Susan's encouragement he probably would have quit right then. She agreed that

one lap wasn't very far, but she reminded... it would take time to undo the years of ina... smoking, and that he should have patie... decided to give his new routine time to wo... the goal of running one mile by the e... month's running.

STUDENT REFLECTIONS
- What barriers was Frank up against aft... day of running, and how did he overco...
- Have you recently set an exercising goa... self? If so, what is it? How difficult has... reach this goal? How have you overcome... cles in your way of reaching this goal?

FEAR OF AGING AND DYING

Nobody wants to grow old or die. When we are young, we never think about becoming old, nor can we imagine what it is like not to be strong, vigorous, and active. With few exceptions, the media in the United States and elsewhere portray aging as a time of life beset with sickness, inactivity, and slow deterioration of physical and mental functions. These negative views of aging are used to sell products and do not truthfully portray the experiences of most older Americans.

Fear of aging and death may lead to anxiety and stress that may hasten aging processes. A few of the many fears that people associate with aging are illness, poverty, being attacked or victimized, falling and being injured while alone, loss of responsibility for one's life, memory loss, and sexual inadequacy. Most of these fears are unfounded, but may turn out to be self-fulfilling prophesies. However, chronological age often does not correlate with biological age. Some people lose very little in biological functions as they get older, and look and act young almost until the time of death. Generally, older people have about half as many acute illnesses as younger people, although they do suffer more from chronic health problems.

> *I used to believe in reincarnation, but that was in a past life.*
> Paul Krassner,
> humorist

APPROACHING DEATH WITH DIGNITY

Death can strike without warning in the form of an accident or an unexpected heart attack. However, for most people thoughts of death do not occupy their daily lives until old age. People in their 20s are too busy living to think about dying. But people in their 70s and 80s realize the inevitability of death and may modify their lives and affairs accordingly. Younger people who acquire a life-threatening disease such as cancer also are forced to face the possibility of dying.

Most people would prefer to die peacefully in their sleep after living a full, satisfying life. Some may be fortunate to die like this but others may have to endure considerable pain and suffering. In addition to wondering how they are going to die, people usually wonder what will happen to them after death. Christianity provides a heaven where one's "soul" can exist in the grace of God for all eternity. Buddhism embraces a belief in reincarnation; after a series of deaths and rebirths a person can attain "Buddhahood," a perpetual state of enlightenment.

Whatever one's fears or beliefs about death, understanding the process of dying and the preparations that can be made for it can help ensure experiencing a death with peace and dignity (Table 22.2).

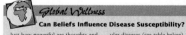
Global Wellness
Can Beliefs Influence Disease Susceptibility?

Just how powerful are thoughts and feelings in influencing health? Can beliefs affect the duration of a person's life? A recent survey of the causes and ages of death among Chinese-Americans shows that strongly held beliefs can affect the cause of death and how long a person lives (Phillips et al., 1993).

In Chinese astrology a particular phase—metal, water, wood, fire, or earth—is associated with the year of a person's birth. Also associated with each phase is susceptibility to partic-

ular diseases (see table below). According to Chinese astrology and medicine, being born in a particular year make a person more likely than usual to succumb to diseases associated with the phase of their birth year. An analysis of almost 30,000 death certificates of Chinese-Americans showed that people with the predicted combination of birth year and disease susceptibility died one to five years younger than white Americans with the same diseases and phases.

The more traditional the Chinese life-style of the person, the shorter their life was once they contracted the disease associated with their birth year. The most plausible explanation of the findings is that Chinese-Americans who believe in the predictions of Chinese astrology are the most likely to succumb to the disease that they expect will kill them. It appears that beliefs not only affect health through the onset and progression of disease, but beliefs even affect life span.

Association between phases of a person's birth year with susceptibility to certain diseases according to Chinese astrology and medicine. Persons born in years corresponding to a particular phase are more susceptible to certain diseases.	Birth year ends in	Phase	Susceptibility to
	0 or 1	Metal	Pulmonary diseases
	2 or 3	Water	Kidney disease
	4 or 5	Wood	Cirrhosis of liver
	6 or 7	Fire	Heart attack
	8 or 9	Earth	Cancer, diabetes, ulcers

Appendices include relaxation exercises and stress management techniques, a list of health agencies that can provide useful information to students, and a list of health and wellness sites on the Internet.

Teaching and Learning Aids

Available with *Health and Wellness, Fifth Edition,* is a comprehensive package of supplementary materials that enhance both teaching and learning. The following ancillaries are complimentary:

Instructor's Guide: The *Instructor's Guide* includes for each chapter: 1) suggestions for incorporating student activities and assessment from the student workbook, *Managing Your Health*; 2) suggestions for incorporating the *Health and Wellness Journal* by Brian Luke Seaward; 3) tips for integrating the new boxed materials into the classroom; 4) learning objectives; 5) a list of key terms; and 6) an outline of the chapter.

Transparencies: Full set of transparencies to complement the text material, carefully selected by the authors.

Test Bank: Revised comprehensive test-item file. Contains true/false and multiple choice test questions and answers.

Computerized Test Bank: A computerized testing software package containing the revised test questions written specifically for *Health and Wellness, Fifth Edition,* available for IBM, IBM-compatible, and Macintosh computers.

Berkeley *Wellness Newsletter*, University of California: This highly respected newsletter is offered to all adopters of *Health and Wellness, Fifth Edition.* The *Wellness Newsletter* is an excellent resource for instructors in providing up-to-date health information.

Health and Wellness On-Line: Health information provided through the information superhighway. Each adopter of the book receives updates via electronic mail. Those without on-line access can receive a hard copy.

Healthy People 2000: A Midcourse Review and 1995 Revisions: This report will demonstrate how far we have come as a nation in achieving the disease prevention and health promotion goals mapped out at the beginning of this decade. This document can be easily cross-referenced to the Healthy People 2000 goals listed throughout the text. An excellent resource for the instructor.

Additional Adoption Options: Also available are a variety of support items that will enhance the teaching and learning experiences with *Health and Wellness, Fifth Edition.* The following ancillaries are available on a complimentary basis to all qualified adopters depending upon annual course enrollment. The instructor will have an opportunity to select from the following supplement options:

Videotapes: As an adopter of *Health and Wellness, Fifth Edition,* you will be able to select videotapes on various health-related topics. These videotapes are selected to enhance teaching and learning. Jones and Bartlett offers 32 nationally acclaimed, broadcast-quality videos to accompany *Health and Wellness, Fifth Edition.* Carefully chosen by the authors, these videos correspond to topics in the text to provide flexibility.

Health Risk Appraisal Software: Developed by the CDC, this computerized instrument evaluates complex information about an individual's family history, health status, and life-style. Students receive a risk assessment based on their personal data.

Instructor's Teaching Package for *Stress Management*: Written by the National Safety Council. *Stress Management* addresses the relationship between stress and the work environment, and provides the latest, most comprehensive approach to identifying and controlling stress. Many college students who work part time will find this material relevant to their lives. The package consists of an *Instructor's Resource Manual, Video, and Instructor's Slide Set* to accompany the student text on stress management.

Managing Stress: A Creative Journal: Contains over 40 thought-provoking exercises that stimulate students to write creatively on how to increase awareness of the causes of stress and to develop effective coping skills.

Stress Reduction Audio Tape: Designed to teach students stress reduction techniques such as meditation, autogenic training, progressive relaxation, and mental imagery.

First Aid Pocket Guide: Provides students with easy-to-follow, step-by-step instructions that tell exactly what emergency care to administer for virtually all injuries or sudden illnesses.

The following books are integrated and cross-referenced with the *Instructor's Manual* and are sold separately:

Managing Your Health: Assessment and Action: Written by David Birch, Indiana University, and Michael Cleary, Slippery Rock University. This workbook includes activities designed to involve students in personal health promotion. The activities focus on self-assessment, issues examination, and skill development. The *Health and Wellness, Fifth Edition Instructor's Guide* refers to this workbook to facilitate teaching and learning.

Health and Wellness Journal: Written by Brian Luke Seaward, University of Northern Colorado. One of the best ways to integrate the material from the text is to personally engage in the process of the concepts highlighted. Journal writing allows the student to explore his or her own thoughts on specific health attitudes and behavioral changes. The *Instructor's Guide* refers to the journal to facilitate behavioral change and self-awareness.

For more detailed information on all of the ancillaries, please contact the marketing department or your Jones and Bartlett representative at 1-800-832-0034.

A NOTE OF THANKS

Throughout all five editions of *Health and Wellness,* many people have contributed support and guidance. This book has benefited greatly from their comments, opinions, thoughtful critiques, expert knowledge, and constructive suggestions. We are most appreciative for their participation in this project.

We would specifically like to thank several people who assisted with the fifth edition of *Health and Wellness:* Debra Connelly, Andrew Wise, Nichelle Goetsch, and Janice Morris.

Fifth Edition Reviewers

David Birch, Ph.D., Indiana University

Donald L. Calitri, Ed.D., Eastern Kentucky University

Judy C. Drolet, Ph.D., Southern Illinois University at Carbondale

Philip Duryea, Ph.D., University of New Mexico

Mal Goldsmith, Ph.D., Southern Illinois University at Edwardsville

Allan C. Henderson, Dr. Ph.H., California State University, Long Beach

William M. Kane, Ph.D., University of New Mexico

Mark Kittleson, Ph.D., Southern Illinois University at Carbondale

Beverly Saxton Mahoney, Ph.D., The Pennsylvania State University

Roberta Ogletree, HSD, Southern Illinois University at Carbondale

Larry K. Olsen, Dr. P.H., The Pennsylvania State University

Bruce Ragon, Ph.D., Indiana University

Janet S. Reis, Ph.D., University of Illinois at Urbana-Champaign

Brian Luke Seaward, Ph.D., Inspiration Unlimited, Longmont, Colorado

David R. Stronck, Ph.D., California State University, Hayward

Bryan Williams, Ph.D., University of Arkansas

Carol A. Wilson, Ph.D., University of Nevada at Las Vegas

Richard W. Wilson, D.H.Sc., Western Kentucky University

Fifth Edition Specialty Area Reviewers

Chapter 6 **Managing Your Weight**

Nicole B. Gegel, M.S., Employee Fitness Director, Illinois State University

Chapter 7 **Achieving Physical Fitness**

Nicole B. Gegel, M.S., Employee Fitness Director, Illinois State University

Chapter 8 **Developing Healthy Intimate and Sexual Relationships**

Susan Sprecher, Ph.D., Department of Sociology, Illinois State University

Chapter 9 **Understanding Pregnancy and Parenthood**

M. Dawn Larsen, Ph.D., Department of Health Sciences, Mankato State University

Chapter 10 **Choosing a Fertility Control Method**
Patti Alsader, B.S., Youth and Community Education Coordinator, Planned Parenthood of West Central Illinois

Chapter 12 **Reducing the Risk of Infectious Disease: Knowledge Encourages Prevention**

M. Dawn Larsen, Ph.D., Department of Health Sciences, Mankato State University

Chapter 13 **Cancer: Understanding Risks and Measures of Prevention**

Geoffrey M. Cooper, Ph.D., Dana Farber Cancer Institute, Harvard Medical School

Chapter 14 **Cardiovascular Diseases: Understanding Risks and Measures of Prevention**

Dwayne Reed, M.D., Ph.D., Buck Center for Research in Aging, Novato, CA

Chapter 16 **Using Drugs Responsibly**

Chapter 17 **Eliminating Cigarette and Tobacco Use**

Chapter 18 **Using Alcohol Responsibly**

Marion Micke, Ph.D., Department of Health Sciences, Illinois State University

Chapter 24 **Working toward a Healthy Environment**

Anne Nadakavukaren, M.S., Department of Health Sciences, Illinois State University

This book could not have been published without the efforts of the staff at Jones and Bartlett Publishing Company and the *Health and Wellness* team: Joseph E. Burns, Vice President and Publisher of the health science program; Maxine Effenson Chuck, Editorial Specialist; Judy Songdahl, Assistant Production Manager; Tina

Samaha, Copy Editor; Nancy Benjamin of Books By Design, Editorial Production Coordinator; and Suzanne Crane, Editorial Assistant. To all we express our appreciation.

Finally, this book could not have been written without the understanding and support of family and friends. Last but not least is the great amount we have learned from our students as we have explored health and wellness issues together.

Gordon Edlin
John A. Burns School of Medicine
University of Hawaii
Honolulu, Hawaii 96822

Eric Golanty
Las Positas College
Livermore, California 94550

Kelli McCormack Brown
Department of Health Sciences
Illinois State University
Normal, Illinois 61790

Achieving Wellness

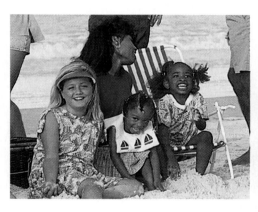

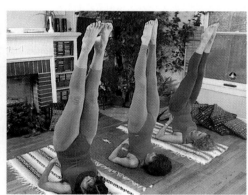

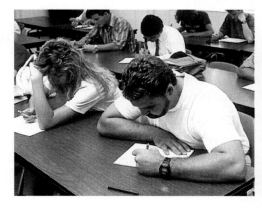

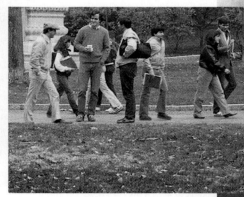

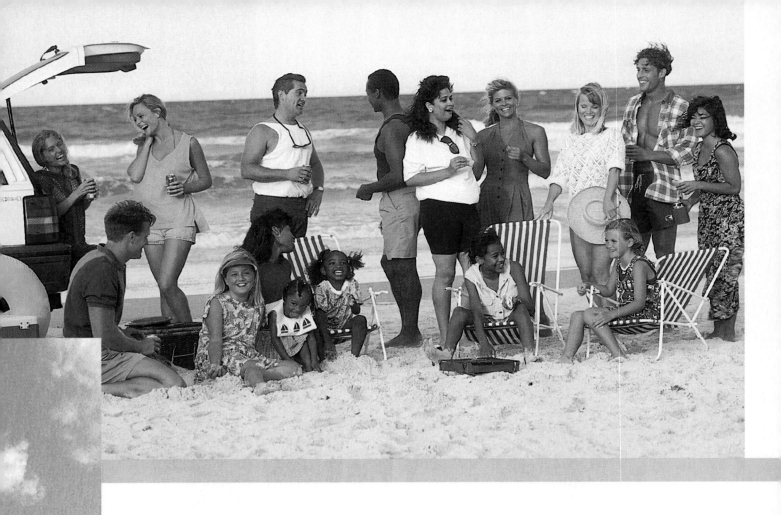

LEARNING OBJECTIVES

After reading this chapter you should be able to:

1. Describe what it means to be healthy.
2. Describe the medical, environmental, and holistic/wellness models of health.
3. Explain the wellness continuum and its impact on your health.
4. Identify and describe the six dimensions of wellness.
5. Explain how over the past century the nature of most illness has changed from infectious/communicable to chronic disease.
6. Describe how life-style diseases affect morbidity and mortality.
7. Explain how you can practice a holistic life-style.
8. Explain the importance of the Year 2000 Objectives.

1

Achieving Personal Health

Ask people what they mean by "being healthy" or "feeling well" and you probably will get different answers depending on whom you ask. Most people usually think of health in terms of disease; that is, people who are well have no disease. But what about someone who has a relatively harmless genetic disorder such as an extra toe? Is this individual less healthy than a person with the usual number of toes? Different perhaps, but not necessarily less healthy. Are you less well when you are struggling with a personal problem than when you are out having fun? Finding an acceptable, generally useful definition of health or wellness is not a simple task.

It is true that not feeling sick is one important aspect of health. Just as important, however, is the idea that health is a sense of optimum well-being—a state of physical, mental, emotional, social, and spiritual wellness. Contained in this view is the idea that health can be obtained by living in harmony with yourself, with other people, and with the environment. Health is gained and maintained by exerting self-responsibility for reducing exposure to health risks and for maximizing things such as good nutrition and exercise.

Throughout this book, we show you ways to maximize your health by understanding how your mind and body function, how to avoid harmful chemicals, how to make informed decisions about health and health care, and how to be responsible for your actions and behaviors. Learning to be responsible while young for the degree of health and energy you want helps to ensure life-long wellness and the capacity to cope with sickness when it does occur.

DEFINING HEALTH AND WELLNESS

To be responsible for your well-being, you must understand what **health** and **wellness** are. Health is defined differently among experts, but all definitions have a common theme: self-responsibility and life-style.

> Health is a state of complete physical, mental, and social well-being and not merely the absence of disease or infirmity.
> —World Health Organization, 1947

> (Health is) an integrated method of functioning which is oriented toward maximizing the potential of which the individual is capable. It requires that the individual maintain a continuum of balance and purposeful direction with the environment where he/she is functioning.
> —Dunn, 1967

Wellness has been defined as

> an approach to personal health that emphasizes individual responsibility for well-being through the practice of health-promoting lifestyle behaviors.
> —Hurley and Schlaadt, 1992

Wellness is many times referred to in a broader context than health, which sometimes means only physical health. For the purposes of this book, we consider health multidimensional, involving the whole person's relation to the total environment. We refer to wellness as a process of moving toward optimal health.

MODELS OF HEALTH

Various models help us understand health and wellness. They include the medical model, the environmental model, and the holistic or wellness model, as well as others.

The Medical Model

The **medical model** is excellent for gathering numerical data (called **vital statistics**) on the **prevalence** (predominance) and **incidence** (occurrence) of diseases, which are interpreted to measure health (Table 1.1). Thus, counting cases of disease in populations becomes a measure of health. In the medical model disease is measured by **morbidity** and **mortality**.

TABLE 1.1 Differences in Causes of Death Age-adjusted death rates for 1992 and percent changes in age-adjusted death rates for the ten leading causes of death for the total population from 1991 to 1992 and 1979 to 1992 in the United States.

Causes of death	Percent change from	
	1991–1992	1979–1992
1. Diseases of heart	−2.6	−27.7
2. Malignant neoplasms (including neoplasms of lymphatic and hematopoietic tissues)	−1.0	1.8
3. Cerebrovascular diseases	−2.2	−37.0
4. Chronic obstructive pulmonary diseases	−1.0	36.3
5. Accidents and adverse effects	−5.2	−31.5
Motor vehicle accidents	−7.1	−31.9
All other accidents and adverse effects	−1.4	−30.1
6. Pneumonia and influenza	−5.2	13.4
7. Diabetes mellitus	0.8	21.4
8. Human immunodeficiency virus infection	11.5	—
9. Suicide	−2.6	−5.1
10. Homicide and legal intervention	−3.7	2.9

Source: Adapted from U.S. Department of Health and Human Services, *Monthly Vital Statistics Report* (Washington, D.C.: U.S. Government Printing Office, December 8, 1994).

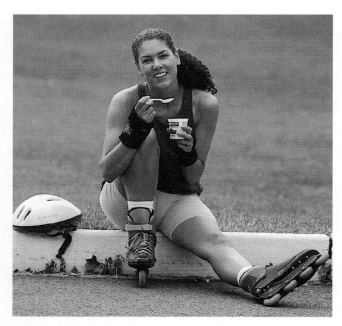

A healthy life-style depends on exercise and good nutrition.

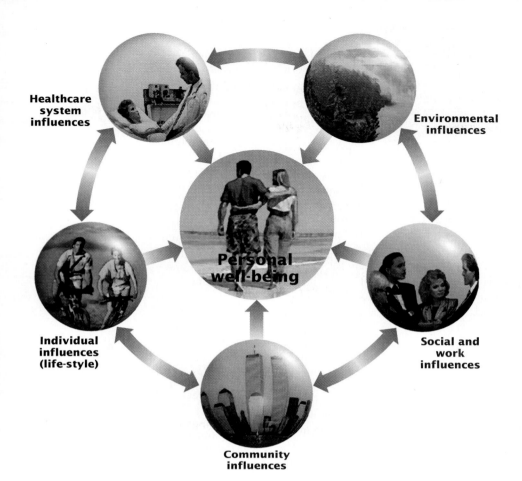

Healthcare system influences

Environmental influences

Personal well-being

Individual influences (life-style)

Social and work influences

Community influences

FIGURE 1.1 Environmental Health Model This model takes into account all factors that interact with one another and their effects on one's health.

The medical model does not deal with social problems that affect health and has difficulty integrating mental and behavioral problems that do not derive from diseased organs. In the medical model health is restored by curing the disease or by restoring function to a damaged body part. Because of its exclusive focus on biological processes, the medical model is of limited value. It does not help us understand psychological and/or social factors that affect health and contribute to disease.

The Environmental Model

The **environmental model** of health emerged with modern analyses of ecosystems and environmental risks to human health. In this model health is defined in terms of the quality of a person's adaptation to the environment as conditions change. This model (Figure 1.1) includes the effects on personal health of socioeconomic status, education, and multiple environmental factors.

Unlike the medical model, which focuses on diseased organs and biological abnormalities, the environmental model focuses on conditions outside the individual that affect his or her health. These conditions include the

Exploring Your Health

How Well Are You?

Complete the following health and wellness inventory to gauge your present degree of wellness. For each of the questions, circle the number

5 if the statement is ALWAYS true
4 If the statement if FREQUENTLY true
3 if the statement is OCCASIONALLY true
2 if the statement is SELDOM true
1 if the statement is NEVER true

1. I am able to identify the situations and factors that overstress me. 5 4 3 2 1

2. I eat only when I am hungry. 5 4 3 2 1

3. I don't take tranquilizers or other drugs to relax. 5 4 3 2 1

4. I support efforts in my community to reduce environmental pollution. 5 4 3 2 1

5. I avoid buying foods with artificial colorings. 5 4 3 2 1

6. I rarely have problems concentrating on what I'm doing because of worrying about other things. 5 4 3 2 1

7. My employer (school) takes measures to ensure that my work (study) place is safe. 5 4 3 2 1

8. I try not to use medications when I feel unwell. 5 4 3 2 1

9. I am able to identify certain bodily responses and illnesses as my reactions to stress. 5 4 3 2 1

10. I question the use of diagnostic X-rays. 5 4 3 2 1

11. I try to change personal habits that are risk factors for heart disease, cancer, and other life-style diseases. 5 4 3 2 1

12. I avoid taking sleeping pills to help me sleep. 5 4 3 2 1

13. I try not to eat foods with refined sugar or corn sugar as ingredients. 5 4 3 2 1

14. I accomplish goals I set for myself. 5 4 3 2 1

15. I stretch or bend for several minutes each day to keep my body flexible. 5 4 3 2 1

16. I support immunization of all children for common childhood diseases. 5 4 3 2 1

17. I try to prevent friends from driving after they drink alcohol. 5 4 3 2 1

18. I minimize my salt intake. 5 4 3 2 1

19. I don't mind when other people and situations make me wait or lose time. 5 4 3 2 1

20. I climb four or fewer flights of stairs rather than take the elevator. 5 4 3 2 1

21. I eat fresh fruits and vegetables. 5 4 3 2 1

22. I use dental floss at least once a day. 5 4 3 2 1

23. I read product labels on foods to determine their ingredients. 5 4 3 2 1

24. I try to maintain a normal body weight. 5 4 3 2 1

25. I record my feelings and thoughts in a journal or diary. 5 4 3 2 1

26. I have no difficulty falling asleep. 5 4 3 2 1

27. I engage in some form of vigorous physical activity at least three times a week. 5 4 3 2 1

28. I take time each day to quiet my mind and relax. 5 4 3 2 1

29. I am willing to make and sustain close friendships and intimate relationships. 5 4 3 2 1

30. I obtain an adequate daily supply of vitamins from my food or vitamin supplements. 5 4 3 2 1

31. I rarely have tension or migraine headaches, or pain in the neck or shoulders. 5 4 3 2 1

32. I wear a safety belt when driving. 5 4 3 2 1

33. I am aware of the emotional and situational factors that lead me to overeat. 5 4 3 2 1

34. I avoid driving my car after drinking any alcohol. 5 4 3 2 1

35. I am aware of the side effects of the medicines I take. 5 4 3 2 1

36. I am able to accept feelings of sadness, depression, and anxiety, ing that they are almost always transient. 5 4 3 2 1

37. I would seek several additional professional opinions if my doctor recommended surgery for me. 5 4 3 2 1

38. I agree that nonsmokers should not have to breathe the smoke from cigarettes in public places. 5 4 3 2 1

39. I agree that pregnant women who smoke harm their babies. 5 4 3 2 1

40. I feel I get enough sleep. 5 4 3 2 1

41. I ask my doctor why a certain medication is being prescribed and inquire about alternatives. 5 4 3 2 1

42. I am aware of the calories expended in my activities. 5 4 3 2 1

43. I am willing to give priority to my own needs for time and psychological space by saying "no" to others' requests of me. 5 4 3 2 1

44. I walk instead of drive whenever feasible. 5 4 3 2 1

45. I eat a breakfast that contains about one-third of my daily need for calories, proteins, and vitamins. 5 4 3 2 1

46. I prohibit smoking in my home. 5 4 3 2 1

47. I remember and think about my dreams. 5 4 3 2 1

48. I seek medical attention only when I have symptoms or feel that some (potential) condition needs checking, rather than have routine yearly checkups. 5 4 3 2 1

49. I endeavor to make my home accident free.   5 4 3 2 1

50. I ask my doctor to explain the diagnosis of my problem until I understand all that I care to.   5 4 3 2 1

51. I try to include fiber or roughage (whole grains, fresh fruits and vegetables, or bran) in my daily diet.   5 4 3 2 1

52. I can deal with my emotional problems without alcohol or other mood-altering drugs.   5 4 3 2 1

53. I am satisfied with my school/work.   5 4 3 2 1

54. I require children riding in my car to be in infant seats or in shoulder harnesses.   5 4 3 2 1

55. I try to associate with people who have a positive attitude about life.   5 4 3 2 1

56. I try not to eat snacks of candy, pastries, and other "junk" foods.   5 4 3 2 1

57. I avoid people who are "down" all the time and who bring down those around them.   5 4 3 2 1

58. I am aware of the calorie content of the foods I eat.   5 4 3 2 1

59. I brush my teeth after meals.   5 4 3 2 1

60. (for women only) I routinely examine my breasts.   5 4 3 2 1
    (for men only) I am aware of the signs of testicular cancer.   5 4 3 2 1

How to Score

Enter the numbers you've circled next to the question number and total your score for each category. Then use the wellness status key to determine your degree of wellness for each category.

Emotional health	Fitness and body care	Environmental health	Stress	Nutrition	Medical self-responsibility
		4 ___	1 ___	2 ___	8 ___
6 ___	15 ___	7 ___	3 ___	5 ___	10 ___
12 ___	20 ___	17 ___	9 ___	13 ___	11 ___
25 ___	22 ___	32 ___	14 ___	18 ___	16 ___
26 ___	24 ___	34 ___	19 ___	21 ___	35 ___
36 ___	27 ___	38 ___	28 ___	23 ___	37 ___
40 ___	33 ___	39 ___	29 ___	30 ___	41 ___
47 ___	42 ___	46 ___	31 ___	45 ___	48 ___
52 ___	44 ___	49 ___	43 ___	51 ___	59 ___
55 ___	58 ___	54 ___	53 ___	56 ___	60 ___
57 ___	59 ___				
Total ___	Total ___	Total ___	Total ___	Total ___	Total ___

Wellness Status

To assess your status in each of the six categories, compare your total score in each to the following key: **0–34** Need improvement; **35–44** Good; **45–50** Excellent.

Contracting with Yourself

Based on your wellness status results, make appropriate changes in categories you would like to improve. List the changes you wish to make, set a time to begin making them, and decide when you want the change to be fully integrated into your life. For example:

Change Desired
- quit smoking
- take up meditation
- record dreams

Begin Change
- in one week
- immediately
- after quitting smoking

Time Allotted
- one month
- two weeks
- one week

Do not try to make all the changes on your list at the same time. Begin with either the one or two most important, or the one or two you know you can accomplish. Then make one or two changes at a time after that.

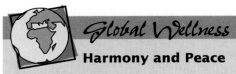
Harmony and Peace

Many Native American cultures and tribes incorporate the idea of harmonious interactions with nature, animals, and other people in their religions.

The first peace,
which is the most important,
is that which comes from
within the souls of men when they
realize their relationship,
their oneness, with the universe
and all its powers,
and when they realize that

at the center of the universe dwells
Wakan-Tanka, and that
this center is really everywhere,
it is within each of us.
This is the real peace, and the
others are
but reflections of this.
The second peace is that which is
made between two individuals,
and the third is that
which is made between two nations.
But above all you should
understand that there can never be
peace

between nations until there is
first known that true peace which
. . .
is within the souls of men.

—Black Elk
The Sacred Pipe

Source: From *The Sacred Pipe: Black Elk's Account of the Seven Rites of the Oglala Sioux,* by Joseph Epes Brown. Copyright © 1953, 1989 by the University of Oklahoma Press.

quality of air and water, living conditions, exposure to harmful substances, socioeconomic conditions, social relationships, and the health-care system.

In many respects the environmental model of health is similar to ancient Eastern and Native American philosophies that associate health with harmonious interactions with fellow creatures and the environment. In particular, as the environment changes, one's interaction with it must change to remain in harmony. Illness is interpreted as disharmony of human and environmental interactions.

> *Far from being simply the absence of disease, health is a dynamic and harmonious equilibrium of all the elements and forces making up and surrounding a human being.*
> Andrew Weil, M.D.

The Holistic Model

The holistic, or wellness, model defines health in terms of the whole person, not in terms of diseased parts of the body. The holistic model encompasses the physiological, mental, emotional, social, spiritual, and environmental aspects of individuals and communities. It focuses on optimal health, prevention of disease, and positive men-

tal and emotional states. The holistic model has been criticized as too idealistic, but in recent years has gained credibility and acceptance.

The holistic model incorporates the idea of spiritual health, which is not considered in the medical model. Unlike the medical model, which assumes that a person who is not sick or not suffering from a disease is as healthy as possible, the holistic model proposes that health is a state of optimum or positive wellness.

Wellness is much more than physical health; it addresses mental, emotional, and spiritual aspects of a person, as well the relationships among these dimensions. The wellness continuum helps delineate between the medical concept of health and the wellness concept (Figure 1.2). Most people find themselves in the neutral area of the continuum. Most of us, however, can remember moving toward disability and also moving toward optimal health or high-level wellness.

One may move from a state of illness or disease back to the neutral point many times with the help of medical

| Pursuit of high-level wellness | Growth | Education | Awareness | Neutral point | Signs | Symptoms | Disability | Premature death |

FIGURE 1.2 The Wellness Continuum The wellness continuum allows you to visualize the difference between wellness and the medical approaches to health.

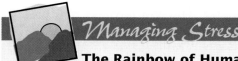

The Rainbow of Human Energy

In truth, we know that we cannot separate the mind from the body, nor can we separate the mind from emotions, or the body from the soul. All aspects are integrated. Through the recent insights of quantum physics, we know that everything, including our thoughts and feelings, consists of energy. This is what the wisdom keepers and shamans have known for millennia. Renowned physicist David Bohm addressed the spiritual nature of health in terms of quantum physics. He used the term *coherence* to describe the harmony among the energies of body, mind, and spirit, which gives a sense of wholeness that can only be described as "inner peace." As we continue to explore the issues of health and illness, some interesting facts come to light which support the holistic concept that the whole is greater than the sum of the parts. Spontaneous remissions and healing through prayer are two of many phenomena that cannot be explained by the mechanistic model. In fact, the new paradigm suggests that we are not a mind in a body, but a body in a mind.

Try the following exercise: Keeping in mind the concept of coherence in this new paradigm, take a moment to reflect on your whole being—all that you are, not just your body. You can begin by thinking about your physical body—your senses, organs, bones, tissue, and fluids. Visualize all the organs, tissues, and fluids working in cooperation with each other (coherence). Imagine that every cell in your body, like the needle of a compass, is headed north. Next imagine that a layer of energy surrounds and permeates your body. This layer of energy is aqua. This represents what is known as your emotional body. Imagine this layer of blue energy around your body like warm Caribbean water. Imagine what it would feel like to sense harmony between your emotions and physical body. Next, imagine that superimposed over this aqua-blue layer is a layer of energy deeper in color—indigo blue. This color represents your intellect and the powers of the mind. When all thoughts are focused in the same direction, you have coherence at this level of energy as well. Finally, visualize that superimposed on the layer of indigo blue is a layer of violet, a color that often represents the spiritual nature of humanity. As you envision these colors, think and sense coherence—the integration, balance, and harmony of your mind, body, spirit, and emotions. Know that there is no separation of body, mind, and spirit and the whole is truly greater than the sum of the parts.

---

care. The wellness continuum also includes prevention, which means taking positive actions to prevent acute and chronic illnesses.

Wellness is not static; it is a dynamic process. It is a process that takes into account all the decisions we make daily such as which foods we eat, the amount of exercise we get, and whether we wear safety belts, smoke cigarettes, or drink alcohol before driving. Every choice we make potentially affects health and wellness.

In this book we discuss aspects of all of the different models of health wherever appropriate. The models themselves are abstractions of ideas, but in real life one needs to use whatever is practical to optimize health. Health depends very much on each person's perception. People with a disease may live joyful, positive, healthy lives; people without a disease may be despondent, unhappy, and feel sick. People need attainable goals to promote wellness and to live harmoniously with family, friends, and the environment.

Although the medical model has been extremely successful in describing, diagnosing, and treating diseases, it has not been very successful in fostering health or in preventing death caused by heart disease or cancer, both of which are often preventable diseases. The medical model has also been unsuccessful in curing many chronic diseases such as arthritis, allergies, psoriasis, and mental illness.

Truth does not change over time. Jesse Williams (1937), one of the founders of modern health education, described health as "that condition of the individual that makes possible the highest enjoyment of life, the greatest constructive work, and that shows itself in the best service to the world. . . . Health as freedom of disease is a standard of mediocrity; health as a quality of life is a standard of inspiration and increasing achievement." This is a goal we believe in, and the content of this book reflects this view.

DIMENSIONS OF HEALTH AND WELLNESS

Because wellness is dynamic and continuous, no dimension of wellness functions in isolation. When you have a high level of wellness or optimal health, all dimensions are integrated and functioning together. The person's environment (including work, school, family, community), and his or her physical, emotional, intellectual, occupational, spiritual, and social dimensions of wellness are in tune with one another to produce harmony.

Experts commonly refer to six dimensions of health and wellness: emotional, intellectual, spiritual, occupational, social, and physical. We will discuss each briefly.

- **Emotional wellness** requires understanding emotions and coping with problems that arise in everyday life.
- **Intellectual wellness** involves having a mind open to new ideas and concepts. If you are intellectually healthy you seek new experiences and challenges.
- **Spiritual wellness** is the state of harmony with yourself and others. It is the ability to balance inner needs with the demands of the rest of the world.
- **Occupational wellness** is being able to enjoy what you are doing to earn a living and/or contribute to society, whether it be going to college, working as a secretary, doctor, construction manager, or accountant. In a job, it means having skills such as critical thinking, problem solving, and communicating well.
- **Social wellness** refers to the ability to perform social roles effectively, comfortably, and without harming others.
- **Physical wellness** is a healthy body maintained by eating right, exercising regularly, avoiding harmful habits, making informed and responsible decisions about health, seeking medical care when needed, and participating in activities that help prevent illness.

HEALTH AS POSITIVE WELLNESS

If freedom from sickness isn't all there is to health, then what else is involved? The World Health Organization (WHO) defines health so broadly and covers so much that some people find it meaningless. Its universality, however, is exactly right. Peoples' lives, and therefore their health, are affected by every aspect of life: environmental influences such as climate; the availability of nutritious food, comfortable shelter, clean air to breathe, and pure water to drink; and other people, including family, lovers, employers, coworkers, friends, and associates of various kinds.

The WHO's definition of health takes into account not only the condition of your body but also the state of your mind. Your mental processes are perhaps the most important influences on your health, because they determine how you deal with your physical and social surroundings, what attitudes about life you have, and how you interact with others.

Health as the totality of a person's existence is the holistic view. It recognizes the interrelatedness of the physical, psychological, emotional, social, spiritual, and environmental factors that contribute to the overall quality of a person's life. No part of the mind, body, or environment is truly separate and independent.

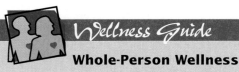

Wellness Guide

Whole-Person Wellness

A person with **emotional wellness** is able to:

- Maintain a sense of humor.
- Recognize feelings and appropriately express them.
- Strive to meet emotional needs.
- Take responsibility for his or her behavior.

A person with **intellectual wellness** is able to:

- Communicate effectively verbally and in written form.
- See more than one side of an issue.
- Keep abreast of global issues.
- Exhibit good time-management skills.

A person with **spiritual wellness** is able to:

- Examine personal values and beliefs.
- Search for meanings that help explain the purpose of life.
- Have a clear understanding of right and wrong.
- Appreciate natural forces in the universe.

A person with **occupational wellness** is able to:

- Feel a sense of accomplishment in his or her work.
- Balance work and other aspects of life.
- Find satisfaction in being creative and innovative.
- Seek challenges at work.

A person with **social wellness** is able to:

- Develop positive relationships with loved ones.
- Develop relationships with friends.
- Enjoy being with others.
- Effectively communicate with others who may be different.

A person with **physical wellness** is able to:

- Exercise regularly and select a well-balanced diet.
- Participate in safer, responsible sexual behavior.
- Make informed choices about medicinal use and medical care.
- Maintain a positive, health-promoting life-style.

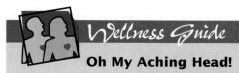

Oh My Aching Head!

Headaches are one of the most common causes of human discomfort. Although headaches can be a symptom of a brain disease or injury, the vast majority of headaches are caused by anxiety, tension, and emotional distress.

Tension headache is the most common type of headache. It is caused by persistent contractions of the muscles in the neck and scalp, brought on by anxiety, stress, or allergic reactions to drugs and foods. Tension headaches may last for hours, may occur frequently, and may be a problem over the course of several years. The pain of a tension headache often can be relieved by experiencing a few minutes of deep mental relaxation or by massaging the tense muscles in the neck and scalp.

Migraine headache, or vascular headache, is characterized by throbbing pain that can last for hours and even days. Migraine headaches are accompanied by altered blood flow to the brain's blood vessels. Massaging the neck and scalp can help relieve the pain, as can mental relaxation and visualizing normal blood flow to the head. Autosuggestion and visualizing the hands becoming warmer may also help relieve pain because some blood flow is diverted from the brain to the hands, thereby reducing blood pressure in the brain.

Identifying and eliminating the sources of tension and anxiety in your life is the surest way to prevent headaches. Some people have learned to use "having a headache" as a means of avoiding unpleasant situations, such as school or work obligations. As children they may have observed their parents coping with tension and stress by "getting a headache," and so they too learned that "having a headache" can be used to avoid anxiety-provoking experiences. Have you developed such an avoidance mechanism?

The philosophy of holistic health is not incompatible with the practice of conventional medicine. Rather, it emphasizes a view that has gained wide acceptance among members of the medical community—that each person has the capacity and the responsibility for optimizing his or her sense of well-being, for self-healing, and for the creation of conditions and feelings that help prevent disease. Holistic health is hardly a revolutionary idea; the Old English root of our word *health* (*hal,* meaning sound or whole) implies that there is more to health than freedom from sickness.

Positive wellness involves (1) being free from symptoms of disease and pain as much as possible, (2) being active, able to do what you want and what you must at the appropriate time, and (3) being in good spirits most of the time. These characteristics indicate that health is not something suddenly achieved at a specific time, like getting a college degree. Rather, health is a *process*—indeed, a way of life—through which you develop and encourage every aspect of your body, mind, and feelings to interrelate harmoniously as much of the time as possible.

The Philosophy of Holistic Health

The philosophy of holistic health emphasizes the unity of the mind, spirit, and body. Therefore, symptoms of illness and disease may be viewed as an imbalance in a person's total state of being and not simply as the malfunction of a particular part of the body. Consider, for example, a common minor illness: the headache. About 80 to 90 percent of American adults experience at least one headache each year. Although a headache can be the result of brain injury or the symptom of another illness, more often it is caused by emotional stress that produces a tightening of the muscles in the head and neck. These contracting muscles increase the blood pressure in the head, thereby causing the pain of headache.

Most people try to relieve a headache by taking aspirin or some other analgesic drug that can alter the physiological mechanisms that produce the pain. In contrast, someone using the holistic approach would first try to determine the *source* of the tensions—such as worry, anger, or frustration—and then work to reduce

T E R M S

emotional wellness: understanding emotions and knowing how to cope with problems that arise in everyday life, and how to endure stress

intellectual wellness: having a mind open to new ideas and concepts

spiritual wellness: state of balance and harmony with yourself and others

occupational wellness: enjoyment of what you are doing to earn a living and/or contribute to society

social wellness: ability to perform the expectations of social roles effectively, comfortably, and without harming others

physical wellness: maintenance of your body in good condition by eating right, exercising regularly, avoiding harmful habits, and making informed responsible decisions about your health

or eliminate the tensions. Similarly, an upset stomach cannot be regarded as simply the result of excessive secretion of stomach acid, requiring an antacid to bring relief. In many cases, the upset results from unexpressed hostility or fear. You are probably aware that such common events as taking an examination or having a dispute with someone can cause uncomfortable feelings in the stomach.

The holistic approach emphasizes self-healing, the maintenance of health, and the prevention of illness rather than the treatment of symptoms and disease. A holistic approach integrates medical technology into a broader treatment that looks not only at a person's symptoms, but also at the sources of disharmony. From the holistic point of view, illness is the result of some imbal-

ance in the harmonious interaction of the body, mind, and environment. Thus, to the extent that we can follow a program of positive wellness and create a healthy environment, we can be free of disease.

Some of the great advances in medicine have resulted from considering illness solely in terms of the affected bodily organ. Indeed, devoting medical attention to one specific ailing part of the body is sometimes the most efficient way to treat a medical problem, which is why we have specialists who are experts in treating diseases of different body parts, such as heart specialists, gastrointestinal specialists, podiatrists, gynecologists, and so on.

Some health professionals have criticized those who advocate holistic health practices and holistic medicine,

Practicing Holistic Medicine

Sometimes a holistic approach to symptoms must consider the life situation of the distressed person as a first step in reducing or eliminating the problem that is creating the stress or fear. Consider the case of Eileen M., a 29-year-old married social worker. While on a two-week stay with her husband's parents in another city, she had to be rushed to a hospital for emergency treatment of sudden and unexpected bleeding from her gastrointestinal tract. Fortunately, the surgeon on duty was able to stop the bleeding and to give proper medical treatment so that Eileen was able to leave the hospital within a few days. Upon her return home, Eileen visited a specialist in gastrointestinal illness who diagnosed her problem as ulcerative colitis. The specialist prescribed certain foods as well as medications, and he carefully monitored her recovery. He found no underlying physical problem associated with Eileen's colitis, and within a few weeks she seemed fully recovered.

The specialist advised Eileen to visit her family physician periodically to be sure her recovery was permanent. On one of these visits, the physician asked her, "Do you want this bleeding business to happen again?" Of course, Eileen said she didn't. The two women began to talk about what might have caused or contributed to Eileen's illness, and the doctor quickly learned that Eileen had been nervous and worried about visiting her in-laws for several months before the trip. She had always felt that her mother-in-law was severely critical of her, and she had once overheard the woman say that Eileen wasn't good enough for her son. Eileen had dreaded spending two

weeks with a person she had grown to dislike intensely but had said nothing for fear of hurting her husband's feelings.

After talking about this situation for a while, Eileen and her physician agreed that the suppression of her hostile feelings for her mother-in-law had probably caused her gastrointestinal problems. Eileen's physician pointed out that unless she learned to deal with her hostile feelings for her mother-in-law, the next time she paid a visit the sudden bleeding might recur—possibly with fatal results. Eileen agreed. She acknowledged that these feelings made her unhappy and that she would like to overcome them. Eileen's physician recommended that she see a psychological counselor who could help her find ways of dealing with the problem.

Fortunately for Eileen, her doctor was not content merely with her recovery from her physical symptoms but instead insisted on determining their underlying cause. In so doing, the physician was practicing holistic medicine.

STUDENT REFLECTIONS

- Do you believe that this approach was the most effective under these circumstances? If not, what alternative(s) would you suggest?
- Has there been a time when holistic medicine should have been used rather than only the traditional medical model when treating symptoms you have had? If so, explain.

arguing that the concepts and methods are antiscientific and hence harmful. Holistic medicine is not antiscientific. By encouraging individuals to take personal command of their health, including how they use medical services, holistic health practices are likely to be less harmful than some traditional medical practices, including much unnecessary surgery (Chapter 19). Criticism is useful but some people resist changes that are perceived as threats to their personal convictions or financial security.

TAKING RESPONSIBILITY FOR YOUR HEALTH

Not so many years ago, people were subject to a variety of diseases over which they had little or no control. In the early part of the twentieth century, infectious diseases caused by organisms were the leading causes of death in the United States. Modern public health methods and modern drugs, such as antibiotics, were not available. In 1918 millions of people around the world died from influenza, whose cause was unknown at that time (Table 1.2).

Today, the leading causes of illness and death are not due to infections, but to "life-style diseases." These diseases, such as heart disease and cancer, result from envi-

TABLE 1.2   The Ten Leading Causes of Death for All Ages, All Races, and Both Sexes, 1900, 1987, and 1992

	1900	1987	1992*
1.	Tuberculosis	Heart disease	Heart disease
2.	Pneumonia	Cancer	Cancer
3.	Diarrhea and enteritis	Stroke	Stroke
4.	Heart disease	Injuries	Chronic obstructive pulmonary disease (COPD)
5.	Liver disease	Bronchitis and emphysema	Accidents, including motor vehicle accidents
6.	Injuries	Pneumonia and influenza	Pneumonia and influenza
7.	Stroke	Diabetes	Diabetes
8.	Cancer	Suicide	HIV infection
9.	Bronchitis	Chronic liver disease	Suicide
10.	Diphtheria	Arteriosclerosis	Homicide

*Source: Adapted from U.S. Department of Health and Human Resources, *Monthly Vital Statistics Report* (Washington, D.C.: U.S. Government Printing Office, December 8, 1994).

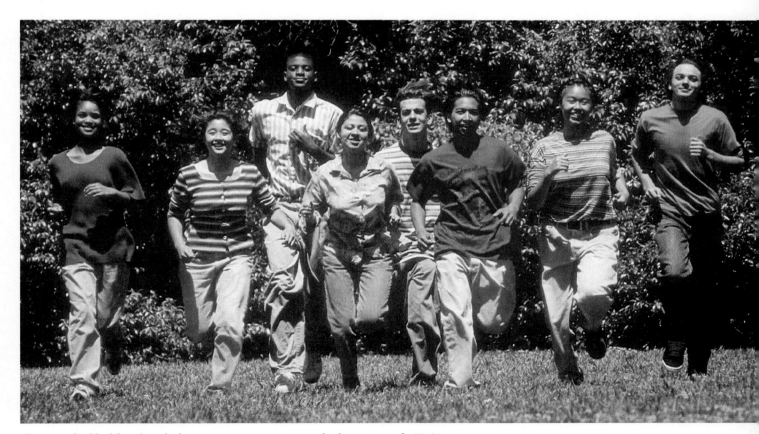

Choosing a healthy life-style is the best way to prevent premature death among people 15–24.

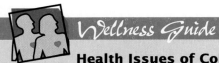

Health Issues of College Students

What health issues face North America's 15 million college students as we approach the next century? Here's what college and university health educators and medical professionals think the answers are (Guyton et al., 1990).

Sexual health. More than any others, sexual issues have the potential to affect the health of college students. These include sexually transmitted diseases (7 to 10 percent of college students carry an undiagnosed STD), unintended pregnancy, and sexual assault, especially acquaintance or date rape.

Sexuality is also related to issues of self-esteem, peer acceptance, loneliness, and relieving academic stress with superficial sexual relationships, all of which have the potential to produce psychological harm and establish negative attitudes and behavior that may impair future sexual and intimate relationships.

Substance abuse. The abuse of alcohol, drugs, tobacco, and food is related to trying to gain peer acceptance, unhealthy role modeling in families and in society-at-large, and trying to cope with psychological distress. Students whose parents abuse substances often have a tendency for substance abuse. Alcohol abuse is related to the majority of sexual assaults, unintended pregnancies (from not using contraceptives properly or at all), and the transmission of STDs from not practicing safer sex.

Mental health. Failure to achieve, academic stress, lack of social support, difficulty adjusting to young adulthood, and pressures to fit in socially all contribute to emotional problems (especially anxiety and depression) that may impair a student's academic performance and sense of well-being. They can also lead to stress-related physical ill-

nesses. Competitive academic environments can create feelings of inferiority, insecurity, and emotional distress.

Food and weight. Many students are highly concerned about their body size and shape and may become malnourished to meet their perceptions of social ideality. Eating disorders such as bulimia and anorexia nervosa affect a large number of students (see Chapter 6).

Health care. A large proportion of college students in the United States have limited access to health care because their colleges do not have comprehensive services for students or they do not have private health insurance.

Accidents and injuries. Many students are susceptible to automobile accidents (often alcohol-related) and sports injuries.

---

ronmental factors and people's behaviors and ways in which they choose to live. The idea that life-style is a major cause of disease and death in modern societies is not new. A generation ago Lewis Thomas, an eminent physician and author, observed that our life-styles were killing us.

> The new theory is that most of today's human illnesses, the infectious ones aside, are multifactoral in nature, caused by two great arrays of causative mechanisms: the influence of things in the environment; and one's personal lifestyle. For medicine to become effective in dealing with such disease, it has become common belief that the environment will have to be changed, and personal ways of living also have to be transformed, and radically.
>
> —Thomas, 1978

There is no "bacterium" that causes heart disease. Heart disease results from today's life-styles, which include overeating (Chapter 6), cigarette smoking (Chapter 17), lack of exercise (Chapter 7), high levels of stress (Chapter 3), and high blood pressure (Chapter 14). Cancer is associated with both life-style and environmental factors

(Chapter 13). Improper nutrition, smoking cigarettes, and exposure to hazardous substances in the environment initiate biological changes that can result in cancer. Unhealthy life-style is also at the root of suicide and homicide (alcohol, drugs, and stress), accidents (alcohol use and stress), and cirrhosis of the liver (alcohol abuse).

Table 1.3 shows that of the ten leading causes of death for young adults 15 to 24 years old, six of the top ten for all races and both sexes can be directly related to personal behavior (accidents, homicide, suicide, cancer, heart disease, HIV infection). If we were to wear seat belts, not carry firearms, deal appropriately with stress and anger, and be sexually responsible, a list of the top ten causes of death for 15- to 24-year-olds might be completely different.

A survey of the actual causes of death (as opposed to the causes reported on the death certificates) revealed that approximately half of all deaths in the United States each year are due to life-style factors (McGuiness and Foege, 1993). Leading the list of risk factors is tobacco use, which was responsible for 400,000 deaths in 1990; other life-

> *If my soul exists without my body, I am convinced all my clothes will be loose-fitting.*
> Woody Allen

TABLE 1.3   The Ten Leading Causes of Death for 15 to 24 Year Olds

All races, both sexes	Males only, all races	Females only, all races
1. Accidents, including motor vehicle accidents	Accidents, including motor vehicle accidents	Accidents, including motor motor vehicle accidents
2. Homicide	Homicide	Homicide
3. Suicide	Suicide	Cancer
4. Cancer	Cancer	Suicide
5. Heart disease	Heart disease	Heart disease
6. HIV infection	HIV infection	Congenital anomalies
7. Congenital anomalies	Congenital anomalies	HIV infection
8. Pneumonia and influenza	Pneumonia and influenza	Complications of pregnancy and childbirth
9. Stroke	Stroke	Pneumonia and influenza
10. Chronic obstructive pulmonary disease (COPD)	COPD	COPD

Source: Adapted from U.S. Department of Health and Human Services, *Monthly Vital Statistics Report* (Washington D.C.: U.S. Government Printing Office, December 8, 1994).

style risk factors that caused death were alcohol, firearms, motor vehicle accidents, illegal drug use, and unsafe sexual behaviors. These scientific studies should convince us that great improvements in health are possible. All we need to do is change our behaviors so we can avoid sickness and achieve wellness.

THE YEAR 2000 NATIONAL HEALTH OBJECTIVES

In 1979 the first *Surgeon General's Report on Health Promotion and Disease Prevention* was released. Its purpose was to create a public health revolution. The strategy was to emphasize prevention of disease. The focus was on personal responsibility for one's own health by reducing risky habits. The report indicated that for the public health revolution to succeed, social changes must also take place to deal with poverty, lack of education, inadequate housing, hunger, drug use, and so on. The report identified five public health goals that were measurable and could be achieved by 1990 (Table 1.4).

In 1980 the United States Department of Health and Human Services (USDHHS) published *Promoting Health/Preventing Disease: Objectives for the Nation,* which provides quantifiable objectives necessary to obtain the broad goals set in the *Surgeon General's Report* of 1979. A total of 226 specific objectives were established for fifteen priority areas identified in the *Surgeon General's Report.* Within each priority, the nature and extent of

TABLE 1.4   1990 Health Status Goals for the U.S. Population Set in 1979

Age group (years)	1990 goal*	Special focus
Healthy infants (birth to 1 year)	35% fewer deaths	Low birth weight Birth defects
Healthy children (ages 1–14)	20% fewer deaths	Growth and development Injuries
Healthy adolescents/ young adults (ages 15–24)	20% fewer deaths	Motor vehicle injuries Alcohol and drug use
Healthy adults (ages 25–64)	25% fewer deaths	Heart attacks Strokes, cancers
Healthy older adults (ages 65+)	20% fewer sick days	Functional independence Influenza/pneumonia

*Relative to 1977
Source: U.S. Department of Health, Education, and Welfare, *Healthy People: The Surgeon General's Report on Health Promotion and Disease Prevention* (Washington, D.C.: U.S. Government Printing Office, 1979), pp. ix–x.

Diabetes Is Caused by Modern Life-styles

Diabetes is a disease in which the level of sugar in the blood cannot be regulated, causing a variety of symptoms including degeneration of some organs in the body and even death. There are two forms of diabetes: type I, or insulin-dependent diabetes, requires injections of insulin to control symptoms of the disease; type II, or insulin-independent diabetes, generally can be controlled by diet, exercise, or drugs other than insulin. Type I diabetes was formerly called "juvenile onset" because it tends to occur in children and adolescents. Type II diabetes was formerly called "maturity onset" because it tends to occur in adults.

Evidence that diabetes is a disease of life-style comes from studies of populations that have dramatically altered their life-style over a brief time span. For example, Yemenite Jews who emigrated to Israel in 1949 had one of the lowest rates of diabetes in the world—less than 1 per 1,000 individuals. Thirty years later, the same population, now adapted to a western lifestyle in Israel, had a rate of almost 12 cases of diabetes per 1,000 individuals.

Another dramatic example is the prevalence of diabetes among the Pima Indians of the southwestern United States. In the last century, these Native Americans lived mostly on maize, beans, wild game, and vegetables. They were active, lean, and strong. Today many Pima Indians are sedentary, corpulent, and suffer the highest rate of diabetes in the world—341 cases per 1000 individuals (Eaton, 1990). As a result of their changed life-style, more than one out of three Pima Indians suffers from diabetes.

Diabetes seems to be a life-style disease that has been increasing recently. Type II diabetes is associated with being overweight: for every 20 percent increase in overweight, the chance of diabetes doubles. Improving nutrition, maintaining normal body weight, reducing stress, and not smoking can help prevent diabetes and other life-style diseases.

TABLE 1.5 Healthy Youth 2000 Priority Areas and Number of Objectives for 10 to 24 Year Olds

Priorities	Health status	Risk reduction	Services and protection	Total
Health promotion				
1. Physical activity and fitness	0	1	2	3
2. Nutrition	1	1	0	2
3. Tobacco	0	2	0	2
4. Alcohol and other drugs	1	7	0	8
5. Family planning	1	3	2	6
6. Mental health and mental disorders	4	0	0	4
7. Violent and abusive drugs	4	2	0	6
8. Educational and community-based programs	0	1	1	2
Health protection				
9. Unintentional injuries	2	0	0	2
10. Environmental health	1	0	0	1
11. Oral health	2	1	0	3
Preventive services				
12. HIV infection	0	2	0	2
13. STDs	1	0	0	1
14. Clinical preventive services	0	1	0	1
				43

Source: American Medical Association, *Healthy Youth 2000* (Chicago: AMA, 1990).

problem, prevention/promotion measures, specific objectives, principal assumptions, and data sources were outlined and discussed.

Efforts by local, state, and federal governments have led to *Healthy People 2000* (U.S. Department of Health and Human Services, 1990), the nation's vision for a new century characterized by enhancing quality of life, reducing preventable death and disability, and reducing the disparity in the health status of people within American society. The purpose of *Healthy People 2000* was "to commit the Nation to the attainment of three broad goals that will help bring us to our full potential" (USDHHS, 1990, p. 6):

1. increase the life span of healthy life for Americans,
2. reduce health disparities among Americans, and
3. achieve access to preventive services for all Americans.

Health Update

The Year 2000: A Profile of the American People

Over the course of the 1990s, the profile of the American population will change. Barring unforeseeable major events, the demographic contrasts between 1990 and 2000 will be evident, if not dramatic. Based on the best available information:

- By the year 2000, the overall population of the United States will have grown about 7 percent to nearly 270 million people, with the slowest rate of growth in the Nation's history projected between 1995 and 2000. Average household size is expected to decline from 2.69 in 1985 to 2.48 in 2000, with husband-wife households decreasing from 58 to 53 percent of all households.

- By the year 2000, the American population will be older, continuing the aging trend of the present century, with a median age of more than 36 years, compared to 29 years in 1975. The number of children under age 5 will actually decline from more than 18 million to fewer than 17 million between 1990 and 2000. By 2000, the 35 million people over age 65 will represent about 13 percent of the population, in contrast to 8 percent in 1950. The population of the "oldest old"— those over age 85—will have increased by about 30 percent to a total of 4.6 million by 2000.

- By the year 2000, the racial and ethnic composition of the American population will form a different pattern. Whites, not including Hispanic Americans, will represent a smaller proportion of the total, declining from 76 to 72 percent of the population. One particularly fast-growing population group will be Hispanics, some estimates forecasting a rise from 8 to 11.3 percent, to more than 31 million Hispanic people by 2000. Blacks will increase their proportion from 12.4 to 13.1 percent. Other racial groups, including American Indians and Alaska Natives and Asians and Pacific Islanders, will increase from 3.5 to 4.3 percent of the total.

- By the year 2000, economic expansion will create up to 18 million new jobs, but the number of young job seekers will decline due to a shift in birthrates. Reflecting changes in racial and ethnic populations, the entry rate of blacks, Hispanics, Asians and Pacific Islanders, and American Indians and Alaska Natives into the workforce will be higher than for whites. Women of all racial and ethnic groups will be the major source of new entrants into the labor force, comprising 47 percent of the total workforce by 2000, compared to 45 percent in 1988. Half of women in the workforce will be between the ages of 35 and 54, a shift from 1986 when the majority were between 25 and 44. Between 1988 and the year 2000, white men will comprise only 25 percent of the net growth of the labor force. Occupations most likely to grow include service, professional, technical, sales, and executive and management positions.

- By the year 2000, the American population may increase by up to 6 million people through immigration. Certain states and cities, especially those on the east and west coasts, can be expected to receive a disproportionately large number of these immigrants.

While 10 years in the history of a nation seems a comparatively short time, it is long enough to alter population patterns in ways that are of great importance to current and future decision makers seeking to design an effective program of health promotion and disease prevention. Informed estimates about the changes in households and family constellations, age groups, racial and ethnic populations, the workforce, and immigration can provide a context that is crucial to decisions and programs to achieve a nation of healthy people.

Source: U.S. Department of Health and Human Services, *Healthy People 2000: National Health Promotion and Disease Prevention Objectives* (Washington D.C.: U.S. Government Printing Office, 1990), pp. 2–3.

Healthy People 2000 presents opportunities in the form of measurable objectives to be achieved by the year 2000, organized into twenty-two priority areas. The first twenty-one areas are grouped into three broad categories: health promotion, health protection, and preventive services. The twenty-second priority is surveillance and data systems. Within each area are health status objectives, risk reduction objectives, services and protection objectives, personnel needs, surveillance and data needs, research needs, related objectives from other priority areas, and baseline data sources. Table 1.5 shows objectives for youth ranging from 10 to 24 years of age.

In each chapter, applicable Year 2000 Objectives are presented to provide a better understanding of what each of us can do to help accomplish these national goals. A brief statement accompanies each selected Year 2000 Objective.

> *The trouble with our times is that the future is not what it used to be.*
>
> Paul Valery,
> author

HEALTH IN REVIEW

- Health means different things to different people.
- The definition of health generally accepted by the medical profession and health professionals that monitor sickness and death in populations is "the absence of disease."
- Wellness includes not only the absence of disease but living in harmony with oneself, with friends and relatives, and with the environment (including school, work, and the community).
- Health means being responsible for preventing illness and injuries as well as knowing when to seek medical help.
- Three common models are used to describe health: the medical model, the environmental model, and the holistic/wellness model.
- The wellness continuum ranges from high-level wellness to death, with many areas in between. Most of us stay in the neutral area, however, at different points in time we move up and down the continuum.
- A holistic approach to health emphasizes prevention of disease and injury, and self-responsibility for nutrition, exercise, and other aspects of life-style that promote wellness.
- Positive wellness is a dynamic process.
- The holistic/wellness and environmental approaches to health are the best paths to life-long wellness.
- The commonly stated dimensions of wellness are emotional, intellectual, spiritual, occupational, social, and physical.
- Taking responsibility for one's health is the best way to prevent chronic diseases, which are the most common causes of death in the United States today.
- Many chronic diseases (e.g., diabetes, heart disease, cancer, etc.) are primarily attributable to personal life-style.
- *Healthy People 2000* is the nation's vision for a new century characterized by enhancing quality of life, reducing preventable diseases and premature deaths, and reducing disparity in health status among different populations.

REFERENCES

American Medical Association (1990). *Healthy Youth 2000.* Chicago: American Medical Association.

Dunn, H. (1967). *High Level Wellness.* Arlington, Va.: Charles B. Slack.

Eaton, S. B. (1990). "Other Worlds." *Longevity,* February.

Guyton, R., S. Corbin, C. Zimmer, M. O'Donnell, D. Chervin, B. Conant Sloane, and M. Chamberlain (1990). "College Students and National Health Objectives for the Year 2000: A Summary Report." *Journal of American College Health,* 38(1): 9–14.

Hurley, J. S., and R. G. Schlaadt (1992). *The Wellness Life-Style.* Guilford, Conn.: The Dushkin Publishing Group, Inc.

McGuiness, J. M., and W. H. Foege (1993). "Actual Causes of Death in the United States." *Journal of the American Medical Association,* 270(18): 2207–2212.

Sumatriptan Study Group (1991). "Treatment of Migraine Attacks with Sumatriptan." *New England Journal of Medicine,* August 1.

Thomas, L. O. (1978). "On Magic in Medicine." *New England Journal of Medicine,* August, 31.

United States Department of Health and Human Services (1979). *Healthy People: The Surgeon General's Report on Health Promotion and Disease Prevention.* (PHS 79-55071). Washington, D.C.: U.S. Government Printing Office.

United States Department of Health and Human Services (1994). *Monthly Vital Statistics Report*. Washington, D.C.: U.S. Government Printing Office.

United States Department of Health and Human Services (1990). *Healthy People 2000: National Health Promotion and Disease Prevention Objectives*. (PHS 91-50212). Washington, D.C.: U.S. Government Printing Office.

Williams, J. (1937).

World Health Organization (1947). *Constitution of the World Health Organization*. Geneva, Switzerland.

SUGGESTED READINGS

Hurley, J. S., and R. G. Schlaadt (1992). *The Wellness Life-Style*. Guilford, Conn.: The Dushkin Publishing Group, Inc. A book that helps you think critically about your life-style and offers suggestions for change.

Papazian, R. (1994). "Trace Your Family Tree." *American Health* (May): 80–84. Many illnesses have a hereditary link. This article discusses how to become more aware of your family medical history.

Segal, B. (1986). *Love, Medicine and Miracles*. New York: Harper & Row. A cancer physician describes how he learned to practice healing as well as medicine.

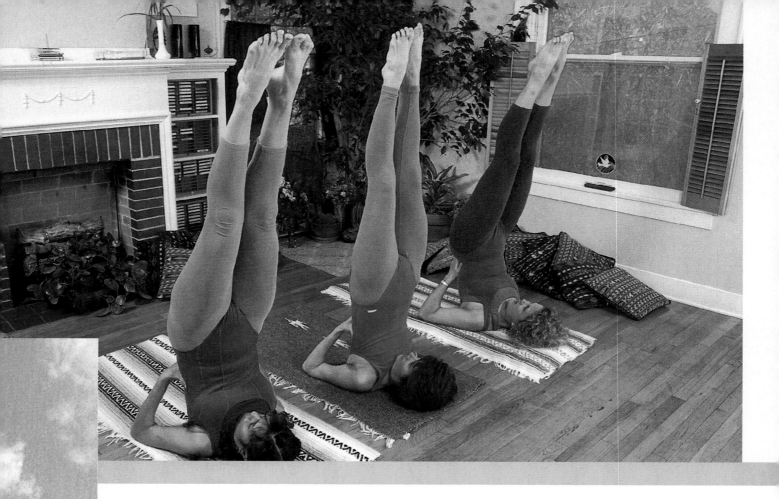

LEARNING OBJECTIVES

After reading this chapter you should be able to:

1. Briefly describe how the mind and body communicate to enhance physical and mental well-being.
2. Explain the importance of homeostasis and the role it plays in maintaining health.
3. Describe the function(s) of the autonomic nervous system.
4. Briefly explain the galvanic skin response and how your mental state can influence the autonomic nervous system.
5. Describe the relationship between hormones and certain body functions.
6. Compare and contrast how Western medicine handles psychosomatic illnesses with how Chinese medicine handles psychosomatic illnesses.
7. Identify several ways you can relieve test anxiety.
8. Describe how faith and hypnosis are used in healing.
9. Describe how visualization can promote wellness and behavioral change.

Promoting Wellness through Mind-Body Communications

$\mathscr{E}$veryone can learn to control, at least to some degree, supposedly unconscious mental and physiological processes. Although some people learn to control stress, pain, and healing processes without understanding the mechanisms that connect the mind and the body, most people need some knowledge of the nervous and hormone (endocrine) systems to improve health. Understanding how the organs of the body respond to thoughts and feelings can help you make healthy changes. The brain, the nervous system, and the endocrine system coordinate the body's physiological activities and responses. Brain and body chemistry help determine wellness and sickness.

No human body exists without a mind; no mind exists without a body. That our mind and body communicate with one another by means of hormones and signals from the nervous system has great significance for our health and well-being. What goes on in the mind affects physiological processes such as digestion, blood pressure, breathing, muscle tension, sexual arousal, and the functions of many organs. Thought and feeling centers in the brain influence the activities of the nervous, hormone, and immune systems, which interact to maintain health or to invite disease. People affect their health by what they think and feel as well as by what they eat and how they live. No medicine or treatment is more capable of healing than the human mind.

In Western culture we are accustomed to thinking about sickness and healing in terms of drugs, surgery, or other medical treatments. In other cultures, past and present, healing has been accomplished by magic, ritual, faith, and other nonmedical methods. Nontraditional approaches to healing do work and do cure people of many illnesses. Even in our culture we recognize that a patient's attitude plays an important role in the success of a treatment and in recovery. Nonmedical healing practices are effective because thoughts, beliefs, faith, and convictions *do* change body chemistry and physiology. Each one of us can learn to use positive thoughts, healthy feelings, and faith to prevent disease and to promote healing in time of sickness.

HOMEOSTASIS AND HEALTH

Many of the vital functions in the body such as breathing, heartbeat, blood circulation, digestion, and elimination require no conscious effort. Rarely do you think about how often to breathe, or whether your heart needs to beat faster or slower to accomplish a task. Your body has mechanisms for controlling and integrating its functions without conscious control, so that it maintains a relatively constant internal chemical environment. The tendency for body systems to interact and to maintain a constant physiological state is called **homeostasis.**

Homeostatic mechanisms maintain blood pressure in most people within the normal limits of 70 to 130 millimeters of mercury, a temperature of 98.6°F, a heart rate between 50 and 90 beats per minute, and blood glucose (sugar) levels around 80 milligrams per 100 milliliters of blood. Although these processes are regulated automatically, they can be deregulated by stress, anger, emotional upset, and thoughts.

Homeostatic mechanisms also prompt many of our behaviors by indicating needs such as hunger, thirst, or sleep. Centers in the brain monitor the amount of nutrients in the blood and the amount of water in the body's tissues. When nutrients are low or the body is in need of water, these centers become activated, and you feel hungry or thirsty. When the body is cold, the brain tells the body to shiver in order to generate heat; if the body is overheated, the brain tells it to perspire in order to reduce its temperature.

When you are well and healthy, your body systems function harmoniously. It is similar to the members of a

Global Wellness

Yin and Yang: Finding Balance

Taoist philosophy and traditional Chinese medicine embody ideas of balanced energy and internal harmony that are, in many respects, analogous to the Western concept of homeostasis. Harmony is expressed by a balance between the forces of Yin and Yang (Figure 2.1). Yin and Yang represent the opposing and complementary aspects of the universal *ch'i* that is present in everything, including our bodies. Yang forces are characterized as light, positive, creative, full of movement, and with the nature of heaven. Yin forces are characterized as dark, negative, quiet, receptive, and with the nature of earth.

Chinese medicine classifies the organs of the body as predominantly Yin or Yang. Hollow organs such as the stomach, intestines, and bladder are Yang; solid organs such as the heart, spleen, liver, and lungs are Yin. Food and herbs are also classified as having mostly Yin or Yang properties. When Yin and Yang forces are in balance in an individual, a state of harmony exists, and the person experiences health and wellness. However, if either Yin or Yang forces come to predominate in a person, a state of disharmony is produced and disease may result.

In Asian philosophies and medicine body and mind are regarded as inseparable. Yin and Yang apply to both mental and physical processes. Thus, illness and its treatment involve the whole person and are designed to reestablish total harmony of the mind and body. The balance of Yin and Yang forces must be restored so that health returns. In Western medicine treatments are designed to correct an imbalance in the function of a particular organ so as to restore homeostasis.

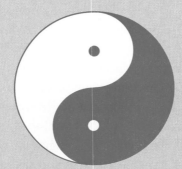

FIGURE 2.1 The Yin/Yang Symbol This symbol represents the harmonious balance of forces in nature and in people. The white and dark dots show that there is always some Yin in a person's Yang component and vice versa. The goal in life and nature, according to the Chinese view, is to maintain a harmonious balance between Yin and Yang forces.

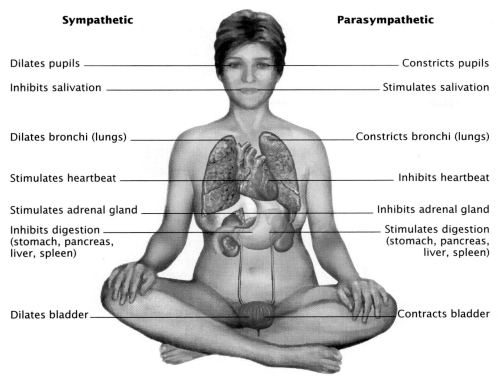

Sympathetic

Dilates pupils

Inhibits salivation

Dilates bronchi (lungs)

Stimulates heartbeat

Stimulates adrenal gland

Inhibits digestion
(stomach, pancreas,
liver, spleen)

Dilates bladder

Parasympathetic

Constricts pupils

Stimulates salivation

Constricts bronchi (lungs)

Inhibits heartbeat

Inhibits adrenal gland

Stimulates digestion
(stomach, pancreas,
liver, spleen)

Contracts bladder

FIGURE 2.2 Functions Controlled by the Autonomic Nervous System The sympathetic nerves and the parasympathetic nerves act in opposition to regulate functions that normally are not under conscious control such as breathing, digestion, and heart rate.

team playing together in a coordinated way to accomplish the goals of the game. If one of your organs is not functioning properly, however, the other organs may not be able to function correctly either, and you become ill. Thus, disease may be regarded as the disruption of homeostasis, or internal disharmony. Chinese and other Asian cultures embody the idea of physiological balance by defining an energy called **ch'i**, which must be distributed harmoniously throughout the mind and body to maintain health.

> *Your daily life is nothing but an expression of your spiritual condition.*
> Thaddeus Golas,
> *The Lazy Man's Guide to Enlightenment*

THE AUTONOMIC NERVOUS SYSTEM

The brain influences health and healing through a special group of nerves that control virtually all of the body's organs and functions. This group of nerves is the **autonomic nervous system** (ANS) and regulates many physiological processes (Figure 2.2). The ANS is divided into two sets of nerves called the *sympathetic* and the *parasympathetic* that tend to work in opposition to one another. For example, sympathetic nerve activity increases heart rate; parasympathetic nerve activity reduces it. Sympathetic nerves decrease digestive activity; parasympathetic nerves increase it.

The autonomic nervous system derives its name from the fact that its activities normally operate without conscious control. For example, a person in a deep coma due to damage of the outer layers of the brain will maintain a heartbeat, continue to breathe, digest food, and carry out other body functions controlled by the ANS. Centers in the brain, well below the conscious level, send signals to the body that maintain functions vital to life.

Although the ANS functions without conscious control, the signals it sends to the body can be changed by thoughts and feelings. Emotional upset can bring on an upset stomach, panic has an immediate effect on breathing and heart rate, and tension can constrict blood vessels causing headaches or elevating blood pressure.

T E R M S

homeostasis: the tendency for body systems to interact in ways that maintain a constant physiological state

ch'i: a Chinese term referring to the balance of energy in the body

autonomic nervous system: the special group of nerves that automatically control some of the body's organs and their functions

A well-investigated example of how mental processes influence the ANS and change physiology is the **galvanic skin response** (GSR), which is the basis of lie detector tests. To monitor GSR, two wires are attached to a person's skin—usually to a finger—and a tiny electric current is passed through the skin separating the two wires, and is recorded. Although the amount of electricity is too small to be felt, it is sufficient to measure the resistance of the skin. The resistance of skin is changed by emotional states such as anger, excitement, or fear which change the moisture content of the skin.

After a person's normal GSR is established by a series of standard questions, others are asked that may provoke an emotional response. Lying tends to produce changes in skin resistance in many people but not in everyone. Many people become upset simply from the nature of the questions being asked, even if they have nothing to hide. Although lie detector tests are used in a number of circumstances to establish the truth of peoples' statements, the test is not regarded as scientific and evidence obtained from lie detectors is not admissible in many courts (Steinbrook, 1992).

The ability to use the mind to alter physiological processes under the control of the ANS is not restricted to a few exceptional people. With **biofeedback training,** almost anyone can learn to change the temperature in one hand as compared to the other or to alter the electrical pattern of the brain's activity. In biofeedback training, the person observes his or her physiological response on a monitor and tries to adjust thought processes in any way that change the response in the desired direction.

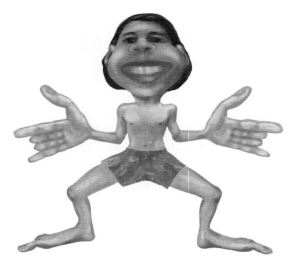

FIGURE 2.3 The amount of the cerebral cortex that the brain devotes to different parts of the body reflects their relative importance. Many more nerves are present in the hands and lips, which gives them increased sensitivity. Mapping parts of the body in the brain produces this image.

Some areas of the body such as the head, hands, or lips have many more nerve connections than other, less sensitive areas of the body (Figure 2.3). Larger areas of the brain are devoted to receiving and sending information to the more sensitive parts of the body. The significance of demonstrating scientifically that people can mentally alter physiology should encourage you to use your mind to help heal yourself in time of sickness or injury.

Wellness Guide

Using Your Mind to Heal Your Body

Everyone has accidentally cut or burned his or her hands at one time or another. Perhaps you were chopping vegetables and the knife slipped, or perhaps you reached for a pan on the stove forgetting that the handle was hot. The usual response to such accidents is anger at being careless or forgetful and anger at the sudden pain. We jump around, curse, and generally act in ways that exacerbate the injury and delay healing.

A much better response to minor accidental injuries that do not require immediate medical attention is the following. In case of a cut, place a clean cloth over the wound and press gently to help stop the bleeding. Then, as quickly as possible, sit or lie down. Close your eyes and allow yourself to become mentally and physically quiet. Visualize the injured part with your mind and see it as it was just *before* the accident. See the skin coming back together. Feel the pain recede. Notice that there is no bleeding. Continue doing this for 5 minutes or longer until you feel calm. If the accident caused a burn, place an ice bag or cool, wet cloth over the wound. Then lie down and visualize the skin becoming cooler and looking like the normal skin around the burn.

By immediately calming the mind after an injury, inflammation and other harmful physiological reactions in the area are reduced. Healing processes begin immediately when you send positive, healthy thoughts and images to the injured area. Many people use this exercise successfully. Healing begins in the mind.

HORMONES

Hormones are chemicals produced in the body that affect a wide range of body functions such as growth, development of male or female sexual organs, the menstrual cycle, digestion in the stomach, the level of sugar in the blood, to mention just a few (Table 2.1). Hormones are synthesized and released from special glands located throughout the body (Figure 2.4). The synthesis

TABLE 2.1   The Functions of Various Glands and Organs That Produce Hormones

Gland and hormones	Function
Hypothalamus and pituitary glands	
Growth hormone	Stimulates growth of bones and other structures
Adrenocorticotropic hormone (ACTH)	Stimulates release of hormones from the adrenal glands
Thyroid-stimulating hormone	Stimulates growth of the thyroid gland and release of thyroxin
Luteinizing hormone	Stimulates ovaries and the release of ovarian hormones in women; stimulates testes to produce hormones in men
Follicle-stimulating hormone	Stimulates ovum production in women; stimulates sperm production in men
Prolactin	Stimulates milk production in breasts
Testes	
Testosterone	Controls maleness
Ovaries	
Estrogen	Controls aspects of female sexuality and reproduction
Progesterone	Controls aspects of female sexuality and reproduction
Pancreas	
Insulin	Regulates blood sugar levels
Thyroid gland	
Thyroxin	Regulates metabolism
Parathyroid glands	
Calcitonin	Regulates calcium and phosphorus levels
Adrenal glands	
Aldosterone	Regulates water balance in the body
Cortisol	Increases blood glucose
Adrenalin (Epinephrine)	Increases heart rate; activates muscles

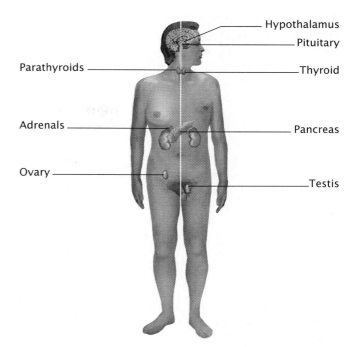

FIGURE 2.4   Where Hormones Are Released Throughout the Body Hormones are released from different glands throughout the body. The synthesis and release of these hormones are regulated by the mind and autonomic nervous system. Hormones carry chemical messages that tell the body how to respond to certain stimuli.

of hormones and their release in the body is regulated by the mind and nervous system. The mind, in turn, responds to the environment; to what a person is thinking, experiencing, and feeling.

Your five senses (sight, hearing, touch, taste, and smell) constantly record whether the environment is safe or hostile, familiar or unfamiliar, pleasurable or painful. In order to be able to respond appropriately to environmental stimuli, the mind must interpret the experiences moment by moment and send chemical signals to the organs of the body. Hormones carry the chemical messages that tell the body how to respond.

For example, when the mind interprets a situation as threatening or frightening, regardless of whether the danger is real or imagined, hormones are released that

T E R M S

galvanic skin response: changes in the skin's electrical resistance in response to changes in a person's emotional state or arousal level

biofeedback training: adjustment of a physiological process by using a monitor that feeds back information allowing the mind to move the response in the desired direction

hormones: chemicals produced in the body that regulate body functions

make the body alert and ready for action. Fear produces an increased heart rate and blood pressure, sweaty palms, changes in breathing, tension in muscles, and so forth. That is why fear, especially if it is prolonged or ongoing, can damage health and increase the risk of sickness.

When people commonly mention stress, they are usually referring to experiences that the mind has difficulty resolving. As a result, the "stress" is converted to hormonal and other chemical changes that affect how the body functions; homeostasis is disturbed. Feelings such as anger, anxiety, frustration, hostility, and guilt may cause adverse hormonal changes. For example, anxiety or guilt can block the release of hormones that are necessary for a sexual response. By governing the overall chemistry of the body, the mind is the most important determinant of wellness or illness.

THE MIND CAN CREATE ILLNESS AND HEALTH

The power of the mind to affect the health of the body is illustrated by **psychosomatic illnesses.** When a person is subjected to stress, emotional upset, or negative mental states, this can cause harmful changes in the body that may manifest as diseases (Figure 2.5). The terms *psycho* ("mind") and *soma* ("body") emphasize the connection between the mind and the body with respect to health.

Many people believe that if a person has a psychosomatic illness, he or she is imagining it, that it is "all in the mind." This is not true. The symptoms of a headache brought on by stress can be just as severe as one brought on by being hit over the head with a bat. In one case, stress has caused a change in the flow of blood through the head, and in the other case, blood vessels may have been damaged by the injury. Psychosomatic illnesses are as real as a cold brought on by a virus. The difference is that the factors causing psychosomatic illnesses are social, psychological, and environmental.

Western medicine is not well equipped to deal with psychosomatic illnesses. Although physicians can treat the symptoms, they are not well trained to help with the underlying mental states that cause the illness. On the other hand, Buddhist and Chinese medicine take the position that all sickness, to some degree, is brought on by a person's state of mind. In Western medicine, if a physician cannot find an organic cause for symptoms, the patient usually is advised to see a psychologist or a psychiatrist.

This view should not be interpreted to mean that sickness is brought on *just* by a person's state of mind, but that our psychological state, at any time, may invite illness. In order for an emotional or mental state to change physiology, a process called **somatization** must occur. Somatization refers to the occurrence of physical symptoms in a person without the presence of disease or injury that can be detected medically. Physicians believe that somatization is the most common way for people to express stress and emotional disorders. Thus, it should come as no surprise that physicians estimate that half of their patients suffer to some extent from somatization of their worries and emotional upsets.

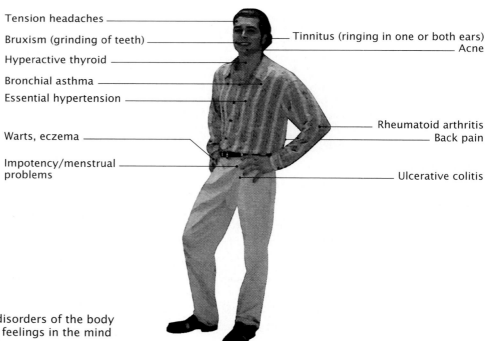

FIGURE 2.5 Many diseases and disorders of the body are partly caused by thoughts and feelings in the mind that produce psychosomatic illnesses.

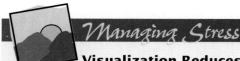

Visualization Reduces Exam Anxiety

The following exercise can reduce the stress and anxiety of taking exams. It can result in improved scores and a reduction in symptoms produced by stress.

1. Find a comfortable place in your house or room and a time when you will not be disturbed by other people. Sit in a comfortable chair or lie down on a couch or floor. The main thing is to get physically comfortable. If music helps you relax, play some of your favorite music softly.

2. Close your eyes and ask your mind to recall a place and time where you felt content. It might be a vacation time, being with someone, or being alone in a beautiful environment. Use your imagination and memory to reconstruct the scene where you felt happy and healthy. Notice that you had no concerns there at that time. Let yourself become involved with the scene. The process is similar to having a daydream or a fantasy. While your mind is focused on pleasurable memories, your body automatically relaxes.

3. When you feel quite relaxed, refocus your mind on the upcoming exam. See yourself taking the exam while feeling relaxed and confident. Because your mind and body are relaxed and comfortable, your mind automatically associates the same feelings with the image of taking the exam. Visualize the exam room, the other students, yourself answering the questions; let your mind focus on as many details as possible.

4. Now project your mind into the future to the actual day and place of the exam. Notice how relaxed you feel as you take the exam; the anxiety you used to experience seems to have vanished. Continue with the visualization until you see yourself turning in the exam and feeling confident and pleased with your performance.

5. Do this exercise for several days prior to any exam that causes anxiety. You will be surprised at the absence of nervousness and stress on exam day. You will be even more surprised at the improvement in your grades.

Exam Anxiety

People in American society equate educational success, academic degrees, and professional licenses with the attainment of important life goals, particularly financial ones. As a consequence, competition among students at all levels has become intense. Students believe that grades and exam scores will determine how successful their lives will be in terms of jobs, careers, and money.

Because of academic pressures and anxiety about exams, many students experience health problems. They may suffer from frequent headaches, stomach and bowel problems, eating disorders, recurrent infections, and other symptoms of stress (Chapter 3). Students whose exam anxiety affects their health need to make personal adjustments to reduce the anxiety while they pursue their goals.

The first thing to realize is that exam anxiety is learned behavior and probably began very early in school. Perhaps parents or teachers scolded you or warned you about the consequences of poor performance. Like any undesirable learned behavior, exam anxiety can be unlearned or the response to taking an exam can be changed. The anxiety a student feels about an exam is often related to the importance he or she attaches to the exam or grade (*If I get a B in this course, my life is ruined!*). The first step to reduce exam anxiety is to realize that life does not hinge on the results of one exam or one course, or even several. Another powerful technique to reduce anxiety is to practice a visualization exercise before taking an exam.

THE PLACEBO EFFECT

The healing that results from a person's belief in a harmless substance or a treatment that has no medical value is called a **placebo effect.** The term *placebo* first appeared in the 116th Psalm in the Old Testament. The English translation of the biblical word is "I shall please." In 1785 *placebo* appeared in a medical dictionary where it was defined as "a commonplace medicine or treatment." Later the term came to mean a make-believe medicine or a sugar pill. Today anything that a person takes or believes in that has a healing effect can be called a placebo. Prayer, meditation, suggestion, hypnosis, good luck charms, laughter, elixirs, and sugar pills may all act in the placebo effect to heal and cure people of all forms of illnesses.

T E R M S

psychosomatic illnesses: physical illnesses brought on by negative mental states such as stress or emotional upset

somatization: occurrence of physical symptoms without any bodily disease or injury being present

placebo effect: healing that results from a person's belief in a treatment that has no medicinal value

How powerful is the placebo effect? What kinds of sickness and disease respond to placebos? Although the curative power of placebos has been demonstrated scientifically in many experiments, few people really appreciate what placebos can accomplish in curing diseases. Remember that in any placebo effect, it really is the mind of the person that is changing physiology and causing the cure. To be sure medications are effective, all new drugs approved by the Federal Drug Administration (FDA) must be tested for efficacy in a double-blind, placebo-controlled clinical trial.

Drugs or Placebos: Which Are More Effective?

Consider peptic ulcers, a common ailment among Americans. Long regarded as a psychosomatic illness, peptic ulcers recently have been shown to be caused primarily by bacteria that infect cells in the lining of the stomach (Chapter 12). Peptic ulcers can be cured, or at least the symptoms relieved, by antacid drugs such as cimetidine (trade name, Tagamet). Even more remarkable than the efficacy of antacid drugs is the finding that 70 percent of people with peptic ulcers are cured with a placebo pill (Figure 2.6). Tagamet, one of the most widely used drugs in the United States, is only 19 percent more effective in curing ulcers than a placebo.

Another interesting placebo experiment tested nicotine patches as a cure for ulcerative colitis, a serious intestinal disease. This disease occurs primarily among nonsmokers, which led to the hypothesis that a substance in cigarettes such as nicotine might act to protect nonsmokers from ulcerative colitis. Patches that released nicotine continuously were attached to the skin of patients with ulcerative colitis. After six weeks, 50 percent of the patients had complete remission of their symptoms. However, among patients who had placebo patches attached to their skin, 24 percent also were cured. In other words, a placebo cures half as many patients of ulcerative colitis as does the drug (Pullan et al., 1994).

We do not see things as they are,
We see things as we are.
Talmud

Why Placebos Often Work

Other biological processes or illnesses that respond to a placebo include postoperative pain, seasickness, headaches, coughs, rheumatoid arthritis, blood cell counts, hay fever, hypertension, and warts. The number of people responding to placebos for any kind of symptom range from about 30 to 70 percent; most studies report about a 50 percent response. What does this mean? For almost any disease or symptom, a person has a 50 per-

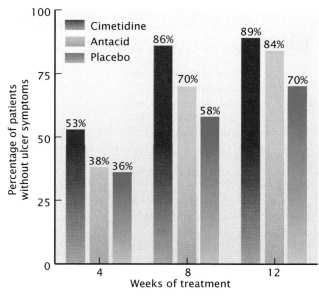

FIGURE 2.6 Effects of cimetidine, an antacid drug, and placebo pills in the treatment of peptic ulcers. Although cimetidine is effective in curing ulcers, it is only 19 percent more effective than a placebo pill. Seventy percent of patients with ulcers are cured when their minds believe they have been given a medicine for them.

cent chance of being cured by believing in the power of a placebo pill, prayer, a suggestion from a physician, an herbal tea, or magic.

Because the placebo effect is so powerful in healing, we discuss it in other chapters to emphasize the power of the mind in overcoming many diseases and conditions. For example, placebos are almost as effective as antidepressant drugs in treating serious depression (Chapter 4), and placebos have reversed tumor progression in some cancer patients (Chapter 13).

You might be wondering why, if placebos are so effective, they are not used more by physicians. One reason is that pharmaceutical companies do not make money from selling placebos; their profits come from selling drugs. Another reason is an ethical (and legal) dilemma for the physician who would like to prescribe a placebo that may or may not work for a particular patient. Because medicine is regarded as a science, a physician must have proof of the effectiveness of a drug or treatment before he or she can prescribe it for a patient.

Yet another reason physicians do not prescribe placebos is that they can be dangerous. Patients have become addicted to placebo pills and have had withdrawal symptoms when they stopped using them. Placebo pills cause side effects just like prescription drugs do. Such reactions show quite convincingly the power of the mind to affect physiology, for better or for worse.

FAITH AND HEALING

Thousands of years ago the priest-healers of ancient civilizations and the shamans of primitive tribes used the beliefs of their people to heal by incantation, to exorcise evil spirits, and to vanquish demons who were thought to cause disease. The existence of shamans, faith healers, and medicine men in cultures throughout human history suggests that their healing methods must have been generally successful. Egyptian papyri show that although the priest-physicians of ancient Egypt prescribed herbs and performed surgeries, their treatments relied on the belief of the people in the healing power of the gods. Priests would put patients into a trance in a temple and tell them that when they awakened, they would be healed. And often they were.

> The man who fears suffering is already suffering from what he fears.
> Montaigne

The Greeks and Romans also had gods, oracles, and temples of healing. Their priests also used trance and sleeplike mental states to impart healing suggestions to receptive minds. Sometimes "miraculous cures" resulted. Greek and Roman emperors and priests also healed by the "laying on of hands" because they were believed to have divine powers. King Pyrrhus of Epirus is reputed to have cured sick patients solely by the touch of his big toe.

All religions believe divine persons have the power of healing. The New Testament recounts many examples of the healing power of Jesus.

> That evening they brought him many who were possessed with demons, and he cast out the spirits with a word, and healed all who were sick.
> —Matthew 8:14

> And he said to her, "Daughter, your faith has made you well; go in peace and be healed of your diseases."
> —Mark 5:34

Over the centuries, faith and prayer have healed many people. Some ascribe healing to the power of God; others explain it by the power of a placebo.

Today's patients have faith in the knowledge of their physicians and the drugs they prescribe just as people of ancient civilizations believed in their priests and herbs. The improvement in any patient's condition is a combination of faith in the healer and the efficacy of the treatment.

HYPNOSIS AND HEALING

The modern use of hypnosis as a medical technique began with the Viennese physician, Franz Anton Mesmer, who practiced in the late eighteenth and early nineteenth centuries. History has preserved the term *mesmerism* for the trancelike state that Mesmer produced in his patients. Many years later, a Scottish physician, James Braid, introduced the term *hypnosis* (from the Greek *hypnos,* meaning sleep) and began to practice **hypnotherapy,** the use of hypnosis to cure sickness.

Mesmer called his technique for healing "animal magnetism" because he had his patients hold onto metal rods that supposedly transmitted healing energy while they were in trance. Mesmer was so successful that other physicians in Vienna forced the authorities to order him to stop using his unorthodox methods. In 1778 Mesmer moved to Paris where he again was successful in attracting patients. Eventually, the French authorities appointed a scientific panel, which included Benjamin Franklin (a U.S. Ambassador to France at the time), to investigate Mesmer and his methods. The panel concluded that there was no scientific basis to animal magnetism and that Mesmer was a fraud. This conclusion was reached even though the panel did not dispute Mesmer's success in curing many patients. Discredited by physicians and scientists, Mesmer died in obscurity in 1815.

Despite being discredited officially, mesmerism (now called hypnotism) flourished throughout England, Europe, and the United States in the nineteenth century. In 1847 J. W. Robbins, a Massachusetts physician, reported using hypnotherapy to treat eating disorders and to help people stop smoking (Gevitz, 1988). Dr. Robbins used aversive suggestions while patients were in trance and also gave them posthypnotic suggestions. Many of the same procedures are used today in treating these and other behavioral disorders.

In the late nineteenth century two French physicians showed that healing could be accomplished solely by suggestion and that cures resulted from the patient's expectation of being cured. Hippolyte-Marie Bernheim, who used hypnotherapy successfully with thousands of patients, argued that almost all healing resulted from suggestions he gave receptive patients while they were in trance.

Effective use of suggestion in healing seems to depend on the degree of mental relaxation involved. For reasons that are not entirely clear, a mind engaged in the conscious thoughts of daily living is not so open to suggestion as one that is internally relaxed by hypnosis or an equivalent mental relaxation technique.

In 1975 Herbert Benson and his colleagues at Harvard Medical School (Benson et al., 1975) studied the

T E R M

hypnotherapy: the use of hypnosis to treat sickness

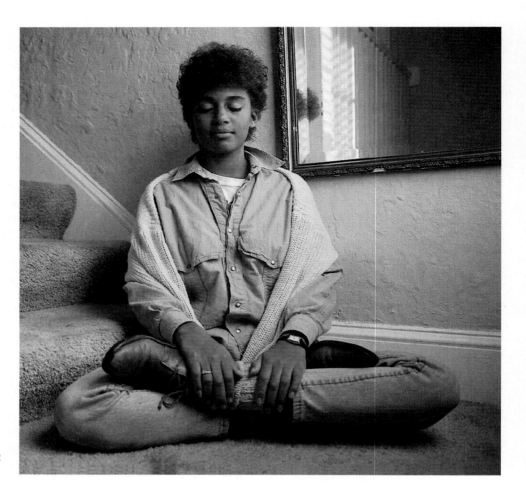

Meditation can be done anywhere that is quiet and convenient.

Managing Stress

The Relaxation Response

In the technique called progressive relaxation, you lie on your back in quiet, comfortable surroundings with your feet slightly apart and palms facing upward. Before beginning the exercise allow the thoughts of the day and any worries to leave your mind. Then you are ready to begin.

1. Close your eyes; squeeze your lids shut as tightly as you can. Hold them shut for a count of five; then slowly release the tension. Notice how your eyes feel as they relax. Keep your eyelids lightly closed; breathe slowly and deeply.

2. Turn your palms down. Bend your left hand back at the wrist, keeping your forearm on the floor. Bend your hand as far as it will go until you feel tension in your forearm muscles. Hold for a count of five; then release the tension. Notice the warm, relaxed sensation that enters your wrist. Repeat with your right hand.

3. With palms up, make a tight fist in your left hand by tightening the muscles of the arm and fingers. Hold for a count of five; release the tension. Notice the tingling, relaxed sensation in your hand and arm. Repeat with your right hand.

4. Focus your attention on your left leg; slowly bring the top of your foot as far forward as you can while keeping your heel on the floor. Notice the tension in the muscles of your lower leg. Hold for a count of five; release the tension. Repeat with your right leg.

5. Point the toes in your left foot away from you as far as you can. Notice the tension in your calf muscles. Release the tension slowly. Repeat with your right foot.

Similar exercises can be performed to tense and relax other muscles.

I have learned to relax through meditation and I have learned the basic elements I need to meditate. The first element is a quiet environment. I have found a quiet room in my home and a place outdoors where I can go to be alone with myself. The second element is a scene to dwell on with my mind. I have a special memory of a peaceful sensation I experience when I am in the mountains, lying in a floating chair in a cool pool of water with the warm sun on me and the sight of green trees in the distance. This is a strong image for me, since I have actually been there and will return often. The third element is a passive attitude. I can empty my mind of all thoughts and distractions. Thoughts drift in and out of my mind, until I have reached a state of total relaxation, a kind of not-feeling. The fourth element is a comfortable position. I find that lying down on my back is most comfortable for me; I feel freer to let go.

I meditate soon after I awaken. In the past I found it difficult to face preparing the children for their day and planning my day's activities while trying to make breakfast. Now I begin the day feeling energetic and really tuned in to what everyone in the family is saying, and more important, what they are feeling. My meditations help me deal with the distressing aspects of my life, and they seem to have a positive effect on the rest of my family, too.

STUDENT REFLECTIONS

- Describe the elements needed for you to meditate. You may wish to include environment, sensory perceptions, attitude, and position.
- Explain how meditation could help you get through the stresses of the first month at college or the week of final exams.

effects of various relaxation techniques on human physiology. Techniques such as hypnosis, **meditation,** in which the person focuses on an internal sound or image, and **yoga,** a combination of physical movements and mental focusing exercises that relax the mind and the body, all produce similar physiological responses. They found that persons practicing these techniques had lower blood pressure, reduced oxygen consumption, more relaxed muscles, and a reduced heart rate.

Benson called the sum of these physiological effects the **relaxation response.** He found that, regardless of the relaxation technique used, the relaxation response was produced by four common elements: (1) a quiet environment; (2) repetition of a specific word, phrase, or exercise that focuses the mind's attention; (3) a passive, accepting mood; and (4) a comfortable physical position. One simple, relaxation technique that anyone can learn quite easily is **progressive relaxation.**

MEDITATION FOR RELAXATION

People meditate to relax the mind and body and to attain spiritual awakening. In some forms of Buddhist or Hindu meditation, the meditator focuses by internally repeating a sound called a **mantra.** Keeping the mind focused on a specific sound or phrase induces relaxation and beneficial physiological changes. Among Western religions, singing, chanting, and prayer play a similar role in focusing the mind and reducing stress.

Other techniques for meditation focus the mind's attention on the process of breathing or on a visual symbol such as the **mandala,** an artistic, religious design used in Buddhist meditation practices. Daily meditation or relaxation exercises can be of great benefit in reducing stress and improving health.

The Power of Suggestion

Anytime the mind becomes focused and relaxed, it also becomes more open to suggestion. This can be very beneficial or it can create problems, depending on the kind of suggestions being received by the mind. Suggestions given as warnings, especially when they are given to children who are particularly vulnerable to suggestion,

T E R M S

meditation: relaxed state of mind produced by focusing the mind on internal images, sounds, or passing thoughts

yoga: a combination of physical movements and mental exercises that relax the mind and the body

relaxation response: the physiological changes in the body that result from mental relaxation techniques

progressive relaxation: a specific technique that produces relaxation by tensing and relaxing muscles

mantra: the sound or phrase that is repeated in the mind to help produce a meditative state

mandala: an artistic religious design used as an object of meditation

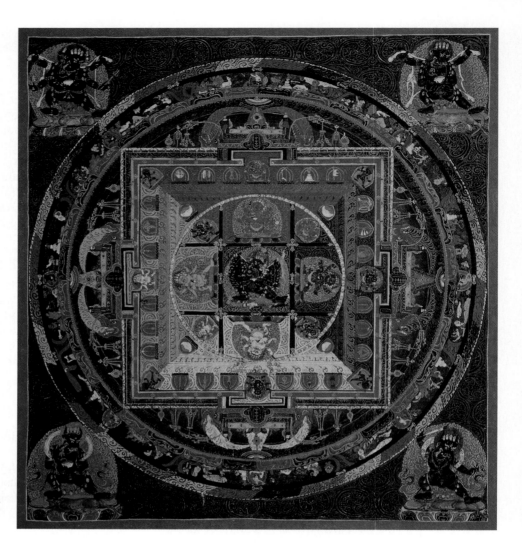

A mandala is a complex visual image used to focus attention and facilitate meditation. (Asian Art Museum of San Francisco, The Avery Brundage Collection, B63D5+)

CASE STUDY

Visualization Eliminates the Pain

Everyone can learn to reduce or eliminate the pain of minor surgery and dental procedures. One way to reduce pain is to imagine it as a *discomfort;* most people can handle discomfort even if they have difficulty coping with pain. Self-induced deep mental relaxation, or self-hypnosis, can effectively control most pain, even that of terminal cancer. One woman describes her use of visualization to control the pain of dental surgery.

Just two days ago, before going for extraction of a molar, I relaxed and imagined painless, bloodless surgery. It came to pass just as I had programmed it. No bleeding and no pain, in spite of having the bone scraped and the gum stitched. The prescription given me for codeine was not necessary. Prior to my recent understanding, my threshold for pain was practically nonexistent. For years I bled excessively at the dentist's office or while having minor surgery. Now I am no longer a "bleeder" but a believer.

STUDENT REFLECTIONS

- Describe two other instances in which image visualization could prevent pain.
- Describe an incident in which you used visualization to decrease pain (e.g., sports, injury, doctor's office visit).

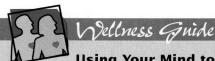

- Become more aware of the power your mind has to improve health, hasten healing, and help you perform better in school and in other activities. Belief in yourself, in prayer, or in a particular treatment can facilitate healing and help prevent sickness.

- Use mental images that feel right to you to reduce exam anxiety and to improve performance in sports or other activities. Avoid negative mental images and thoughts such as "I feel lousy," or "I'm too tired to run," or "I just know I can't do that." Use your mind to create positive images and thoughts. You can reverse what seems to be a "bad" day by suggesting to yourself that things are going to change and improve.

- Practice a daily mental relaxation technique in a place that is comfortable and quiet. Use the time to "talk" to your body to promote healing or to change behaviors. Visualize scenes from the past or the future that you know are healthy and constructive. As you become more adept at using your mind, you will find new ways to use mental relaxation in all aspects of your life. (*Notice how we inserted a positive suggestion.*)

affect behaviors and can cause health problems throughout life. For example, here are some common admonitions given to children that can cause health problems.

- Put on your boots when you go out in the snow or you will catch cold.
- If you keep eating cookies, you'll get fat.
- If you don't try harder, you'll be a failure in life.
- If you climb those trees, you'll fall and get hurt.
- If you go out at night, the ghosts will get you.

Each of these suggestions predicts a negative outcome. To a child's mind, which is usually in a trancelike, suggestible state, these negative suggestions become fixed in the unconscious mind and may have a harmful effect even many years later.

A physician's recollection of a frequent warning he received as a child shows how the negative effects persisted in his life.

> As a child en route to a Saturday movie on a rainy afternoon, I was frequently admonished by my mother to remove my galoshes in the theater or else suffer a severe headache and premature blindness. To this day, the neglect of that ritual in a darkened motion picture house gives me a troublesome pain behind the eyes and a slight blurring of vision.
>
> —Weisse, 1989

The mind can be made more open to suggestion by many things we are exposed to in daily life. For example, movies and television focus attention with both images and sound. As a consequence, they can induce a trancelike state and cause us to cry, laugh, and become angry or upset; they can actually manipulate our emotions

> *Pain has an element of blank;*
> *it cannot recollect*
> *When it began, or if there were*
> *A day when it was not.*
> Emily Dickinson

through light and sound. No one dies on a movie screen, but we often react as if they did. The violence and horror people watch at movies and on TV often do affect both physical and emotional states. As a result of watching some frightening scene, people may actually become sick days, weeks, or years later when something reminds them of the scene and brings back the fear.

Advertisers know how to take advantage of viewers' suggestible, hypnotic states of mind. Television programs usually are interrupted at an emotional peak to advertise a product by flashing it onto the screen while viewers' are still in a suggestible state of mind. Many people believe they are not influenced by advertising, but marketing studies indicate otherwise. Most advertisers try to persuade people to buy products they may not need or that may damage health. It is important to become more aware of how suggestible you are and to protect yourself from obvious and subtle suggestions that can damage your health.

IMAGE VISUALIZATION

One of the most effective ways to promote wellness and change undesirable behaviors is through the use of **image visualization.** Many healing techniques employ some form of image visualization. For example, frighten-

T E R M

image visualization: use of mental images to promote healing and to change behaviors

ing scenes from the past, especially from early childhood, can be reexperienced while a person is in a state of mental relaxation brought on by hypnotherapy or some other technique. As the scenes and emotional upsets are visualized in the mind, they can be reinterpreted and reprogrammed to change their negative effects on health and behaviors. Mental imagery can also be used to reduce pain, hasten healing, improve performance in sports, change smoking, drinking, or eating behaviors, and help control compulsive urges to gamble. At one time or another in our lives we all daydream or run an "internal movie," fantasizing our hopes and fears. During such fantasies we visualize experiences and create feelings. Image visualization can change body temperature, blood flow, heartbeat, breathing rate, production of hormones, and other body processes regulated by the brain.

Most psychologists who work with athletes to improve physical performance use image visualization. The so-called inner games of tennis, golf, skiing, and skating are based on image visualization. Baseball players in a batting slump use relaxation and visualization to "see" themselves getting hits. Basketball players use the technique to "see" their free throws going cleanly through the hoop.

Image visualization is also the secret to improved sexual responses and enjoyment. Sexual arousal begins in the mind and negative thoughts or fears can stifle the sexual responses. The sex organs are particularly sensitive to images generated in the mind. Most sex therapists use relaxation techniques and image visualization to help clients improve their sexual experiences. Tension related to sexual performance is usually the main reason for not experiencing the desired sexual sensations. In all areas of your life, begin to use your mental powers more to enhance health and improve performance in daily tasks.

> *Miracles seem to rest not so much upon faces or voices or healing power coming suddenly near to us from far off, but upon our perceptions being made finer so that for a moment our eyes can see and our ears can hear that which is about us always.*
> Willa Cather

HEALTH IN REVIEW

- The human mind can cause changes in body chemistry through thoughts and feelings, which may have a positive or negative effect on your health.
- Optimal health is achieved when the mind and body function harmoniously.
- The unconscious regulation of all vital processes in the body is called homeostasis.
- Dis-ease can be regarded as disruption of homeostasis or disruption of the harmonious interaction of mind and body.
- The mind and organs of the body communicate continuously via the autonomic nervous system, which maintains vital body functions such as heart rate, level of blood sugar, and temperature.
- Psychosomatic illnesses are physical symptoms caused by stress, anxiety, and emotional upsets.
- Image visualization and meditation can play a positive role in reducing psychosomatic illnesses.
- Belief, faith, and suggestion all have the power to heal because the mind can change disturbed body functions and reestablish homeostasis.
- A key to maintaining or improving health and wellness is to learn and practice a mental relaxation technique.

REFERENCES

Benson, H., M. Greenwood, and H. Klemchuk (1975). "The Relaxation Response: Psychophysiologic Aspects and Clinical Applications." *International Journal of Psychiatry Medicine* 6(1–2): 87–98.

Gevitz, N., ed. (1988). *Other Healers: Unorthodox Medicine in America.* Baltimore: Johns Hopkins University Press.

Pullan, B. M., et al. (1994). "Transdermal Nicotine for Active Ulcerative Colitis." *New England Journal of Medicine,* 330(12): 811–815, March 24.

Steinbrook, R. (1992). "The Polygraph Test—A Flawed Diagnosis Method." *New England Journal of Medicine,* 327(2): 122–123, July 9.

Weisse, A. B. (1989). "On Chinese Restaurants, Prolapsing Heart Valves, and Other Medical Conundrums." *Hospital Practice,* 24(2): 275–276, February 15.

SUGGESTED READINGS

Achterberg, J. (1985). *Imagery in Healing: Shamanism and Modern Medicine.* Boston: Shambhala. A classic book on mental imagery and its various uses in healing.

Afrika, L. O. (1993). *African Holistic Health.* Brooklyn, N.Y.: A and B Books. A guide to traditional views of health in Africa and natural remedies that can be used today.

Asimov, I. (1994). *The Human Mind.* New York: Mentor Books. The famous science and science fiction writer explains the chemistry of the brain and the body. Good explanation of hormones.

Benson, H. and E. M. Stuart (1993). *The Wellness Book.* New York: Fireside. Describes how to use the mind to enhance healing. Good exercises and instructions.

Moyers, B. (1992). *Healing and the Mind.* Public Broadcasting Videotape. A videotape series on the role the mind plays in healing.

Turner, J. A. et al. (1994). "The Importance of Placebo Effects in Pain Treatment and Research." *Journal of the American Medical Association,* May 25. Explains how placebo effects can influence the outcome of any treatment.

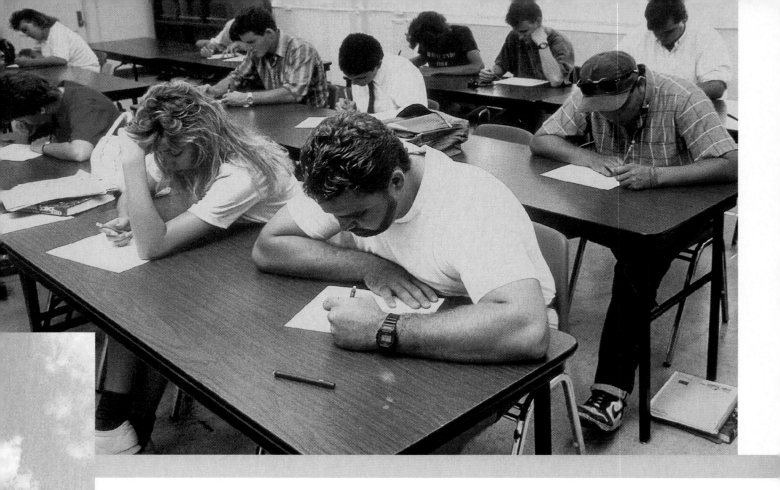

LEARNING OBJECTIVES

After reading this chapter you should be able to:

1. Define the terms stress, stressor, eustress, distress, and stress-related illness.
2. Describe the changes in behavior, autonomic nervous system, and immune system that are due to stress.
3. Name several stress-related illnesses.
4. Identify and explain the three components of stress.
5. Explain how situations in one's life activate stress.
6. Explain how daily hassles such as frustration, inner conflict, and social pressures can cause stress.
7. Explain three common reactions to stress.
8. Identify and briefly explain several factors that influence the degree of stress a person experiences.
9. Explain the fight-or-flight response.
10. Explain the three phases of the General Adaptation Syndrome.
11. Briefly explain how stress affects the immune system.
12. Explain a stressful situation that might confront a college student.
13. Explain how you can and will manage stress.

Managing Stress
Mind over Body

*L*ife is filled with a never-ending array of challenges, some of which present themselves as obstacles to accomplishing necessary daily tasks or life goals. Other challenges provide opportunities for positive and unplanned changes in our lives.

When confronted with a particular challenge—whether it be earning good grades in school, obtaining a well-paying job, becoming a parent, becoming involved in an intense relationship, or living with an uncompromising room-mate—we may feel anxiety, sadness, depression, anger, and fear. Such feelings may cause symptoms like sleeplessness, gastrointestinal upset, headache, and muscular tension, which signal a disruption of psychobiological balance. Usually this disruption is brief, because we find ways to meet the challenge and to restore our well-being. And often confronting and resolving a challenge becomes a positive growth experience. Other times, however, disruption in mind-body harmony is prolonged or severe, and we are said to be "under stress" or "stressed out." Prolonged, unresolved stress can contribute to the development of several kinds of disorders.

In this chapter we discuss the various definitions of *stress* and how the manifestation of stress may lead to illness. We also suggest ways to reduce stress and to prevent stress-related illness.

THE DEFINITION OF STRESS

Although most people have at some time considered themselves "under stress" or "stressed out," it is important to recognize a significant difference in use of the word *stress*. In the phrase "under stress," *stress* refers to the *cause* of the disruption of psychological and/or physiological balance; for example, "She was under stress from having to take five final exams in two days." It does not describe the person's response to the stress. On the other hand, "stressed out" refers to the consequences of a stressful situation; for example, "During final exams she was so stressed out that she suffered from stomach cramps, diarrhea, and insomnia."

Because it is confusing to use the word *stress* to represent both causes and results of challenging or disruptive life experiences, we use the term **stressor** in this chapter to refer to circumstances and events that produce disruptions in mind-body harmony. We use the term **stress** to refer to the symptoms resulting from stressors.

> To most individuals, the word Buick is not stressful, but it is to a thief who has just stolen one.
> *Seymour S. Kety, M.D.*

Defining stress in terms of a person's response focuses attention on an individual's experience rather than on external factors (the stressors) in the relationship between stress and illness. This distinction places the avoidance or prevention of stressful experiences under the control of the individual, and suggests that stress-related illnesses can be prevented by reducing stressful interactions or by coping with them in ways that do not cause a breakdown of mind-body harmony. In many instances, people can minimize or avoid a stressor—they can change how they perceive a challenging situation and thereby lessen their degree of distress; and they can bring forth physical, mental, and social resources to help them meet the challenge without incurring a stress-related illness.

STRESS CONTRIBUTES TO ILLNESS

Stress-related illnesses such as high blood pressure (hypertension), asthma, ulcers, and skin problems are considered psychophysiological or psychosomatic disorders. These illnesses are not phantoms, as the term *psychosomatic* is sometimes thought to mean, but are real physical conditions.

When we experience stress, the nervous, endocrine (hormone), and immune systems produce a host of physiological changes intended to meet the challenge (Figure 3.1). These are normal changes meant to deal with short-term stressful situations. Illness arises when our stress-response mechanisms are continually activated, and organs wear down and become diseased, and lowered immunity leads to increased susceptibility to infections and other diseases.

Stress also contributes to illness by inducing individuals to engage in unhealthy behaviors in order to manage stressful feelings. Some people smoke cigarettes, drink alcohol or take other drugs, overeat, undereat, or overwork. People with high levels of stress may not engage in regular health-promoting activities, such as exercising regularly, eating properly, and getting enough sleep.

Stress has three components: activators, stress response, and consequences (Figure 3.2). **Activators** are occurrences, situations, and events that are potential stressors. They become actual stressors when a person's reac-

Wellness Guide

Disorders That Can Be Caused or Aggravated by Stress

Gastrointestinal disorders
Constipation
Diarrhea
Duodenal ulcer
Anorexia nervosa
Obesity
Ulcerative colitis

Respiratory disorders
Asthma
Hay fever
Tuberculosis

Skin disorders
Eczema
Pruritus
Urticaria
Psoriasis

Musculoskeletal disorders
Rheumatoid arthritis
Low back pain
Migraine headache
Muscle tension

Metabolic disorders
Hyperthyroidism
Hypothyroidism
Diabetes

Cardiovascular disorders
Coronary artery disease
Essential hypertension
Congestive heart failure

Menstrual irregularities

Cancer

Accident proneness

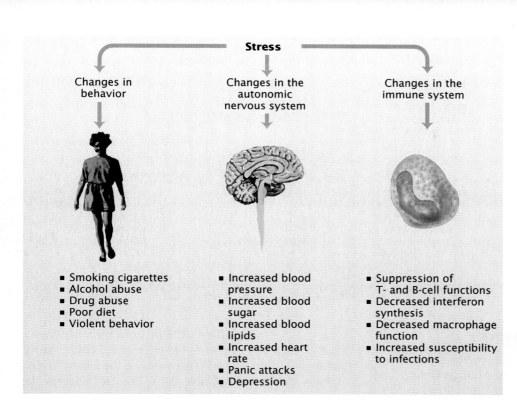

Stress

Changes in behavior

- Smoking cigarettes
- Alcohol abuse
- Drug abuse
- Poor diet
- Violent behavior

Changes in the autonomic nervous system

- Increased blood pressure
- Increased blood sugar
- Increased blood lipids
- Increased heart rate
- Panic attacks
- Depression

Changes in the immune system

- Suppression of T- and B-cell functions
- Decreased interferon synthesis
- Decreased macrophage function
- Increased susceptibility to infections

FIGURE 3.1 Stress Causes Physiological Changes
Relationships between stress and changes in behaviors, the autonomic nervous system, and the immune system.

tion (stress response) is to interpret them as taxing or exceeding her or his mental, physical, and social resources. For example, taking six courses in a school term becomes an activator when the student interprets that course load as potentially overwhelming and becomes anxious about completing the work successfully. This work load would not be an activator of stress to someone who did not interpret it as overwhelming. The **stress response** depends on the mind of the beholder.

Consequences are the effects of a reaction to stress. These can include minimizing the stressful situation, trying to quell stressful feelings with alcohol, drugs, cigarettes, tranquilizers, overwork, or other unhealthy behav-

iors, or, if unable or unwilling to alter interaction with the activator or reaction, facing the possibility of a stress-related illness.

STRESS ACTIVATORS

Activators are situations that have the potential to disrupt a person's emotional or mental state. Activators or stressors can be major external events (war, flood, famine) or unpleasant interactions with people (divorce, job loss), or they may result from changes in the body resulting from accidents, disease, or aging. An unmet emotional need or happy events such as marriage or winning a lottery can also activate stress.

T E R M S

stressor: any physical or psychological event or condition that produces stress

stress: the sum of physical and emotional reactions to any stimulus that disturbs the organism's homeostasis

activators: potential stressors; occurrences, situations, or events one may perceive as stressful

stress response: the physiological changes associated with stress

consequences: the effect of one's action; the effect of stress response

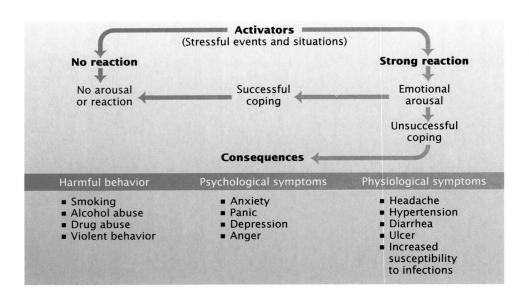

FIGURE 3.2 The Stress-Illness Relationship It is through one's reaction that a given situation is experienced as stressful.

Life Changes as Activators

In an attempt to identify and measure the potential for certain experiences to be activators, Thomas Holmes and Richard Rahe (1967) devised the Social Readjustment Rating Scale (SRRS). The SRRS lists common life events, and for each event a corresponding number of life change units (LCUs) is assigned. They measure the relative stressfulness of the event (Table 3.1). The SRRS scores the

Exploring Your Health

How Susceptible Are You to Stress?

Some persons are more susceptible to the harmful effects of stress than others. The following inventory can give you an indication of your susceptibility. Score each item from 1 (almost always) to 5 (never) as it applies to you. Any number lower than 50 indicates you are not particularly vulnerable to stress. A score of 50–80 indicates moderate vulnerability, and higher than 80, high vulnerability and time to make some changes.

_____ 1. I eat at least one hot, nutritious meal a day.

_____ 2. I get seven to eight hours sleep at least four nights a week.

_____ 3. I am affectionate with others regularly.

_____ 4. I have at least one relative within 50 miles on whom I can rely.

_____ 5. I exercise to the point of sweating at least twice a week.

_____ 6. I smoke fewer than ten cigarettes a day.

_____ 7. I drink fewer than five alcoholic drinks a week.

_____ 8. I am about the proper weight for my height and age.

_____ 9. I have enough money to meet basic expenses and needs.

_____ 10. I feel strengthened by my religious beliefs.

_____ 11. I attend club or social activities on a regular basis.

_____ 12. I have several close friends and acquaintances.

_____ 13. I have one or more friends to confide in about personal matters.

_____ 14. I am basically in good health.

_____ 15. I am able to speak openly about my feelings when angry or worried.

_____ 16. I discuss problems about chores, money, and daily living issues with the people I live with.

_____ 17. I do something just for fun at least once a week.

_____ 18. I am able to organize my time and do not feel pressured.

_____ 19. I drink fewer than three cups of coffee (or tea or cola drinks) a day.

_____ 20. I allow myself quiet time at least once during each day.

TOTAL _____

Source: Adapted from a test developed by L. H. Miller and A. D. Smith.

Managing Stress

Letting Go of Stress

The creation of a stress-management program is a very personal undertaking because no two people are alike. The following are some of the most well-recognized ways to make changes in your behavior. You can learn some or all of them to prevent stress from setting the stage for disease and illness, to make life less troublesome and more enjoyable.

1. **Respond** rather than react to situations that upset you or that violate your rights as an individual.

2. **Refine your expectations.** Build a healthy tolerance toward situations that often disturb your inner balance. Reasonable and realistic expectations avoid the extremes of shock and utter disappointment that result when unrealistic expectations are not met or fulfilled.

3. **Pat yourself on the back.** Randomly give yourself positive feedback by way of daily affirmations to recognize and validate your worthiness. Self-esteem, like a house plant, needs regular attention. This practice may seem awkward at first, but give it a try.

4. **Exercise.** Make it a habit to get out and burn off residual stress hormones that may be circulating in your body from a stressful day (at the office, at school, with the family). When your motivation is low, remember, walking is a great form of exercise that requires no fee, no sign-up, no equipment, no training.

5. **Laugh.** Balance your scale of emotions with some comic relief by incorporating humor and mirth into your daily routine.

6. **Try to relate.** Nurture your connectedness with friends and family. If you feel that your personal network doesn't support you enough, then take the time to meet new people with similar interests and build new relationships.

7. **Diversify.** Broaden your interests and try new activities so that your whole identity is not wrapped up in one aspect of your life such as career, grade point average, children, or paycheck. This will make a bad day tolerable and can actually improve your attitude.

8. **Feel your feelings.** Learn to recognize and become comfortable with all your emotions, spanning the spectrum from anger to love. Learn to express them creatively, productively, and effectively—with respect and regard for the rights and feelings of other people.

9. **Imagine!** Exercise your sense of creativity. Use your imagination, playfulness, and other inner resources to relieve stress.

10. **Do it now.** Learn to resolve issues and concerns with others *when they arise,* through peaceful and diplomatic confrontation rather than avoidance or aggression.

11. **Give yourself some breaks.** Take short breaks in the course of each day to relax. Your body needs a chance to return periodically to a normal resting state, as does your mind.

12. **Take your time.** Make it a habit every day to dedicate personal time for you and you alone—without feeling guilty. Take a few moments at the start or end of each day to sit quietly and meditate or reflect on who you are and where you are going in your life. Start with 5 minutes and build from there.

death of a spouse as requiring the most adjustment (arbitrary numerical LCU value of 100), marriage carries a value of 50 LCUs, and a vacation has a value of 13 LCUs.

Research using the SRRS has shown that the accumulation of more than 150 LCUs in one year correlates with a high probability that a person will experience a negative health change within that year or soon thereafter. The likelihood of negative health changes increases as the number of LCUs accumulate. Negative health changes include heart attacks, accidents, infectious diseases, worsening of a previous illness, injuries, and metabolic disease. Table 3.2 is a modified version of the SRRS designed to assess stressors in the lives of students. Note that the general SRRS and the student version both include the stress of positive events such as taking a vacation or beginning a new relationship.

Recognizing that people's reactions to various life situations differ in intensity, Irwin Sarason and his colleagues (1985) developed the Life Experience Survey (LES) for students. The LES lists forty-seven life events that are potential activators of stress, thirty-four of which appear on the SRRS. The LES does not assign a value to events; rather, each respondent is asked to rate the degree of distress experienced with each event. Results of research with the LES are similar to the results obtained with the SRRS.

It is important to remember that surveys such as the SRRS and LES are culture bound, that is, their effectiveness in predicting health problems associated with activators depends on the similarity of the people in the group being surveyed. The potential for health changes depends on the meaning and importance people place on certain events. Because individuals from different

TABLE 3.1 The Holmes-Rahe Social Readjustment Rating Scale

Rank	Event	Life change units
1	Death of spouse	100
2	Divorce	73
3	Marital separation	65
4	Jail term	63
5	Death of close family member	63
6	Personal injury or illness	53
7	Marriage	50
8	Fired from job	47
9	Marital reconciliation	45
10	Retirement	45
11	Change in health of family member	44
12	Pregnancy	40
13	Sexual difficulties	39
14	Gain of new family member	39
15	Business adjustment	39
16	Change in financial state	38
17	Death of close friend	37
18	Change to different line of work	36
19	Change in no. of arguments with spouse	35
20	Mortgage over $10,000	31
21	Foreclosure of mortgage or loan	30
22	Change in responsibilities at work	29
23	Son or daughter leaving home	29
24	Trouble with in-laws	29
25	Outstanding personal achievement	28
26	Wife begins or stops work	26
27	Begin or end school	26
28	Change in living conditions	25
29	Revision of personal habits	24
30	Trouble with boss	23
31	Change in work hours or conditions	20
32	Change in residence	20
33	Change in schools	20
34	Change in recreation	19
35	Change in church activities	19
36	Change in social activities	18
37	Mortgage or loan less than $10,000	17
38	Change in sleeping habits	16
39	Change in no. of family get-togethers	15
40	Change in eating habits	15
41	Vacation	13
42	Christmas	12
43	Minor violations of the law	11

Source: T. H. Holmes and R. H. Rahe (1967). "The Social Readjustment Rating Scale," *Journal of Psychosomatic Research,* 11(2): 213–218. Reprinted with permission, Elsevier Science Ltd., Pergamon Imprint, Oxford, England.

TABLE 3.2 Stress Units Associated with Common Life Changes Experienced by Students

Event	Life change units
Death of close family member	100
Death of a close friend	73
Divorce between parents	65
Jail term	63
Major personal injury or illness	63
Marriage	58
Fired from job	50
Failed important course	47
Change in health of family member	45
Pregnancy	45
Sex problems	44
Serious argument with close friend	40
Change in financial status	39
Trouble with parents	39
Change of major	39
New girlfriend or boyfriend	38
Increased workload at school	37
Outstanding personal achievement	36
First quarter/semester in college	35
Change in living conditions	31
Serious argument with instructor	30
Lower grades than expected	29
Change in sleeping habits	29
Change in social activities	29
Change in eating habits	28
Chronic car trouble	26
Change in number of family get-togethers	26
Too many missed classes	25
Change of college/change of work	24
Dropped more than one class	23
Minor traffic violations	20

Source: I. G. Sarason, B. R. Sarason, and J. H. Johnson, "Stressful Life Events: Measurement, Moderators, and Adaptation," in Susan R. Burchfield, ed., *Stress* (Washington, D.C.: Hemisphere, 1985).

social strata or ethnic groups have different values, beliefs, and attitudes, they often respond differently to the same activator.

Daily Events as Activators

Stress results from the cumulative effects of daily hassles, which irritate us, cause us to worry, and create psychic and bodily tension. Hassles include frustrations, inner conflicts, and social pressures and demands.

What Are Your Stress Reactions?

Many people experience particular physical reactions to excessive stress. Here's a list of some common stress reactions. Which ones do you frequently experience? Can you add some reactions that are not on the list?

	Once a day	Once every 2–3 days	Once a week	Once a month	Not in the last 2 months
Headaches	___	___	___	___	___
Nervous tics and twitches	___	___	___	___	___
Blurred vision	___		___		
Dizziness	___				
Fatigue	___				
Coughing			___		
Wheezing	___				
Backache	___	___			
Muscle spasms	___	___			
Itching			___		
Excessive sweating	___	___			
Palpitations	___	___			
Constipation		___		___	
Jaw tightening	___		___	___	
Rapid heart rate	___	___	___		
Impotence	___				___
Pelvic pain	___	___			
Stomachache		___			
Diarrhea	___				
Frequent urination			___		___
Dermatitis (rash)				___	___
Hyperventilation	___				___
Irregular heart rhythm	___	___	___	___	___
High blood pressure	___	___		___	
Delayed menstruation	___			___	
Vaginal discharge	___			___	___
Nail biting	___	___	___		
Heartburn	___	___	___		

Frustration is the feeling resulting from being blocked from attaining a personal goal, like getting stuck in a traffic jam when you're trying to get somewhere. Besides being uncomfortable, frustration produces potentially illness-causing physiological changes (increased heart rate, changes in hormone levels, and lowered immune function). Frustration can lead to feelings of aggression (the motivation to overcome an obstacle). Acting on feelings of frustration and aggression, a stuck motorist might honk the horn, yell at other stopped

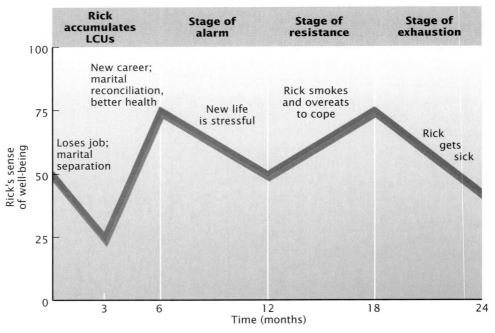

The Plunge (132 LCUs)

It all started one unfortunate Wednesday when Rick got the news that he was being laid off from work (47 LCUs). The architectural firm he worked for, while innovative and well regarded, did not have enough business to keep Rick, their newest architect, on staff. And if that weren't enough, a week later, Rick got another shock: his wife Marilee—for reasons unrelated to losing his job—decided to move out of the house (65 LCUs). At first Rick was devastated by the double-barreled loss, and his friends worried as they watched him sink into lethargy and depression.

The Climb Back (235 LCUs)

After about three months, Rick suddenly snapped out of it, claiming that he was sick of feeling down. Determined to improve his life, he gave up his longtime habit of smoking (24 LCUs), and began eating healthfully and exercising, resulting in a loss of 25 unneeded pounds of fat (24 LCUs). His surprised friends said Rick never looked better.

Rick felt better, too. His self-confidence regained, he decided to start his own business (29 LCUs) in partnership with his cousin, a stockbroker. Rick knew little about stock trading (36 LCUs), but his cousin

motorists, be angry with himself or herself for choosing this particular route, or pound on the steering wheel. None of these actions are likely to get traffic moving again; instead, they are likely only to increase frustration. It would be healthier to reduce frustration by changing the importance of the goal ("The world won't end because I'm late for work") or changing the goal to something that can be accomplished ("I'm stuck so I'm going to listen to this relaxation audiotape or enjoy a few

minutes of meditation.") Releasing frustration healthfully is better than "bottling it up inside," which tends to make people sick.

Inner conflict is represented by having to choose between two incompatible goals. The choice can be between two desired goals (approach-approach conflict), two undesirable goals (avoidance-avoidance conflict), or a goal that has both desired and undesired outcomes (approach-avoidance conflict). Having to choose between

assured him he could easily learn "the tricks of the trade." They bought a small firm in Chicago, for which Rick had to borrow $100,000 (31 LCUs). As all this was unfolding, Rick and Marilee reconciled (45 LCUs). Two weeks later they sold their house (25 LCUs) and moved to Chicago (20 LCUs).

In the four months between losing his job at the architectural firm and starting work in Chicago, Rick had accumulated 367 LCUs, more than double the 150 LCUs that predict a negative health change. Even though he was enjoying one of the most exhilarating times of his life, Rick was at risk.

The Stage of Alarm

Rick's cousin was correct in predicting that Rick could master stock trading. After a few months, however, Rick began to suffer. With an hour commute to work by train each way, Rick had to get up at 4 A.M. so he could be in the office by 6:30, when trading began. He never returned home before 6 P.M. On weekends he was exhausted. Furthermore, although he was good with clients and able to earn decent money, Rick didn't like stock trading. He longed for the quiet, creative hours he devoted to designing interesting buildings. Marilee did her best to adjust to their new life, but she resented that Rick was tired and grumpy all the time, and the frequency of their arguments began to increase. Rick was tense and frustrated.

The Stage of Resistance

In order to cope with his tension and frustration, Rick resorted to his familiar coping mechanisms: he began smoking again, he began overeating, and he distanced himself from Marilee by going to bed as soon as he got home and sleeping or watching TV nearly all weekend.

The Stage of Exhaustion

Within six months, Rick was smoking two packs of cigarettes a day and weighed forty pounds more than he should. He had constant heartburn and what seemed like a never-ending cold. A trip to the doctor revealed high blood pressure and the beginnings of diabetes. Rick began taking medications for the heartburn and high blood pressure, and was told to lose weight to stave off the impending diabetes.

Recovery

Marilee's response to Rick's problems was to pack up and leave Chicago. Although he was relieved at first, the separation quickly made Rick reevaluate his life. He easily saw that he had to make some radical changes or he would get very much sicker. And he didn't want to lose his marriage. Fortunately, Rick's cousin was able to buy Rick's half of the business, and released of this financial burden, Rick followed Marilee back home.

Eventually Rick became the manager of his parents' hardware business, where helping customers solve their home building and repair problems enabled him to combine his knowledge of building and his knack for business. Rick stopped smoking and began eating healthfully. He didn't exercise much, so he remained plump, but not dangerously so; the heartburn, high blood pressure, and diabetes went away. The marriage stayed on track.

After nearly two years Rick's wild roller-coaster ride with stress was over, fortunately with good result.

STUDENT REFLECTIONS

- Outline a recent life experience. Identify the stages of the General Adaptation Syndrome for this experience.

two desired goals, like deciding which film to see or what toppings to put on a pizza, causes little stress. Having to choose between two undesirable goals—"being between a rock and a hard place"—is very stressful.

Approach-avoidance situations often produce vacillation, inaction, or procrastination. For example, someone wanting to ask someone out may vacillate because of fear of rejection. To get unstuck from approach-avoidance conflict, psychologists generally advise lessening focus on the negative ("Rejection might hurt but I'm still a nice person") and increasing focus on the positive ("It'll be great if she or he says yes"). Procrastinators can stop judging themselves as inferior and instead focus on lessening the reason they avoid pursuit of their goal.

Pressure is the expectation or demand that we behave in a certain way. Pressure can be external (social or peer pressure) or internal (the perfectionist inside you). Pressure is stressful because it increases anxiety.

Life Changes and Stress

Indicate any life changes you've experienced in the previous year and calculate the Life Change Units you've accumulated in that time. If you have accumulated more than 300 LCUs, you may be susceptible to a health change in the near future. How can you modify your life-style to decrease the number of life changes you encounter in the near future?

Event	LCU value	LCUs accumulated
1. Death of close family member	100	——
2. Death of a close friend	73	——
3. Divorce between parents	65	——
4. Jail term	63	——
5. Major personal injury or illness	63	——
6. Marriage	58	——
7. Fired from job	50	——
8. Failed important course	47	——
9. Change in health of family member	45	——
10. Pregnancy	45	——
11. Sex problems	44	——
12. Serious argument with close friend	40	——
13. Change in financial status	39	——
14. Trouble with parents	39	——
15. New girlfriend or boyfriend	38	——
16. Change of major	38	——
17. Increased workload at school	37	——
18. Outstanding personal achievement	36	——
19. First quarter/semester in college	35	——
20. Change in living conditions	31	——
21. Serious argument with instructor	30	——
22. Lower grades than expected	29	——
23. Change in sleeping habits	29	——
24. Change in social activities	29	——
25. Change in eating habits	28	——
26. Chronic car trouble	26	——
27. Change in number of family get-togethers	26	——
28. Too many missed classes	25	——
29. Change of college/change of work	24	——
30. Dropped more than one class	23	——
31. Minor traffic violations	20	——
Total		

Failure to conform risks rejection from the group, and failure to perform risks loss of self-esteem.

Antidotes to the negative effects of the frustration and inner conflict associated with daily hassles are daily uplifts from the things in life that give you pleasure: spending time with someone you like, having fun, enjoying a good movie, taking a walk, or reading a good book.

REACTIONS TO ACTIVATORS

Reactions depend largely on the individual's personality and emotional makeup and not on the nature of the activator. Everyone interprets the world and events differently. Each of us is born with a capacity for certain behaviors, which are greatly modified and shaped by what we learn and experience. Each of us reacts to a particular situation according to individual values, beliefs, and attitudes.

Because of these differences, a situation that may be stressful and upsetting to one person may not even bother another. Experiencing stress requires that an individual interpret a given situation as significant ("This situation is important to me.") and that he or she decide what to do with the situation ("What can I do about it?"). For most people, situations that are interpreted as stressful include (1) harm and loss, (2) threat, and (3) challenge.

Harm-and-loss situations include the death of a loved one, theft or damage to one's home, physical injury or loss of an organ, physical assault, or loss of self-esteem. Harm-and-loss situations create stress because an important physical or psychological need is not satisfied. Emotions that signal harm or loss include sadness, depression, and anger. Note that eight of the first ten items on the SRRS involve harm and loss.

Threatening situations are perceived and interpreted as likely to produce harm or loss whether any harm or loss actually occurs. The experience is one of continually warding off demands that tax one's abilities to cope with life. Emotions associated with threat include anger, hostility, anxiety, frustration, and depression.

Challenging situations are perceived and interpreted as opportunities for growth, mastery, and gain. Very often such situations involve major life transitions such as leaving one's family to start life on one's own, graduating from college, or getting married. Even though they are interpreted as good, life transitions can be stressful because they require considerable psychological and physical adjustment. Often a life transition involves both sadness and excitement: sadness for the loss of what is familiar and excitement in anticipation of the new. Psychologists refer to the stress that comes from positive

> *I never look at the consequences of missing a big shot. Why? Because when you think about the consequences you always think of a negative result.*
> Michael Jordan,
> basketball star

H E A L T H Y   P E O P L E   2 0 0 0

Increase to at least 40 percent the proportion of worksites employing 50 or more people that provide programs to reduce employee stress.

Worksite programs can be important in reducing stress-related disorders. Two specific means of addressing this are (1) identify key risk factors for occupational stress for the most populous occupations, and (2) conduct and evaluate job redesign and organizational changes that will reduce stress in major occupations.

challenges as **eustress** and the stress associated with negative life challenges or the anticipation of them as **distress.**

Interpreting a situation as threatening or challenging often leads to asking oneself, "what can I do about it?" The degree of stress may depend on your answer. Believing we can manage a stressful situation is more likely to lessen stress than believing that the situation is overwhelming. In laboratory experiments, for example, animals given the opportunity to avoid or delay a mild electric shock develop only slightly more ulcers than do animals who receive no shock at all. People who work in jobs that involve a lot of pressure to perform but allow little opportunity for deciding how the tasks of the job are to be accomplished experience greater stress than do workers who have more control over decision making (Karasek and Theorell, 1989). Efforts to manage a situation are called **coping.** This definition differs from the popular idea that coping means success at solving a problem.

Several factors influence the degree of distress a person experiences. Among them are predictability, control, belief in the outcome, and social support.

Predictability   Research shows that knowing when a stressful situation will occur produces less stress than not knowing. Individuals may be just as stressed when the event occurs, but knowing when it will occur allows them to relax afterward. Knowing that something stressful may occur but not knowing when (like a "pop" quiz

T E R M S

eustress: stress resulting from pleasant stressors

distress: stress resulting from unpleasant stressors

coping: the ability to manage yourself in a difficult situation

in a class) puts the individual on constant alert. For example, during World War II, London was bombed every night, but the London suburbs were not. Londoners had fewer ulcers than suburbanites, presumably because they knew bombings would occur.

Control Individuals who believe they can influence the course of their lives (internal locus of control) are likely to suffer less stress than individuals who believe their destiny is influenced largely by factors outside of themselves (external locus of control). The crucial factor is not whether the locus of control is internal or external, but the belief that one can influence one's destiny.

Belief in the Outcome People who believe that things are improving (optimistic) experience less stress than do people who believe that things are getting worse (pessimistic).

Social Support Having someone to talk to and believing that that person can be supportive with physical, emotional, and intellectual resources lessens stress. For example, patients who talk with their surgeons about their fears before surgery require less anesthetic during the operation and have a smaller stress response than patients who go through such procedures feeling uninformed and unsupported.

THE CONSEQUENCES OF OUR REACTIONS

Although the human mind interprets a given situation as harmful, threatening, or challenging, the nervous and endocrine systems, which link the brain and the rest of

---

T E R M S

fight-or-flight response: a defensive reaction that prepares the organism for conflict or escape by triggering hormonal, cardiovascular, metabolic, and other changes

sympathetic nervous system: a division of the autonomic nervous system that reacts to danger or challenges by almost instantly putting the body processes in high gear

parasympathetic nervous system: a division of the autonomic nervous system that tones down the excitatory effects of the sympathetic nervous system; slows metabolism and restores energy reserves

epinephrine: a hormone secreted by the medulla (inner core) of the adrenal gland; also called adrenaline

cortisol: a steroid hormone secreted by the cortex (outer layer) of the adrenal gland

hypothalamus: a part of the brain that activates, controls, and integrates the autonomic nervous system, the endocrine system, and other bodily functions

---

the body, bring about the changes in physiology that lead to harmful behaviors or to disease. The feelings associated with stressful experiences (fear, anger, sadness, etc.) activate the nervous and endocrine systems, which in turn produce changes in the immune system and in physiology. Illnesses arise when the nervous and endocrine systems are continually activated or overstimulated. Anxiety, sadness, frustration, and other emotions alter the functions of the heart, blood vessels, immune system, and other organs. If prolonged, such alterations can produce heart disease, high blood pressure, and an increased susceptibility to infectious disease and possibly cancer (Chapters 12, 13, and 14).

The Fight-or-Flight Response

The challenge-response systems activate the **fight-or-flight response**. All mammals, including humans, are capable of displaying this particular response when con-

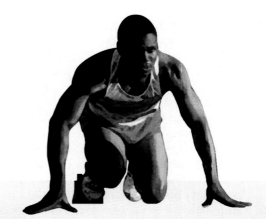

Heart
Increases in heart rate and force of contractions

Blood vessels
Constriction in abdominal viscera and dilation in skeletal muscles

Eye
Contraction of radial muscle of iris and relaxation of ciliary muscle

Intestines
Decreased motility and relaxation of sphincters

Skin
Contraction of pilomotor muscles and contraction of sweat glands

Spleen
Contraction

Brain
Activation of reticular formation

FIGURE 3.3 The Fight-or-Flight Response All humans display this response when confronted with challenges they interpret as frightening or threatening.

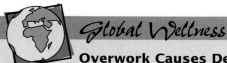
Overwork Causes Death in Japan

Stress not only can increase a person's susceptibility to infections and sickness, but it is even recognized in Japan as a cause of death. Many people in Japan work long hours and sometimes are asked to take on more work than they can handle. The stress from overwork can raise blood pressure, lower immune system functioning, and cause changes in some peoples' bodies that result in sudden death. In Japan sudden death from overwork is called *karoshi*.

The Japanese Labor Ministry officially recognizes *karoshi* as a cause of death. In 1992 and 1993 the ministry recorded forty-nine cases of *karoshi*, but it is thought that the actual number of deaths from overwork is far greater. Families that have lost someone to *karoshi* can sue the employer who imposed the stressful workload. In 1994 the Shimbi Gakuen School was ordered by the courts to pay $123,000 to the family of a 44-year-old teacher who suffered a brain hemorrhage brought on by overwork, and died (*New York Times*, March 12, 1994).

fronted with challenges they interpret as frightening or as a threat to survival. The response is characterized by a coordinated discharge of the **sympathetic nervous system** and portions of the **parasympathetic nervous system** and by the secretion of a number of hormones, especially **epinephrine** and **cortisol**. When a person (or other animal) experiences a threatening situation, the associated emotions (usually fear or rage) that arise in the limbic system portion of the brain are translated automatically into the appropriate physiological responses through nervous and hormonal pathways mediated by the **hypothalamus**.

As Figure 3.3 shows, some prominent aspects of the fight-or-flight response are an elevation of the heart rate

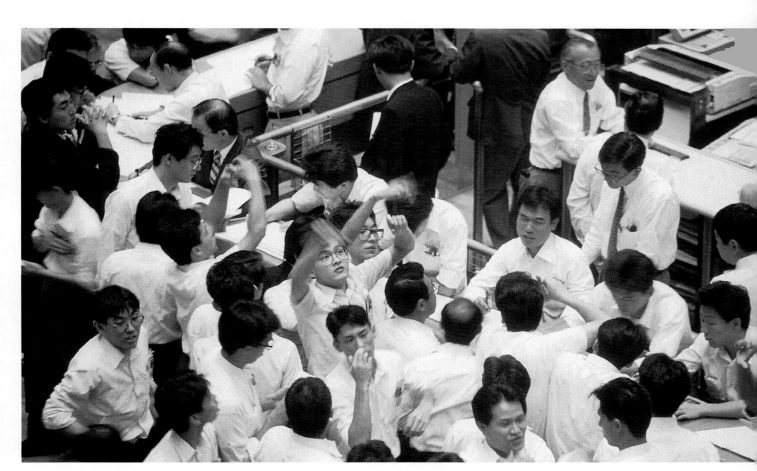

Stressful jobs can bring on illness—even a life-threatening one.

and blood pressure (to provide more blood to muscles), constriction of the blood vessels of the skin (to limit bleeding if wounded), dilation of the pupil of the eye (to let in more light, thereby improving vision), increased activity in the reticular formation of the brain (to increase the alert, aroused state), and liberation of glucose and free fatty acids from storage depots (to make more stored energy available to the muscles, brain, and other tissues and organs).

> To endure uncertainty is difficult, but so are most of the other virtues.
> Bertrand Russell, philosopher

Everyone is capable of the fight-or-flight response; it is part of the human biological makeup. Individuals display this reaction to some extent when they narrowly escape from a dangerous mishap or when they get angry or frustrated and lose their tempers. The heart rate quickens, the person becomes more alert and tense, and he or she experiences a rush of excitement from increased secretion of epinephrine into the blood. In short, the person becomes ready to take action to deal with the situation.

In our modern civilized society, however, literally fleeing from a threatening situation or engaging in physical combat is often an inappropriate—and sometimes impossible—response. Social norms dictate that people handle many difficult situations "civilly." Moreover, many threats are symbolic. The fear of losing a job, social status, or a lover is not the same as being confronted by a ferocious animal or thug, but the anxiety can produce similar stress-related physiological responses. Thus, one of the consequences of having a highly evolved brain with the ability for symbolic thought and the intellectual capacity to produce a "civilized" society is the existence of social norms that make people unwilling or unable to take direct action when confronted with threatening situations. Civilized humankind has, in most situations, outgrown the original usefulness of the fight-or-flight reaction, which was essential to survival in more primitive times. Unfortunately, human biological changes have not kept pace with cultural and social changes. Thus, we are left with a biological response that is inappropriate for most stressful situations we encounter.

The General Adaptation Syndrome

Hans Selye, a pioneer in researching stress, found that continued physiological responding to stressors led to a characteristic response called the General Adaptation Syndrome (GAS). The GAS is a three-phase response to a stressor (Figure 3.4). The three phases are stage of alarm, state of resistance, and stage of exhaustion.

1. *Stage of alarm:* A person's ability to withstand or resist any type of stressor is lowered by the need to deal with the stressor, whether it is a burn, a broken arm, the loss of a loved one, the fear of failing a class, or losing a job.

2. *Stage of resistance:* The body adapts to the continued presence of the stressor by producing more epinephrine, raising blood pressure, increasing alertness, suppressing the immune system, and tensing muscles. If interaction with the stressor is prolonged, the ability to resist becomes depleted.

3. *Stage of exhaustion:* When the ability to resist is depleted, the person becomes ill. Because many months or even years of wear and tear may be required before the body's resistance is exhausted, illness may not appear until long after the initial interaction with the stressor.

Experiments with laboratory animals performed by Selye and others have demonstrated that profound changes in vital body organs—principally the adrenal glands, the thymus gland, the lymph nodes, and the lining of the stomach—can be caused by activation of the GAS. For example, stomach ulcers often result in humans or other animals from a prolonged interaction with a stressor. In a study of more than one hundred air traffic controllers, more than half were found to be suffering from gastrointestinal illnesses. Among those who were ill, more than one-half were diagnosed as having peptic ulcers. The constant stress from worrying about airplane crashes and collisions caused ulcers in many of the persons engaged in this kind of job.

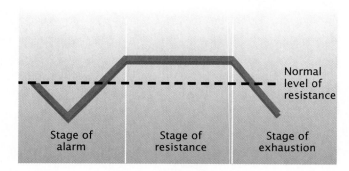

FIGURE 3.4 The Three Phases of the General Adaptation Syndrome In the stage of alarm, the body's normal resistance to stress is lowered from the first interactions with the stressor. In the stage of resistance, the body adapts to the continued presence of the stressor and resistance increases. In the stage of exhaustion, the body loses its ability to resist the stressor any longer and becomes exhausted.

Exploring Your Health

Do You Have "Hurry Sickness"?

	Almost always	Only sometimes	Almost never
1. Do you interrupt other people before they have finished speaking?	____	____	____
2. Are you irritated when you have to wait in line?	____	____	____
3. Do you eat fast?	____		
4. Do you try to do more than one thing at a time?	____		
5. Are you annoyed if you lose at sports or games?	____		
6. How often do you forget what you were going to say?	____		____
7. Do you tap your fingers or bounce your feet while sitting?	____		____
8. Do you speed up and drive through yellow caution lights at intersections?	____		____
9. Do you race the car engine while waiting for the signal to change?	____		____
10. Do you fall behind in the things you need to accomplish?	____	____	____

Here's how to determine your score. If you checked *Almost always*, give yourself 3 points; if you checked *Only sometimes*, 2 points; and for *Almost never*, 1 point. Add up all the points. If you scored 25–30, you probably have hurry sickness (don't worry, it's not fatal) and need to work on slowing down or relaxing more. If you scored 16–24, you have a potential for hurry syndrome. If you scored less than 16, you are probably pretty laid back.

STRESS AND THE IMMUNE SYSTEM

A variety of studies have shown that stress can impair the functions of the immune system. For example, students who experience considerable stress prior to taking exams show reduced blood levels of immune system cells (natural killer cells, T-cells, etc.) (Chapter 12), thus making exam-stress a risk factor for colds and flu (Van Rood et al., 1993). Stress also slows the body's ability to mount an immune response to a vaccine (Glaser et al., 1992). Also, men whose wives have recently died have been shown to have lower-than-normal levels of immune cells. This finding may explain the observation that among older adults a surviving spouse has a higher-than-expected risk of death during the period of bereavement. In addition to bereaved spouses, unhappily married, never married, and recently divorced people have reduced immune functioning, as do individuals experiencing job loss.

Stress-related impairment of the immune system is mediated by hormonal and neurological responses to stress. A variety of hormones secreted by the hypothalamus in the brain, the pituitary gland, and the adrenal glands bind to cells of the immune system and alter their functions. Activation of the sympathetic nervous system fibers that connect the brain to tissues and organs that produce immune-system cells and molecules also can alter immune functions. The immune system responds negatively to stress; it responds positively to relaxation.

MANAGING STRESS

The best way to manage stress is to replace stressful ways of living with beliefs, attitudes, and behaviors that promote peace, joy, and mind-body harmony. That does not mean you must become reclusive or try to eliminate all sources of conflict and tension from your life. People need tension to be creative and grow psychologically and spiritually. It may mean, however, changing some self-harming ways of thinking and behaving. Seeking help from a teacher, counselor, psychotherapist, clergyman, or coach can help you recognize sources of stress and ways to deal with them.

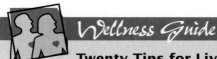

Twenty Tips for Living with Stress

Once you have recognized the fact that you are under too much stress, you are well on your way to coping with it. Although there are no pat answers, no instant solutions, no one-day stress-off programs, there are a number of ways you can manage stress. Here are some suggestions, compiled with the assistance of a noted psychologist:

1. **Work off stress.** If you're angry or ready to blow up, physical activities are a terrific outlet. This is a time to vent that energy. Whether you go out and chop wood, take a run, wash the floor, or tackle a time-and energy-consuming project you've put off, chances are that you'll feel better and also will have accomplished something useful.

2. **Talk to someone you truly trust.** Confiding in another person and talking out your problem, even if there is no immediate solution, usually makes you feel better. If there is no one you trust, not even a relative or clergyperson, then call one of the hotlines that operate around the country twenty-four hours a day. They are staffed with counselors who can listen and/or discuss any problem with a great deal of understanding and compassion. Look them up in a telephone directory under such listings as Alcoholics Anony-

mous, Gamblers Anonymous, Help.

3. **Learn to accept what you cannot change.** Sometimes problems simply cannot be avoided or solved right now. Whether it's a serious illness in the family, a divorce, an economic setback, or even a death, simply accepting what has happened will lessen the stress.

4. **Avoid self-medication.** Many easily available substances, from aspirin to alcohol, are often abused in an effort to avoid the stress by blotting out pain. They are not a solution to a problem, and if taken in excess, become a problem in themselves. Think about what you are doing if you have an urge to "drown your sorrows."

5. **Get enough sleep and rest.** Sometimes we are so busy we tend to cut down on things we need most. Sleep is a wonderful cure-all, a time to recharge your body's batteries, and usually one of the first things sacrificed to stress. Keep in mind that lack of sleep makes you cranky and irritable. If you find that you can't sleep, after a week or ten days, consult your family physician.

6. **Take time to play.** All work won't make you dull, it's more likely to make you a nervous wreck. Working extra hours tends to be counterproductive

past a certain point. Make the time to relax, even if it's only to take a short nap. Schedule a sanity break. If you are too busy to take a weekend off, schedule minivacations during the day. Treat yourself to an hour or two off whether it's to play racquetball, shop for something personal, or take a walk around the block.

7. **Do something for others.** It may sound Pollyannaish but doing some good things for others makes you feel good and helps you put your life into perspective.

8. **Take one thing at a time.** Sometimes we are so overwhelmed that we try to do everything at once—and nothing gets accomplished. Take a few minutes to make a list of what has to be done, establish priorities, and tackle one project at a time, the most essential thing first. Completing the most important, pressing project will give you a sense of accomplishment, relieve some stress, and give you the strength to dive back into your workload.

9. **Agree with someone.** Sometimes we get so irritable that we wind up fighting with everyone. If life has turned into a battleground—from the bedroom to the boardroom—stop and agree with someone. Let someone have his or her way, even if you

One way to manage stress is to alter or eliminate interaction with the stressor, for example, by changing jobs, changing a college major, accepting that a career that makes you happy is more important than one that promises a large income. Because stress is mediated by beliefs and attitudes, another way to manage it is to alter your perception of the situation. Ask yourself, "Am I seeing this potentially stressful situation realistically? And even if I am, is it really that threatening?" By perceiving

a situation as less difficult (turning a mountain into several molehills), you lessen the chance of feeling overwhelmed.

Another way to lessen stress is to change beliefs and goals. Winning may be an athlete's highest goal, but worrying about losing may bring about an ulcer. The solution is not to give up sports but to change priorities, perhaps by emphasizing the joy of participation and not the outcome of competition.

really don't agree. He or she may turn around and agree with you on something else and the sense of working together, of cooperation, will change the emotional environment from one of hostility and stress to one of teamwork. Feeling like you are besieged by an army of enemies and idiots hurts you more than it hurts anyone else.

10. **Manage your time better.** The overwhelming feeling that there simply aren't enough hours in the day can defeat you before you begin. Perhaps it means take-out food instead of cooking; maybe it means asking your spouse to work out a new system of sharing; maybe you've really taken on too much. You need to develop a system that works *for* not against you.

11. **Plan ahead.** If you see a period of increased stress coming—a big project, holidays, vacation, moving, even a promotion— plan now to rest and be ready. Or postpone what can be delayed.

12. **If you become sick, don't carry on as if you're not.** No matter how pressing your work, don't be a martyr. Stay home. Get enough rest until you can resume your duties. If you go back prematurely, you risk a relapse. If you don't take off, you risk a breakdown. If your work is so vital that noth-

ing can function without you, have work sent to your home.

13. **Develop a hobby.** Even if you are either totally happy and work is a thrill or you are too busy to have a hobby, you aren't indulging yourself but doing yourself a favor by changing the focus of your interest. It lessens stress to have a hobby. Quite simply, it's good therapy.

14. **Believe the answer lies within you.** No one can give you a stress-free life, although they can offer advice. It is up to you to take that advice and incorporate it into your life-style. Just as no one can tell you what happiness or peace is or describe chocolate to you, so you have to search out your own inner desires and needs and make them work for you.

15. **Eat well and exercise.** You can't simply relax and hope stress will go away. A liveable stress level is only attainable if you integrate stress management with proper nutrition (Chapter 5) and exercise (Chapter 7).

16. **Don't put off relaxing.** Some people promise themselves that "tomorrow" or "next week" I'll take care of myself and take a break. That simply won't work. You have to relax every single day, even if it's for a few minutes between appointments or some deep breathing on your way home from work.

17. **Don't be afraid to say no.** If you are asked to do someone a favor, or complete an extra project, if it really is too much say so. Taking on too much can in itself be the stress that breaks you down.

18. **Know when you are tired.** Being able to stop work when you are fatigued rather than pushing yourself beyond your limits will reduce unnecessary stress.

19. **Learn to delegate responsibility.** Sometimes you can't do everything yourself and yet the work must get done. Don't be afraid to ask for help.

20. **Be realistic about perfection.** When there is a tremendous amount of work to be done, don't dwell on doing and redoing it until it is perfect. This isn't to advocate being slipshod, but to accept that a fourth or fifth draft of a report that was due yesterday is putting an unnecessary amount of stress on yourself.

Source: What You Should Know About Stress, Diet and Exercise, Now!: The RIA Guide to Feeling Good (New York: The Research Institute of America, Inc., 1984). Reprinted with permission by the Research Institute of America, 90 Fifth Avenue, New York, N.Y. 10011. For information about RIA Services, call (800)431-9025, extension 4.

You can also change beliefs about yourself. Give yourself credit for things you have done that have lessened stress in your life rather than thinking it was blind luck. This will increase your sense of **self-efficacy,** the belief and confidence that you can master many situations that you encounter. Some stressful situations cannot be overcome, but be aware of tendencies toward needlessly feeling helpless in the face of a challenge.

Stress can be reduced by seeking support from peo-ple you trust. Talk to friends, teachers, counselors— whomever you believe can understand, lend a sympathetic ear, and offer sound feedback and advice if you request it.

T E R M

self-efficacy: your belief that you are capable of handling the situation; self-esteem

The Two-Minute Stress Reducer

Stressed Out?
Be still.
  And take a
        D
         E
          E
           P
            Breath.

Center Yourself
Focus your attention inward to unite your body, mind, and spirit. Allow thoughts, ideas, and sensations to pass through your mind without attaching to any one of them. You will notice them pass out of your mind, only to be replaced by new thoughts and sensations. Continue to breathe normally and watch the passing of the thoughts that stress you.

Empty Your Mind
Acknowledge that you have preconceived ideas and ingrained habits of perceiving, all of which are products of the programming of your mind. Know that you can empty your mind of old, worn-out, dysfunctional thoughts and replace them with attitudes and beliefs that create greater wisdom and inner and outer harmony.

Ground Yourself
Feel the sensation of your body touching the earth. Place your feet (or your bottom if you are sitting, or your entire body if you are lying down) firmly on the earth. Let your awareness come to your point of contact with the earth, and feel gravity connecting you to Mother Earth and stabilizing you.

Connect
Allow yourself to feel your physical and spiritual connection with all things. Remind yourself that with every breath, even though in a small way, you reestablish your connection with all the matter and energy in the universe.

HEALTHY PEOPLE 2000

Decrease to no more than 5 percent the proportion of people aged 18 and older who report experiencing significant levels of stress who do not take steps to reduce or control their stress.

Most adult Americans report having a great deal of stress in their lives. More than one-fourth of those who acknowledge a great deal of stress say they do not consciously take steps to control or reduce it. Emotional denial, physical exercise, and stress avoidance are the most popular measures in controlling or reducing stress.

Still another way to manage stress is to alter the mental and physical experience of stress. Many people do this by consuming alcohol, smoking cigarettes, taking tranquilizers and sleeping pills, and over- or undereating. Because these behaviors do not focus on the problem causing stress, at best they offer only short-term relief of symptoms and can lead to drug addiction to a powerful drug or an eating disorder. Replace destructive behaviors with a stress-reduction technique that produces a psychophysiological condition opposite of the fight-or-flight response, called the relaxation response (Chapter 2).

People use a variety of strategies to manage stress. In general, practical problems and situations perceived as high threats call forth active strategies and social support. Situations perceived as involving loss tend to call forth strategies using religion, faith, and passive acceptance.

Frequently individuals use more than one strategy (versatile coping) and occasionally they use none (passive coping). Versatile coping tends to be effective in situations involving practical events (taking an exam, losing a job, legal problems). Passive coping tends to be

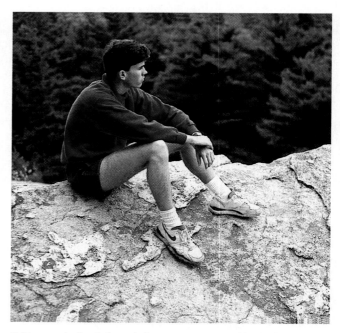

Taking a quiet break from daily activities is, in itself, a healthy activity.

effective when action is unlikely to change the situation, such as dealing with the ravages of a flood or earthquake. In such instances, passivity is adaptive inasmuch as one accepts one's fate and "cruises" with the situation until an opportunity for change presents itself. Avoidance and thinking a lot about a stressful situation without actively doing anything about it tend to be ineffective means of coping.

HEALTH IN REVIEW

- Life presents situations that can disrupt mind-body harmony. Such situations and events are called stressors.
- Prolonged stress can impair functioning of the body's organs and the immune system and result in illness.
- Activators are situations and events that have the potential to become stressors depending on how a person interprets them.
- Stress responses are an individual's responses to activators. The nature and degree of a person's reactions depends on how threatening or challenging she or he perceives a situation to be.
- Consequences are the psychological and physiological effects of a reaction. An appraisal of how difficult it is to deal with a situation determines how well a person is able to cope.
- The onset of stress-related illness is the result of interpreting a situation as personally disruptive, threatening, or challenging and believing that personal resources to meet the challenge are insufficient, including frustrations, inner conflicts, and social pressures and demands.
- Stress results from the cumulative effects of daily hassles including frustrations, inner conflicts, and social pressures and demands.
- The fight-or-flight response is the body's way of dealing with the challenges it encounters.
- The General Adaptation Syndrome has three phases: (1) stage of alarm, (2) stage of resistance, and (3) stage of exhaustion.
- Stress can be reduced by disengaging from stressors, by altering perceptions and goals, and/or by reducing the experience of stress and, hence, the potential for stress-related illness.
- Stress can be reduced by techniques that produce a peaceful state of being: image visualization, meditation, exercise, yoga, and just taking it easy.

REFERENCES

Glaser, R., J. Keicolt-Glaser, R. H. Bonneau, and W. Malarkey, et al. (1992). "Stress-Induced Modulation of the Immune Response to Recombinant Hepatitis B Vaccine." *Psychosomatic Medicine,* 54(1): 22–29.

Holmes, T. H., and R. H. Rahe (1967). "The Social Readjustment Rating Scale." *Journal of Psychosomatic Research,* 11(2): 213–218.

Karasek, R., and T. Theorell (1989). *Healthy Work.* New York: Basic Books.

Kiecolt-Glaser, J. K., and R. Glaser (1992). "Psychoneuroimmunology: Can Psychological Interventions Modulate Immunity?" *Journal of Consulting and Clinical Psychology,* 60: 569–575.

Sarason, I. G., B. R. Sarason, and J. H. Johnson (1985). "Stressful Life Events: Measurement, Moderators, and Adaptation." In S. R. Burchfield (ed.), *Stress.* Washington, D.C.: Hemisphere.

Van Rood, Y. R., M. Bogaards, E. Goulmy, and H. C. van Houweligen (1993). "The Effects of Stress and Relaxation on the Invitro Immune Response in Man: A Meta-analytic Study." *Journal of Behavioral Medicine,* 16: 163–181.

SUGGESTED READINGS

Davis, M., E. Eshelman, and M. McKay. (1988). *The Relaxation and Stress Reduction Workbook.* Oakland, Calif.: New Harbinger. Exercises for self-managed stress reduction.

Sapolsky, R. M. (1994). *Why Zebras Don't Get Ulcers.* New York: W. H. Freeman. A highly readable report by a renowned scientist on the mental and physical aspects of stress.

Seaward, B. L. (1994). *Managing Stress.* Boston: Jones and Bartlett. A thorough text on the theory of stress and methods of stress reduction.

Tart, C. (1988). *Waking Up.* Boston: Shambhala. A guide to various spiritual practices and ways to resolve obstacles to inner peace.

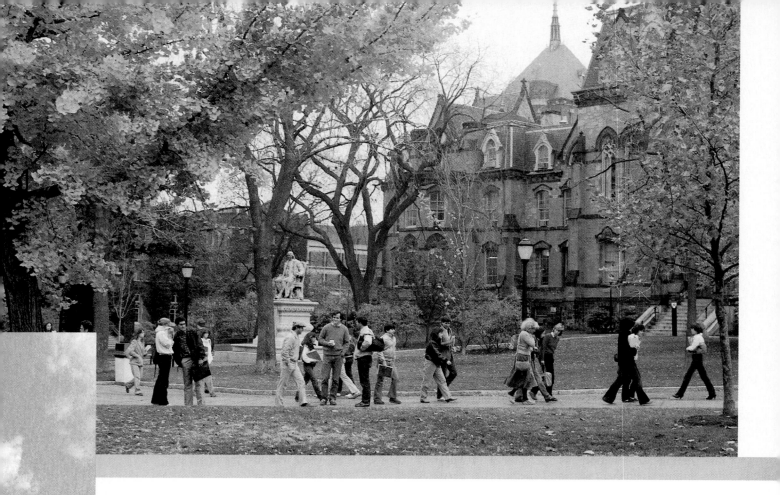

LEARNING OBJECTIVES

After reading this chapter you should be able to:

1. Explain Maslow's hierarchy of needs and the role it plays in your emotional wellness.
2. Identify several strategies for coping with emotional distress.
3. Identify several defense mechanisms.
4. Identify and explain five phobias.
5. Identify four characteristics of depression.
6. Discuss the prevalence of and several signs of suicide.
7. Discuss the importance of sleep for your mental well-being.
8. Identify characteristics of schizophrenia.

Maintaining Emotional Wellness

$\mathcal{M}$uch of human behavior is motivated by basic human needs. When individuals succeed in meeting their basic needs, they experience pleasant emotions such as joy, pleasure, satisfaction, and contentment. When they do not, however, they experience unpleasant emotions such as frustration, anger, sadness, grief, and shame.

Although basic needs are intrinsic to humans, the ways in which people satisfy them are not. Everyone may need to eat, but not everyone obtains food in the same way. Neither does everyone choose to eat the same kind of food. Similarly, people engage in a variety of activities, occupations, relationships, and recreational pursuits to meet their needs.

Infants have a limited need-fulfilling repertoire. A child can cry when wanting to be fed or comforted, and can smile or coo to invite touching and play. Beginning in childhood, individuals learn to understand the nature of their needs and they develop strategies for interacting with the environment to meet them.

There are two types of basic human needs: **maintenance needs** involve physical safety and survival; **growth needs** involve social belonging, self-esteem, mental, psychological, and spiritual stimulation. Mental and emotional health are functions of how successfully a person meets her or his basic needs and deals with circumstances in which they are not met. This involves thoughts, beliefs, and attitudes that help us appropriately interpret and respond to internal needs,

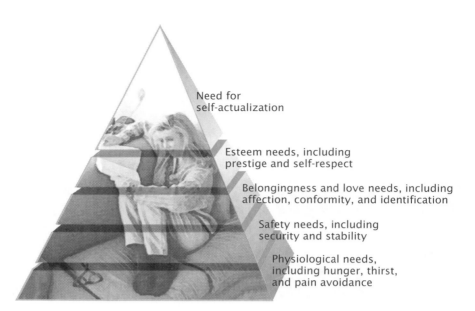

Need for
self-actualization

Esteem needs, including
prestige and self-respect

Belongingness and love needs, including
affection, conformity, and identification

Safety needs, including
security and stability

Physiological needs,
including hunger, thirst,
and pain avoidance

**FIGURE 4.1   Maslow's
Hierarchy of Human Needs**

as well as environmental challenges. It means having emotional experiences that accurately help us interpret the environment and our interactions with it. It also means having a biologically healthy brain and nervous system, not one that is undernourished, diseased, or disequilibrated with drugs or alcohol.

According to psychologists, there is a **hierarchy of needs** that describes a process through which people gravitate throughout life. These include physiological needs, safety, love, self-esteem, and self-actualization (Figure 4.1). When the needs for food, clothing, and shelter have been met, less urgent needs become a priority. As people meet their needs, they move up the hierarchy. A person attains **self-actualization** (the highest level), by living to the fullest. People who are self-actual-

ized have met their basic needs and reached their human potential (Maslow, 1970).

To be emotionally healthy, we do not necessarily have to be like everyone else. Being true to ourselves leads to greater satisfaction in life than social conformity. Also,

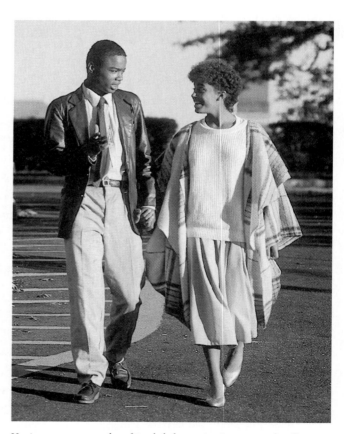

Having one or more close friends helps maintain emotional wellness.

T E R M S

maintenance needs: human needs that include physical safety and survival requirements such as food and water

growth needs: a human need that includes social belonging, self-esteem, and spiritual growth

hierarchy of needs: a progression of human requirements, including physiological needs, safety, love, self-esteem, and self-actualization

self-actualization: a state in which a person has achieved the highest level of growth in Maslow's hierarchy of needs

cognition: the act or process of knowing in the broadest sense

conscious: knowing or perceiving something within oneself

unconscious: whatever is in the mind but out of the awareness

being mentally healthy does not mean that we never feel angry, anxious, lonely, depressed, confused, or overwhelmed. These are normal human emotions. Furthermore, being mentally healthy does not mean that we never need support, advice, or other kinds of help. In fact, inner strength is being able to recognize our limits and to seek and accept help so we can restore harmony when our mental and emotional resources are taxed.

UNDERSTANDING THOUGHTS AND EMOTIONS

One foundation of mental health is seeing the world realistically. This perspective helps people devise strategies to meet their needs.

How we see the world is determined by the mental process called **cognition,** (from the Latin *cogito,* meaning "I know"). Cognition includes the following mental processes:

> *I don't know the key to success, but the key to failure is trying to please everybody.*
> Bill Cosby

- *perception,* interpreting data gathered by the sensory receptors (sight, smell, hearing, taste, touch, movement)
- *learning,* integrating new perceptions with prior ones and storing them in memory as values, beliefs, and attitudes

- *reasoning and problem solving,* formulating plans of action

Some thoughts, beliefs, and attitudes are **conscious,** which means that an individual can be aware of them. Others are **unconscious,** which means that they are not in our everyday awareness. Unconscious thoughts can be accessed through hypnosis, dreams, fantasies, and other experiences.

Cognitions are usually associated with emotions. Emotions are patterns of energy in the body that can arise spontaneously or in response to cognitive evaluations of what we experience, have experienced, or believe we may experience. Emotions provide a sense of what is pleasant or unpleasant, which helps evaluate an experience. This sets the stage for appropriate behavior. Emotions also provide the energy or motivation for behavior, and they play a part in evaluating the outcome of behavior.

Here is an example of how cognition and emotions affect behavior. An exam is scheduled in an economics course. If a student believes that success on the exam is beneficial (i.e., doing well meets a need), the student is likely to feel challenged and/or anxious. These emotions motivate her to study. If she does well on the exam, she is likely to feel happy. If she attributes her success to the fact that she studied, she is likely to study for the next exam and feel good about herself and her ability to master schoolwork.

 Wellness Guide

Hints for Emotional Wellness

People who have a positive self-image

. . . are not incapacitated by their emotions of fear, anger, love, jealousy, or guilt.

. . . can take life's disappointments in stride.

. . . have a tolerant attitude toward themselves and others; they can laugh at their shortcomings and mistakes.

. . . respect themselves and have self-confidence.

. . . are able to deal with most situations that come along.

. . . get satisfaction from simple, everyday pleasures.

People who feel positive about other people

. . . are able to give love and accept others the way they are.

. . . have personal relationships that are satisfying.

. . . expect to like and trust others and take it for granted that others will like and trust them.

. . . respect the many differences they see in people.

. . . do not need to control or push other people around.

. . . feel a sense of responsibility to friends and society.

People who are able to meet life's demands

. . . do something about their problems as they arise.

. . . accept their responsibilities.

. . . shape their environment whenever possible; otherwise they adjust to it.

. . . plan ahead but do not fear the future.

. . . welcome new ideas and experiences.

. . . use their natural capacities and talents.

. . . set attainable and realistic goals for themselves.

. . . get satisfaction from what they accomplish.

Another student in the same class believes that performance on the exam will determine all future success in school and in life. This erroneous belief is likely to produce anxiety to the point of panic, which may be so intense that she is unable to concentrate; she may even be sick or psychologically incapacitated on the day of the test (Chapter 2). This experience may be so unpleasant that the student may drop economics or even drop out of school. In the end, she may be unable to master this particular course. She might have helped herself by changing her belief about the significance of the test, which would have altered her emotional experience. This could have produced a different set of behavioral choices. With a different perspective, she might have done quite well on the exam.

> *Your health is bound to be affected if day after day you say the opposite of what you feel.*
>
> Boris Pasternak,
> *Doctor Zhivago*

DEVELOPING COPING STRATEGIES

There are times in life when everything seems to be going well, and it is possible to experience reasonably long periods of great joy. Change is a fact of life, however, and satisfaction is rarely permanent. Even if all your physical needs were met, you lived in harmonious relationships, and your work were meaningful and fulfilling, you would still probably experience some degree of frustration and conflict because you would initiate changes in your life in the pursuit of new and enriching experiences to satisfy your growth needs.

Coping strategies are ways of dealing with the emotional distress that comes from not having your needs met. In general, there are three categories of coping strategies: you can alter (1) the interaction with the cause of the distress, (2) thoughts and beliefs regarding the significance of the need that is not being met, or (3) the distressing feeling without changing the situation or how you think about it.

HEALTHY PEOPLE 2000

Reduce the prevalence of mental disorders (exclusive of substance abuse) among adults living in the community to less than 10.7 percent.

Mental disorders include a variety of conditions that interfere seriously with people's interpersonal relationships as well as with their productivity. These disorders include cognitive, emotional, and behavioral disorders that can interfere with one's life and productivity at school, work, and home.

One way to change the situation that is causing emotional distress is to attack the situation head-on. If you are anxious about asking someone out, just go ahead and do it. Another way is to avoid the situation ("I'm too nervous about possible rejection. I'll do it some other time"). A third way is to adapt to the situation ("I get nervous every time I ask someone out, but that's normal, so what").

Reducing emotional distress by changing the way you think about a situation could involve:

- judging your situation to be less distressing than someone else's ("At least I'm meeting people. Poor John works so much he doesn't get to meet anyone")
- seeing your distress as necessary or temporary ("This is the way it is" or "Eventually I'll find somebody and I won't have to go through this anymore")
- focusing on positive aspects of a situation and minimizing the negatives ("If she says yes, I'm sure we'll have a great time")
- devaluing the goal and believing you will do fine no matter the outcome ("If he says no, it won't be the end of the world").

Reducing emotional distress by changing or reducing the intensity of the feeling could involve releasing emotional energy through an alternative activity:

- Exercise helps with frustration and anger.
- Meditation helps with sadness and anger.
- Talking to a receptive and empathic person can help with grief, shame, and anxiety.

Defense Mechanisms

Defense mechanisms are strategies people use to distort the perception and awareness of reality in order to avoid unpleasant thoughts, memories, emotions, and situations. A common defense mechanism is denial, which is not believing a truth. An example of denial is a smoker not believing she is at risk for lung cancer even though she knows that smoking causes cancer. This person denies reality to prevent awareness of the truth, possibly to avoid the fear of death.

Defense mechanisms protect us from thoughts and beliefs that we find threatening. The distorted reality feels safe because of the distortion. Strategies for meeting needs that are based on a faulty foundation result in needs not met. This may lead to disappointment, depression, self-blame, and withdrawal or avoidance of involvement in similar situations.

Distorting reality is not always bad. Sometimes it is healthy or fun to take a mental vacation. From the per-

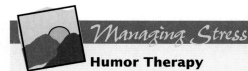
Humor Therapy

It's true that laughter is the best medicine. On average, the typical person laughs about 15 times per day. This number can shrink dramatically, however, when people are influenced by emotions such as anger or fear or grief. Just as unresolved emotions can ultimately have a negative effect on the body, positive emotions can also influence our state of health. The importance of humor on health has been recognized as far back as ancient Greece. Plato was a strong advocate of humor as a means to lighten the burdens of the soul and to improve one's state of health. From medieval court jesters to circus clowns, humor has long been an influencing factor of mind-body healing wisdom. Only now is medical science learning what people have known intuitively for centuries—laughter is good medicine.

Thanks to the pioneer work of Norman Cousins and others who have followed in his footsteps to develop the field of psychoneuroimmunology, we know that our emotions can trigger physiological responses, including the release of special neuropeptides which seem to have a healing effect all their own. The result of several bouts of laughter can actually bring about a sense of homeostasis to help calm the body, in effect, bringing a sense of inner peace.

The real message of humor therapy is that we must learn to establish a sense of emotional balance, to feel the range of feelings—anger, fear, joy, love, and so on. Shortly before he died, Norman Cousins said that it wasn't humor that healed him; it was love. Humor, he said, was a way in which compassion could do its healing work.

Here are some ways to tickle your funny bone and get your quota of 15 laughs per day.

1. Create a tickler notebook of cartoons, stories, photographs, and other items that bring a smile to your face. Refer to it often, especially when you're down in the dumps.

2. Walk into a greeting card shop and buy five of the funniest cards you find.

3. Tell a close friend the most embarrassing event that has ever happened to you.

4. Buy ten red roses and go to the nearest hospital or nursing home and distribute them to the first ten people you see.

5. Over the weekend, go to a video store and pick up three comedy videos and have a humorfest at home.

6. Read a Tom Robbins novel.

7. Listen to a Steven Wright audiotape or CD.

8. Hang out at a children's playground and watch little kids play for a half hour.

9. Fill your tub with hot water, bubble bath, and a rubber duck. And play!

10. Call some old friends you haven't talked to in a while, catch up on their lives; tell them a funny joke; then tell them you love them.

spective of mental health, however, the key is knowing when you are "on a fantasy trip" and when you are not, and not letting certain defensive ways of thought become habitual. You can do this by learning to observe how your mind works. Such self-knowledge is a goal of meditation, yoga, modern psychotherapies, and other practices that help to focus on awareness and engage one's consciousness.

Facilitating Coping

Even when emotions make us aware that something in our lives is not going well, we do not always know what the problem is, or what is the best way to deal with it, or how to overcome fear of change or longstanding inertia. People should not suffer in silence or believe themselves to be flawed or "crazy." Support and advice are available from trusted family members, friends, teachers, and mental health professionals such as clergy, counselors, psychotherapists, and physicians. Reaching out to such people helps those in distress gain a new perspective on their problems, and to see a workable solution.

Psychotherapists are professionals who have undergone considerable training to help people deal with their emotional distress. Whether a person has feelings of inferiority, is troubled by painful dependency in a love relationship, or is immobilized by fear, a therapist can facilitate change that can make a person's life better. The change comes about not only by talking, but also by helping the distressed person recognize and understand the changes. It is one thing to know intellectually the source of a personal problem and even what to do about it, but it may be quite another to face these unpleasant

T E R M S

coping strategies: ways people devise to prevent, avoid, or control emotional distress from unfulfilled needs

defense mechanisms: mental strategies for controlling anxiety

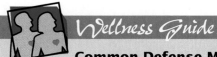
Common Defense Mechanisms

Recognizing the following defense mechanisms will help you in maintaining emotional wellness.

Repression: keeping distressing thoughts and feelings unconscious
Example: A rape victim has no memory of the assault.

Projection: attributing one's own thoughts and feelings to someone else
Example: A student dislikes her roommate but feels the roommate dislikes her.

Displacement: diverting an emotion from the original target or source to another
Example: You are angry with your parents but yell at your best friends.

Reaction formation: believing and experiencing the opposite of how you really feel
Example: You are friendly to someone you dislike.

Rationalization: creating a plausible but false reason for your behavior
Example: Failing the course was due to the teacher's poor teaching methods.

Identification: imagining that someone's or some group's attributes are your own
Example: People connect with a winning football team by wearing the team's colors, singing the team's song, and talking about the plays "we" made.

Isolation/dissociation: compartmentalizing thoughts and emotions in different parts of awareness
Example: A man gives successful and lucrative seminars to teach negotiation skills to business people, but he is always feuding with his neighbors.

Denial: absolute rejection of a truth or of objective reality
Example: A college student drinks a six-pack of beer every day but believes he/she has no problem with alcohol addiction.

---

emotions and adopt new behaviors ("the map is not the road").

The value of psychotherapy, regardless of the method, is that the distressed person has faith in the professional's ability to facilitate change. This faith produces a situation of trust that enables the distressed person to be honest about himself or herself and to disclose painful and unflattering thoughts, memories, and emotions that would not likely be shared with a friend or relative.

COPING WITH FEARS AND PHOBIAS

Everybody experiences fear at some time or another. Some fears we learn to overcome and others we learn to live with. Specific things may cause fear, but usually are not severe enough to cause illness. For example, a person may fear snakes, but anxiety about encountering a snake while hiking won't bring on an illness.

A **phobia**, on the other hand, involves intense fear that can seriously disrupt a person's life. Some common phobias are fear of heights (**acrophobia**), fear of open spaces (**agoraphobia**), fear of closed spaces (**claustrophobia**), fear of dirt and germs (**mysophobia**), fear of snakes (**ophediophobia**), and fear of animals (**zoophobia**). Phobias produce severe, often incapacitating anxiety and even panic reactions.

Panic attacks are extreme reactions to fear. In some instances, a panic attack is a response to a life situation that seems overwhelming; for example, some people experience panic when a lover breaks up with them (separation panic). In other instances, panic attacks seem spontaneous, that is, they happen without a situation a person deems threatening. Panic attacks are generally so debilitating that individuals require help to overcome them, and sometimes they are helped by medications.

Chogyam Trungpa, a Tibetan Buddhist teacher, believes that true fearlessness is not the absence of fear but accepting and understanding it, what he refers to as "going beyond fear."

> Acknowledging fear is not a cause for depression or discouragement. Because we possess fear we are potentially entitled to experience fearlessness (which) is not a reduction of fear but going beyond fear. Going beyond fear begins when we examine our fear: our anxiety, nervousness, concern, and restlessness. If we look into our fear, if we look beneath its veneer, we find sadness . . . which is gentle and calm. Sadness hits you in your heart, and your body produces a tear.

> This is the first step of fearlessness. Discovering fearlessness comes from working with the softness of the human heart.

> Fear comes in many forms: as mild or moderate body tension, restlessness, anxiety, panic, and terror. Some of us face our fears head-on by doing things we think will keep them from coming true. Some of us try to keep them from our awareness through over-activity, watching TV, smoking cigarettes, overusing alcohol and drugs. Some of us try to become heroes in the belief that the courageous person is fearless, that is, has no fear.

> —C. Trungpa, 1977

Exploring Your Health

Identify Your Fears or Phobias

Frightening situations or objects	No fear	Mild fear	Strong fear
Airplanes	——	——	——
Birds	——	——	——
Bats	——	——	——
Blood	——	——	——
Cemeteries	——	——	——
Dead animals	——	——	——
Insects	——	——	——
Crowds of people	——	——	——
Dark places	——	——	——
Dentists/doctors	——	——	——
Hospitals	——	——	——
Dirt and/or germs	——	——	——
Lakes or oceans	——	——	——
Dogs/cats	——	——	——
Other animals	——	——	——
Guns	——	——	——
Closets or elevators	——	——	——
Heights	——	——	——
Public presentations	——	——	——
Loud noises	——	——	——
Driving in a car	——	——	——
Being shouted at	——	——	——
Being rejected	——	——	——
Walking alone at night	——	——	——
Other fears			

DEPRESSION

According to the National Institute of Mental Health, each day approximately one person in seven experiences **depression,** characterized by feelings of dejection, guilt, hopelessness, self-recrimination, loss of appetite, insomnia, loss of interest in sex, reduced interest in previously enjoyable activities, withdrawal from social contacts, inability to concentrate and make decisions, lowered self-esteem, and a focus on negative thoughts and the bad things in life. If asked how they feel, depressed people usually say something like, "Life's a drag" or "What's the use of doing anything?"

Depression is a normal response to the loss of something that a person values or is attached to, such as a loved one, a job, good health, or self-esteem (e.g., when a person does not succeed at a task she or he deems important). When individuals experience a loss, it is "normal" for them to feel sad and depressed, and to grieve the loss. Sadness and grief are the human spirit's way to heal the hurt of loss and open the way for new attachments. Individuals who are actively "processing" a

T E R M S

phobia: a powerful and irrational fear of something

acrophobia: fear of heights

agoraphobia: fear of open spaces

claustrophobia: fear of closed spaces

mysophobia: fear of dirt and germs

ophediophobia: fear of snakes

zoophobia: fear of animals

panic attacks: severe anxiety accompanied by physical symptoms

depression: a mental disorder characterized by sadness, feelings of inadequacy, and low self-esteem

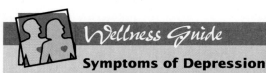

Wellness Guide

Symptoms of Depression

Symptoms you may recognize as depression:

- You don't feel pleasure in anything—you don't enjoy doing the things you used to do.
- You don't have the energy to complete tasks, do your homework, dress well, or get involved in any activities.
- You frequently cry or have crying jags for no real reason.
- You don't feel good about yourself and often don't even like yourself.
- You feel isolated or apart from others, both physically and emotionally. You are very lonely.

- You feel unloved and unwanted by your friends and even your family.

If you are experiencing a combination of any of these symptoms and they have lasted for two weeks or more, ask for professional help. You may be experiencing depression; get help now before the depression increases and becomes dangerous.

You may also be depressed and not realize it if you experience many of these symptoms:

- You are irritable most of the time.
- You have trouble sleeping and wake up unrested.

- You have difficulty concentrating and your mind often wanders—nowhere.
- You feel an underlying anxiety.
- You have no appetite and get no enjoyment from eating—even the pizza and other snacks you used to love.
- You have other physical complaints like stomachaches and constipation.

Source: S. F. Smith and C. M. Smith, *Personal Health Choices* (Boston: Jones and Bartlett Publishers, Inc., 1990), p. 71. Reprinted with permission from Jones and Bartlett Publishers, Inc.

loss with grief, sadness, and depression often are simultaneously aware that the experience is transitory; along with their grief they have hope for the future.

Depressive states also occur in response to not grieving the loss of a valued person, goal, or object. Depression can occur in response to situations in the present that trigger memories or emotions associated with not grieving past losses. Not grieving the loss may bring up intense fear, anxiety, and panic as well as intense anger from feeling abandoned. Unable to cope with these intense feelings, the person may turn the anger inward, where it may manifest as harsh self-blame and self-criticism. The sense of being abandoned may lead to

feelings of helplessness, and the onslaught of self-criticism may lead to feelings of worthlessness and shame, which generate a sense of hopelessness—all of which makes the depression worse.

A third reason for depression is injury, disease, or biological malfunctions of some part of the brain. When depression has an organic basis, medications can often help.

Some individuals are susceptible to depression during the winter months because a lack of sunlight disturbs the production of neurotransmitters in the brain that affect mood. This "Seasonal Affective Disorder" (SAD) is sometimes remedied by increased exposure to

Health Update

Long-Term Blues: Dysthymia

Some people suffer for years from a milder form of depression, known as dysthymia, without ever knowing the problem. Its analogy is a low-grade infection that just doesn't go away. An estimated 3 to 4 percent of Americans, two out of three of them women, experience dysthymia. Like

victims of major depression, they may have problems concerning sleep, appetite, energy, and concentration. The disorder often strikes early in life, usually beginning in childhood or adolescence. Only about 10 to 15 percent of the cases

actually go away with treatment.

Prior to 1980, when the disorder was first identified, dysthymics were typically dismissed as dark, gloomy people. Today, however, mental health practitioners treat dysthymia like depression with positive results.

stronger-than-normal indoor lighting that mimics sunlight or relocation to southern latitudes where there is more light.

One of the characteristics of depression is that it can intensify itself, thus creating a depressive cycle. The depressed person's negative thoughts, social withdrawal, and loss of interest in pleasurable experiences serve to reinforce feelings of worthlessness, helplessness, gloom, and doom. Recovery from depression requires both interrupting the depressive cycle and correcting the life situation that brought on the depression.

One way to deal with depression is to get life moving again. This is accomplished by establishing and achieving simple, attainable goals that can be done in a brief period of time. The goals should involve movement that restores fundamental breathing and other mind-body rhythms and may alter the chemistry of the brain to facilitate pleasant feelings instead of unpleasant moods.

To alleviate depression, it is important to interact with people who offer support. Remaining in seclusion only reinforces feelings of loss and worthlessness. It is also helpful to partake in recreational activities rather than engage in long conversations about what's wrong. Physical and social activity can divert attention from the negative inner dialogue and break the depressive cycle.

> *Madness is a relative state. Who can say which of us is truly insane?*
> Woody Allen,
> *The Lunatic's Tale*

Because depression involves inactivity, withdrawal, hopelessness, and self-defeating thoughts and behaviors, it is often difficult for individuals to activate themselves on a program of self-healing. At such times, the encouragement of a caring friend or family member and the guidance of a therapist, counselor, or other helper can be invaluable. Others can help a depressed person confront the causes of the depression and become aware of and try to minimize negative self-talk—negative views about the self, the world, and the future; self-critical inner dialogue, and logic errors in the assessment of self and events. Becoming aware of and stopping negative self-talk opens the way to adopting positive self-images and more realistic appraisals of the world.

Suicide

One of the most worrisome aspects of depression is the risk of suicide. In the United States, suicide ranks among the ten most frequent causes of death, accounting for approximately 30,000 deaths per year. The number of reported suicides is thought to represent only 10–15 percent of suicide attempts. People over 65 make up the largest age group of suicides. Among young people

Wellness Guide

Talking to a Friend Who Is Depressed

Showing that you care by taking the time to talk to a depressed friend is very important. This kind of conversation can be uncomfortable and draining for you, especially if you feel uneasy talking about feelings. Here are some general interventions that may make your job of being a friend easier.

- Allow your friend to express feelings. Don't cut him or her off or try to minimize the depth of the feeling. Just be there, in word and body language, so that your friend feels safe to talk. You may be providing a psychological lifeline.
- Acknowledge your friend's distress. Perhaps this validation of

how terrible and painful life is will help your friend avoid making the point by trying to kill himself or herself.

- Reinforce positive thinking or responses. If your friend mentions any positive thought or action, talk about it. Any hopeful thought is the beginning of a positive trend in thinking.
- Don't play amateur psychiatrist. For example, don't reflect back what your friend says or why he feels this way. Just being present and really listening is enough. If possible, discuss the reality of the problem and possible solutions.
- One of the most effective and therapeutic actions on your part

would be to suggest that you and your friend do something. Help change the pattern of immobilization and get your friend moving. Go to dinner or the movies; better yet, exercise or get outside. Any physical action will help lift the depression.

- Don't become depressed yourself. You can only do what you can do—set limits on your own time and energy, then seek outside assistance.

Source: S. F. Smith and C. M. Smith, *Personal Health Choices* (Boston: Jones and Bartlett Publishers, Inc., 1990), p. 73. Reprinted with permission of Jones and Bartlett Publishers, Inc.

(15–24 years old), suicide ranks third behind accidents and murder as a cause of death (USDHHS, 1994).

Suicide is not a disease, nor is it a disorder that can be inherited. Suicides are not caused by the weather or a full moon. Generally people consider suicide because they feel overwhelmed and painfully distressed by life and they believe suicide to be their only option. Sometimes people attempt suicide not because they really want to die but because they want to express anger at others or signal others for help. In such instances, suicides are characterized by limited self-destructive acts, such as taking less than a lethal dose of sleeping pills or arranging that the suicide attempt be discovered in time to be saved.

Occasionally a person expresses thoughts of suicide to a friend or relative. This can be extremely distressing to the listener, who may react with disbelief, panic, or avoidance. In attempting to deal with his or her own uncomfortable feelings, a listener might say things like, "Cheer up, you've got a lot to live for," or "You're better off than I am," or "You can't be serious!" These and similar statements have the effect of denying the distressed person's feelings. Psychologists recommend instead that listeners speak directly to suicidal thoughts—("Tell me more about why you want to kill yourself") and offer the

distressed person nonjudgmental sympathy and concern, and firmly but patiently direct the distressed person to professional help immediately.

Often suicidal individuals offer excuses for not seeing a professional and may even try to blackmail a friend into silence with threats ("I'll kill myself if you tell anyone"). The friend must hold firm and, if necessary, make an appointment with a counselor or psychiatrist at the student health center or hospital emergency room, and

Wellness Guide

If a Friend Is Considering Suicide

If you suspect that a friend is considering suicide, how can you help? You can take any of several possible courses of action. All involve your making a concrete intervention. Intervention is tough. It is much easier to tell yourself that things will get better, or tomorrow is another day. Rationalization and procrastination are not useful behaviors in a situation that involves depression or potential suicide. Let's look at some options available to you.

- Talk to your friend. Tell him or her that you are concerned. Describe the behavior that is causing you to worry. Ask if you can help (but don't give up if your friend says no).

- Ask your friend directly if he or she is thinking about suicide. You may be shocked if your friend

answers yes, but, remember, even someone who sees suicide as a potential solution always has a wish to live. If your friend admits thinking of suicide, ask if he or she has thought of a plan.

- Negotiate a "no-suicide" agreement before leaving your friend. Ask your friend to agree not to commit suicide at any time. If your friend will not agree to this contract or tries to change it to a certain time, then he or she is at increased risk. Report this situation to a professional counselor at once. Stay with your friend or arrange for someone else to stay with him or her until professional help arrives.

- If your friend agrees to a "no-suicide" pact, go to your college health service or residence hall

advisor, speak with a counselor or physician, and describe your friend's behavior. The professional will know the best way to handle the situation. And remember, even if you feel you are interfering or breaking a confidence, you may be saving a life. An intervention made now can prevent suicide.

- Talk to other friends, a residence hall advisor, or even a teacher—anyone who will assist you to verbalize your concerns and decide how to help. The most important action is to do something after you become aware of the potentially dangerous outcome.

Source: S. F. Smith and C. M. Smith, *Personal Health Choices* (Boston: Jones and Bartlett Publishers, Inc., 1990), p. 78.

deliver the distressed person there, or telephone a suicide prevention hotline.

At the time a person contemplates suicide, life seems absolutely hopeless. But few life problems are beyond solution. Life crises improve and distressing emotions pass. Time does heal many hurts. And the experience gained by working through a distressing time of life can bring confidence, insight, and understanding. Acquiring experience and understanding, a person is better able to cope with life's problems and is better able to help others deal with their challenges.

ANGER

Anger occurs when we've been attacked, blamed, hurt, or have experienced a loss; when we imagine we've been attacked, blamed, hurt, or have experienced a loss; when we imagine we *may* be attacked, blamed, hurt, or experience a loss; or when the pursuit of an important goal is blocked. Anger is an excitatory emotion, providing the motivational energy to protect ourselves or things we care about or to overcome obstacles to our goals. We use anger to stop physical or psychological abuse and to protect ourselves from the hurt of loss. Sometimes we get angry because we perceive something as threatening that really isn't. In this case, we make ourselves angry by what we think.

Many people have difficulty dealing with anger in themselves or in others. They fear the intensity of the emotion. They fear the possibility of violence that may accompany its expression. They fear retaliation or rejection.

One constructive way to work with anger is to understand the source of the emotion. For example, to deal with frustration you can reassess the merits of the goal you cannot attain or reconsider the strategy you've employed for attaining it. It may feel right to blame someone else for your troubles, but a reevaluation of how you contribute to the situation may be more productive.

The next time you feel angry, take a "time out" for a few seconds, minutes, or days if necessary. Ask yourself what you've experienced that's led you to be angry. Are you really being harmed or threatened or are you making yourself angry because you've interpreted a situation as such? If you feel frustrated about not being able to accomplish a goal, is your goal realistically attainable? Have you expected too much of yourself? Have you expected too much of someone else? Is your strategy for attaining your goal workable? Is something else better? Did you communicate your goals, needs, plans, and desires to people whose help you wanted or expected?

SLEEP AND DREAMS

All living things exhibit cycles of rest and activity, which in humans is represented by the daily sleep-wake cycle. Everyone has a sleep-wake cycle that corresponds to her or his optimum degree of physical, mental, and spiritual well-being. Studies show that adequate sleep enhances

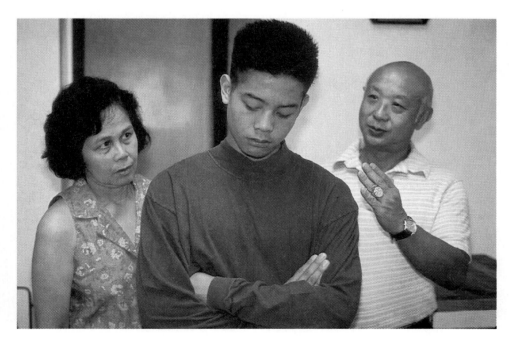

Family arguments disrupt the emotional well-being of parents and children.

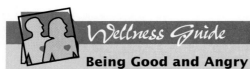

Being Good and Angry

Here are some suggestions for expressing anger constructively.

1. **Recognize your anger.** Pay attention to anger in yourself when you become aware of it. Then take some time to determine which of your thoughts are causing it. Are you hurt, frustrated, frightened? What happened that made you angry?

2. **Own your anger.** Try not to blame someone else for your angry feeling with thoughts or statements like, "It's all your fault!" or "If it weren't for you," or "If only you'd have . . ." Don't put it on to someone else unless you're sure it belongs there.

3. **Find anger's origins.** Even if you are very angry, try not to act immediately on those feelings. Instead, set aside a time to think about them, and how best to express them.

4. **Resolve the anger.** Try not to let anger build up over time. If you do, you may become resentful, which may cause you to distance emotionally or physically or to displace the anger on to someone else, like a child or a co-worker.

5. **Don't ambush.** Attacking with anger when it's least expected is unfair and invites resentment or a counterattack, not reconciliation.

6. **Be specific.** When you're talking about emotional conflicts, name exactly what's causing the anger and stick to that issue. Don't bring up past hurts. Don't discuss second and third topics until the first one is settled. If other issues arise, write them down so you can discuss them later. Make it a habit to keep pencil and paper handy when issues are discussed. Don't give in to the temptation to bring up secondary issues in order to retaliate for hurt feelings or as a way to avoid resolving the issue at hand.

7. **Don't hit below the belt.** Don't attack your partner with something you know will hurt because you think you're losing an argument.

8. **Attack the problem, not each other.** Don't engage in character assassination with put-downs and accusations. Use "I statements" to communicate resentments. If someone attacks with a put-down, rather than retaliate, the recipient can say "Ouch, that hurt." This can be a cue to redress the attack and go on with the issue under discussion. If this doesn't happen, the discussion will probably be sidetracked from the main point to the put-down, and a fight about hurt feelings may ensue.

9. **Be respectful and respectable.** When working to resolve an issue, try to maintain an attitude of respect. Try to understand the other's point of view. Ask the other person to respect you and your feelings, even though you disagree.

10. **Take some time.** Sometimes you can sense that an anger-causing issue isn't getting resolved in the discussion. It's all right to acknowledge that and to take a few hours or days to reconsider things, then discuss the issue again. Sometimes emotions are too high and it's not possible to think clearly. Sometimes you just need time to reflect and figure things out.

11. **Physical affection is okay.** Sex or any other affectionate behavior before an issue is resolved is acceptable, as long as it's not taken as a sign that the issue is resolved. Both of you must understand this. Affectionate behavior shows that arguing about something can be accommodated within a caring relationship.

12. **Both sides win.** After a issue has been discussed and the partners seem agreed on the outcome, if one or both feels a grudge, then the argument has produced a winner and a loser, and the relationship has been harmed. Holding a grudge is a sign that the issue is not resolved. Try again.

---

attentiveness, concentration, mood, and motivation. Sleep deprivation, on the other hand, impairs a person's ability to be productive, good-humored, satisfied with life, and even to laugh at a joke! Lack of sleep can gravely impair judgment; sleeplessness is second only to drunkenness as a cause of automobile accidents. Long-term sleep deprivation can be fatal.

Sleep researchers believe that a majority of Americans are sleeping 60 to 90 minutes a night less than the seven, eight, or nine hours that would leave them refreshed and energetic during the day. Individuals "cheat on their sleep" to create time for other things in the busy schedules that characterize modern life. Sleep is considered expendable, and *not* sleeping a sign of ambition and

T E R M
insomnia: prolonged inability to obtain adequate sleep

drive. Furthermore, around-the-clock TV and radio entertainment can distract people from sleeping. Before the advent of the electric light bulb about 100 years ago, people tended to sleep about nine hours a night. When it got dark, people slept. Because sleep is so strongly linked to one's total state of being, focusing on healthy sleep habits can produce greater mind-body harmony.

Sleep Problems

Because of life's never-ending array of challenges, just about everyone has trouble sleeping once in a while. Experiences that commonly disrupt sleeping patterns include being sick, jet-lagged, nervous about an upcoming exam, or excited about something new; having consumed too much food, alcohol, or caffeine; or losing a loved one. Fortunately, most people tend to adjust to these situations and their sleep rhythms return to normal (for them) in a few days. A large percentage of Americans, however, have problems with sleeping that last sev-

eral weeks to years. The most common sleep problems are not sleeping enough (insomnia), sleeping during the day (excessive daytime sleepiness), and unusual activities associated with sleep (parasomnias).

Insomnia

The majority of people with long-term sleep problems have **insomnia.** They have trouble falling asleep or staying asleep, or they awaken after a few hours sleep and cannot go back to sleep. The daytime results of insomnia are fatigue, the desire to nap, impaired ability to concentrate, impaired judgment, and a lack of zest for life. Although insomnia may be related to disease or injury in the brain's sleep centers, most often it is the result of a physical illness, chronic pain, stress, depression, anxiety, obsessive-compulsive ruminations, panic attacks, post-traumatic stress disorder, and drug or alcohol abuse.

Sometimes as a result of insomnia, some individuals have a difficult time staying awake during the day. They

 Wellness Guide

Getting a Good Night's Sleep

How can you create healthful sleeping habits for yourself? Here are some suggestions for getting a good night's sleep.

1. **Establish a regular sleep time.** Give your own natural sleep cycle a chance to be in synchrony with the day-night cycle by going to bed at the same time each night (within an hour more or less) and arising *without being awakened by an alarm clock.* This will mean going to bed early enough to give yourself enough time to sleep. Try to maintain your regular sleep times on the weekend. Getting up early during the week and sleeping late on weekends may upset the rhythm of your sleep cycle.

2. **Create a proper (for you) sleep environment.** Sleep occurs best when the sleeping environment is dark, quiet, free of distractions, and not too warm. If you use radio or TV to help you fall asleep, use an autotimer to shut off the noise after falling asleep.

3. **Wind down before going to bed.** About 20 to 30 minutes before bedtime, stop any activities that cause mental or physical arousal, such as work or exercise, and take up a "quiet" activity that can create a transition to sleep. Transitional activities could include reading, watching "mindless" TV, taking a warm bath or shower, meditation, or making love.

4. **Make the bedroom for sleeping only.** Make the bedroom your place for getting a good night's sleep. Try not to use it for work or for discussing problems with your partner.

5. **Don't worry while in bed.** If you are unable to sleep after about 30 minutes in bed because of worry about the next day's activities, get up and do some limited activity such as reading a magazine article, doing the dishes, or meditating. Go back to bed when you feel drowsy. If you cannot sleep because of thinking

about all that you have to do, write down what's on your mind and let the paper hold onto the thoughts while you sleep. You can retrieve them in the morning.

6. **Avoid alcohol and caffeine.** Some people have a glass of beer or wine before bed in order to relax. Large amounts of alcohol, while sedative, block normal sleep and dreaming patterns. Because caffeine remains in the body for several hours, people sensitive to caffeine should not ingest any after noon.

7. **Exercise regularly.** Exercising 20 to 30 minutes three or four times a week enhances the ability to sleep. You should not exercise vigorously within three hours of bedtime, however, because of the possibility of becoming too aroused to sleep.

Source: Adapted from M. L. Reite, K. E. Nagel, and J. R. Ruddy, *The Evaluation and Management of Sleep Disorders* (Washington, D.C.: American Psychiatric Press, 1990).

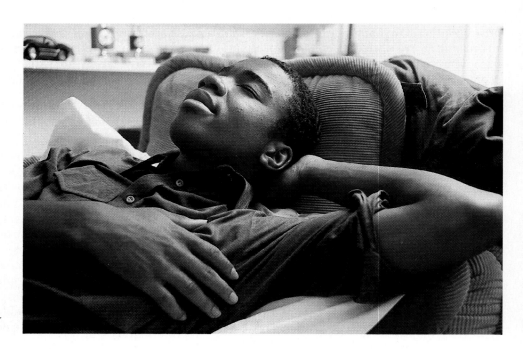

Sufficient sleep and dreams are essential to mental health.

may feel sleepy most of the time, may "nod off" easily during a routine activity, or may nap at the slightest opportunity. Because they get insufficient sleep at night, about 20 percent of college students can fall asleep almost instantaneously if permitted to lie down in a darkened room. Extreme tendency to fall asleep during the day is called **narcolepsy.**

Parasomnias

Parasomnias present themselves in many forms and have the potential to interrupt restful sleep. Nightmares are dreams that arouse feelings of fear, terror, panic, or anxiety. Sleepwalking, or **somnambulism,** is a condition occurring primarily in children and often associated with anxiety, fatigue, or stress. The person performs motor activity, usually leaving bed and walking around, while sleeping and has no memory of it on awakening. Other vigorous behaviors such as punching, kicking, and night terrors (episodes that begin with a loud cry followed by

rapid heart rate, sweating, and feelings of panic) will also interrupt sleep. Another abnormality is **sleep apnea,** in which individuals stop breathing while sleeping; typically, breathing resumes within 30 seconds.

Since the majority of sleep problems represent some form of disharmony within ourselves and/or with our surroundings, restoring harmony is a way to return to our natural rest-activity cycle. This can be accomplished by employing mind-body health practices such as meditation, exercise, and proper nutrition. For extreme sleep disorders, help should be sought.

Some people turn to alcohol, sleeping pills, tranquilizers and other drugs, however, they offer only short-term symptomatic relief for sleep disorders. Without a holistic approach and fundamental changes in one's lifestyle and attitudes, relying on drugs to restore natural sleep rhythms may be harmful; and may lead to physical dependency and habituation on the drugs.

Understanding Our Dreams

We all dream while we sleep. Even animals dream. Although some people deny they dream, this is because they do not recall their dreams when awake. On the other hand, some people have vivid recall of the several dreams they have each night (a skill that can be learned).

Dreams tend to occur in the stage of sleep called **rapid eye movement sleep,** or **REM** sleep (Figure 4.2). While asleep, people cycle through the four stages several times. Dreams usually occur between Stage 4 (deep sleep) and the return to Stage 1 (light sleep) of the ensuing cycle.

Exploring Your Health

Keep a Sleep and Dream Record

Each morning for one week, assess your sleep behavior with the aid of a chart like the one here; also record the details of your dreams in your journal or notebook. Hints for dream recording:

1. Keep a pen or a pencil and a pad of paper near your bed.

2. Remind yourself before going to sleep that you want to remember your dreams.

3. Write down your dreams immediately upon awakening.

Sleep Assessment Chart

	Sun.	Mon.	Tues.	Wed.	Thurs.	Fri.	Sat.
Time to bed							
Time fell asleep (estimated upon waking)							
Feelings before falling asleep							
Trouble falling asleep? (yes/no)							
Take sleeping aid? (milk/pills)							
Number of times awake in the night							
Time woke up							
Time arose							
Feelings upon awakening							
Dreams? (yes/no)							
Total sleep time							

No one knows why we dream. Some researchers have suggested that REM sleep states are necessary for brain growth, daily information processing, and cellular rejuvenation. Others believe that dreams are the brain's way of processing and eliminating information and memories that are no longer useful. Whatever the reasons, studies indicate that dreams are necessary for health. Experimental subjects who were deprived of the chance to dream (they were awakened by experimenters during REM sleep) developed bizarre behaviors and psychotic symptoms. The individuals returned to normal after at least one night of catching up on the missed REM time.

For thousands of years dreams have been used in many cultures to restore mental and physical health. The temples of Asclepius were used by ancient Greeks for

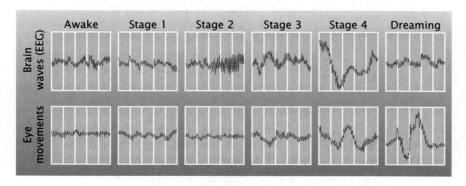

FIGURE 4.2 **Tracings of the Electrical Signals (EEGs) Produced during the Various Stages of Sleep**
Tiny electrodes are placed on a person's scalp and eyelids. They detect electrical signals within the brain and movements of the eyes. Notice that rapid eye movement (REM) occurs during a dream period.

over a thousand years as places where people went to have healing dreams and to have them interpreted by the priests and priestesses.

Indications that dreams can be healthy come from studies of the Senoi, a Malaysian tribe known as the "dream people." The Senoi live in a nonaggressive, noncombative, communal society. The tribe's members have a remarkable degree of mental and emotional health, which is attributed by some to the daily ritual of discussing and interpreting their dreams. Both children and adults gather each morning to recount their dreams to one another, singly and in groups. According to Senoi custom, the events, anxieties, and people in a dream are real and must be acknowledged and dealt with. Such behavior is similar to our custom of looking for meaning in dreams, especially as a component of psychotherapy.

> People who don't have nightmares don't have dreams.
> Robert Paul Smith, researcher

Interpreting Your Dreams

In our culture, numerous theories of dream interpretation have been proposed. Perhaps the best known are those of Sigmund Freud and Carl Jung, who proposed universally applicable rules for uncovering the meaning of symbols and events in dreams. Most modern dream researchers do not believe in universal symbolism, however. Instead, they believe that the symbolism and meaning in a dream are unique. Dreams are private conversations with ourselves, communicated in a private language of images that often are bizarre, dramatic, emotional, and exaggerated.

Much dream research suggests that dreams are reflections of recent happenings, thoughts, and feelings that are not dealt with in our daily consciousness. Many people are too busy to attend to everything they experience, think, and feel. Sometimes, they purposely do not deal with reality because it is unpleasant. In a dream, however, you "come clean" with yourself. You bring forth subtle feelings and impressions that were not attended to while awake. You engage your innermost thoughts and feelings about fears, worries, conflicts, and problems that you chose not to deal with when awake. Thus, many problems (and sometimes their solutions!) are presented in dreams.

Dreams may also be a literal representation of reality that went unattended. For example, if you dream of a mouse, perhaps you saw a mouse in your kitchen, or perhaps you noticed some movements out of the corner of your eye and thought of a mouse. In either case, your discomfort of the thought of a mouse in your house caused you to block the thought from consciousness.

Another device for finding the message in a dream is to focus on the emotions in the dream and not on the dream's content. Although you may have dreamed of dancing an incredibly brilliant solo on a stage to an audience's wild applause, the actual emotion in the dream may have been fear. The dream, therefore, is probably about fear and not pride or accomplishment.

MENTAL DISORDERS

The brain, like all other body organs, is composed of molecules and cells whose functioning is controlled by biological processes. It is possible, therefore, for brain tissue to be affected by chemical imbalance, injury, infection, toxins, and genetic disorders. When brain injury or disease occurs, thoughts, mood, and behaviors can be impaired. In most cases, the biological basis for mental disorders is unknown.

Schizophrenia is a debilitating mental disorder characterized by hallucinations, delusions, an inability to maintain logical and coherent thought patterns, diminished emotional and social experience, and a diminished sense of purpose. Typically schizophrenia manifests in teenage years and progresses into adulthood. The disease occurs at the same rate (0.85 percent) in virtually all societies in the world; it is responsible for 2.5 percent of total U.S. health expenditures. The cause of schizophrenia is unknown, although scientists believe that biological (possibly inherited) factors are partially responsible. While medications and psychosocial rehabilitation can help lessen symptoms, there is no cure. About one third of schizophrenics become well spontaneously, but many individuals with a diagnosis of schizophrenia require ongoing medical and psychological support.

T E R M

schizophrenia: a mental disorder that involves a disturbance in thinking, in perceiving reality, and in functioning

H E A L T H Y   P E O P L E   2 0 0 0

Increase to at least 20 percent the proportion of people aged 18 and older who seek help in coping with personal and emotional problems
Most of the adult population reports experiencing personal or emotional problems in the course of a year. Half of these people report they are unable to solve their problems, and about one-third indicate they are unable to do anything that makes their problems more bearable. Mental health professionals, physicians, and religious counselors are the most likely choices of those who seek professional help.

TABLE 4.1 Signs of Schizophrenia

Aspect of life	Typical symptoms
Emotions	Inappropriate responses to stimuli Blunted or flat emotions Fear of warmth or closeness Erratic and negative feelings
Thought	Inability to tell real from unreal Delusions and hallucinations Disorganized and confused thoughts Tangential or circumstantial conversation Bizarre ideas and language
Interpersonal relationships	Thoughts only of self, autistic Unpredictable responses when approached Social isolation Lack of response Withdrawal Impaired role functioning
Behavior	Deteriorated level of functioning, immobilized Inability to make decisions Poor judgment Bizarre or peculiar behavior Lethargy, loss of initiative Poor personal hygiene and grooming

Source: S. F. Smith and C. M. Smith, *Personal Health Choices* (Boston: Jones and Bartlett Publishers, Inc., 1990), p. 79. Reprinted with permission of Jones and Bartlett Publishers, Inc.

HEALTH IN REVIEW

- Mental and emotional health depend on how well individuals meet their maintenance and growth needs and cope with situations in which their needs are not met.

- People understand their needs by interpreting what they sense from the environment and in their bodies. As they mature, people develop ideas about and learn strategies to meet their emotional needs.

- Emotions tell us whether we are satisfied by, and the level of satisfaction from, our experiences, plans, and outcomes of behavior.

- Emotional distress occurs when needs are not met. People cope with emotional distress by changing their modes of interaction with the environment, changing the importance of their unmet needs, and/or changing the distressing feelings.

- Counselors, therapists, and others can help clarify the source of emotional distress and find healthy ways to cope with it.

- Fears, anxieties, and depression are common emotional problems.

- Common phobias include acrophobia, agoraphobia, claustrophobia, mysophobia, ophediophobia, and zoophobia.

- Depression is often characterized by feelings of dejection, guilt, hopelessness, self-recrimination, loss of appetite, insomnia, loss of interest in sexual activity, withdrawal from friends, inability to concentrate, lowered self-esteem, and a focus on the negative.

- Suicide is the third leading cause of death among youth 15–24 years of age, all races, both genders.

- Many of the signs of depression occur in someone suicidal. Many suicidal people talk about suicide when life appears hopeless.

- Sleep and dreams are fundamental to human health. Sleep has four stages. REM sleep, when dreams occur, happens during the cycle of sleep from deep to lighter stages.

- Many people use their dreams to help them understand and deal with distressing situations and confusing emotions.

- Schizophrenia is a mental disorder characterized by delusions, inability to think logically and coherently, diminished social and emotional experiences, and loss of sense of purpose.

REFERENCES

Maslow, A. L. (1970). *Motivation and Personality*. New York: Harper & Row.

Smith, S. F., and C. M. Smith (1990). *Personal Health Choices*. Boston: Jones and Bartlett Publishers, Inc.

Trungpa, C. (1977). "Acknowledging Death." In P. Olson and J. L. Fosshage, eds., *Healing: Implications for Psychotherapy*. New York: Human Science Press.

U.S. Department of Health and Human Services (Dec. 8, 1994). *Monthly Vital Statistics Report*. Washington, D.C.: U.S. Goverment Printing Office.

SUGGESTED READINGS

Braiker, H. B. (1989). "The Power of Self-Talk." *Psychotherapy Today:* 23-27. A concise guide to monitoring and eliminating inner negative self-talk and enhancing self-esteem.

Kirschstein, R. (1993). "Sleep Research Has Broad Sweep." *Journal of the American Medical Association,* 270(10): 1172. Discusses the research that is currently being done on sleep and its impact on health and well-being.

Papolos, D. F., and J. Papolos (1992). *Overcoming Depression*. New York: HarperCollins.

Eating and Exercising toward a Healthy Life-style

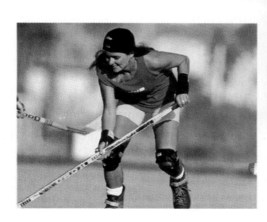

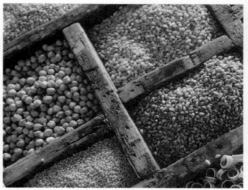

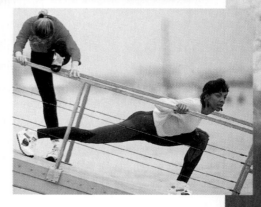

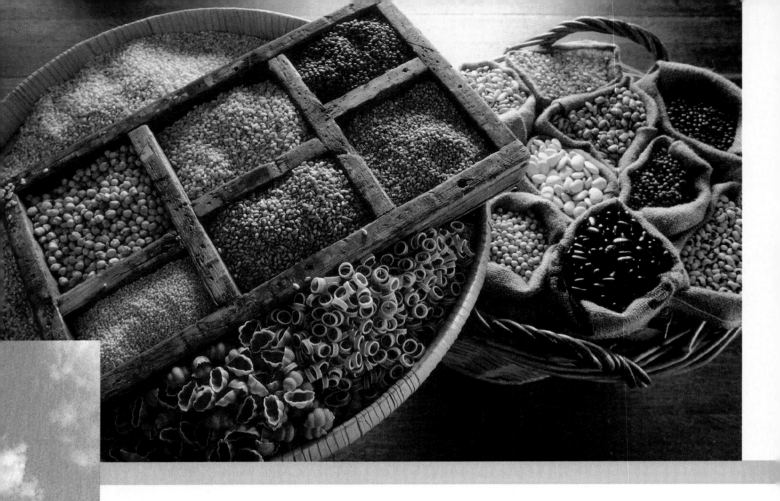

LEARNING OBJECTIVES

After reading this chapter you should be able to:

1. Discuss the various factors that influence your dietary choices.
2. Describe the different dietary guidelines proposed by various organizations.
3. Properly read a food label.
4. Describe how the human body receives essential nutrients from food.
5. Explain the nature of dietary supplements and food additives.
6. Describe how major fast-food establishments have responded to consumer concerns.
7. Describe the three kinds of vegetarian diets and several reasons for vegetarianism.
8. Describe the relationship between good nutrition and health.

Choosing a Nutritious Diet

*O*f the many things you can do to enhance your well-being, none is more important than maintaining proper nutrition. Many people are aware that good nutrition is essential and sincerely want to eat healthfully. But the plethora of claims and counterclaims about nutrition and health and the aggressive marketing of food products tend to confuse rather than enlighten.

Moreover, many factors other than knowledge of nutrition influence a person's dietary choices. Nutritious food (except perhaps for those with very low incomes) tends to be accessible to most U.S. residents and people in other industrialized countries. For these people, dietary choices are influenced by family, ethnic, and cultural eating patterns, social factors (eating what friends eat), and time pressures that limit thoughtful food shopping, meal preparation, and making convenience foods attractive. Current food fads *and* stress also influence food choices; frequently, they encourage consumption of foods high in fat and sugar to soothe jangled nerves and emotions.

DIETARY GUIDELINES FOR EATING RIGHT

To encourage and promote healthy dietary choices, the U.S. government, the World Health Organization, and organizations such as the American Heart Asso-

Eat for Good Nutrition

Are you "in action"? Are you ready to stay in shape—for a lifetime? From these statements, check (√) seven best guidelines for smart eating that can help keep you healthy.

_____ Use salt and sodium only in moderation.

_____ Choose a diet low in fat, saturated fat, and cholesterol.

_____ Avoid snacking.

_____ Eat an apple a day for good health.

_____ Use sugars only in moderation.

_____ Avoid desserts.

_____ Maintain healthy weight.

_____ Avoid alcoholic beverages.

_____ Eat green vegetables every day.

_____ Avoid candy, chips, and soft drinks.

_____ Choose a diet with plenty of vegetables, fruits, and grain products.

_____ Eat a variety of foods.

_____ Avoid fast foods.

I want to follow the Dietary Guidelines so I stay healthy. Here's how I'll eat smart:

_____

_____

_____

_____

_____

SIGNED _____

DATE _____

Source: U.S. Department of Agriculture, _Dietary Guidelines and Your Health: Health Educator's Guide to Nutrition and Fitness_ (Washington, D.C.: U.S. Government Printing Office, 1992).

ciation and the American Cancer Society (Table 5.1) promote guidelines for good nutrition. These guidelines are based on the latest scientific evidence for good nutrition obtained by examining the biological effects of specific dietary components and by comparing the dietary patterns and disease frequencies in different populations. For example, compared to the standard American diet with its associated high levels of heart disease and cancer, the high-carbohydrate/low-fat diet of rural China is associated with less heart disease and fewer cancers of all kinds (Campbell and Junshi, 1994). Seventh Day Adventists, who consume high-carbohydrate/low-fat diets, also have less heart disease and cancer than other Americans. The same is true of Mediterranean countries (Greece,

TABLE 5.1   American Heart Association and American Cancer Society's Dietary Guidelines

American Heart Association's Dietary Guidelines with your heart in mind	American Cancer Society's Dietary Guidelines for reducing your risk of cancer
• Total fat intake should be less than 30 percent of calories	• Maintain a desirable body weight
• Saturated fatty acid intake should be less than 10 percent of calories	• Eat a varied diet
• Polyunsaturated fatty acid intake should be no more than 10 percent of calories	• Include a variety of both vegetables and fruits in the daily diet
• Monounsaturated fatty acids make up the rest of the total fat intake, about 10 to 15 percent of total calories	• Eat more high-fiber foods, e.g., whole grain cereals, legumes, vegetables, fruits
• Cholesterol intake should be no more than 300 mg/day	• Cut down on total fat intake
• Sodium intake should be no more than 3000 milligrams (3 grams) per day	• Limit consumption of alcoholic beverages, if you drink at all
	• Limit consumption of salt-cured, smoked, and nitrate-preserved foods

southern Italy), whose traditional diet is high in fruits, vegetables, and legumes and low in animal fat (Willett, 1994).

In 1988 the first *Surgeon General's Report on Nutrition and Health* offered comprehensive documentation for recommended dietary changes. The report's main conclusion stated "overconsumption of certain dietary components is now a major concern for Americans. While many food factors are involved, chief among them is the disproportionate consumption of foods high in fats, often at the expense of foods high in complex carbohydrates and fiber that may be more conducive to health." The report also issued five recommendations for most people and four recommendations for some people.

The current dietary guidelines for Americans (Figure 5.1), published by the U.S. Departments of Agriculture and Health and Human Services, are recommendations to help healthy Americans maintain and possibly improve their health. The first two guidelines form a framework for a healthy diet; the other five underscore qualities of a good diet. The dietary guidelines offer flexibility; they encourage wise food choices from a variety of foods.

The Food Guide Pyramid

To help implement the dietary guidelines, the U.S. government created the "Food Guide Pyramid," which promotes diets emphasizing grains, fruits, and vegetables, with moderate to little consumption of meat and dairy

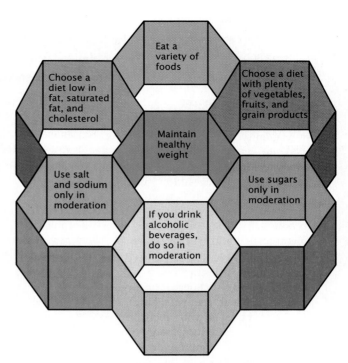

FIGURE 5.1 Current Dietary Guidelines for Americans These guidelines call for moderation—avoiding extremes in diets. The guidelines reflect recommendations of nutrition authorities who agree that enough is known about diet's effect on health to encourage these dietary practices by Americans.

Source: U.S. Department of Agriculture and U.S. Department of Health and Human Services, *Nutrition and Your Health: Dietary Guidelines for Americans* (Washington, D.C.: U.S. Government Printing Office, 1990).

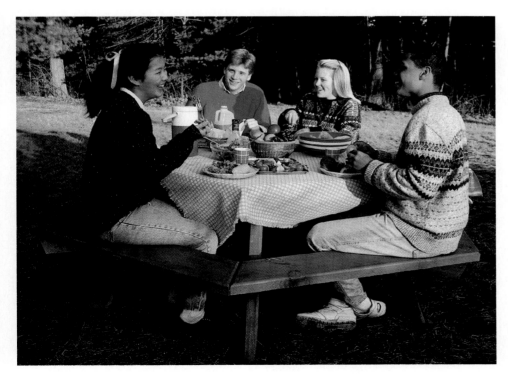

Natural, unprocessed foods provide the best nutrition.

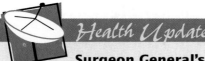

Surgeon General's Report on Nutrition and Health: Recommendations

Issues for Most People

- *Fats and cholesterol:* Reduce consumption of fat (especially saturated fat) and cholesterol. Choose foods relatively low in these substances, such as vegetables, fruits, whole grain foods, fish, poultry, lean meats, and low-fat dairy products. Use food preparation methods that add little or no fat.

- *Energy and weight control:* Achieve and maintain a desirable body weight. To do so, choose a dietary pattern in which energy (caloric) intake is consistent with energy expenditure. To reduce energy intake, limit consumption of foods relatively high in calories, fats, and sugars, and minimize alcohol consumption. Increase energy expenditure through regular and sustained physical activity.

- *Complex carbohydrates and fiber:* Increase consumption of whole grain foods and cereal products, vegetables (including dried beans and peas), and fruits.

- *Sodium:* Reduce intake of sodium by choosing foods relatively low in sodium and limiting the amount of salt added in food preparation and at the table.

- *Alcohol:* To reduce the risk for chronic disease, take alcohol only in moderation (no more than two drinks a day), if at all. Avoid drinking any alcohol before or while driving, operating machinery, taking medications, or engaging in any other activity requiring judgment. Avoid drinking alcohol while pregnant.

Other Issues for Some People

- *Fluoride:* Community water systems should contain fluoride at optimal levels for prevention of tooth decay. If such water is not available, use other appropriate sources of fluoride.

- *Sugars:* Those who are particularly vulnerable to dental caries (cavities), especially children, should limit their consumption and frequency of use of foods high in sugars.

- *Calcium:* Adolescent girls and adult women should increase consumption of foods high in calcium, including low-fat dairy products.

- *Iron:* Children, adolescents, and women of childbearing age should be sure to consume foods that are good sources of iron, such as lean meats, fish, certain beans, and iron-enriched cereals and whole grain products. This issue is of special concern for low-income families.

Source: U.S. Department of Health and Human Services, *The Surgeon General's Report on Nutrition and Health* (Washington, D.C.: U.S. Government Printing Office, 1988).

FIGURE 5.2 Food Guide Pyramid: A Guide to Daily Food Choices Each of these food groups provides some, but not all, of the nutrients you need. No one food group is more important than another—for good health, you need them all. Go easy on fats, oils, and sweets, the foods at the small tip of the Pyramid.

Source: U.S. Department of Agriculture and U.S. Department of Health and Human Services.

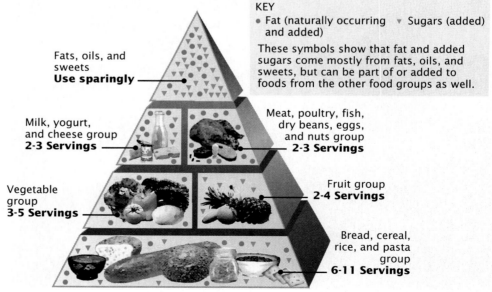

products, and only the sparest consumption of sweets and fats (Figure 5.2). The Food Guide Pyramid has been criticized because it accommodates politically powerful meat and dairy industries, and it does not offer sufficient information to guide healthy food choices. For example, meat and dairy products, which can contain high percentages of fat, are lumped together with beans and other legumes, which are high in fiber and contain little or no fat. Some products in the grain group are manufactured with considerable sugar and salt, but these additives are not reflected in the recommendations.

On the other hand, the Pyramid's proponents point out that the pictorial display placing the most healthful food at the broad base and the least healthful at the tip is easy to remember. They believe it allows people to stop counting calories and grams and build diets based on foods found at the bottom of the Pyramid: these include whole grains, fresh fruits, and fresh vegetables, which provide adequate nutrients and calories for good health.

Making daily food choices can be frustrating and confusing. However, using the Food Guide Pyramid

Wellness Guide

How to Use the Daily Food Guide

What Counts As One Serving?

Breads, Cereals, Rice, and Pasta
1 slice of bread
1/2 cup of cooked rice or pasta
1/2 cup of cooked cereal
1 ounce of ready-to-eat cereal

Vegetables
1/2 cup of chopped raw or cooked vegetables
1 cup of leafy raw vegetables

Milk, Yogurt, and Cheese
1 cup of milk or yogurt
1-1/2 to 2 ounces of cheese

Fruits
1 piece of fruit or melon wedge
3/4 cup of juice
1/2 cup of canned fruit
1/4 cup of dried fruit

Meat, Poultry, Fish, Dry Beans, Eggs, and Nuts
2-1/2 to 3 ounces of cooked lean meat, poultry, or fish
Count 1/2 cup of cooked beans, or 1 egg, or 2 tablespoons of peanut butter as 1 ounce of lean meat (about 1/3 serving)

Fats, Oils, and Sweets
LIMIT CALORIES FROM THESE especially if you need to lose weight

> The amount you eat may be more than one serving. For example, a dinner portion of spaghetti would count as two or three servings of pasta.

How Many Servings Do You Need Each Day?

	Women and some older adults	Children, teenage girls, active women, most men	Teenage boys and active men
Calorie level*	about 1,600	about 2,200	about 2,800
Bread group	6	9	11
Vegetable group	3	4	5
Fruit group	2	3	4
Milk group	**2–3	**2–3	**2–3
Meat group	2, for a total of 5 ounces	2, for a total of 6 ounces	3, for a total of 7 ounces

*These are the calorie levels if you choose lowfat, lean foods from the 5 major food groups and use foods from the fats, oils, and sweets group sparingly.
**Women who are pregnant or breastfeeding, teenagers, and young adults to age 24 need 3 servings.

Source: U.S. Department of Agriculture/ U.S. Department of Health and Human Services, 1992.

How Does Your Diet Rate for Variety?

A varied diet is a healthful diet. How would you describe the variety in your food choices?

How often do you eat:	Seldom or never	1 or 2 times a week	3 to 4 times a week	Almost daily
1. At least six servings of breads, cereals, rice, crackers, pasta, or other foods made from grains (a serving is one slice of bread or a half cup cereal, rice, etc.) per day?	☐	☐	☐	☐
2. Foods made from whole grains?	☐	☐	☐	☐
3. Three different kinds of vegetables per day?	☐	☐	☐	☐
4. Cooked dry beans or peas?	☐	☐	☐	
5. A dark-green vegetable, such as spinach or broccoli?	☐	☐	☐	☐
6. Two kinds of fruit or fruit juice per day?	☐	☐	☐	☐
7. Three servings of milk, yogurt, or cheese per day?	☐	☐	☐	☐
8. Two servings of lean meat, poultry, fish, or alternates, such as eggs, dry beans, or nuts per day?	☐	☐	☐	☐

Count the number of check marks in each column. _____ _____ _____ _____

To eat a varied diet, I will: _____

_____

My Eating Habits: Some Clues to Calories?

Calories come from food—all kinds of food. Do you get enough? Or more than you need? Think about your eating patterns—and why you eat what you eat. Check all the answers that describe your eating patterns.

What do I usually eat?

_____ A varied and balanced diet.
_____ A diet with only moderate amounts of fats and sugars.
_____ Deep-fat-fried and breaded foods.
_____ "Extras," such as salad dressings, potato toppings, spreads, sauces, and gravies.
_____ Sweets and rich desserts, such as candies, cakes, and pies.
_____ Snack foods high in fat and sodium, such as chips and other "munchies."
_____ Soft drinks.

When do I usually eat?

_____ At mealtime.
_____ While studying.
_____ While preparing meals or clearing the table.
_____ When spending time with friends.
_____ While watching TV or participating in other activities.
_____ Anytime.

Where do I usually eat?

_____ At home at the kitchen or dining room table.
_____ In the school cafeteria.
_____ In fast-food places.
_____ In front of the TV or while studying.
_____ Wherever I happen to be when I'm hungry.

Why do I usually eat?

_____ It's time to eat.
_____ I'm hungry.
_____ Foods look tempting.
_____ Everyone else is eating.
_____ Food will get thrown away if I don't eat it.
_____ I'm bored or frustrated.

Changes I want to make:

1. _____
2. _____
3. _____

Source: U.S. Department of Agriculture, *Dietary Guidelines and Your Health: Health Educator's Guide to Nutrition and Fitness* (Washington, D.C.: U.S. Government Printing Office, 1992).

when shopping, planning, and preparing meals for yourself and others can provide a varied and nutritious diet. A pattern for daily food choices includes:

- Choosing daily from breads, cereals, and other grain products, fruits, vegetables, meat, poultry, fish, and milk, cheese, and yogurt.
- Including different foods from within the groups.
- Having the smaller number of servings suggested from each group.
- Limiting total amount of food eaten to that needed to maintain desirable body weight.

- Choosing foods that are low in fat and sugars.
- Managing your intake of fats, sweets, and alcoholic beverages.

READING THE "NEW" FOOD LABEL

In 1990, when the Nutritional Labeling and Education Act (NLEA) became law, the Food and Drug Administration (FDA) took on food labeling education as an important challenge for the 1990s. The NLEA is responsible

Wellness Guide

Special Diets and Label Information

Label information can help individuals select foods appropriate for their special dietary needs, determined by a physician, registered dietitian, or nutritionist. Some medical conditions that require special attention to diet are:

Kidney Disease

For many people whose kidneys have failed or are failing, protein, potassium, and sodium are restricted. The nutrient phosphorus also may be restricted.

People undergoing dialysis may be encouraged to eat 20 to 25 grams (g) of fiber daily because fluid restrictions, lack of exercise, and some kidney medications can cause constipation. The Daily Value for fiber, which is based on a 2,000-calorie diet, is 25 g.

Daily Values are reference numbers based on recommended dietary intakes to help consumers use label information to plan a healthy diet.

Liver Disorders

People with hepatitis, cirrhosis, and other liver diseases often need a high-calorie, low-protein diet to help rejuvenate the damaged liver and maintain adequate nutrition. They also may need to increase their intake of vitamins—particularly folic

acid, vitamin B_{12}, and thiamin—and minerals.

Food Sensitivities

According to the Food Allergy Network (a national nonprofit organization), the most common food allergens are milk, eggs, wheat, peanuts and other nuts, and soy. The treatment: avoiding the food or foods containing them.

Celiac Disease

This is a genetic disorder in which the body cannot tolerate gliadin, the protein component of the gluten in wheat, barley, rye, and oats. So, people with celiac disease must avoid all products containing these grains —even foods that may contain only small amounts of the protein, such as vinegar, bouillon, and alcohol-containing flavorings. The intolerance leads to malabsorption—not only of the offending food but virtually all nutrients.

Cancer

Because weight loss is common during cancer treatment, many cancer patients need to increase their calories and protein intake.

In the case of bowel obstruction— either from surgery, radiation or the tumor—cancer patients may need to

eat less fiber. But, they may need more if they become constipated.

To help reduce their risk of developing cancer again, following treatment, patients may want to choose foods and nutrients whose role in reducing cancer risk has been borne out by significant scientific evidence.

Bowel Disease

Increased fiber is often recommended for people with chronic constipation, irritable bowel syndrome, and diverticulosis. Low-fiber diets may be called for during flare-ups of these and other bowel diseases, such as Crohn's disease and ulcerative colitis.

Osteoporosis

In osteoporosis, bone mass decreases, causing bones to become brittle and easily broken, especially in later life. A low-calcium intake throughout life is thought to be a major risk factor. The Daily Value for calcium, based on calcium needs for all ages, is 1,000 milligrams. Vitamin D also is important because it aids calcium absorption. The Daily Value for vitamin D is 400 International Units.

Source: FDA Consumer (January–February, 1995): 24.

Total Fat

Aim low: Most people need to cut back on fat! Too much fat may contribute to heart disease and cancer. Try to limit your calories from fat. For a healthy heart, choose foods with a big difference between the total number of calories and the number of calories from fat.

Saturated Fat

A new kind of fat? No — saturated fat is part of the total fat in food. It is listed separately because it's the key player in raising blood cholesterol and your risk of heart disease. Eat less!

Cholesterol

Too much cholesterol — a second cousin to fat — can lead to heart disease. Challenge yourself to eat less than 300 mg each day.

Sodium

You call it "salt," the label calls it "sodium." Either way, it may add up to high blood pressure in some people. So, keep your sodium intake low — 2,400 to 3,000 mg or less each day.*

*the AHA recommends no more than 3,000 mg sodium per day for healthy adults.

Daily Value

Feel like you're drowning in numbers? Let the Daily Value be your guide. Daily Values are listed for people who eat 2,000 or 2,500 calories each day. If you eat more, your personal daily value may be higher than what's listed on the label. If you eat less, your personal daily value may be lower.

For the fat, saturated fat, cholesterol and sodium, choose foods with a low % Daily Value. For total carbohydrate, dietary fiber, vitamins and minerals, your daily value goal is to reach 100% of each.

g = grams (About 28 g = 1 ounce)
mg = milligrams (1,000 mg = 1 g)

Nutrition Facts

Serving Size 1/2 cup (114 g)
Servings Per Container 4

Amount per Serving

Calories 90	Calories from Fat 30
	% Daily Value*
Total Fat 3g	5%
Saturated Fat 0g	0%
Cholesterol 0mg	0%
Sodium 300g	13%
Total Carbohydrate 13g	4%
Dietary Fiber 3g	12%
Sugars 3g	
Protein 3g	

Vitamin A	80%	•	Vitamin C	60%
Calcium	4%	•	Iron	4%

* Percent Daily Values are based on a 2,000 calorie diet. Your daily values may be higher or lower depending on your calorie needs:

	Calories	2,000	2,500
Total Fat	Less than	65g	80g
Sat Fat	Less than	20g	25g
Cholesterol	Less than	300mg	300mg
Sodium	Less than	2,400mg	2,400mg
Total Carbohydrate		300g	375g
Fiber		25g	30g

Calories per gram:
Fat 9 • Carbohydrate 4 • Protein 4

More nutrients may be listed on some labels.

Serving Size

Is your serving the same size as the one on the label? If you eat double the serving size listed, you need to double the nutrient and calorie values. If you eat one-half the serving size shown here, cut the nutrient and calorie values in half.

Calories

Are you overweight? Cut back a little on calories! Look here to see how a serving of the food adds to your daily total. A 5'4", 138-lb. active woman needs about 2,200 calories each day. A 5'10", 174-lb. active man needs about 2,900. How about you?

Total Carbohydrate

When you cut down on fat, you can eat more carbohydrates. Carbohydrates are in foods like bread, potatoes, fruits and vegetables. Choose these often! They give you nutrients and energy.

Dietary Fiber

Grandmother called it "roughage," but her advice to eat more is still up-to-date! That goes for both soluble and insoluble kinds of dietary fiber. Fruits, vegetables, whole-grain foods, beans and peas are all good sources and can help reduce the risk of heart disease and cancer.

Protein

Most Americans get more protein than they need. Where there is animal protein, there is also fat and cholesterol. Eat small servings of lean meat, fish and poultry. Use skim or low-fat milk, yogurt, and cheese. Try vegetable proteins like beans, grains and cereals.

Vitamins & Minerals

Your goal here is 100% of each for the day. Don't count on one food to do it all. Let a combination of foods add up to a winning score.

FIGURE 5.3 Knowing What to Look For in a Label

for most of the food labeling changes taking place today; but, as the name implies, education is also a major emphasis. In particular, the law calls for activities to educate consumers about the availability of nutrition information in food labeling and the importance of using that information to make healthy dietary choices (Kurzweil, 1995). Consumers with certain medical conditions need to pay close attention to label information.

Until recently, food labels were difficult to read, understand, and comprehend. Today all food labels must follow a simple and consistent format to let you know the nutritional facts about the product you are buying.

Food labels have two important parts: the nutrition information and the ingredient lists (Figure 5.3). Also, some labels have different claims, such as "low-fat" or "light." All food labels list the product's ingredients in order by weight. The ingredient in the greatest amount is listed first; the ingredient in the least amount is listed last.

Reading the label will help you choose healthy foods. Eating a healthy diet can help reduce your risk factors for some diseases. For example, too much sodium may be linked to high blood pressure, a risk factor for heart attack and stroke.

 Health Update

Food Label Key Words

You Can Rely on the New Label

Rest assured, when you see key words and health claims on product labels, they mean what they say as defined by the government.

Key Words	What They Mean
Calorie Free	Fewer than 5 calories per serving
Light (Lite)	1/3 less calories or no more than 1/2 the fat of the higher-calorie, higher-fat version; or no more than 1/2 the sodium of the higher-sodium version
Fat Free	Less than 0.5 gram of fat per serving
Low Fat	3 grams of fat (or less) per serving
Reduced or Less Fat	At least 25% less fat per serving than the higher-fat version
Lean	Less than 10 grams of fat, 4 grams of saturated fat, and 95 milligrams of cholesterol per serving
Extra Lean	Less than 5 grams of fat, 2 grams of saturated fat, and 95 milligrams of cholesterol per serving
Low in Saturated Fat	1 gram saturated fat (or less) per serving and not more than 15% of calories from saturated fatty acids
Cholesterol Free	Less than 2 milligrams of cholesterol and 2 grams (or less) of saturated fat per serving
Low Cholesterol	20 milligrams of cholesterol (or less) and 2 grams of saturated fat (or less) per serving
Reduced Cholesterol	At least 25% less cholesterol than the higher-cholesterol version, and 2 grams (or less) of saturated fat per serving

Key Words	What They Mean
Sodium Free (No Sodium)	Less than 5 milligrams of sodium per serving, and no sodium chloride (NaCl) in ingredients
Very Low Sodium	35 milligrams of sodium (or less) per serving
Low Sodium	140 milligrams of sodium (or less) per serving
Reduced or Less Sodium	At least 25% less sodium per serving than the higher-sodium version
Sugar Free	Less than 0.5 gram of sugar per serving
High Fiber	5 grams of fiber (or more) per serving
Good Source of Fiber	2.5 to 4.9 grams of fiber per serving

You don't have to try to remember all these! **But notice that the key words follow the same pattern for each nutrient:**

- "Free" has the least amount.
- "Very Low" and "Low" have a little more.
- "Reduced" or "Less" always means that the food has 25% less of that nutrient than the reference (or standard) version of the food.

And all these terms are based on standard serving sizes.

Source: American Heart Association, *Facts About the New Food Labels,* 1993. Reprinted with permission from the American Heart Association.

Achieve useful and informative nutrition labeling for virtually all processed foods and at least 40 percent of fresh meats, poultry, fish, fruits, vegetables, baked goods, and ready-to-eat carry-away foods.

To facilitate the selection of foods consistent with *Dietary Guidelines for Americans,* food labels should be easy to read and understand, and contain information that is important to the consumer. Food selection can be made easier for consumers through universal labeling with the major food processing categories.

There are four primary messages health officials hope you will gain when you read the new food label:

1. You can believe the claims on the package.
2. You can more easily compare products because serving sizes will be more comparable for similar products.
3. By using the percent daily value, you can quickly determine whether a product is high or low in a nutrient.
4. By consulting the daily values, you can determine

how much, or how little, of the major nutrients you should eat daily.

By taking the time to read the new labels, health professionals hope you will be able to make informed decisions about food.

THE FUNCTIONS OF FOOD IN YOUR BODY

Food provides the physical material that makes up the body and the chemicals that help regulate body functions. Food also provides chemical energy for life.

Body Structure and Function

Your body is made up of billions of atoms and molecules arranged in particular combinations and proportions. Most of the atoms and molecules that now make up your body were not part of you even a few weeks ago, because living things continually exchange their chemical constituents with the environment. Food provides the "raw materials" for your body's cells to manufacture the specific chemical substances that make you *you.*

Adequate amounts of 40 chemical substances, called the **essential nutrients** (Table 5.2), must be supplied

TABLE 5.2   The Essential Nutrients*

Amino acids	Fats	Water	Vitamins	Minerals
Isoleucine	Linoleic acid		Ascorbic acid (vitamin C)	Calcium
Leucine	Linolenic acid		Biotin	Chlorine
Lysine			Cobalamin (vitamin B_{12})	Chromium
Methionine			Folic acid	Cobalt
Phenylalanine			Niacin (vitamin B_3)	Copper
Threonine			Pantothenic acid	Iodine
Tryptophan			Pyridoxine (vitamin B_6)	Iron
Valine			Riboflavin (vitamin B_2)	Magnesium
Arginine[†]			Thiamine (vitamin B_1)	Manganese
Histidine[†]			Vitamin A	Molybdenum
			Vitamin D	Phosphorus
			Vitamin E	Potassium
			Vitamin K	Selenium
				Sodium
				Sulfur
				Zinc

*Must be obtained from food.

†Not essential for adults; needed for growth of children.

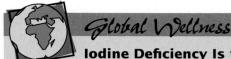
Iodine Deficiency Is the Most Common Cause of Mental Deficits Worldwide

Iodine is an essential trace element in the human diet. Supplementing table salt with iodine in most countries of the world has eliminated the terrible effects of iodine deficiency in most populations. However, in many areas of Africa, Asia, Latin America, and parts of Eastern Europe, people's diets are deficient in iodine. The most severe consequence of iodine deficiency is severe mental retardation called *cretinism.*

Conclusive proof of the importance of iodine in the diet comes from an experiment carried out in Papua, New Guinea. Over a four-year period, some families received an injection of iodine and other families received placebo injections. Only one case of cretinism occurred among 412 newborns of mothers who had received iodine injections. Among women who had not received iodine injections, 21 of 406 babies were born with cretinism.

The primary sign of iodine deficiency is the presence of a *goiter,* an enlarged thyroid gland that is observable as a large external bulge in the throat. Almost all of the iodine in the body is concentrated in the thyroid gland, where it regulates the production of essential thyroid hormones. In 1990 the World Health Organization estimated that 200 million people had goiter and another 20 million had mental deficits resulting from iodine deficiency. In most areas of the world the soil does not contain iodine, and plants grown in these regions are also deficient. Efforts are underway to supply everyone in the world with iodized salt or oil to prevent cretinism and other iodine-deficiency diseases.

Source: Adapted from B. S. Hetzel, "Iodine Deficiency and Fetal Brain Damage," *New England Journal of Medicine* (December 29, 1994).

---

continually to the body. Failure to do so can result in a nutritional deficiency disease, such as **goiter** from lack of iodine. Some forms of **anemia** result from insufficient dietary iron and blindness results from vitamin A deficiency. The most common cause of blindness in children worldwide is lack of vitamin A.

Researchers have determined how much of the essential nutrients are required to prevent deficiency diseases. Many countries and the World Health Organization have produced dietary standards based on that research. In the United States, these requirements are called the **Recommended [Daily] Dietary Allowances,** or **RDA,** which lists values for protein, eleven vitamins, and seven minerals (Table 5.3). The RDA assumes that if the listed nutrients are consumed in recommended amounts, all other necessary nutrients will be too. The RDA also lists values for pregnant women, lactating women, and children. The RDA is set for people in reasonably good health, that is, not suffering from a major disease or under undue stress.

Surveys indicate that many Americans do not consume recommended RDA amounts of calcium, vitamin B_6, magnesium, zinc, copper, and potassium. People can determine if their diets contain the RDA of particular nutrients by consulting tables listing the composition of foods. Packaged food labels also carry information on the nutrient composition of the product.

TERMS

essential nutrients: chemical substances obtained from food and needed by the body for growth, maintenance, or repair of tissues. Essential nutrients are not made by the body; they must be obtained from food

goiter: an enlargement of the thyroid gland resulting from lack of iodine, causing a swelling in the front part of the neck

anemia: a deficiency of red blood cells; often caused by insufficient iron

Recommended [Daily] Dietary Allowances (RDA): levels of nutrients recommended by the Food and Nutrition Board of the National Academy of Sciences for daily consumption by healthy individuals, scaled according to gender and age

calorie: the amount of energy required to raise one gram of water from 14.5 to 15.5 degrees Celsius. The energy released from food is too enormous to be described in these units, so nutritionists use the term kilocalorie

Energy for Life

Food also provides energy to the body. The ultimate source of energy for complex organisms is sunlight, which is captured by green plants and converted to chemical energy that is stored as plant material. When humans eat plant matter or tissue from plant-eating animals, they use this stored chemical energy. Biological energy is used most efficiently when liberated in the presence of oxygen, which is one reason you breathe. In the process, the food material is converted to carbon dioxide, water, and other waste products and eliminated from the body in expired air, urine, feces, and sweat.

Energy transformations in living things are discussed in terms of calories. A **calorie** is the amount of heat

TABLE 5.3   Recommended Daily Dietary Allowances, Revised 1989

		Water-soluble vitamins						
Category	Age (years) or condition	Vitamin C (mg)	Thiamin (mg)	Riboflavin (mg)	Niacin (mg NE)	Vitamin B_6 (mg)	Folate (mg)	Vitamin B_{12} (µg)
Infants	0.0–0.5	30	0.3	0.4	5	0.3	25	0.3
	0.5–1.0	35	0.4	0.5	6	0.6	35	0.5
Children	1–3	40	0.7	0.8	9	1.0	50	0.7
	4–6	45	0.9	1.1	12	1.1	75	1.0
	7–10	45	1.0	1.2	13	1.4	100	1.4
Males	11–14	50	1.3	1.5	17	1.7	150	2.0
	15–18	60	1.5	1.8	20	2.0	200	2.0
	19–24	60	1.5	1.7	19	2.0	200	2.0
	25–50	60	1.5	1.7	19	2.0	200	2.0
	51+	60	1.2	1.4	15	2.0	200	2.0
Females	11–14	50	1.1	1.3	15	1.4	150	2.0
	15–18	60	1.1	1.3	15	1.5	180	2.0
	19–24	60	1.1	1.3	15	1.6	180	2.0
	25–50	60	1.1	1.3	15	1.6	180	2.0
	51+	60	1.0	1.2	13	1.6	180	2.0
Pregnant		70	1.5	1.6	17	2.2	400	2.2
Lactating	1st 6 months	95	1.6	1.8	20	2.1	280	2.6
	2nd 6 months	90	1.6	1.7	20	2.1	260	2.6

		Minerals						
Category	Age (years) or condition	Calcium (mg)	Phosphorus (mg)	Magnesium (mg)	Iron (mg)	Zinc (mg)	Iodine (µg)	Selenium (µg)
Infants	0.0–0.5	400	300	40	6	5	40	10
	0.5–1.0	600	500	60	10	5	50	15
Children	1–3	800	800	80	10	10	70	20
	4–6	800	800	120	10	10	90	20
	7–10	800	800	170	10	10	120	30
Males	11–14	1,200	1,200	270	12	15	150	40
	15–18	1,200	1,200	400	12	15	150	50
	19–24	1,200	1,200	350	10	15	150	70
	25–50	800	800	350	10	15	150	70
	51+	800	800	350	10	15	150	70
Females	11–14	1,200	1,200	280	15	12	150	45
	15–18	1,200	1,200	300	15	12	150	50
	19–24	1,200	1,200	280	15	12	150	55
	25–50	800	800	280	15	12	150	55
	51+	800	800	280	10	12	150	55
Pregnant		1,200	1,200	320	30	15	175	65
Lactating	1st 6 months	1,200	1,200	355	15	19	200	75
	2nd 6 months	1,200	1,200	340	15	16	200	75

TABLE 5.3 Recommended Daily Dietary Allowances, Revised 1989, continued

Category	Age (years) or condition	Protein (g)	Fat-soluble vitamins			
			Vitamin A (µg RE)	Vitamin D (µg)	Vitamin E (mg α-TE)	Vitamin K (µg)
Infants	0.0–0.5	13	375	7.5	3	5
	0.5–1.0	14	375	10	4	10
Children	1–3	16	400	10	6	15
	4–6	24	500	10	7	20
	7–10	28	700	10	7	30
Males	11–14	45	1,000	10	10	45
	15–18	59	1,000	10	10	65
	19–24	58	1,000	10	10	70
	25–50	63	1,000	5	10	80
	51+	63	1,000	5	10	80
Females	11–14	46	800	10	8	45
	15–18	44	800	10	8	55
	19–24	46	800	10	8	60
	25–50	50	800	5	8	65
	51+	50	800	5	8	65
Pregnant		60	800	10	10	65
Lactating	1st 6 months	65	1,300	10	12	65
	2nd 6 months	62	1,200	10	11	65

Source: Food and Nutrition Board, National Academy of Sciences National Research Council.

energy required to raise one gram of water from 14.5 to 15.5 degrees Celsius. A **nutritional calorie,** which is what weight watchers watch, is 1,000 calories, or a **kilocalorie.** Books that discuss human nutrition and physical fitness frequently use the word "calorie" when actually referring to a kilocalorie. This book follows the same convention.

Energy requirements for individuals vary depending on a number of factors including: body size and composition; physical activity; growth needs during adolescence and young adulthood; pregnancy or breast feeding; and injury or illness. The RDA for adult American men is 2,800 calories per day; for nonpregnant, nonlactating adult American women, it is about 2,200. Energy from food is derived from the breakdown of proteins (4 calories per gram), carbohydrates (4 calories per gram), and fats (9 calories per gram). Nutritionists recommend that carbohydrates from grains, vegetables, and fruits be the principal source of energy, supplying about 60 to 80 percent of total calories consumed. Fats should make up 1 to 30 percent of total calories consumed. Protein is generally not recommended as a source of energy, but only as a source of building blocks for the body's tissues and organs.

THE COMPOSITION OF FOOD

Food is composed of seven kinds of chemical substances: proteins, carbohydrates, lipids (fats), vitamins, minerals, phytochemicals, and water. Dietary proteins, most types of carbohydrates, and most lipids cannot be used by the body until they are broken down in the digestive system into smaller chemical units (Figure 5.4). In fact, only a few kinds of carbohydrates, vitamins, minerals, and water are absorbed into the body as is.

Proteins

Proteins make up about 20 percent of body mass. The main function of protein is to provide your body with

T E R M S

nutritional calorie: unit of energy; often used interchangeably with the term kilocalorie

kilocalorie: unit of energy. The amount of heat needed to raise one kilogram of water one degree centigrade. A kilocalorie is equivalent to 1,000 calories

proteins: the foundation of every body cell; biological molecules composed of chains of amino acids

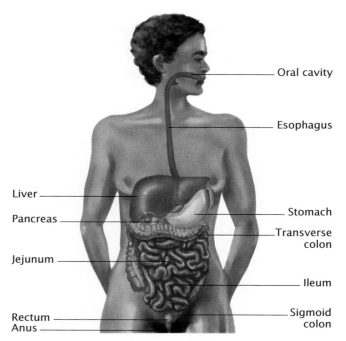

Oral cavity

Esophagus

Liver

Pancreas

Stomach

Transverse colon

Jejunum

Ileum

Rectum

Sigmoid colon

Anus

FIGURE 5.4 The Human Digestive System Teeth and glandular secretions in the mouth help break up food, which the esophagus transports to the stomach. The stomach breaks down some of the food molecules and passes it to the rest of the digestive tube: the duodenum, the jejunum, the ileum, the colon, and the rectum. The pancreas secretes enzymes and fluid into the duodenum to help the digestive process. The liver controls the release of absorbed nutrients into the body. Undigested material is eliminated from the body at the anus.

the amino acids necessary for growth and maintenance of body tissues. Cells, enzymes, hormones, antibodies, muscles, blood, all tissues and fluid (except urine and bile) require amino acids obtained from protein.

Proteins are made up of chemical units call **amino acids,** which come in twenty different forms. Amino acids are classified as **essential** and **nonessential.** Eight essential amino acids are required by adults, and nine are required by infants. Animal sources of protein include milk and milk products, meat, fish, poultry, and eggs. Plant sources include breads and cereal products, legumes, nuts, and seeds. The primary sources of protein for the majority of the world's population are cereal grains. Animal sources of protein will become less available as the world's population increases and land to raise animals becomes scarcer.

Amino acids are not stored in the body in any appreciable amounts; therefore, proper nutrition requires eating enough protein every day to meet the body's needs for essential amino acids. Adult women

should consume about 45 grams per day and adult men about 55 to 60 grams. The average North American adult consumes about twice that amount; the unneeded protein is broken down by the body and excreted in urine or stored as fat.

Because the amino acid composition of most animal protein is similar, people tend to acquire adequate amounts and proportions of the essential amino acids from various sources, such as fish, meat, eggs, and dairy products. Most vegetable proteins, however, are deficient in one or more of the essential amino acids, so individuals who eat little or no meat and/or dairy products must eat foods in which an amino acid deficiency in one food is compensated for by an amino acid surplus in another. For example, wheat, rice, and oats contain very little lysine, but have large amounts of methionine and tryptophan. Soybeans and other legumes are relatively high in lysine, but are low in methionine and tryptophan. Meals consisting of both grains and legumes (rice and beans, corn and beans, wheat and soybeans, for example) can supply adequate amounts of these essential amino acids.

Meat, dairy products, and eggs provide the essential amino acids, but are also high in fat, and thus contribute to the health problems associated with a high-fat diet (Table 5.4). For this reason, nutritionists recommend consuming nonfat or low-fat dairy products, using butter as a spread and not as an ingredient for cooking, being mindful of the amount of ice cream eaten, and limiting egg consumption to a few eggs per week. Nutritionists also favor trimming fat from meat before cooking, selecting meat with a low-fat content, and eating poultry (with skin removed because it contains fat) and fish, which have proportionately less fat than red meats. They also recommend using meat sparingly by adding it to grain- or bean-based dishes, rather than making it the center of the meal.

> *Vegetables aren't my meat and potatoes.*
> Yogi Berra,
> former New York Yankee catcher

Another reason for avoiding a lot of meat is its association with colorectal cancer. Countries with the highest per capita meat consumption—New Zealand, Canada, and the United States—also have the highest rates of colon cancer. The reasons for this association are not clear. One pos-

T E R M S

amino acids: compounds containing nitrogen, which are the building blocks of protein

essential amino acids: amino acids that cannot be synthesized by the body and must be provided by food

nonessential amino acids: eleven amino acids required for protein synthesis that are synthesized by humans and are not specifically required in the diet

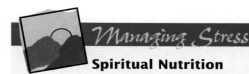

Managing Stress

Spiritual Nutrition

The Ayurvedic principles of India suggest that people eat certain foods, specifically fruits and vegetables, which correspond to the colors of the body's energy centers, called *chakras*. Chinese Taoist philosophy also advocates balance in the foods that are eaten, specifically in terms of their acidity or alkalinity. Imbalance in the foods that are eaten can create an energy disturbance that may result in illness.

In his book *Spiritual Nutrition,* physician Gabriel Cousens highlights several ways to make our eating habits more conducive to healthy living. These include:

1. Avoid eating big meals prior to meditation as the stomach and brain compete for blood flow and when the stomach is full, more blood is needed for digestion. As a rule, undereat.
2. Drink plenty of water to cleanse the body of nutrients and toxins no longer needed.
3. Good nutrition consists not only of digesting quality foods, but also requires sunlight (vitamin D), plenty of fresh air (oxygen), and plenty of fresh drinking water.
4. Learn what foods are associated with the acid/alkaline balance and make an effort to achieve good balance in your daily diet.
5. Learn to concentrate on the food you are eating, noting taste, texture, and temperature. Be mindful that eating is also a spiritual experience.

TABLE 5.4 Fat and Cholesterol Content of Various Meats and Fish

Food (100 grams)	Total fat (grams)	Polyunsaturated fat (milligrams)	Cholesterol (milligrams)
Ground beef, extra lean	16.0	600	82
Ground beef, lean	18.0	700	78
Ground beef, regular	21.0	800	87
Top round	8.8	400	85
T-bone steak	25.0	900	84
Bacon	7.0	800	48
Ham—cured, lean	4.6	400	38
Ham—cured, regular	13.0	1,400	54
Beef liver	4.9	1,100	389
Bologna (slice)	6.6	300	13
Cod	0.6	200	37
Crab	1.0	400	47
Frozen fish sticks (1 stick)	3.4	900	31
Haddock	0.6	200	49
Salmon	2.9	1,200	44
Shrimp	1.5	600	130
Tuna (in water)	.2	200	0
Tuna (in oil)	7.0	2,500	15
Chicken breast without skin, roasted	3.6	810	85
Chicken breast with skin, fried	8.7	1,900	88

Source: J. A. T. Pennington, *Food Values of Portions Commonly Used,* 16th ed. (Philadelphia: J. B. Lippincott: 1989).

sibility is that commercially grown and distributed meats may contain cancer-causing/cancer-promoting pesticide residues (DDT), industrial chemicals (PCBs), hormone growth promoters (DES), dyes for color enhancement, and preservatives such as **nitrates** and **nitrites,** often found in hot dogs, ham, sausage, and other cured meats. Another possibility is that bacteria in the colon convert substances necessary for the digestion of fats (bile acids) into cancer-causing agents. A third possibility is that charring meats in cooking converts substances in the meat into cancer-causing heterocyclic amines (HCAs).

Carbohydrates

Carbohydrates are the principal source of the body's energy, and also are used to manufacture some cell components, such as the hereditary material, **DNA.** Because the body can manufacture them from other substances, carbohydrates are not considered essential nutrients. However, not eating enough carbohydrates, recommended by some ill-conceived reducing diets, can force the body to break down muscle tissue to supply energy necessary for life functions.

There are two principal types of carbohydrates: **simple sugars,** found predominantly in fruit, and **complex carbohydrates,** found in grains, fruit, and the stems, leaves, and roots of vegetables. Simple sugars contribute about 20 percent of calories in the average American diet. Except for increasing the risk of tooth decay, simple sugars in themselves are not harmful. Problems can arise when simple sugars are consumed in high-fat/low-nutrient snack foods (cakes, candies) and/or when they replace the more healthful complex carbohydrates in the diet.

Simple Sugars   **Glucose** is the most common simple sugar; it is found in all plants and animals. Glucose circulates in the bloodstream and is commonly referred to as "blood sugar." Another simple sugar is fructose, which is found in fruits and honey. **Fructose** is one of the sweetest sugars, which means you can eat less fructose than other simple sugars and taste an equivalent amount of sweetness.

Sucrose, which is common table sugar (the "refined" sugar added to many packaged foods), is a combination of glucose and fructose. Sucrose is digested by breaking down the glucose and fructose portions. Because fructose is sweeter than sucrose, you can reduce the amount of sugar in your diet without cutting out sweet tastes by replacing pastries with fresh fruit and table sugar with honey. Furthermore, you will be gaining other nutrients in the fruit and honey that are not present in refined sucrose.

Lactose, found principally in dairy products, is a sugar consisting of glucose combined with the simple

T E R M S

nitrates: preservatives containing any salt or ester of nitric acid. Some individuals are sensitive to nitrates and may suffer from headache, diarrhea, or urticaria after ingesting them

nitrites: preservatives containing any salt or ester of nitrous oxide acid

carbohydrates: the most economical and efficient source of energy; biological molecules consisting of one or more sugar molecules

DNA: deoxyribonucleic acid; a nucleic acid of complex molecular structure occurring in cell nuclei; carrier of the genes; DNA is present in all body cells of every species

simple sugars: a class of carbohydrates called monosaccharides; all carbohydrates must be reduced to simple sugars to be digested

complex carbohydrates: a class of carbohydrates called polysaccharides; foods composed of starch and cellulose

glucose: the principal source of energy in all cells; also called dextrose

fructose: a simple sugar found in fruits and honey

sucrose: common refined "table" sugar; a molecule of glucose and a molecule of fructose chemically bonded together

lactose: a molecule of glucose and galactose chemically bonded together; found primarily in milk

galactose: a monosaccharide derived from lactose, found in many gums and seaweeds

lactase: enzyme secreted by glands in the small intestine that converts lactose (milk sugar) into simple sugars

starch: long chain of glucose molecules

fiber: a group of compounds that make up the framework of plants; fiber cannot be digested

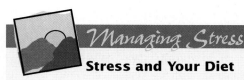

Managing Stress

Stress and Your Diet

Believe it or not, some see eating as a technique to reduce the symptoms of stress. The feeling of food in the stomach sends a message to the brain to calm down. Yet there are certain foods that can send your stress levels off the charts and most people are completely unaware of them. Moreover, repeated bouts of stress can deplete necessary nutrients, vitamins, and minerals creating a cycle of poor health. Here are some examples:

Sugar

An excess of simple sugars tends to deplete vitamin stores, particularly the vitamin B-complex (niacin, thiamine, riboflavin, and B_{12}). White sugar and even bleached flour flushed of its vitamin and mineral content require additional B-complex vitamins to be metabolized. These and other vitamins are crucial for optimal function of the central nervous system. A depletion of the B-complex vitamin may manifest in signs of fatigue, anxiety, and irritability. In addition, increased amounts of ingested simple sugars can cause major fluctuations in blood glucose levels resulting in pronounced fatigue, headaches, and general irritability.

Caffeine

Food sources that trigger the sympathetic nervous system are referred to as *sympathomimetic agents*. There is a powerful substance in caffeine called *methylated xanthine*. This chemical stimulant with amphetamine-like characteristics triggers in the sympathetic nervous system a heightened state of alertness and arousal; it can also stimulate the release of several stress hormones. The result is a intensified alertness which makes the individual more susceptible to perceived stress. Caffeine can be found in many foods, including chocolate, coffee, tea, and several other beverages. Current estimates suggest that the average American consumes three 6-ounce cups of coffee per day. A 6-ounce cup of caffinated coffee contains approximately 250 milligrams of caffeine, half the amount necessary to provoke adverse arousal of the central nervous system.

Salt

It seems that Americans have a love affair with salt. Many people add salt to their food without even tasting it. High sodium intake is associated with high blood pressure, as sodium acts to increase water retention. As water volume increases in a closed system, blood pressure increases. If this condition persists it may contribute to hypertension.

Vitamin and Mineral Deficiency

Chronic stress can deplete several vitamins necessary for energy metabolism and for the stress response. The synthesis of cortisol requires vitamins. The stress response activates several hormones that mobilize and metabolize fats and carbohydrates for energy production. The breakdown of fats and carbohydrates requires vitamins, specifically vitamins C and B-complex. Inadequate amounts of these vitamins may also affect mental alertness, and promote depression and insomnia. Stress is also associated with depletion of calcium and the inability of bones to properly absorb calcium, setting the stage for the development of osteoporosis, the demineralization of bone tissue. Vitamin supplementation is a controversial issue. A balanced diet usually provides an adequate supply of vitamins and nutrients for energy metabolism. However, the majority of Americans do not maintain a balanced diet. Vitamin supplements may be useful for individuals prone to excessive stress.

---

sugar **galactose.** When lactose is digested, the glucose and galactose are separated and the galactose is converted to glucose. Whereas almost all babies have the capacity to digest lactose (it is the major sugar in mother's milk), many older children and adults, particularly of black and Asian heritage, are not able to digest it because they lack a required enzyme **lactase,** which splits lactose into glucose and galactose. Lack of this enzyme causes gastrointestinal upset, diarrhea, and, occasionally, severe illness when lactase-deficient people consume dairy products. These individuals can supplement their diets with products containing lactase (e.g., Lactaid) or by eating yogurt, cheese, and other dairy products in which the lactose has been broken down by the fermentation process. Because dairy products are a major source of calcium in the North American diet, people who avoid dairy products should consume calcium-rich vegetables (e.g., broccoli and peas) and possibly take calcium supplements.

Complex Carbohydrates These come primarily from grains (wheat, rice, corn, oats, barley); legumes (peas, beans); the leaves, stems, and roots of plants; and some animal tissue. There are two main classes of complex carbohydrates: **starch,** which is digestible, and **fiber,** which is not digestible.

Starch consists of many glucose molecules linked together. It is a way organisms store glucose until it is needed. In plants, starch is usually contained in granules within seeds, pods, or roots. Wheat flour, for example, is

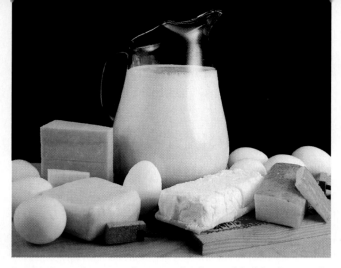

People who are lactose intolerant need to be careful of the dairy products that they eat.

made by crushing wheat grain, which separates the outer husk (the bran) from the middle, starch-containing portion (the endosperm), and the inner germ. The white flour commonly used in baking is "70 percent extraction," which means that 70 percent of the original grain remains after crushing. In the milling of 70 percent extraction flour, many nutrients in the wheat grain are lost, so flour manufacturers add back several vitamins and minerals to produce "enriched flour." A "whole-grain flour," on the other hand, is 90 to 95 percent extraction and does not have to be enriched. In a reasonably varied diet, whatever nutrients not present in flour are obtained in other foods. Those wanting all the nutrients in wheat can choose whole-wheat flour.

> *He who doesn't mind his belly will hardly mind anything else.*
> Samuel Johnson

HEALTHY PEOPLE 2000

Increase calcium intake so at least 50 percent of youth aged 12 through 24 and 50 percent of pregnant and lactating women consume 3 or more servings daily of foods rich in calcium, and at least 50 percent of people aged 25 and older consume 2 or more servings daily.

Dairy products, including milk, yogurt, and hard and soft cheeses, provide about 55 percent of calcium in American diets. Calcium is essential for the formation and maintenance of teeth and bones. Various subgroups of our population have special needs for calcium based on growth, milk production, and absorption of calcium (children, pregnant and lactating women, and older adults).

Bread made with whole-wheat flour is brown, but not all brown bread is whole-wheat bread. Some manufacturers add molasses or honey to white-flour dough to give it a brown color, and they are allowed to label the product "wheat bread." For this reason, it is important to read the package label before buying.

Starch is also found in potatoes, vegetables that have an undeserved reputation for being fattening. Potatoes are no more fattening than any other starchy food unless they are cooked in large amounts of fat or oil, used in making french fries and potato chips. One large potato has about 100 calories, less than a medium-sized soft drink. French fries made from a medium potato, however, contain over 300 calories.

Animals and humans produce a starch in muscle and liver tissue called **glycogen.** When energy is needed, the glycogen breaks down and its constituent glucose molecules are liberated. Athletes sometimes eat large quantities of carbohydrates the day before competition to build up their supply of glycogen, a practice known as "carbohydrate loading."

Contrary to popular belief, athletes do not need special diets, supplements, formulas, concoctions, or excess protein intake. The basic nutrients you need are the same basic nutrients needed by an athlete. The amount of energy an athlete expends determines the *amount* of food needed, not the necessary basic nutrients. Carbohydrates are the most efficient energy source for athletes and nonathletes, and should be used to meet increased energy needs. The practice of carbohydrate loading can be risky, and is particularly dangerous for diabetics.

Fiber is the second main class of complex carbohydrates. There are two kinds of fiber, **insoluble fiber,** which cannot dissolve in water, and **soluble fiber,** which can. Insoluble fiber is made up of **cellulose** and **hemicellulose,** substances that offer rigidity to plant material (wood; stems; the outer coverings of nuts, seeds, grains; the peels and skins of fruits and vegetables). Soluble fiber is composed of pectins, gums, and mucilages. The differences in insoluble and soluble fiber are not significant for health. Nutritionists recommend that individuals consume 20 to 35 grams of fiber daily, regardless of its type (Table 5.5).

Fiber adds bulk to the feces, thereby preventing constipation and related disorders such as hemorrhoids and hiatal hernia, which can result from prolonged increase in intra-abdominal pressure while defecating. Fiber also facilitates the transport of waste material through the digestive tract, lessening the risk of appendicitis, diverticular disease (out pocketings in the wall of the lower intestine), and cancer of the colon and rectum. High fiber diets may also help to lessen the risk of heart disease and some cancers (Anderson, Smith, and Gustafson, 1994).

TABLE 5.5 Fiber Content of Various Foods

Food	Amount	Fiber (grams)
Whole-wheat bread	1 slice	1.6
Rye bread	1 slice	1.0
White bread	1 slice	0.6
Brown rice (cooked)	½ cup	2.4
White rice (cooked)	½ cup	0.1
Spaghetti (cooked)	½ cup	0.8
Kidney beans (cooked)	½ cup	5.8
Lima beans (cooked)	½ cup	4.9
Potato (baked)	medium	3.8
Corn	½ cup	3.9
Spinach	½ cup	2.0
Lettuce	½ cup	0.3
Strawberries	¾ cup	2.0
Banana	medium	2.0
Apple (with skin)	medium	2.6
Orange	small	1.2

Lipids (Fats)

Lipids consist of a diverse group of substances that have the common property of being relatively insoluble in water. Some of these substances include **cholesterol** (a fatlike compound occurring in bile, blood, brain and nerve tissue, liver, and other parts of the body) and **lecithin,** which are essential constituents of cell membranes; the steroid hormones produced by the reproductive organs and adrenal glands; vitamins A, D, E, and K; and bile acids, which aid the digestion of fats. Despite the current antifat trend, fats are an essential part of the diet. They supply calories, they provide flavor and texture to food, and digesting fat provides feelings of satiety and well-being. One kind of fat, **linoleic acid,** found in vegetable oils such as safflower, sunflower, and corn, is essential, and must be obtained in food. Deficiencies in this substance can produce skin lesions.

A fat is classified as **saturated, monounsaturated,** or **polyunsaturated,** depending on the type of fatty acids it contains in greatest quantity. Saturated and unsaturated fats are made up of **fatty acids;** saturation refers to the number of hydrogen atoms in the fatty acids. A saturated fatty acid carries all the hydrogen atoms it can. Saturated fats are found in whole milk and products made from whole milk; egg yolks; meat; meat fat; coconut and palm oils; chocolate; regular margarine; and hydrogenated vegetable shortenings. Unsaturated fats, of which there are monounsaturated and polyunsaturated fats, are derived from plants. Sources of monounsaturated fats are olive oil and some nuts. Polyunsaturated fats are found

primarily in safflower, cottonseed, corn, soybean, and sesame seed oils; salad dressings made from oil; and fatty fish (Figure 5.5).

Diets high in cholesterol and saturated fat are believed to increase the risk of coronary heart disease, some cancers, and obesity (Chapter 6). Many nutritionists therefore recommend that we consume no more than 300 mg of cholesterol per day and limit saturated fat intake to 10 percent or less of total calories. "Visible" dietary fats include butter, cream, and whole milk. "Hid-

TERMS

glycogen: the form in which carbohydrate is stored in humans and animals

insoluble fiber: cannot be dissolved in water

soluble fiber: can be dissolved in water

cellulose: a carbohydrate forming the skeleton of most plant structures and plant cells. It is the most abundant polysaccharide in nature and is the source of dietary fiber, preventing constipation by adding bulk to the bowels

hemicellulose: substances found in plant cell walls that are composed of various sugars chemically linked together

lipids: fats such as cholesterol and triglycerides

cholesterol: a fatlike compound occurring in bile, blood, brain and nerve tissue, liver and other parts of the body

lecithin: an essential component of cell membranes

linoleic acid: an essential fat that must be obtained from food

saturated fat: generally solid at room temperature; comes from animal sources

monounsaturated fat: generally liquid at room temperature; common sources are olive oil and nuts

polyunsaturated fat: generally liquid at room temperature; common sources are safflower, sunflower, soybean, and sesame oils

fatty acids: naturally occurring in fats, either saturated or unsaturated (monounsaturated or polyunsaturated)

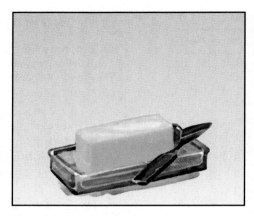 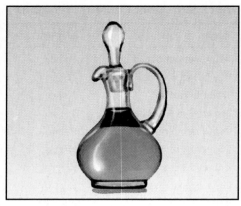

FIGURE 5.5 Healthy and Unhealthy Fats Fats that are solid are considered unhealthy. Fats that are liquid are considered healthier.

den" dietary fats include egg yolks, nuts, seeds, olives, avocados, cakes, pies, snack foods, and even lean meat, which can be 4 to 12 percent fat. Conversely, polyunsaturated fats tend to lower blood cholesterol, which is why nutritionists recommend **polyunsaturated fatty acid (PUFA)** containing vegetable oils.

Food manufacturers use a chemical process to transform natural polyunsaturated fatty acids derived from vegetable oils into artificial trans fatty acids, which tend to be solid at room temperature. This is how margarine and vegetable shortenings are made. Because margarine contains no cholesterol or saturated fat, many people believe it is a healthier food than butter. In recent years, the fast-food industry switched from beef tallow to vegetable shortening for deep frying, because vegetable shortening was purported to be healthier than animal fat, and is less expensive. The bakery industry uses vegetable shortening for the same reasons to manufacture cookies, donuts, and cakes. There is no evidence, however, that margarine or vegetable shortenings are healthier than animal fats.

Indeed, analysis of dietary patterns of more than 87,000 American nurses showed that those with the highest intake of trans fatty acids (3.2 percent of total energy) had the highest risk for heart disease (Willett and Ascherio, 1994). While you do not need to give up eating margarine, french fries, or donuts to be healthy, you need to practice moderation. Since the amount of trans fatty acids in food products is not listed on the product label, intake of these artificial substances can be limited by using liquid vegetable oils that contain PUFAs whenever possible. Vegetables oils are naturally devoid of cholesterol.

Two specific types of blood cholesterol are called **low-density lipoproteins (LDL)** and **high-density lipoproteins (HDL).** LDL cholesterol, sometimes referred to as "bad" cholesterol, causes cholesterol to build up in the walls of your arteries. Therefore, the more LDL you have in your blood, the greater your risk of heart disease. In contrast, HDL cholesterol, or "good" cholesterol, helps your body get rid of the cholesterol in your blood. The higher your HDL the better, as this decreases your risk of heart disease (Chapter 14).

Vitamins

Vitamins are substances that facilitate a variety of biological processes. The body cannot manufacture vitamins; they must be obtained from food (Table 5.6). Vitamins are classified as **water-soluble** or **fat-soluble,** depending on their chemistry.

Vitamins A (and its dietary precursor, Beta-carotene), C, and E are classed as **antioxidants** because they have the capacity to neutralize the effects of chemicals called free radicals, which can damage biological structures via chemical oxidation. Consumption of antioxidants is associated with a lower risk of cancer of the upper gastrointestinal tract (vitamin C), colon (B-carotene), breast, and lung (vitamin A). Antioxidants are also associated

---

T E R M S

polyunsaturated fatty acid (PUFA): a saturated fat except for two or more parts that are unsaturated

low-density lipoproteins (LDLs): plasma protein that is relatively rich in fat; it facilitates deposit of cholesterol in the walls of arteries

high-density lipoproteins (HDLs): plasma protein that contains relatively more protein and fewer fats; it serves to transport cholesterol and other lipids from plasma to tissues

vitamins: essential organic substances needed daily in small amounts to perform specific functions in the body

water-soluble: soluble in water; there are nine water-soluble vitamins

fat-soluble: soluble in fat; there are four fat-soluble vitamins

antioxidants: substances that in small amounts inhibit the oxidation of other compounds.

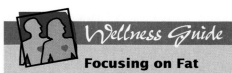

Wellness Guide

Focusing on Fat

Some higher fat choices in a fast-food lunch are balanced with lower fat items at breakfast and dinner.

1,600 calories		2,500 calories
Breakfast		
3/4 cup	Orange juice	3/4 cup
2 biscuits	Shredded wheat	2 biscuits
None	with sliced banana	1/2 medium
None	and sugar	2 teaspoons
1 cup	Milk, lowfat (2%)	1 cup
Fast-Food Lunch		
	Regular hamburger	
2 ounces	Ground beef patty	
1 bun	Hamburger bun, enriched	
	"Quarterpound" cheeseburger*	
	Ground beef patty	3 ounces
	Hamburger bun, enriched	1 bun
	American process cheese	3/4 ounce
1 tablespoon	Catsup	1 tablespoon
1 regular order	French fries	1 regular order
8 fluid ounces	Cola	12 fluid ounces
Dinner		
	Chicken cacciatore:	
3 ounces	Chicken breast, no skin	4 ounces
1/2 cup	Stewed tomatoes	3/4 cup
1/2 cup	Rice	1 cup
1/2 cup	Summer squash, fresh, cooked	3/4 cup
1 1/2 cups	Mixed green salad	1 1/2 cups
	(iceberg lettuce, spinach,	
	green onions, cucumbers)	
1 tablespoon	Italian dressing	1 tablespoon
1 slice	Italian bread	2 slices
1 teaspoon	Margarine, soft	2 teaspoons
None	Poached pear	
	Pear, fresh	1 medium
	Granola	1/8 cup
	Sugar	1 teaspoon
Snacks		
1 medium	Apple	1 medium
None	Oatmeal cookies	2 medium
1 cup	Milk, lowfat (2%)	1/2 cup

The kind of milk is your choice. When you use higher fat milks, be more moderate in your use of other fats.

The skin is removed to lower the fat content. No oil or fat is used in cooking.

No salt or fat is added to the summer squash. For added zest, try lemon juice, onion, caraway seed, or marjoram.

Salad dressings and fatty spreads add calories and sodium as well as fat. Be moderate.

*"Quarterpound" refers to raw weight, which equals 3 ounces cooked weight.
Source: U.S. Department of Agriculture, "Preparing Foods and Planning Menus," *Home and Garden Bulletin,* 232 (Washington, D.C.: U.S. Government Printing Office, 1992).

with lessening the risk of heart disease. Vitamins C and E protect against cataracts. Antioxidants are found in a variety of vegetable and fruits (not in beans), and can be obtained in supplements.

Minerals

Many body functions require one or more chemical elements: these elements are referred to as **minerals** (Table 5.7). Sodium, potassium, and chlorine, for example, are

TABLE 5.6   Water-Soluble and Fat-Soluble Vitamins

Water-soluble vitamin	Why needed?	Primary source	Deficiency results
Ascorbic acid (vitamin C)	Tooth and bone formation; production of connective tissue; promotion of wound healing; may enhance immunity	Citrus fruits, tomatoes, peppers, cabbage, potatoes, melons	Scurvy (degeneration of bones, teeth, and gums)
Biotin	Involved in fat and amino acid synthesis and breakdown	Yeast, liver, milk, most vegetables, bananas, grapefruit	Skin problems; fatigue; muscle pains; nausea
Cobalamin (vitamin B_{12})	Involved in single carbon atom transfers; essential for DNA synthesis	Muscle meats, eggs, milk and dairy products (not in vegetables)	Pernicious anemia; nervous system malfunctions
Folacin (folic acid)	Essential for synthesis of DNA and other molecules	Green leafy vegetables, organ meats, whole-wheat products	Anemia; diarrhea and other gastrointestinal problems
Niacin	Involved in energy production and synthesis of cell molecules	Grains, meats, legumes	Pellagra (skin, gastrointestinal, and mental disorders)
Pantothenic acid	Involved in energy production and synthesis and breakdown of many biological molecules	Yeast, meats and fish, nearly all vegetables and fruits	Vomiting; abdominal cramps; malaise; insomnia
Pyridoxine (vitamin B_6)	Essential for synthesis and breakdown of amino acids and manufacture of unsaturated fats from saturated fats	Meats, whole grains, most vegetables	Weakness; irritability; trouble sleeping and walking; skin problems
Riboflavin (vitamin B_2)	Involved in energy production; important for health of the eyes	Milk and dairy foods, meats, eggs, vegetables, grains	Eye and skin problems
Thiamine (vitamin B_1)	Essential for breakdown of food molecules and production of energy	Meats, legumes, grains, some vegetables	Beri-beri (nerve damage, weakness, heart failure)

Fat-soluble vitamin	Why needed?	Primary sources	Deficiency results
Vitamin A (retinol)	Essential for maintenance of eyes and skin; influences bone and tooth formation	Liver, kidney, yellow and green leafy vegetables, apricots	Deficiency: night blindness; eye damage; skin dryness. Excess: loss of appetite; skin problems; swelling of ankles and feet
Vitamin D (calciferol)	Regulates calcium metabolism; important for growth of bones and teeth	Cod-liver oil, dairy products, eggs	Deficiency: rickets (bone deformities) in children; bone destruction in adults. Excess: thirst; nausea; weight loss; kidney damage
Vitamin E (tocopherol)	Prevents damage to cells from oxidation; prevents red blood cell destruction	Wheat germ, vegetable oils, vegetables, egg yolk, nuts	Deficiency: anemia, possibly nerve cell destruction
Vitamin K (phylloquinone)	Helps with blood clotting	Liver, vegetable oils, green leafy vegetables, tomatoes	Deficiency: severe bleeding

TABLE 5.7 Essential Minerals

Mineral	Why needed?	Primary sources	Deficiency results
Calcium	Bone and tooth formation Blood clotting Nerve transmission	Milk, cheese, dark green vegetables, dried legumes	Stunted growth Rickets, osteoporosis Convulsions
Chlorine	Formation of gastric juice Acid-base balance	Common salt	Muscle cramps Mental apathy Reduced appetite
Chromium	Glucose and energy metabolism	Fats, vegetable oils, meats	Impaired ability to metabolize glucose
Cobalt	Constituent of vitamin B_{12}	Organ and muscle meats	Not reported in man
Copper	Constituent of enzymes of iron metabolism	Meats, drinking water	Anemia (rare)
Iodine	Constituent of thyroid hormones	Marine fish and shellfish, dairy products, many vegetables	Goiter (enlarged thyroid)
Iron	Constituent of hemoglobin and enzymes of energy metabolism	Eggs, lean meats, legumes, whole grains, green leafy vegetables	Iron-deficiency anemia (weakness, reduced resistance to infection)
Magnesium	Activates enzymes Involved in protein synthesis	Whole grains, green leafy vegetables	Growth failure Behavioral disturbances Weakness, spasms
Manganese	Constituent of enzymes involved in fat synthesis	Widely distributed in foods	In animals: disturbances of nervous system, reproductive abnormalities
Molybdenum	Constituent of some enzymes	Legumes, cereals, organ meats	Not reported in man
Phosphorus	Bone and tooth formation Acid-base balance	Milk, cheese, meat, poultry, grains	Weakness, demineralization of bone
Potassium	Acid-base balance Body water balance Nerve function	Meats, milk, many fruits	Muscular weakness Paralysis
Selenium	Functions in close association with vitamin E	Seafood, meat, grains	Anemia (rare)
Sodium	Acid-base balance Body water balance Nerve function	Common salt	Muscle cramps Mental apathy Reduced appetite
Sulfur	Constituent of active tissue compounds, cartilage, and tendon	Sulfur amino acids (methionine and cysteine) in dietary proteins	Related to intake and deficiency of sulfur amino acids
Zinc	Constituent of enzymes involved in digestion	Widely distributed in foods	Growth failure Small sex glands

essential for maintaining cell membranes, conducting nerve impulses, and muscle contraction. Magnesium, copper, and cobalt facilitate certain biochemical reactions; iron is essential for the oxygen-carrying function of hemoglobin; iodine is needed to produce thyroid hormone; calcium and phosphorus make up bones and teeth.

Minerals are found in almost all food, especially fresh vegetables. Women and growing young people are susceptible to iron deficiency, so they must eat iron-rich foods, such as eggs, lean meats, brans, whole grains, and green leafy vegetables. Most women and elderly people ingest too little calcium, which is found in dairy prod-

ucts and some green leafy vegetables (such as broccoli and turnip greens).

Many people take in excess sodium, which may contribute to high blood pressure. The amounts of sodium naturally present in almost every kind of food pose no problem; excess sodium comes from manufactured and restaurant food, to which salt is added to increase flavor.

T E R M

minerals: inorganic elements found in the body both in combination with organic compounds and alone

Some people consume as many as 20 grams of sodium per day, which is about 10 times the 2 grams per day the body needs. Athletes are often advised to take salt tablets to replace body salt lost in sweat; this advice is misguided. Except in cases of severe fluid loss, which more often accompanies medical therapies involving diuretics than with sports, salt is readily replaced by eating food.

Phytochemicals

Plant matter contains hundreds of chemical substances, called **phytochemicals**, that positively affect human physiology. They often help the body destroy and eliminate toxins acquired from the environment or tissue-damaging substances that are byproducts of metabolism. Cruciferous plants (broccoli, cauliflower, kale, brussels sprouts, cabbage, mustard greens, etc.) are rich in the cancer-preventing phytochemical sulforaphane. A number of fruits, vegetables, cereal grains, and citrus oils contain substances called **isoprenoids,** which are associated with lowering cancer risk. Tea, onions, apples, and wine contain antioxidant substances called **flavonoids,** whose consumption has been associated with reducing the risk of heart disease. Barley, wheat, corn, and a variety of seeds contain **phytosterols** and **tocotrienols,** which can reduce levels of cholesterol in the blood.

Water

Water is the principal constituent of blood and is the major component of all cells. Water provides the medium in which all cell chemical activities take place.

Body water is maintained at a relatively constant level by the nervous, endocrine, and urinary systems. If body water is low, a person experiences thirst, which motivates drinking. Low body water activates hormonal mechanisms that reduce the production of urine. Excess body water activates different hormonal mechanisms that increase the output of urine. Increasing output is the function of diuretics, often given to reduce blood pressure, fluid volume after a heart attack, or feelings of bloatedness. Caffeine and alcohol are diuretics. The popular maxim that you should drink eight glasses of water a day is partially correct. The average adult loses about that much body water through sweat, moisture in expired air, urine, and feces. This loss is partly offset by drinking water and obtaining water in other fluids and foods.

EVALUATING DIETARY SUPPLEMENTS

A varied diet that contains the recommended five-a-day servings of fruits and vegetables and 55 to 80 percent of calories from cereals, whole grains, and legumes is likely to provide most people with the minerals and vitamins they need for good health. Strict vegetarians may need to supplement their diets with vitamin B_{12}. Supplements might also be necessary for people who eat primarily processed foods, since many nutrients are removed during manufacturing. Other people who may need supplements include those who restrict caloric intake, such as weight-conscious people; athletes concerned about body size; people who have a biological need for a particular substance; or people who consume large amounts of alcohol or coffee, which are diuretics and can increase urinary loss of necessary vitamins and minerals. Smoking is associated with a loss of vitamin C.

Those who are concerned that their diets may be nutritionally inadequate may take vitamin, mineral, and amino acid supplements as a form of "dietary insurance." People should be aware, however, that in massive doses (so-called **megadoses**), some dietary supplements can be toxic. More is not always better with vitamins A, D, K, B_3 (niacin), and B_6 (pyridoxine). In fact, when vitamins, minerals, and other nutrients are taken in large quantities for therapeutic reasons, they are considered drugs and not nutrients. This fact is rarely mentioned by proponents of megadosing, sometimes out of a sincere desire to help people and other times because of the drive to increase sales and profits. Before megadosing on vitamins, consumers should educate themselves about any possible risks.

Whether a supplement is "natural" or "synthetic" makes no difference chemically. However, there may be a difference in the purity of a substance depending on the preparation process. In 1990, thousands of Americans

TERMS

phytochemicals: chemicals produced by plants

isoprenoids: fat-soluble vitamins that may reduce the risk of some cancers

flavonoids: antioxidant substance that may reduce the risk of heart disease

phytosterols: sterols of vegetable origin

tocotrienols: have some biological vitamin E activity

megadoses: large doses of a substance; used in reference to excessive vitamin supplementation

sulfites: used as preservatives for salad, fresh fruit and vegetables, wine, beer, and dried fruit; in susceptible individuals, especially those with asthma, they can cause a severe reaction

gamma irradiation: nonchemical method of food preservation

tartrazine: a yellow food dye, referred to by the FDA as "FD&C yellow No. 5"

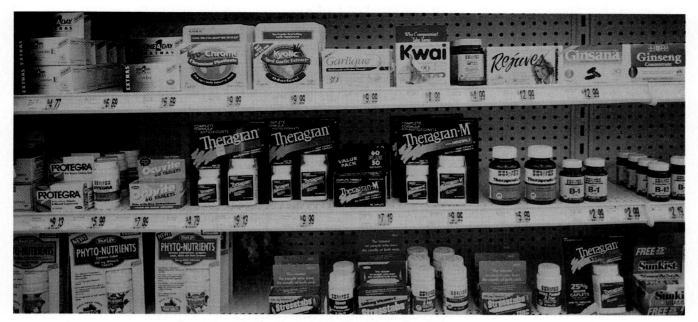

People who eat a variety of nutritious foods do not need dietary supplements; taken in excess, some supplements may be harmful.

became ill and several died from consuming a supplement of the amino acid tryptophan because of impurities in the product.

Supplements containing enzymes, other proteins, and nucleic acids (DNA and RNA) are not absorbed intact from the digestive tract; instead, they are broken down into smaller molecules. Therefore, claims by manufacturers and sellers about the health benefits of ingesting these substances are most likely attributable to placebo effect.

FOOD ADDITIVES

Manufactured foods contain a variety of additives that alter their texture, flavor, color, and stability. These additives, help to increase sales appeal and lengthen shelf life. We'll discuss the two most common additives: preservatives and artificial sweeteners.

Preservatives

About 20 percent of the world's food supply is lost to spoilage each year. Common preservatives include BHA (butylated hydroxyanisole), BHT (butylated hydroxytoluene), and sodium nitrite. Each of these substances can be toxic and damaging to humans if taken in excess; however, in amounts commonly consumed in food, they are presumed safe.

Sulfites in the form of sulfur dioxide, sodium sulfite, sodium/potassium bisulfite, and sodium/potassium metabisulfite are added to many foods to kill bacteria and to slow the food's breakdown. Sulfites are commonly added to wine and to dehydrated soups, vegetables, and fruit (apples, apricots, raisins, pears, and peaches). To keep vegetables looking fresh, they are also used in restaurant salad bars. Some individuals, particularly those with asthma, may be extremely sensitive to sulfite and may experience nausea, diarrhea, respiratory distress, and skin eruptions. Such problems have led to some banning of sulfites in restaurants.

A nonchemical method of food preservation involves exposing food to **gamma irradiation** to destroy fungi, bacteria, and other microorganisms. Some opponents of food irradiation argue that the method has not been proven safe. Their concern is that irradiation may produce cancer-causing or toxic byproducts or mutant strains of toxic, radiation-resistant microorganisms. Furthermore, vitamins can be destroyed by irradiation. Nonetheless, some have proposed that all hamburger meat be gamma irradiated to destroy harmful bacteria.

Many food additives are nutritionally unnecessary and some may adversely affect health. For example, sugar and salt are added to food to enhance taste and increase sales. Food dyes, some of which have been banned, have been implicated in human cancers and allergies. The FDA estimates that as many as 100,000 Americans are intolerant to **tartrazine**, a yellow dye added to hundreds of manufactured foods, such as frozen breakfast pastries, pill coatings, and some soft drinks.

Consumers concerned about additives and gamma irradiation should read product labels. Manufacturers must list all the additives in the order of their relative proportions in the food. Irradiated products carry a small flower-like symbol, or the words "picowaved" or "treated by irradiation." Do not assume that the words "natural," "organic," or "health food" are free from additives or extra sugar and salt. The only sure way to be certain of the contents of a food is to know how it was produced.

Artificial Sweeteners

Fifty to seventy million Americans use artificial sweeteners. As a presumed ally in the continual battle against fat and as a theoretical help to diabetics, artificial sweeteners are in all types of foods. Their widest use, however, is in "diet" soft drinks.

The three major artificial sweeteners—cyclamate, saccharin, and aspartame ("Nutrasweet")—have been associated with health risks. In the 1970s, cyclamates and saccharin were linked to cancer, although the data were not strong enough to cause out-

> *The biggest seller is cookbooks and the second is diet books—how not to eat what you've just learned how to cook.*
>
> Andy Rooney,
> TV commentator

right banning of these substances. Aspartame, made of the amino acids aspartic acid and a modified form of phenylalanine, has been associated with mood changes, insomnia, and seizures. Health-conscious consumers should be aware of the artificial sweeteners used in the products they ingest.

FAST FOOD

Grabbing a fast-food meal is integral to the fast-paced life in America today. Each day approximately 46 million people, or 20 percent of the U.S. population, will eat in a fast-food restaurant. Convenience notwithstanding, fast-food items must be chosen carefully because many contain high quantities of saturated fat, cholesterol, and salt, few complex carbohydrates, and little vitamins A and C (Table 5.8).

The major fast-food companies have responded to consumers' concerns about nutrition by offering salads, baked potatoes, roast beef, and broiled chicken. Roast

Controversy in Health

Food Irradiation: Toxic to Bacteria, Safe for Humans

Irradiating food to prevent illness from food-borne bacteria is not a new concept. Research on the technology began shortly after World War II, when the U.S. Army began a series of experiments irradiating fresh foods for troops in the field. Since 1963, the Food and Drug Administration has passed rules permitting irradiation to curb insects in foods and microorganisms in spices, control parasite contamination in pork, and retard spoilage of fruits and vegetables.

But, to many people, the word irradiation means danger. It is associated with atomic bomb explosions and nuclear accidents such as Cher-

nobyl and Three Mile Island. The idea of irradiating food signals a kind of "gamma alarm." But when it comes to food irradiation the only danger is to the bacteria that contaminate food. The process damages their genetic material, so the organisms can no longer survive or multiply.

Irradiation does not make food radioactive and, therefore, does not increase human exposure to radiation. The process involves exposing food to a source of radiation, such as gamma rays from radioactive cobalt or cesium or to x-rays. However, no radioactive material is ever added to the product. Manufacturers

use the same technique to sterilize many disposable medical devices.

The World Health Organization believes irradiation can substantially reduce food poisoning. According to a 35-year WHO study, there has been a constant increase in the incidence of food-borne diseases, as well the emergence of "new" disease-causing organisms. To date, 35 countries have issued unconditional or provisional clearances allowing irradiation of commercial foods.

Adapted from: D. Blumenthal, "Food Irradiation: Toxic to Bacteria, Sage for Humans," *FDA Consumer* (November, 1990).

STUDENT REFLECTIONS
- Will the fear of nuclear energy prevent this technology from being used to its fullest potential?
- What types of education would be useful to win acceptance of this procedure, which can potentially lower the incidence of food-borne illnesses?

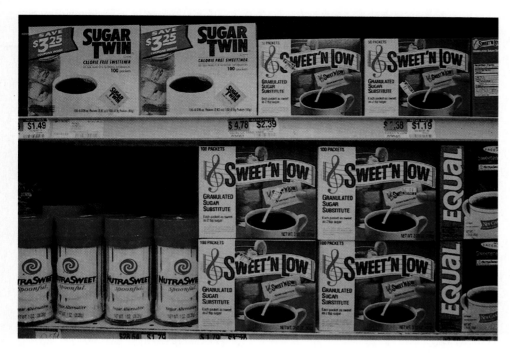

Artificial sweeteners are present in many foods and drinks and may cause health problems for some people.

beef has less fat than hamburger, and broiled chicken breast has less fat than deep fried chicken. Fish, a low-fat food, if breaded and fried, may be 50 percent fat. Salads and baked potatoes can be carriers of high-fat toppings. Consumers, however, have low-fat choices available in the face of temptation (Table 5.9).

VEGETARIAN DIETS

Vegetarianism has existed as long as humankind and has been advocated by such famous people as Leonardo da Vinci, George Bernard Shaw, Mahatma Gandhi, and Albert Einstein (Vegetarian Resource Group, 1990). The practice of vegetarianism in the United States is more

HEALTHY PEOPLE 2000

Increase to at least 90 percent the proportion of restaurants and institutional food service operations that offer identifiable low-fat, low-calorie food choices, consistent with the *Dietary Guidelines for Americans.*

In 1985, 40 percent of all meals were consumed outside the home. On a typical day, 45.8 million people eat in a fast food establishment. If people eat outside the home, they should be offered food choices based on the *Dietary Guidelines for Americans.*

widespread today than at any other time in history (American Dietetic Association, 1988). According to the U.S. Department of Agriculture, meat consumption has decreased during the past decade, while there has been a steady increase in the consumption of fresh fruits and vegetables, and grains.

Many factors have influenced and motivated the increased interest in vegetarianism. Major motivating factors include an increased interest in health, ecology and world issues; an influx of Eastern religions in the United States; and economics. The American Dietetic Association has also identified a certain ethic as a motivator. An example may be someone who does not believe in killing animals or having them slaughtered for the purpose of food consumption.

There are three kinds of **vegetarian** diets: strict or **vegan**, which excludes all animal products including milk, cheeses, eggs, and other dairy products; **lacto-vegetarian**, which excludes meat, poultry, fish, and eggs, but includes dairy products; and **lacto-ovo-vegetarian**,

T E R M S

vegetarian: one who consumes no meat, poultry, or fish

vegan: one who excludes all animal products from the diet including milk, cheese, eggs, and other dairy products

lacto-vegetarian: one who excludes meat, poultry, fish, and eggs but includes dairy products

lacto-ovo-vegetarian: one who excludes meats, poultry, and fish, but includes eggs and dairy products

TABLE 5.8 Nutritional Information from McDonald's, Wendy's, and Burger King

Menu item	Weight (g)	Calories	Calories from fat	Total fat (g)	Saturated fat (g)
Sandwiches					
McDonald's Quarter Pounder	171	420	180	20	8
Wendy's Plain Single	133	350	140	15	6
Burger King's Hamburger	129	330	140	15	6
French Fries					
McDonald's large	147	450	200	22	4
Wendy's biggie	159	420	180	20	4
Burger King's medium	116	400	180	20	5
Chicken Nuggets					
McDonald's 6 piece	109	300	160	18	3.5
Wendy's 6 piece	94	280	180	20	5
Burger King's 6 piece	88	250	110	12	3
Sweet & Sour Sauce					
McDonald's	32	50	0	0	0
Wendy's	28	45	0	0	0
Burger King	28	45	0	0	0
Shakes/Frosty					
McDonald's (ounces)	16	350	50	6	3.5
Wendy's (ounces)	16	460	120	13	7
Burger King (ounces)	16	310	60	7	4
Garden Salad					
McDonald's	234	80	35	4	1
Wendy's	271	110	50	6	1
Burger King	215	90	45	5	3
Blue Cheese Dressing					
McDonald's	60	190	150	17	3
Wendy's	28	180	170	19	3
Burger King	30	160	140	16	4

which excludes meats, poultry, and seafood, but includes eggs and dairy products. Properly planned vegetarian diets can meet the body's nutritional needs, especially by combining sources of protein to assure adequate intake of the essential amino acids. Strict vegetarians may need vitamin B_{12} (cobalamin) supplements if bacteria in the digestive tract do not supply enough.

Scientific evidence indicates that vegetarians are generally at lower risk than nonvegetarians for coronary heart disease, hypertension, some forms of cancer, non-insulin dependent diabetes, and obesity (Vegetarian Resource Group, 1990). Although vegetarians show lower mortality rates from these chronic disease than nonvegetarians, it is still unclear whether it is diet alone that is the major contributing factor. A large number of vegetarians also choose other healthy life-styles such as exercise and stress reduction, which contribute to wellness.

TABLE 5.8 *(Continued)*

Cholesterol (mg)	Sodium (g)	Carbohydrates (mg)	Fiber (g)	Sugars (g)	Protein (g)	Vitamin A	Vitamin C	Calcium	Iron
70	690	36	2	7	23	4	4	15	25
70	510	31	2	5	24	0	0	10	30
55	570	28	1	4	20	2	0	4	15
0	290	57	5	0	6	*	30	2	6
0	260	58	5	0	6	0	20	2	8
0	240	43	3	0	5	*	4	*	6
65	530	16	0	0	19	*	*	2	6
50	600	12	0	N/A	14	0	0	2	4
35	530	14	2	0	16	*	*	*	4
0	160	12	0	11	0	8	*	*	*
0	55	11	N/A	N/A	0	0	0	0	2
0	50	11	0	10	0	*	*	*	*
25	240	62	1	58	13	4	4	35	6
55	260	76	4	63	12	10	0	40	6
20	230	54	3	48	9	6	*	20	10
140	60	7	3	5	6	60	35	6	8
0	320	10	4	4	7	60	60	20	8
15	110	7	3	0	6	110	50	15	6
30	650	8	0	3	2	2	*	6	2
15	180	1	0	0	1	0	0	2	0
30	260	1	<1	0	2	*	*	*	*

HOW NUTRITION AFFECTS YOUR BRAIN

The brain requires nutrients in order to function properly. For example, the amount of the neurotransmitter serotonin in the brain is influenced by levels in the blood of the amino acid, tryptophan, and by the amount of carbohydrate recently eaten. A meal containing tryptophan (derived from dietary protein) and high in carbohydrate increases brain levels of serotonin. Brain levels of the amino acid tyrosine, the precursor of the neurotransmitters dopamine, norepinephrine, and epinephrine, increase after the ingestion of tyrosine-containing protein in a meal. Ingesting choline, a component of lecithin (found in egg yolks, liver, and soybeans), increases the level of the neurotransmitter acetylcholine.

TABLE 5.9 Taco Bell's New Border Light Menu

			Nutritional information					
	Calories	*Fat (g)*	*% Calories from fat*	*% Fat reduction*	*% Calorie reduction*	*Cholesterol (mg)*	*Protein (g)*	*Carbohydrates (g)*
Taco	180	11	55	—	—	32	10	11
LIGHT Taco	144	5	34	51	20	1	11	13
Soft Taco	223	11	44	—	—	32	12	19
LIGHT Soft Taco	181	5	26	52	28	4	12	22
Taco Supreme™	225	15	60	—	—	47	11	12
LIGHT Taco Supreme™	162	5	30	64	19	1	12	16
Soft Taco Supreme®	268	15	50	—	—	47	13	21
LIGHT Soft Taco Supreme®	199	5	24	65	26	4	14	25

Light = 50% less fat per serving.   g = grams   mg = milligrams

To some degree, moods, feelings of vitality, and sleep patterns depend on the amount of neurotransmitter molecules ingested, and depend indirectly on meals (Fernstrom, 1994). The habit of eating cookies and milk at bedtime may be a way someone increases brain serotonin to help induce a peaceful night's sleep. Some preliminary experiments indicate that tyrosine may help to relieve depression and choline may help to modify certain postural and motor disturbances.

The thoughts, moods, and body sensations of some individuals are highly sensitive to the amount of simple sugars they ingest. Shortly after consuming a couple of donuts or a candy bar, they might experience anxiety, trembling, fatigue, weakness, depression, and inability to concentrate. This response, called **reactive hypoglycemia,** is often the result of a sharp drop in blood sugar when insulin is secreted; this drop, in turn, is produced in response to the large load of sugar in the blood. Something akin to reactive hypoglycemia may be at the root of an eating pattern common to many: consumption of a high-sugar food at breakfast, followed two hours later by a reactive blood sugar low, which motivates a midmorning sugar "hit." The cycle is repeated at noon and midafternoon, and at dinner and late in the evening. To break this cycle, it helps to consume high-sugar foods with protein and some fat, thereby moderating the rate at which simple sugars enter the body.

HEALTH IN REVIEW

- For most of us, good nutrition is a matter of informed choice and is not governed by harsh environmental and economic circumstances.

- The U.S. government commissioned nutritionists and other scientists to create dietary guidelines. These guidelines are aimed at preventing undernutrition and a variety of diseases (heart disease, many kinds of cancer), which are associated with the high-fat/low-complex carbohydrate diets of Western industrialized nations.

- The new government-required food label is designed to be easy to understand. Reading the food label will help you choose foods that are healthy and that potentially reduce your risk of some diseases.

- In order to be healthy and well, people must obtain 40 essential nutrients from their food in proper amounts and proportions. Food energy, measured in calories, comes principally from sugars, carbohydrates, and fats.

- Dietary supplements can be a form of "dietary insurance" for those who are concerned their diet may be nutritionally inadequate.

- Food is composed of seven kinds of substances: proteins, carbohydrates, fats, minerals, vitamins, phytochemicals, and water. Nutritionists recommend basing our diets on complex carbohydrates and fresh fruits and vegetables to lessen the consumption of saturated fat, and to ensure consumption of fiber, vitamins, minerals, and micronutrients.

- Manufactured foods contain a variety of additives that alter their texture, flavor, color, and stability. Preservatives keep foods from spoiling through the use of sulfites.

T E R M

reactive hypoglycemia: occurring after the ingestion of carbohydrate, with consequent excessive release of insulin

- A nonchemical method of food preservation involves exposing food to gamma irradiation to destroy microorganisms.
- Artificial sweeteners are widely used, most commonly in "diet" soft drinks.

- There are several reasons for being a vegetarian, including increased interest in health, increased interest in ecology and world issues, economical issues, and the philosophy of not killing animals. A strict vegetarian diet eliminates all animal products, including milk, cheese, eggs, and other dairy products.

REFERENCES

American Dietetic Association (1988). "Position of the American Dietetic Association: Vegetarian Diets." *Journal of the American Dietetic Association*, 88(3): 351–355.

Anderson, J. W., B. M. Smith, and N. J. Gustafson (1994). "Health Benefits and Practical Aspects of High-Fiber Diets." *American Journal of Clinical Nutrition*, 59(May): 1242–1247.

Campbell, T. C., and C. Junshi (1994). "Diet and Chronic Degenerative Diseases: Perspectives from China." *American Journal of Clinical Nutrition*, 59(suppl): 1153–1161.

Fernstrom, J. D. (1994). "Dietary Amino Acids and Brain Function." *Journal of the American Dietetic Association*, 94(1): 71–78.

Kurtzweil, P. (1995). "The New Food Label: Better Information for Special Diets." *FDA Consumer*, January–February: 19–23.

Vegetarian Resource Group (1990). *Lesson Plan*. Baltimore, Md.

Willett, W. C. (1994). "Diet and Health: What Should We Eat?" *Science*, 264: 532–537.

Willett, W. C., and A. Ascherio (1994). "Trans Fatty Acids: Are the Effects Only Marginal?" *American Journal of Public Health*, 84(5): 722–724.

SUGGESTED READINGS

DiSogra, L., B. Abrams, and M. Hudes (1994). "Low Prevalence of Healthful Dietary Behaviors in a California Agricultural County: Emphasis on White and Mexican-American Adults." *Journal of the American Dietetic Association*, 94(5): 544–546. A study that looked at the dietary behaviors of a select group of Californians. The results indicated poor dietary habits.

"Fourteen Dietary Habits You Can Stop Feeling Guilty About" (1993). *Tufts University Diet and Nutrition Letter*, 11(2): 3–5. An enjoyable, simple dietary guideline to help you get through the day.

Kurtzweil, P. (1994). "The New Food Label: Making It Easier to Shed Pounds." *FDA Consumer*, July–August: 10–15.

This article discusses how to use the new food label and how understanding food labels will help you avoid unwanted calories.

Nestle, M. (1994). "The Politics of Dietary Guidance—A New Opportunity" (editorial). *American Journal of Public Health*, 84(5): 713–715. An editorial urging that now is the time to look at our dietary guidelines and move forward.

Willett, W. C. (1994). "Micronutrients and Cancer Risk." *American Journal of Clinical Nutrition*, 59(suppl): 1162–1165. Provides an understanding of cancer risk and nutrition.

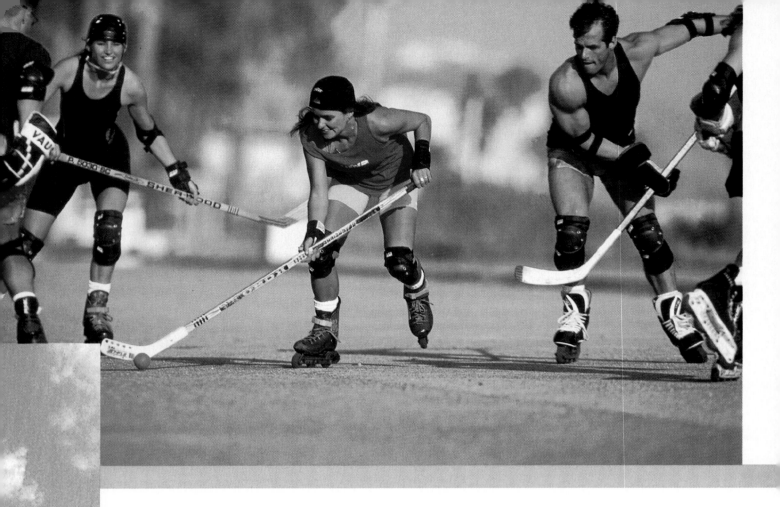

LEARNING OBJECTIVES

After reading this chapter you should be able to:

1. Discuss the difference between obesity and overweight.
2. Describe how to measure overweight.
3. Distinguish between the different theories of overweight: set-point theory, fat-cell theory, dietary-fat theory, and genetics.
4. Identify a recreational eater.
5. Identify several ways you can lose weight sensibly.
6. Briefly discuss body wraps, diet pills, diet programs, and fasting.
7. Define anorexia nervosa and bulimia. Identify several characteristics of both eating disorders.

6

Managing Your Weight

*J*udging from the number of books and magazine articles extolling various "surefire" weight-loss programs, it would appear that the U.S. national pastime is dieting. Indeed, surveys indicate that among adults in the United States 50 to 70 percent of women and 25 to 40 percent of men are on reducing diets. About one-third of the U.S. population is overweight (Figure 6.1), and needs to reduce to lessen its risks of heart disease, diabetes, high blood pressure, gallbladder disease, and some cancers (Kuczmarski, Flegal, Campbell, and Johnson, 1994). Many who are not clinically overweight are caught in the seemingly endless battle with the same five or ten pounds, which they struggle to shed in order to look youthful and attractive (Figure 6.2).

Some individuals who diet are concerned about the possible adverse health consequences of being overweight. The majority of individuals who diet, however, do so more for cosmetic reasons than for health. Their goal is to achieve a body size and shape that meet currently fashionable social models of "perfection." At present, those models call for women to be slim and trim and for men to have a muscular chest and arms and a slim lower body.

Whereas some weight watchers should be concerned about their body size for health reasons, those who diet for cosmetic reasons need to be aware that eating behavior dictated by social pressures can have adverse consequences. In their desire to be slim, individuals may restrict food intake to the degree that they

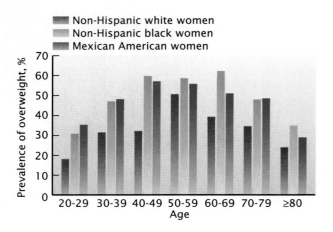

Non-Hispanic white women
Non-Hispanic black women
Mexican American women

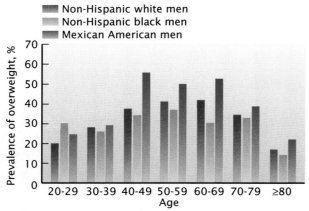

Non-Hispanic white men
Non-Hispanic black men
Mexican American men

FIGURE 6.1   Prevalence of Overweight Adults in the United States
Source: Data from R. J. Kuczmarski, K. M. Flegal, S. M. Campbell, and C. L. Johnson "Increasing Prevalence of Overweight among U.S. Adults," *Journal of the American Medical Association,* 272(1994): 205–211.

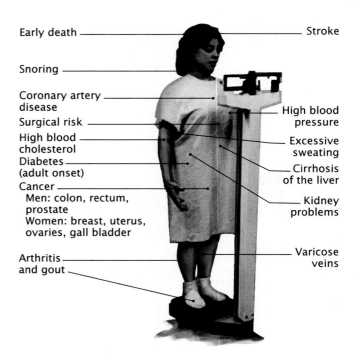

FIGURE 6.2 Overweight people have a greater likelihood of developing certain health problems than do people of normal weight.
Source: A. L. Thygerson, *Fitness and Health* (Boston: Jones and Bartlett Publishers, 1989). Reprinted with permission.

suffer ill health from nutrient imbalance and endanger themselves with eating disorders, such as anorexia nervosa and bulimia.

It is important for you to remember that although many people in contemporary industrialized societies consider fat to be an enemy, the capacity to store energy as fat is a normal physiological function. Thus, health issues related to overfatness are not necessarily associated with physiological or behavioral malfunctions but result from adaptation to an environment in which food is plentiful. In communities in which food is scarce or obtained irregularly, the ability to store calories as fat is highly adaptive. In communities in which food is abundant, this same biological adaptation can cause problems.

In this chapter we discuss weight-control issues. As you read the material, keep in mind that such issues are not solely about an individual's food intake, but in reality are about food intake in relation to a number of other factors central to modern life in the United States: a sedentary life-style, an endless bombardment of advertising pushing food products, lack of guidance regarding proper nutrition, confusing public health information about the effects of food on health and well-being, the custom of using body shape as a measure of social desirability, and a hectic, stressful life-style. In such a complex environment, the overavailability of food allows it to be used for a variety of personal and social reasons other than to provide nutrients and energy for life.

DEFINING OVERWEIGHT AND OBESITY

There are no good definitions for the terms **overweight** and **obesity.** Overweight is generally defined as exceeding an "ideal" weight tied to gender, height, and frame size. Unfortunately, these standards do not take into account differences in body composition, activity level,

T   E   R   M   S

overweight: excessive fat tissue, exceeding the "ideal" weight listed by gender, height, and frame size

obesity: increase in body weight beyond skeletal and physical requirements

or genetics. You may be classified as overweight based on tables, but may have an average or below average amount of body fat. This is common among athletes; they may be overweight due to muscle development but they are not overly fat.

Obesity has traditionally been defined as 20 percent or more above an optimal weight for height derived from actuarial statistics correlated with lowest death rates (*FDA Consumer,* 1991). However, some health experts say that the weight-for-height yardstick is imprecise and overly restrictive.

The social and economic impact of obesity may be as great as its health consequences. Studies show that almost 25 percent of children and adolescents are obese and obesity has increased to 54 percent among children ages 6–11. Childhood obesity has been strongly associated with the parent's being obese. Americans spend almost $35 billion annually in the effort to reduce weight. Unfortunately, much of this money was spent in vain; most people will gain weight back over a period of time.

Recent research indicates the most important issue regarding excess weight is not the *amount* but the *location*

HEALTHY PEOPLE 2000

Reduce overweight to no more than 20 percent among people aged 20 and older and no more than 15 percent among adolescents aged 12 through 19.

Overweight affects a large portion of the U.S. population and has not declined among adults for two decades. Overweight is associated with elevated serum cholesterol levels, elevated blood pressure, and non-insulin diabetes, and is an independent risk factor for coronary heart diseases. Overweight is multifactorial in origin, reflecting inherited, environmental, cultural, and socioeconomic conditions. Overweight acquired during childhood or adolescence may persist into adulthood and increase the risk for some chronic diseases later in life.

of extra weight a person carries. Obesity should be defined in terms of waist-to-hip ratio rather than height-to-weight ratio. Waist-to-hip ratio can be calculated by dividing the number of inches around the waistline by

Exploring Your Health

Body Image

How do you feel about the appearance of these regions of your body?

	Quite satisfied	Somewhat satisfied	Somewhat dissatisfied	Very dissatisfied
Hair	☐	☐	☐	☐
Arms	☐	☐	☐	☐
Hands	☐	☐	☐	☐
Feet	☐	☐	☐	☐
Waist	☐	☐	☐	☐
Buttocks	☐	☐	☐	☐
Hips	☐	☐	☐	☐
Legs and ankles	☐	☐	☐	☐
Thighs	☐	☐	☐	☐
Chest/breasts	☐	☐	☐	☐
Posture	☐	☐	☐	☐
General attractiveness	☐	☐	☐	☐

1. Which of your thoughts and actions enhance your body image?
2. Which of your thoughts and actions are detrimental to your body image?
3. What societal forces (expectations of friends and parents, advertising, celebrities and professional athletes, etc.) influence your body image most strongly?
4. What could you do to become more satisfied with your body image?

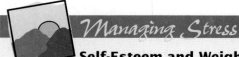

Self-Esteem and Weight Control

Experts agree that for weight control to be effective it must begin in the mind, not the body. And two mental factors are crucial for a weight-control program to be effective: high self-esteem and will power.

One of the most effective ways to build self-esteem is positive self-talk, which in turn helps boost will power. Our minds, like frequency bands on a radio tuner, have many voices or stations. The one frequency people typically tune into is the voice of the *critic*—a negative voice who constantly tells us that we are not good enough, we are too fat, too skinny, too short, badly proportioned, or just plain ugly. But we have a choice. We don't have to listen to this voice of the critic. Like pushing a button of a car radio we can tune out the critic's voice and find another station—one that gives better feedback. Like a distant radio

station with much static, the reception may not come in clearly at first, but with concentration, the voice that honors your being will come in much clearer. With practice, the message of choice will provide positive feedback.

One way you can tune into this frequency is to program your mind with positive affirmations: words, phrases, or expressions that you say to yourself to raise your self-esteem and confidence. These words of encouragement stroke the ego and enhance your sense of well-being. While this notion of giving yourself positive strokes may sound silly, it works. Many Olympic athletes, actors, and successful achievers use positive self-talk to accomplish their goals.

It is important to use the present tense, and even though the statement may not be true, say it as if it

is, so "as if, becomes as is." The following are some examples of positive affirmations that can help you raise your self-esteem, increase your will power, and help you control your weight. If you like one of these, use it regularly three or four times per day (especially near meal times), or if you like, create your own statement. When you use an affirmation statement, say it to yourself, and feel it at the gut level.

- I am at the right weight for my body size
- I am happy with my weight and body composition
- I am coming closer to my ideal body weight and composition
- I have the will power to eat only the amount of food I need to sustain optimal wellness
- I enjoy both quality food and quality exercise

---

the circumference of the hips. For example, someone who has a 28-inch waist and 37-inch hips would have a ratio of 0.75. A woman whose ratio is 0.8 or higher would be at greater risk of weight-related health problems, as would a man whose ratio is 0.95 or above.

Numerous studies have shown that fat in the hips and thighs is less health-threatening than abdominal fat. While other fat cells empty directly into the general circulation, abdominal fat cells go directly to the liver. They interfere with the liver's ability to effectively clear insulin from the bloodstream. This interference in turn causes

the pancreas to produce more insulin, prompting the autonomic nervous system to produce **norepinephrine,** which raises blood pressure. This sets the stage for diabetes, hypertension, and heart disease.

To be a more useful indicator of health risks, we suggest that the definition of obesity be broadened to include the following criteria: 1) weight to age and height ratio rather than gender and height ratio; 2) waist-to-hip ratio; and 3) inclusion of health-related problems such as hypertension and diabetes.

T E R M S

norepinephrine: a neurohormone released by the postganlionic adrenegic nerves and some brain neurons; a major neurotransmitter

lean body mass: structural and functional elements in cells, such as body water, muscle, and bone

body fat: essential fats and storage fats; needed for normal physiological functioning

essential fat: necessary and required fat in the diet; required for normal physiological functioning

storage fat: also called depot fat; excess fat that is deposited in various parts of the body

MEASURING YOUR WEIGHT

In most instances, concerns about being *overweight* are really concerns about being overfat. There is a difference. Some professional male athletes, for example, weigh much more than the recommended weight standards for the normal population. Yet as little as 1 percent of their body weight may be fat. Most of the body weight of a well-conditioned athlete is muscle and bone.

When you consider issues of body weight and body fat, think of the body as being composed of two distinct parts, **lean body mass** and **body fat.** Lean body mass is made up of the structural and functional elements in cells, body water, muscle, and bone. Body fat is composed of two parts: **essential fat**—fat necessary for normal physiological functioning, such as nerve conduction—and **storage fat.** Essential fat comprises about 3 to 7 percent of body weight in men and about 10–12 percent of total body weight in women. This gender difference, which is presumably caused by hormones, is due to the deposition of greater amounts of fat on the hips, thighs, and breasts in females. Female body builders, who are the leanest of all female athletes, have about 8 to 13 percent of their total body weight as fat, which is nearly all essential fat. This probably represents the lower limit of fat for a healthy woman. Storage fat, also called depot fat, constitutes only a small percent of the total body weight of lean individuals and 5 to 25 percent of the body weight of the majority of the population (Figure 6.3). However, storage fat can account for 40 to 50 percent of the body weight of clinically obese persons.

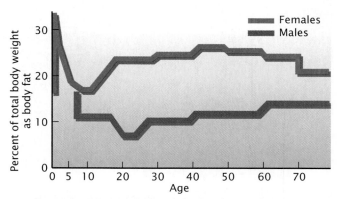

FIGURE 6.3 Body Fat Percentage Percent of total body weight as body fat for men and women, by age.

As yet there are no universally accepted standards for the most "desirable" or "ideal" body weight or body composition (fat percentage). One reason is that social

Whose Image Is It Anyway?

Erica Davis

A recent Gary Larson "Far Side" cartoon showed two mosquitoes stalking prey at a nudist camp full of fat, wrinkled people. "Oops," says one bug to the other, "there goes the appetite."

Larson's creepy critters have the same attitude about the folks they were about to lunch on that I used to have about myself: disgusted by a non-perfect body.

I mean, I didn't like much of anything I had. Well, maybe my feet. A boyfriend once told me I had pretty feet.

To compensate for this less-than-flattering opinion of myself, I strove for the perfect hard body (except my breasts and rear—they had to be soft). No flab. No waist. I became obsessed with food and exercised my butt off.

I wanted to look like Madonna or Cher or all the women at the rec pool with bodies right out of a Cosmo swimsuit ad. I think I actually got close, but I couldn't be satisfied. If I got a compliment, I'd brush it aside. I was in a war against all fat and my natural shape, and was determined to win. Any loafing brought massive guilt.

Do you know how much work that is? And for what? For whom?

When I first started thinking about this I got mad at men because I thought all they wanted from me was a Victoria Secret body to play with. After a while

I got mad at women, too. All that competition and the tsk-tsk-ing if I had a bulge somewhere.

Then I got mad at society for telling me that I had to look a certain way in order to feel good about myself and to be socially and sexually attractive. Advertisers became my most hated enemy.

I'm still a little mad at all those influences, but I'm also mad at myself for trying to please everyone else with how I looked rather than trying to please myself for how I was.

Don't get me wrong. Looking good is important to me. More important, though, is feeling good about myself. When I was working so hard to sculpt my body, I was a tyrant. I'd scold myself for having an ice cream or if I missed a work out.

I've learned that when I feel good about myself, I take care of my body in ways that are more natural for me. It's better for me when my body and I are in harmony and not at war. I may not be asked to be in any swimsuit ads, but I think I look just fine.

Source: Reprinted with permission from the *Penguin League's Health Letter* (Summer 1990).

STUDENT REFLECTIONS

- Why does society play a large role in how we perceive ourselves?
- Does society treat men and women equally regarding body image?

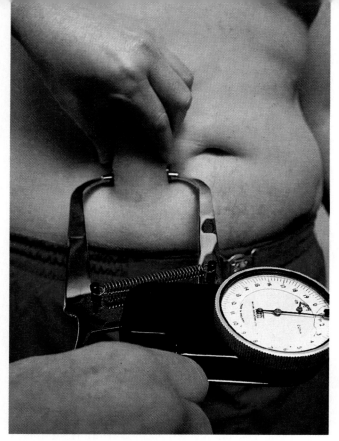

Body fat is measured using a skin-fold caliper.

and psychological factors, as well as health considerations, influence what is considered desirable. For example, fatness, particularly in women and children, is prized in some cultures. In these groups, women with significant storage fat are considered physically attractive and sexually desirable, and fatness in children is considered a sign of robust health. In the United States, attitudes about desirable body configuration tend to fluctuate and are often keyed to fashion trends. During the 1950s, for example, large body size, characterized by "full-figured" women and "he-men," was considered desirable, whereas today it seems that thin is in.

Health-related indexes of desirable body weight are given in tables of "ideal weight for height" issued by both the federal government and insurance companies and are based on statistics for longevity (Table 6.1 and Table 6.2). Good health is associated with weighing no more than 5 percent below or 20 percent (for men) and 30 percent (for women) above the standards. Beyond these levels, people have higher risks for diabetes, gallbladder disease, varicose veins, arthritis, heart disease, stroke, high blood pressure, breathing problems, and accident proneness (due to having a large body). People who are extremely overweight often face stigmas, such as job discrimination, lower social acceptance, and lower self-esteem.

A long-term study of 19,297 men found that at their ideal weights, based on the 1983 Metropolitan Life

TABLE 6.1 Metropolitan Life Insurance Company Weight-for-Height Tables

	Women (with clothing)				Men (with clothing)		
Height (with shoes, 2-inch heels)	Small frame	Medium frame	Large frame	Height (with shoes, 1-inch heels)	Small frame	Medium frame	Large frame
4'10"	92–98	96–107	104–119	5'2"	112–120	118–129	126–141
4'11"	94–101	98–110	106–122	3"	115–123	121–133	129–144
5'0"	96–104	101–113	109–125	4"	118–126	124–136	142–148
1"	99–107	104–116	112–128	5"	121–129	127–139	135–152
2"	102–110	107–119	115–131	6"	124–133	130–143	138–156
3"	105–113	110–122	118–134	7"	128–137	134–147	142–161
4"	108–116	113–126	121–138	8"	132–141	138–152	147–166
5"	111–119	116–130	125–142	9"	136–145	142–156	151–170
6"	114–123	120–135	129–146	10"	140–150	146–160	155–174
7"	118–127	124–139	133–150	11"	144–154	150–165	159–179
8"	122–131	128–143	137–154	6'0"	148–158	154–170	164–184
9"	126–135	132–147	141–158	1"	152–162	158–175	168–189
10"	130–140	136–151	145–163	2"	156–167	162–180	173–194
11"	134–144	140–155	149–168	3"	160–171	167–185	178–199
6'0"	138–148	144–159	153–173	4"	164–175	172–190	182–204

Source: Metropolitan Life Insurance Company. Used by permission.

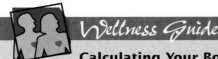

Wellness Guide

Calculating Your Body Mass Index

Body mass is obtained by dividing your weight in kilograms by the square of your height in meters.

To convert to kilograms, divide your weight in pounds (without clothes) by 2.2: _____

To convert to meters, divide your height in inches (without shoes) by 39.4, then square it: _____

Divide your weight by your height.

Body mass = _____

Women Desirable body mass is 21 to 23. Obesity (20 percent above the desirable range) begins at 27.5. Serious obesity (40 percent above) begins at 31.5.

Men Desirable body mass is 22 to 24. Obesity begins at 28.5, and serious obesity begins at 33.

The National Institutes of Health urges those who weigh more than the desirable range to lose weight. The greater one's weight, the more urgent the recommendation becomes.

Insurance Company tables, these men lived significantly longer than those just 2 to 6 percent above ideal. In 1983, Metropolitan Life suggested a 5-foot, 10-inch man over 35 should weigh less than 172 pounds; however, the 1990 U.S. Department of Agriculture's weight-height chart indicated the 5′10″ man could weigh 188 pounds.

TABLE 6.2   U.S. Department of Agriculture Height-Weight Tables

Height	Weight (pounds)	
	Ages 19–34	Ages 35 and greater
5′0″	97–128	108–138
5′1″	101–132	111–143
5′2″	104–137	115–148
5′3″	107–141	119–152
5′4″	111–146	122–157
5′5″	114–150	126–162
5′6″	118–155	130–167
5′7″	121–160	134–172
5′8″	125–164	138–178
5′9″	129–169	142–183
5′10″	132–174	146–188
5′11″	136–179	151–194
6′0″	140–184	155–199
6′1″	144–189	159–205
6′2″	148–195	164–210
6′3″	152–200	168–216
6′4″	156–205	173–222
6′5″	160–211	177–228
6′6″	164–216	182–234″

Note: In each range, the higher weights generally apply to men and the lower weights to women.

Source: U.S. Department of Agriculture, Nutrition and Your Health: Dietary Guidelines for Americans (Washington, D.C.: U.S. Government Printing Office, 1990).

Recently that increase in acceptable pounds per height has been challenged by others. The study also found that men who weighed 157 pounds or less had the lowest mortality rate, while men over 181 pounds had a mortality rate 67 percent greater and were two and one-half times more likely than the leanest men to die of heart disease. Although many agree with these findings, some researchers argue that body-fat distribution is just as important as weight-height in predicting morbidity and mortality (Morice, 1994).

Another measure of overweight is the **body mass index,** or **BMI,** calculated by dividing a person's weight in kilograms by the square of her or his height in meters. Studies show that adults with a BMI between 20 and 30 are in relatively good health, and those with BMIs below 20 and above 30 tend to have health problems and lower longevity. For most people, a BMI of 30 corresponds to weighing about 20 percent more than the "ideal" prescribed by the weight-for-height tables.

REGULATING BODY WEIGHT

Human physiology obeys the first law of thermodynamics, which states that energy is neither created nor destroyed in a closed system. This means that when you consume more food energy than is needed for growth and activity, the unused calories will be stored. In humans, the two principal calorie-storing mechanisms are 1) **glycogen,** the storage form of carbohydrate, and 2) **adipose tissue,** the storage form of fat. One gram of

T E R M S

body mass index (BMI): a measure of overweight

glycogen: polysaccharide that is the principal form in which carbohydrates are stored in the body

adipose tissue: type of connective tissue containing fat cells that forms a layer under the skin; serves as an insulating layer and as an energy reserve

glycogen stores four calories, whereas one gram of fat stores nine. There are several theories regarding how body weight is determined. This chapter will discuss the set-point theory, fat-cell theory, dietary-fat theory, and genetics.

Set-Point Theory

Some researchers suggest that the body has an internal "set point," much like the temperature set point on a thermostat; the amount of body fat supposedly is regulated within a narrow range specific to each individual. Evidence supporting this theory comes from experiments with animals and humans in which, after having gained weight through force-feeding, subjects return to their pre-experiment weight without any effort. Set-point theory is also supported by the observation that the body defends against severe calorie restriction—and thereby avoids lower than set-point body fatness—by lowering the metabolic rate.

One way the "fatness set point" is maintained is through a protein called **adipsin,** which is made by fat cells and released into the bloodstream. The function of adipsin is to signal the brain that fat cells are "full" (that is, that the body has reached its set point), and that further increases in fat are unnecessary. This signal produces feelings of satiety and a reduction in eating in general, and possibly a reduction in the desire to consume fat specifically. Natural biological variations in the efficiency of the adipsin-brain signaling system could be partly responsible for the diversity in fatness set points observed in the population. A very low efficiency or malfunctioning adipsin-brain system could be responsible for at least some instances of very high body fatness.

Another way the fatness set point is maintained is through the activity of an enzyme called **lipoprotein lipase,** whose function is to remove fat that is circulating in the blood. In some individuals, this enzyme becomes very active during times of fat-calorie restriction. The increased enzyme activity is the body's way of increasing the efficiency of fat storage and thus maintaining the fatness set point. The capacity to enhance fat-storage efficiency is highly adaptive in an environment in which food—especially calorie-rich, fat-containing food—is consumed irregularly. In modern society, however, such efficiency is generally unnecessary and can lead to an overfat problem. Indeed, studies show that this particular fat-storing mechanism works with much greater efficiency in obese people than in lean ones.

Set-point theory helps explain many a dieter's complaint that adherence to a very low-calorie diet, while at first successful, eventually produces no further loss in body fat. Severe calorie restrictions put the dieter in a state of continual semistarvation, to which the body responds by lessening its resting metabolic rate. This means fewer calories are needed to fuel basic life functions, so less stored fat is used and further weight loss ceases. The goal in weight loss is to raise resting metabolic rate, which is done by exercising.

Fat-Cell Theory

When adults overeat, fat cells grow larger at first. At some point the enlarged fat cells send a signal that initiates the formation of new fat cells. This process suggests that when a demand for more fat storage is sufficiently compelling, the body increases its fat storage capacity. Once fat cells form they become a permanent part of the body unless great weight loss is maintained for an extended period. The primary way to decrease your weight is through shrinkage of the existing fat cells, because once they are formed they are almost impossible to eliminate.

Dietary-Fat Theory

Obesity is due primarily to the abundance and availability of tasty, fat-rich foods. High sugar diets promote obesity to a lesser extent than diets higher in fat. Excessive fat in foods (dietary fat) produces more fat than overeating carbohydrates.

Genetics

Statistical studies confirm that obesity runs in families. Studies of twins show that a tendency to obesity has a strong genetic component. A strong relationship between the body mass index of adopted children and their biological parents was found in a study of adopted children; no relationship was found to their adoptive parents. Eighty percent of children of two obese parents become obese themselves, compared with only 14 percent of children with both parents of normal weight. However, it is difficult to separate out genetic and environmental components that contribute to obesity.

> *I must've lost a thousand pounds in my life. The same ten pounds over and over again.*
> Student

RECREATIONAL EATING

In contrast to set-point theory, many people are overfat because their eating behavior is triggered by external stimuli. In many cases, eating is unrelated to feelings of hunger or satiety. A good example of such behaviors is the fact many of us eat at predetermined times of the day ("mealtimes") regardless of whether or not we are hungry. The reason may be social conditioning (e.g., among family members) or convenience, such as being on a

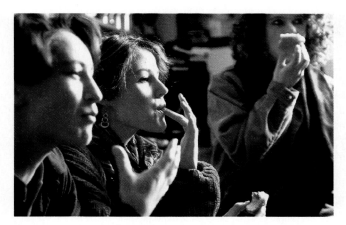
A steady diet of "junk" food will add to your weight and undermine your health.

break from work or school. In addition, the foods that are consumed and their amounts are often based on custom and economic factors, rather than satisfying hunger.

Some people are "recreational" overeaters. This means they ingest food not because they are hungry, but because it is a leisure-time pursuit. Snacking while watching television is a common form of recreational overeating; television advertisers bank on this. That is why so many TV commercials advertise soft drinks, beer, and snack foods. How often do you see a TV commercial for fruits and vegetables?

Another form of recreational overeating is drinking alcoholic beverages. Since alcohol contains the energy equivalent of seven calories per gram, a few beers or mixed drinks per day can lead to an excess of fat rather quickly.

Frequently, people with a weight problem are unaware of the many environmental cues that trigger their eating. When passing a refrigerator or a soft-drink machine, they may habitually succumb to the lure of eating or drinking something. Studies show overfat people who have free access to food tend to eat more than do people of normal weight.

Stress, anxiety, loneliness, boredom, and anger can all motivate overeating. Many people derive emotional comfort from food. One possible explanation is that as children we learn to associate eating (particularly nursing as infants) with receiving love, affection, and comfort. Another possibility is when we consume certain foods, particularly those containing sugar and fat, they contribute to feelings of calm because certain hormones are released that act on the brain.

T E R M S

adipsin: a protein made by fat cells and released into the bloodstream

lipoprotein lipase: an enzyme secreted in the digestive tract that catalyzes the breakdown of fats

yo-yo dieting: repeated cycles of weight loss and gain

LOSING WEIGHT SENSIBLY

Individuals whose body weights are 30 percent or more fat are encouraged to lose weight to avoid a variety of health problems. For unknown reasons, very large bodies resist becoming slim no matter how hard the individual tries to reduce body size. For this reason, some physicians recommend that large individuals stop trying to be slim, stop blaming themselves for lack of self-control, and try to reduce their body weight about 10 percent, which often puts them in the range for good health, if not high fashion.

Many people who are weight conscious are not clinically overfat, but may simply want to be slimmer. Social pressures create stereotypes of attractive body size that most people cannot attain. Sensible weight management begins with being aware of these pressures and not succumbing to them.

Those who wish to lose weight should be aware that no single weight-loss program has been shown to be effective over the medium-to-long term, regardless of advertising claims to the contrary. Rapid weight-loss programs can produce early results, in *weight,* but over time about 95 percent of people regain the weight they had lost. While many of the unusual and sometimes bizarre foods and/or exercises prescribed in rapid weight-loss programs do reduce body fat, people tend to become bored with restrictive diets. As a result, they frequently become obsessed with food and frustrated at not being able to eat what they want. After a time, they give up and return to their former habits. When the weight returns, they blame themselves for being weak-willed failures. They often try to diet again, giving rise to repeated cycles of weight loss and weight gain. This is called **yo-yo dieting,** or weight cycling.

HEALTHY PEOPLE 2000

Increase to at least 50 percent the proportion of overweight people aged 12 and older who have adopted sound dietary practices combined with regular physical activity to attain an appropriate body weight.

Overweight occurs when too few calories are expended and too many are consumed for individual metabolic rates. The results of weight loss programs focused on dietary restrictions alone have not been encouraging. Neither frequent fluctuation in body weight nor extreme restrictions in food intake are desirable. Overweight people should increase their physical activity and should avoid calorie-dense foods, especially those high in fat.

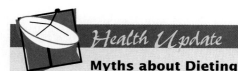
Myths about Dieting

MYTH: Your body knows what it needs.
FACT: Your body does not know what it needs. If you listened to your body, it would probably crave fruits and vegetables as often as sweets.

MYTH: After a certain age, it's inevitable that you put on weight. And it's a lot harder to lose a pound than when you are younger.
FACT: Your caloric needs do decrease as you get older and you may also be less active as well. So you will gain weight if you eat the same amount as when you were younger. In order to maintain your weight as you get older, you need to eat less. It takes the same amount of work to lose a pound no matter what age you are.

MYTH: If I eat a balanced diet there's no reason for me to take a vitamin supplement.
FACT: Despite the fact that you may be eating a well-balanced diet, you may still need to take a vitamin supplement. You may need a supplement if you are under stress, smoke, drink alcohol, take certain drugs, have been recently ill or pregnant, are getting older, or if you are taking an oral contraceptive.

MYTH: Sugar is bad for you.
FACT: Refined sugar is bad for you. It has no nutritive value and only adds calories. Table sugar is a refined sugar. Natural sugars found in fruits and vegetables are part of a balanced diet.

There is no one definition for weight cycling; however, all definitions share certain features. The National Task Force on the Prevention and Treatment of Obesity (1994) reported the following conclusions, after reviewing reports from 1966 through 1994 on weight cycling, yo-yo dieting, and weight fluctuation. First, there is no evidence that weight cycling has adverse effects in humans with regards to energy expenditure, body composition, risk factors for cardiovascular disease, or effectiveness of future weight-loss attempts. Second, the evidence is not clear regarding a connection between body weight variation and increased morbidity and mortality. Third, individuals who are not obese and do not have risk factors for obesity-related illnesses should not attempt weight loss, but should focus on preventing weight gain through physical activity and a healthy diet. Finally, the data is inconclusive regarding long-term effects of weight cycling; as a precaution, however, obese individuals need to commit to life-long behavioral changes in diet and physical activity.

When we eat less to reduce our caloric intake, the resulting weight loss tends to be temporary. To lose weight and keep it off requires a change in dietary and exercise behaviors. The energy equivalent of one pound of body fat is 3,500 calories. Reducing the number of ingested calories per day and increasing the level of physical activity each day to produce a net deficit of 500 calories per day will produce a loss of one pound a week, the recommended amount. This could be done by walking a little more and cutting out a soft drink or a couple of cookies each day.

To plan a 500-calorie per day deficit, you must determine the kinds of foods you can safely reduce or eliminate. One way to do this is to keep a diary of everything you eat for four days and record the circumstances associated with food intake. Everything you eat must be recorded, from a carrot stick to a five-course meal. You can consult tables that show the number of calories for different foods to determine the approximate number of calories you are ingesting. You should also read food product labels (see Chapter 5) to find much of this information.

Some people have the misconception that increasing their level of physical activity will increase their appetite and food consumption. This is true only of individuals who expend large amounts of energy in work (lumberjacks) or play (football players). For most people, however, appetite and calorie consumption tend to decrease as physical activity increases.

There are some rules to successful weight loss. Here are some simple, effective techniques to help stay on a diet and achieve desired results:

- Keep a record of everything you eat.
- Familiarize yourself with how much a particular quantity (1 portion, 1 cup, etc.) really is, not how much you think it is.
- **DO NOT** go food shopping on an empty stomach.
- Drink a glass of water before eating anything.
- Eat only when sitting down.
- **DO NOT** snack between meals.
- **DO NOT** put anything in your mouth while you are preparing meals.
- You can eat out, but insist on no sauce, no butter, low-calorie dressings, and broiled dishes.

> *How many more years do I have to eat stuff that's good for me?*
> Dennis the Menace

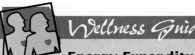

Wellness Guide

Energy Expenditures for Certain Activities

Calories/hour	Activity	Benefits
72–84	Sitting	None
150–240	Golf using power cart	Will not promote endurance
240–300	Cleaning windows Vacuuming Mopping floors	Will condition if done for at least 20 to 30 minutes
	Bowling	Not taxing enough
	Walking, 3 mph Cycling, 6 mph	Adequate if you are just beginning a shape-up condition program
300–360	Scrubbing floors	Good for endurance if done in at least 20 to 30 minutes stints
	Walking, 3.5 mph Cycling, 8 mph	Good aerobic exercise
	Table tennis Badminton Volleyball	Vigorous, continuous play can have benefits; otherwise just helps skills
	Tennis (doubles)	Aids skills but not helpful unless there is continuous play for at least 2 minutes at a time
	Many calisthenics Ballet exercises	Will promote endurance if continuous rhythmic and repetitive. Promotes agility, coordination, and muscle strength
350–420	Walking, 4 mph Cycling, 10 mph Ice or roller skating	Dynamic, aerobic exercise. Skating should be done continuously
420–480	Walking, 5 mph Cycling, 11 mph	Dynamic, aerobic exercise
	Tennis (singles)	Must be played 30 minutes or more with attempt to keep moving for for benefit
	Water skiing	Total isometrics but very risky for people not in good condition
480–600	Jogging, 5 mph Cycling, 12 mph	Dynamic, aerobic endurance-building exercise
	Downhill skiing	Mostly benefits skill
	Paddleball	Promotes skill; if continuous good exercise
600–650	Running, 5.5 mph Cycling, 13 mph	Excellent conditioning
Above 650	Running, 6+ mph	Excellent conditioning
	Handball	Competitive environment in hot room—only for those in good condition. Benefits if played 30 minutes with effort to keep moving
	Swimming	Good conditioning exercise—if continuous strokes

Note: These figures are approximations and are different for each individual. Calories burned are directly related to an individual's metabolic rate.

Source: Adapted and reprinted by permission of the Research Institute of America, 90 Fifth Avenue, New York, N.Y. 10011. For information about RIA services, call 1(800)431-9025, ext. 4.

- Be aware of invisible calories (e.g., mayonnaise, salad dressings, alcohol).
- Avoid eating when you are anxious or unhappy.
- Become familiar with listening to your body's own natural signs of hunger—then feed yourself. When you are hungry, eat. Try not to deprive your natural hunger feelings.

WEIGHT-CONTROL FADS AND FALLACIES

"Lose weight effortlessly, even as you sleep!" "New diet discovery lets you lose excess pounds in just one week!" So claim advertisements for products and eating regimens that are directed to chronic dieters and others con-

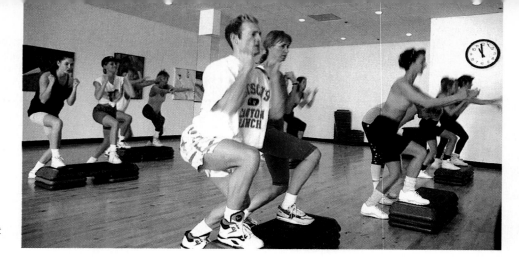

Exercise is essential to effective weight management.

cerned about being overfat. Because current social custom calls for the "slim and fit" look, the weight-control industry is bigger than ever, with annual sales of $35 billion.

Unfortunately for consumers, nearly all of the claims made by the heavily advertised weight-control regimens and products are exaggerated and misleading. By themselves, these programs are not likely to produce a significant reduction in body fat sustained over any long-term period. Whatever weight loss they do bring about is usually a reduction in lean body tissue or in body water. The only proven way to reduce body fat and to maintain normal body weight is life-style modification that includes

changing eating behaviors and increasing the level of physical activity.

Four major faddish, and generally ineffective, weight-control products or schemes are 1) body wraps, 2) diet pills (including vitamins), 3) diet programs, and 4) fasting.

Body Wraps

Body wraps are plastic or rubber garments, ranging from waist belts to entire body suits, that are worn during exercise, routine daily activity, or sleep in order to produce weight loss. A wrap designed for just one part of

Controversy in Health

Product Bans

In the wake of House Committee on Small Business hearings on the $33 billion weight-loss industry, the Food and Drug Administration and the Federal Trade Commission separately announced investigations into the safety and efficacy of diet pills and programs, and how they are promoted in advertising.

In the fall of 1990, the FDA proposed a ban on 111 ingredients in the over-the-counter (OTC) diet

products, including amino acids, cellulose, grapefruit extract, and kelp. The FDA has given manufacturers an opportunity to provide information that demonstrates their products' effectiveness and safety. The FDA recently recalled Cal-Ban 3000, a heavily advertised diet pill containing guar gum, after receiving consumer complaints.

The FTC monitors advertising claims of diet aids and takes legal

action if necessary. Recent targets have been Fat-Magnet (a pill claimed to break up "fat-attracting" particles) and Fibre Trim (a high-fiber supplement that claimed it could aid in weight reduction).

Consumers can get a list of ineffective diet aids by writing to: FDA, HFE-20, 5600 Fishers Lane, Rockville, Md., 20857.

Source: FDA Consumer (October 1991).

STUDENT REFLECTIONS

- Why have manufacturers been able to advertise products despite federal laws and regulations?
- Recognizing that many diet aid products may not do what they claim, how would you convince your roommate not to purchase one of these products?

the body (such as the waist or hips) is supposed to reduce the size of just that body region ("spot reducing").

Body wraps do result in weight loss and a reduction in body size. The catch is that the weight lost is body water and not body fat. These garments increase perspiration; they do not diminish the body's fat stores. The lost body water is quickly regained and so is the lost body weight. Because these products cause a loss of body water, they make dehydration a potential, although not very likely, danger.

The appeal of body wraps stems from the common misconception that fat can be eliminated from the body by heat. The phrase "burning off fat" is part of the professional physiologist's jargon and contributes to this false notion. The process by which body fat is reduced does not involve heat. (Human body temperature is uniformly maintained at 37°C.) The "burning" that physiologists speak of is a chemical breakdown of fat molecules requiring oxygen, not the liquefaction and evaporation that one would expect from high temperatures. Hence, the claim that body wraps reduce body size by "melting away fat" is quite misleading.

Diet Pills and Aids

A number of products that contain drugs and "natural" substances are sold as weight-loss remedies. Often these products are used in conjunction with dieting, modification in eating behavior, and exercise programs, so they appear effective to the naive consumer. However, no single product by itself has been shown to reduce weight.

Amphetamines and amphetamine-like drugs have been used for years as appetite suppressants. However, there is considerable debate as to the wisdom of using amphetamines for weight loss—or of using any other drug for that matter—because of the lack of proven efficacy and because of the potential for drug abuse and dependence.

Phenylpropanolamine (PPA) is an amphetamine-like substance that is the principal ingredient in several weight-loss products sold over the counter (Dexatrim, Appedrine, Control, Dietac). PPA is thought to be an appetite suppressant, but the doses recommended in commercial preparations are probably not effective, and higher doses (greater than 75 mg per day) are likely to cause nervousness, nausea, insomnia, headaches, and elevated blood pressure.

Benzocaine, an anesthetic, is found in candies, lozenges, and chewing gums sold as aids to weight reduction. Benzocaine is supposed to help produce weight loss by numbing the sense of taste and thereby reducing the desire for food. There is no scientific evidence, however, that temporarily reducing the sense of taste leads to weight loss. Because benzocaine is intended as a topical anesthetic, these products are useful (if at all) only if they are not swallowed.

Bulk-producing agents, such as methylcellulose, psyllium, and agar, are supposed to produce a sense of fullness in the gastrointestinal tract, thus suppressing appetite. These agents swell when mixed with water and are much more effective as laxatives than as weight reducers. Glucomannan, a bulk-producing starch derived from konjac tubers, is often touted by health food enthusiasts as a "natural" weight-loss method. There is no evidence that glucomannan or any other bulk producer reduces appetite and produces weight loss.

Hormones, such as human chorionic gonadotropin (HCG) and thyroid hormone, are occasionally offered by unscrupulous clinics as aids for weight loss. Neither of these hormones is effective as a weight reducer. Moreover, because hormones are regulators of the body's homeostatic mechanisms, it is never wise to take them unless monitored closely by a well-trained clinician.

Vitamins, minerals, and some amino acids (including arginine, ornithine, tryptophan, and phenylalanine) are occasionally sold as weight-loss agents. For example, Spirulina, a product made from blue-green algae, is claimed to be effective in reducing weight because it contains the amino acid phenylalanine, which supposedly regulates the body's appetite. Vitamins, minerals, and amino acids have not been shown to be effective in causing weight loss. And in very high doses, some of these substances, although "natural," can be harmful.

Diet Programs

If you want to make some money, get involved in publishing a book that describes a "revolutionary" new diet for weight loss. So many people make a hobby of trying fad diets that the book is virtually guaranteed to sell many copies. Be sure that the diet you invent requires no exercise, is based on some "new" dietary or nutritional discovery, carries an air of authoritativeness, and promises a rapid reduction in body weight, although not necessarily a reduction in body fat. It doesn't matter a bit if the lost weight is regained in a short time. In fact, it's

---

T E R M S

amphetamines: central nervous system stimulant used to decrease appetite

phenylpropanolamine (PPA): active ingredient in over-the-counter weight-control products

benzocaine: an anesthetic sometimes used in over-the-counter weight-control products to numb the sense of taste

bulk-producing agents: agents used to promote a sense of fullness in the gastrointestinal tract, thus suppressing appetite

hormones: complex chemicals produced and secreted by endocrine glands that travel through the bloodstream

A Cure for Obesity on the Horizon?

Almost 50 years ago, a mutant strain of mouse was discovered in a laboratory that causes all mice of this strain to be extremely obese. Now the mouse gene (called *Ob* for obese) has been isolated and its protein product identified as a hormone that acts to control obesity. When this hormone (named leptin) was isolated from normal mice and injected into obese mice, their eating behaviors changed and they lost weight. And of greater significance was the observation that the formerly obese mice were able to maintain the weight loss as long as they were given the hormone.

Leptin is produced by fat cells in mice and released into the blood. It appears that the level of this hormone in the circulation tells the brain how much fat is stored in the body. The brain responds to this chemical signal by controlling the animal's eating behavior. It seems likely that a similar hormone exists in human beings. Scientists now are trying to isolate the human hormone leptin in order to test its effects on controlling human obesity. While the prospects are exciting, it will be several years before researchers know if a comparable human hormone exists and if it can be administered to obese people safely and effectively.

Source: M. Barinaga, "Obese Protein Slims Mice." *Science*, 269, July 28, 1995, p. 475.

---

probably better for the weight-loss industry if your diet does not produce permanent weight loss, since that would reduce the sales of the next crop of diet books.

Many of the weight-loss diets that have come and gone have been based on altering the usual proportions of the three basic types of foods—protein, fat, and carbohydrate. Hence, the high-fat, low-fat, high-carbohydrate, low-carbohydrate, high-protein, and low-protein diets have all had their day and made their proponents wealthy. Occasionally diet regimens require the ingestion of only certain kinds of foods, such as fruits (grapefruit or papaya), cottage cheese, or steak. Fortunately, most of these unusual diets are too expensive, too boring, or too fatiguing to maintain for long, and people give them up before the nutritional deficiencies they can produce cause irreparable harm. Unfortunately, that is not always the case, and a few people have died from unsound dieting practices (such as stringent macrobiotic diets).

A variety of weight-loss programs not only tell clients how to lose weight, but also supply packaged foods and, sometimes, social support to bolster the weight-loser's efforts. Many of these programs are based on severe calorie-restriction regimens. Some plans use "real" food but control the portions and others are based on liquid diets containing sufficient protein, vitamins, and minerals to prevent the loss of lean body tissue. As with other special efforts to lose weight, the dietary plans often fail because they are difficult or expensive to maintain, and also because they often do not include life-style changes that would alter the fatness set point and fat-accumulating eating behaviors.

Fasting

Fasting is the simplest concept of all diets: stop eating and you'll lose weight. Unfortunately, this technique has complications that are far from simple. To deprive the body of all the basic nutrients may present problems.

There is little scientific evidence to support the contention that fasting is physiologically beneficial. Nevertheless, people who go on periodic short-term fasts often claim that fasting makes them feel better. The healthier

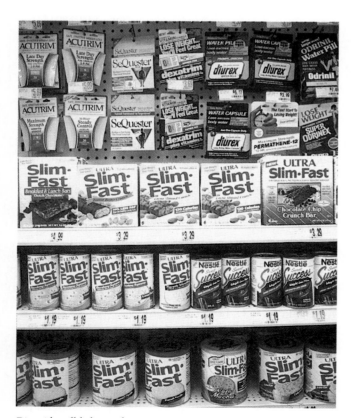

Diet aids will help you lose your money—not your excess pounds.

feeling is often attributed to cleansing the body of toxins, accumulated environmental pollutants, and tissue debris. Feeling better may also be a placebo effect or the result of changes in the brain chemistry brought on by lack of food.

Most fasting regimens call for one-, three-, or sometimes seven- or ten-day fasts, during which only water or occasionally fruit juice is ingested. Long fasts are often monitored by an experienced fasting facilitator. Guidelines for breaking a fast include consuming juice only at first, followed by soft palatable foods. The usual diet is resumed after a day or two of careful eating.

The experience of fasting is often accompanied by altered states of consciousness. Not long after beginning a fast, the person may feel hungry, but after a time, hunger subsides. About five hours after having passed up the usual first meal of the day, the person may feel tired and possibly irritable. This phase tends to pass, and by the end of the first day, the faster experiences a renewed feeling of energy and coincident loss of interest in eating. If the fast continues, similar cycles may occur, with the down phase becoming progressively shorter and the energetic phase longer.

Experienced fasters usually feel refreshed and invigorated after their fasts, and may also claim increased feelings of harmony with their environment and their spiritual selves. This is one reason fasting has been used in many cultures for thousands of years as a way to purify the spirit. Despite its potential to purify the spirit, fasts should only be undertaken under medical supervision, and only if you are healthy to begin with.

BODY IMAGE ISSUES

Body image is a person's mental "picture" of her or his body. Nearly everyone has a body image. Nearly everyone judges that image as good, or less good, by comparing her or his body image to a standard of the "ideal body" communicated to individuals by their culture and people who are important to them, such as lovers, family, and friends. The judgment a person makes about her or his body image is called *body esteem*. Individuals with a positive body image tend to have higher body esteem than do individuals with a less positive body image.

In North America, many women are exceedingly concerned about their body image, and many tend to have low body esteem because they believe themselves to be overweight. Books, films, TV, and popular maga-

zines (especially women's magazines) consistently send messages that our society esteems thin women and disdains the heavy ones. Whereas maintaining appropriate body size is associated with good health, attempting to achieve an unrealistic ideal of slimness is oppressive to many women. Failure to meet unrealistic standards leads many women to judge themselves as unattractive and lowers their self-esteem.

The current emphasis on slimness is partly fad—there have been times (and they surely will return) when thinness was associated with being sickly, and a full body was a sign of robust health and sexual attractiveness—and partly desire to be healthy and fit. A lean body is associated with high status, sexual attractiveness, youthfulness, and a demonstration of the personal power to be trim and fit in a culture in which sedentary habits and overeating are common.

It is important to realize that, for the most part, standards of attractive and healthful appearance are set by companies seeking to sell products and increase profits. Advertisements try to convince women they fall short of an ideal, and that by purchasing a product, dieting, or exercising to change their body size and shape, they can improve themselves and their lives. These messages cause many women to judge themselves on how they look and cause many men to judge women largely by their physical appearance. Overconcern about body image and weight can have adverse health consequences:

- depression from low body esteem and low self-worth
- poor nutrition from extensive dieting
- inadequate calcium and iron intake from undernutrition
- anorexia or bulimia
- musculoskeletal injuries from overexercising
- risks associated with cosmetic surgery
- cigarette smoking to reduce body weight

EATING DISORDERS

For women, a slim body reflects the current trend toward sexual equality: it represents a rejection of the traditional woman's role as homemaker and childbearer and emphasizes a new femininity characterized by individualism, athleticism, and nonreproductive sexuality.

Whereas freedom from traditional sex-role behavior may be praiseworthy, using slimness as a measure of social achievement has become an oppressive standard for many, particularly for young people. In some instances, individuals develop such a morbid fear of becoming fat that they adopt unusual (and very unhealthy) eating behaviors.

Young athletes, who are often obsessed with high achievement in sports, may also be susceptible to an inordinate fear of fatness. Most serious athletes are encouraged to be as lean as possible, and some overreact to the expectations of parents and coaches by restricting their food intake to excessively low amounts. This behavior, called **anorexia athletica**, affects both males and females. According to Nathan J. Smith, an expert in sports medicine, "losing fat becomes a challenge in which the athlete promises himself uncompromised success. Hunger pains become gratifying signals of accomplishment, and food becomes the opponent in a contest that he is dedicated to win by an overwhelming score" (Smith, 1980). Counseling and reassurance that athletic goals can be met without such drastic eating behavior usually alleviate the condition.

Although abnormal eating behavior can be caused solely by the fear of becoming obese, there are instances when a compulsive desire to be slim is a manifestation of more complex psychological stress. Increasing demands on school health services for help with abnormal eating behavior indicate that many young people, especially young women, have problems associated with eating. Two of the most common eating disorders are **anorexia nervosa**, a voluntary refusal to eat, and **bulimia**, binge eating and immediate purging of the ingested food either by vomiting or by using laxatives.

Anorexia Nervosa

Anorexia nervosa is characterized by a relentless pursuit of thinness resulting in progressive weight loss and metabolic disturbances. Most of those affected are young women. Anorexia is not caused by any known disease-causing agent but by self-induced starvation, which can lead to serious illness and even death.

Elizabeth Barrett Browning (1806–1861), one of England's most famed poets, is thought to have suffered from anorexia nervosa. As a teenager, Elizabeth was nagged by her parents to eat and gain weight, yet she stubbornly refused to eat much more than toast. When she met her future husband, poet Robert Browning, she

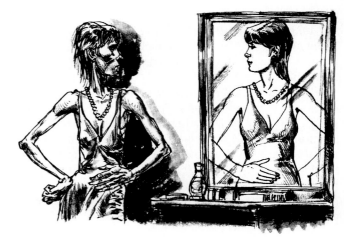

FIGURE 6.4 Reflections of an Anorexic Often anorexics see a different person in the mirror.

weighed merely 87 pounds. Apparently the Barrett family possessed characteristics found in other families with an anorectic member: overprotectiveness, overinvolvement with each other, and inability to express or resolve intrafamilial conflict.

Stubbornness and irony are characteristics of anorexia nervosa. For example, a person with anorexia nervosa is likely to defend her emaciated appearance as normal and will insist that weight gain makes her feel fat. Besides such distortions in normal body image, anorectics tend to have a fanatical preoccupation with food. They may spend an inordinate amount of time planning and preparing elaborate meals for others, while they themselves eat only a few bites and claim to be full. Often they will not eat in the presence of others; when they do, they may dawdle over their food. Some anorectics resort to self-induced vomiting or frequent use of diuretics or laxatives to reduce their body weight. These practices may lead to severe depletion of body minerals, which can precipitate abnormal heart rhythms and even cardiac arrest. Despite the low intake of calories, anorectics are remarkably energetic and tend to be hyperactive.

Another characteristic of anorexia nervosa is a paralyzing sense of powerlessness. The anorectic sees herself as responding to demands of others rather than taking initiative in life. As children, anorectics tend to be obedient, dutiful, helpful, and excellent students. Some psychologists interpret the intense preoccupation with weight loss as an expression of an underlying fear of incompetence. Control of eating and body weight becomes a way of demonstrating general control and competence.

One theory seeks to explain anorexia as a preoccupation with extreme slimness (and associated absence of

In 1988 at the age of 16, Christie Henrich missed making the U.S. Olympic team in women's gymnastics by less than two-tenths of a point. At her performance peak, Christie weighed 93 pounds. During one of the international competitions during 1988, a judge told her that she needed to watch her weight if she wanted to be a champion. According to her coach, Christie perceived herself as being too fat to be an Olympic competitor so she began to starve herself (anorexia) and to vomit when she did eat (bulimia). By 1990 she was too weak to compete even though she was ranked among the top 10 women gymnasts in the U.S. In 1994 Christie Henrich died; she weighed less than 60 pounds.

If someone you know seems to have an eating problem, here are some ways to help.

- Express your concern about any apparent weight loss. Even if the person denies that anything is wrong, your concern may alert him/her that something is wrong.
- Encourage the person to talk about his/her feelings concerning problems or worries even if they are not food related. Listen without making judgments.
- Suggest that the person see a health counselor, physician, or mental health professional.
- Express your own concerns to a professional counselor who may be able to intervene and help.

Anorexia and bulemia are very serious disorders and require professional help.

STUDENT REFLECTIONS

- What resources are available at your college or university for dealing with eating disorders?
- Can you think of any other pressures that might cause someone to deprive herself of food?

---

menstruation) in an attempt to remain a child who is cared for and fed by others, who can be stubborn and obstinate, and who has no sexual identity or desires. Another theory suggests that anorexia is the manifestation of a struggle for a sense of identity and personal effectiveness through controlling the environment; the resulting stubborn, rejecting behavior then becomes reinforced by the attention received from others. Yet another theory sees anorexia as a manifestation of impaired family interaction. The family of the anorectic becomes so engrossed with her symptoms that they avoid dealing with conflicts among themselves.

Three goals characterize the treatment of anorexia nervosa: 1) weight gain, 2) changed attitudes toward food and eating, and 3) resolution of underlying personal and family conflicts. Unfortunately, therapeutic intervention is not always successful and the condition may persist for years. Anorexia nervosa has a 15 to 20 percent mortality rate.

Bulimia

Bulimia is marked by a voluntary restriction of food intake followed by a binge-purge cycle: extreme overeating, usually of high-calorie junk foods, immediately followed by self-induced vomiting, use of diuretics or laxatives, or intense exercise. Like anorexia nervosa, bulimia occurs primarily in young women with a morbid fear of becoming fat, who pursue thinness relentlessly. Most bulimics are model individuals: good students, athletes, extremely sociable and pleasant. Fearing discovery of

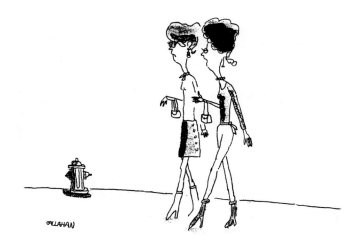

"OF COURSE YOU'RE NOT FEELING WELL—YOU HAVEN'T THROWN UP A THING ALL DAY!"

Courtesy of John Callahan and Levin Represents.

their bulimic behavior, they frequently carry out their binge-purge episodes in private. Bulimics usually are aware that their binge-purge behavior is abnormal; however, they are unable to control it. Many feel guilty and depressed about their problem, leading to a tendency to hide the behavior. Bulimia can pose a serious risk to health for many of the same reasons that anorexia does.

Several theories have been proposed to explain bulimia. One is that bulimia is a maladaptive way of dealing with anxiety, loneliness, and anger. Another suggests that bulimia is a manifestation of the drive to become the "ideal" woman, achieving the societal norm of slimness. Bulimics tend to have low self-esteem and a weak sense of identity.

Recovering from bulimia includes stopping binge-purge cycles and regaining control over eating behavior. Bulimics must also establish more appropriate ways to handle unpleasant feelings and discomfort with close relationships, and their self-esteem must be improved. Often psychological counseling is helpful.

IT'S IN YOUR HANDS

Successful weight control involves reducing intake of calories (often by recognizing the social and psychological reasons that cause one to overeat) and by increasing the level of physical activity. Heavily advertised reducing schemes such as body wraps, diet pills, and fad diets are almost totally ineffective in producing permanent fat reduction and weight loss.

The primary reason that people are overfat is that their life-styles do not include sufficient physical activity to use up the calories ingested in food. You can begin today to consciously watch what you eat and how much you exercise. You need not start out with an all out weight or physical regime; start slowly. When offered a cookie, decline. When you have the choice between the elevator and stairs, take the stairs. These efforts, which appear to be small, can make a difference when made daily and over an extended period of time.

HEALTH IN REVIEW

- Many people are primarily sedentary, behavior that may contribute to ill health, muscular and psychic tension, and overweight.
- Approximately one-third of the U.S. population is overfat and at risk for a variety of illnesses including heart disease, diabetes, hypertension, and gallbladder disease.
- The most important issue is not the amount of extra weight a person carries, but where he or she carries it.
- Obesity is better defined in terms of waist-to-hip ratio rather than height-to-weight ratio.
- A weight problem results when the body stores as fat those calories consumed in food that are not expended in resting metabolism and physical activity.
- There are several theories why people are overweight: set-point theory, fat-cell theory, dietary-fat theory, and genetic explanations.

- People eat for reasons other than hunger, such as social interaction, recreation, and stress.
- Successful weight control involves changing eating and exercise habits.
- There are four major ineffective weight control products/schemes: body wraps; diet pills; diet programs; and fasting.
- Two common eating disorders that occur primarily among young women today are anorexia nervosa and bulimia.
- Anorexia is a voluntary refusal to eat which can lead to disturbances in thought, mood, perception, to amennorrhea, and possibly to death.
- Bulimia is characterized by binge eating followed by self-induced vomiting.

REFERENCES

Barinaga, M. (1995). "Obese Protein Slims Mice." *Science*, 269: 475.

Kuczmarski, R. J., K. M. Flegal, S. M. Campbell, and C. L. Johnson (1994). "Increasing Prevalence of Overweight among U.S. Adults." *Journal of American Medical Association*, 272(3): 205–211.

Morice, L. (1994). "New Weight Guidelines." *American Health*, 13(4): 62.

National Task Force on the Prevention and Treatment of Obesity (1994). *Journal of the American Medical Association*, 272(15): 1196–1202.

"Never say diet." (1991). *FDA Consumer*, 25(8): 8.

Smith, N. J. (1980). "Excessive Weight Loss and Food Aversion in Athletes Simulating Anorexia Nervosa." *Pediatrics*, 66: 139–142.

SUGGESTED READINGS

Eldredge, K. L., W. S. Agras, and B. Arnow (1994). "The Last Supper: Emotional Determinants of Pretreatment Weight Fluctuation in Obese Binge Eaters." *The International Journal of Eating Disorders,* 16(1): 83. A study of obese binge eaters' self-reported tendency to binge eat because of negative emotions of anger, anxiety, and depression.

Emery, E. M., T. L. Schmid, H. S. Kahn, and P. P. Filozof (1993). "A Review of the Association between Abdominal Fat Distribution, Health Outcome Measures, and Modifiable Risk Factors." *American Journal of Health Promotion,* 7(5): 342–353. Examines the relationship between abdominal fat distribution and specific health outcomes, modifiable risk factors, and intervention efforts.

Fraser, L., and D. Weger. (1993). "Nothing to Lose." *Health,* 7(7): 60. Discusses the idea of letting the body decide when it's hungry rather than eating at set times during the day.

St. Jeor, S. T. (1993). "The Role of Weight Management in the Health of Women." *Journal of the American Dietetic Association,* 93(9): 1007–1012. Discusses hormonal, psychological, and environmental influences that place women at an increased risk for overall weight concerns.

Willet, W. C. (1994). "Diet and Health: What Should We Eat?" *Science,* 264: 532, April 22. Explains what people should do to correct suboptimal diets.

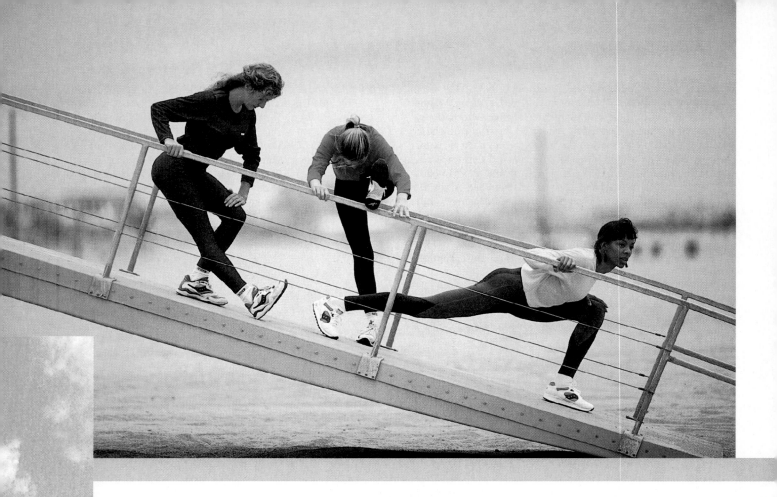

LEARNING OBJECTIVES

After reading this chapter you should be able to:

1. Describe the importance of physical fitness in your life.
2. Identify and briefly explain the physiological benefits of physical activity.
3. Identify and briefly explain the psychological benefits of physical activity.
4. Describe fitness and two means of achieving fitness.
5. Determine your target heart rate zone during exercise.
6. Compare and contrast aerobic training and strength training.
7. Identify several potential goals for an exercise program.
8. Identify four benefits of exercising and the exercise(s) that will help to achieve this benefit.
9. Identify the most common form of exercise abuse.

Achieving Physical Fitness

Our bodies were designed to be used. We were not made to sit behind desks or computers all day. But we often do. Life has become so filled with conveniences that we tend to sit back and "let our fingers do the walking." We slouch in a sofa and "channel surf" rather than getting up and changing the TV channel. We drive our car across campus or just a few blocks rather than walking the distance. We have become a nonphysical society.

However, fitness is not a fad; it's a way of life. To be physically fit you must eat right, make wise health decisions, and exercise. No one factor is more important than the other.

Regular physical activity helps:

- maintain normal blood pressure
- reduce blood pressure in people with hypertension
- maintain body weight within healthful limits
- prevent and alleviate chronic low-back pain
- provide greater energy reserves for work and recreation
- improve posture
- minimize stress
- shorten the recovery period from illness and injury

Physical fitness also increases your ability to overcome fatigue, cope effectively with stress, and fight off colds and other infections by boosting the immune system's defenses. Heart disease, obesity, and high blood pressure may not be an overriding concern today; however, your exercise and fitness behaviors today can affect your health in the future.

WHAT IS PHYSICAL ACTIVITY?

The health club and exercise equipment industries and the advertising and TV infomercials that support them can easily lead people to think that exercising for health requires considerable time, energy, money, and commitment. These investments can seem so overwhelming that some people forego exercising altogether.

Fortunately, physical activity does not require special equipment or spending a lot of money. Physical activity is anything you do when you are not sitting or lying down. Besides jogging, swimming, cycling, and aerobic dancing, physical activity includes yoga, tai chi ch'uan, martial arts training, gardening, and walking. For instance, regular walking strengthens muscles, increases aerobic capacity, clears and quiets the mind, reduces stress, expends calories, and is virtually injury-free. Other than appropriate shoes, walking requires no special clothing, equipment, or money, and it can be worked into a busy schedule. Instead of eating at breaks at work or between classes, you can walk to a job or class. Walk up stairs instead of using elevators. If you need to drive, park and walk the last ten minutes to your destination. Aerobic capacity can be increased by walking briskly enough to increase the heart rate (e.g., walking uphill or up stairs).

Once a commitment is made to an exercise program, other healthy behaviors often follow, such as improved eating habits and a reduction in heavy alcohol consumption. Such programs also may lessen stress so that undesirable stress-reducing behaviors such as cigarette smoking, overeating, or drug consumption are unnecessary.

If none of these points convinces you of the many benefits of exercise, think of it as setting aside time and attention for you. Many people feel overwhelmed by the demands of school, job, and family. Just taking a few hours a week to exercise can give you the chance to relax, reflect, and indulge your imagination.

Physiological Benefits of Physical Activity

Research shows that only moderate, not necessarily extensive exercise is sufficient for good health. For example, for both women and men, the chance of dying from heart disease, cancer, and several other diseases is greater for individuals with sedentary life-styles than those who engage in a daily brisk walk of 30 to 60 minutes (Curfman, 1993). Moderate regular exercise, lasting say 15 to 30 minutes, five times a week also has been found to improve health. In fact, high levels of exercise increase the risk of injuries.

CASE STUDY

Beginning Your Fitness Routine

Frank is a graduate student who took up jogging about a year ago because so many of his friends were runners, including his financée, Susan. Although he wasn't overweight, Frank nevertheless thought he could stand to have firmer muscles, especially in his thighs and abdomen. He began to run with Susan on the college track several times a week.

At first, Frank found running to be very hard. He had never before been physically active. In fact, he had always hated sports because of bad experiences in high school physical education classes. Also, he smoked about a pack of cigarettes a day, which severely limited his breathing ability. On the first day he could barely run one lap of the track—one-fourth of a mile—and without Susan's encouragement he probably would have quit right then. She agreed that one lap wasn't very far, but she reminded Frank that it would take time to undo the years of inactivity and smoking, and that he should have patience. Frank decided to give his new routine time to work, and set the goal of running one mile by the end of one month's running.

STUDENT REFLECTIONS

• What barriers was Frank up against after the first day of running, and how did he overcome them?
• Have you recently set an exercising goal for yourself? If so, what is it? How difficult has it been to reach this goal? How have you overcome the obstacles in your way of reaching this goal?

If you exercise regularly, your overall risk of a heart attack is about 50 percent less than if you are inactive and out of shape. With routine exercise you can reach a level of physical fitness comparable to an inactive person ten to twenty years younger. Regular exercise may also lower your cholesterol and blood pressure, and reduce the risk of diabetes.

Exercise increases the size of your coronary arteries and reduces clogging due to atherosclerosis (Chapter 14). Exercise also increases the efficiency of your blood's oxygen-carrying capacity and your muscles' uptake of oxygen.

Exercise has been linked to increased levels of high-density lipoprotein (good) cholesterol and decreases low-density lipoprotein (bad) cholesterol and triglyceride levels (Chapters 5 and 14). After exercising regularly for 6 to 12 months, lowered cholesterol levels can mean as much as a 30 percent reduction in the risk of coronary artery disease.

A recent study on physical fitness and the risk of death in both men and women revealed that those who had higher fitness levels had lower mortality rates from cardiovascular disease and cancer (Blair et al., 1989). Another study shows that low levels of both leisure-time physical activity and cardiorespiratory fitness are important coronary risk factors for men, suggesting that moderate-to-high-intensity activity may be needed to decrease the risk of heart disease (Lakka et al., 1994).

The Centers for Disease Control and Prevention and the American College of Sports Medicine issued a joint report recommending 30 minutes of physical activity at least five days a week (Pate et al., 1995). The report defines physical activity far more broadly than in the past. Anything from raking leaves to playing with the kids is considered a form of physical activity. Also you don't have to do all your activity at once. You can take the stairs instead of the elevator, walk instead of drive, do a little gardening, play touch football, scrub the kitchen floor or bathtub, and when the day is done you have been physically active (Table 7.1).

Psychological Benefits of Physical Activity

Regular physical activity can result in periods of relaxed concentration, characterized by reduced physical and psychic tensions, regular breathing rhythms, and increased self-awareness. This effect is often compared to meditation and is the aim of all Eastern body work, including Hatha yoga (Figure 7.1), t'ai chi ch'uan, and many martial arts practices. This effect also results from any physical activity in which one focuses the mind to produce a loss of self-consciousness through total concentration on various body movements. T'ai chi ch'uan instructor Sophia Delza (1961) explains:

> The goal of t'ai chi ch'uan is the achievement of health and tranquillity by means of a "way of movement," characterized by a technique of moving slowly and continuously, without strain, through a varied sequence of contrasting forms that create stable vitality with calmness, balances strength with flexibility, controlled energy with awareness. The calmness that comes from harmonious

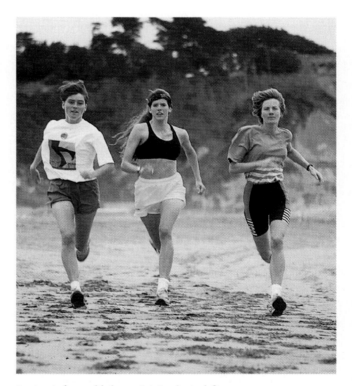

Jogging is fun and helps maintain physical fitness.

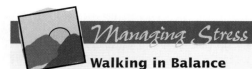

Walking in Balance

Native Americans have an expression that helps when trying to understand our place in the physical world. The expression "walking balance" means becoming aware of engaging your body with your mind in the natural world, feeling a sense of connectedness rather than separation from nature. Many people speak of a runner's high when they exercise, referring to the mind-body integration where there is also a sense of oneness. Walking in balance suggests that we combine the powers of the mind and body to become more aware of ourselves in our environment.

During your next workout try one of these exercises.

1. While you dress and warm up, think of a problem you are dealing with (e.g., term paper topic, roommate difficulties, finding a job). Identify the problem and name it. Once you begin exercising, think of the problem and at least three viable ways to solve it. The best type of activity for this thinking is rhythmical, like running, walking, or swimming. Before you shower and change, write down your solutions and put the paper aside for a few hours. Then refer back to it and see how clearing your mind by exercising can really help to find balance in everyday life issues.

2. While you dress and warm up, remind yourself that you are taking time away from your problems and worries—a mini-vacation, if you will, from daily responsibilities. The mission during this exercise period (preferably walking or running) is to see where you are exercising as if you are seeing it for the first time. Notice the trees, the birds, the clouds in the sky, and so on. Try to feel that you are a part of nature by noticing as much about the natural world as you can.

TABLE 7.1 Calories Burned by Everyday Activities

Burn an average of 200 calories a day by doing these activities and you will decrease your risk of disease and live longer, without ever going near a gym or treadmill.

Activities	Calories burned (10 minutes)	
	Women	Men
Walking fast	45	60
Painting	45	60
Weeding	45	60
Washing a car	45	60
Playing tag with a child	50	67
Mowing the lawn	55	73
Square dancing	55	73
Scrubbing floors	55	73
Hiking off-trail	60	80
Biking to work	60	80
Shoveling snow	60	80
Moving furniture	60	80
Walking upstairs	70	93
Cross-country skiing	80	106
Backpacking	80	106
Running upstairs	150	200

Note: Figures are for a 132-pound woman and a 176-pound man. All values are approximate and will vary from person to person.

physical activity and mental perception, and the composure that comes from deep feeling and comprehension are at the very heart of this exercise.

Several hypotheses have been offered to explain the psychological benefits of exercise:

1. Exercise becomes a means for autohypnosis, which increases the tendency for creative visualization.
2. Exercise increases the body's output of **epinephrine**, which produces feelings of euphoria.
3. Exercise changes the pattern of the secretion of brain neurotransmitters, particularly **norepinephrine**, which produces changes in mood.
4. Exercise increases the secretion of **endorphins** and **enkephalins**, hormone-like substances which can facilitate feelings of inner peace.

T E R M S

epinephrine: hormone secreted principally by the adrenal medulla with a wide variety of functions, such as stimulating the heart, making carbohydrates available in the liver and muscles, and releasing fat from fat cells

norepinephrine: hormone that has many of the same effects as epinephrine

endorphins and *enkephalins:* morphine-like substances that are secreted by the brain which mitigate pain; produced during strenuous exercise and childbirth

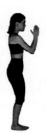

Position 1
Stand erect with your palms together in front of your chest. Inhale and exhale slowly and calmly.

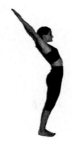

Position 2
Raise your arms high above your head. Inhale, and then slowly bend back, arching your back as far as it will go without discomfort.

Position 3
Bend forward from the waist, keeping your arms extended and your head between them. Keep your legs straight, but relax your head, neck, shoulders, and arms. Exhale.

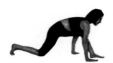

Position 4
Bend both knees and place your palms flat on the floor by the outer sides of your feet. Move your right leg back, touching the knee to the floor. Stretch your chin up toward the ceiling. Inhale.

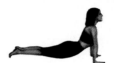

Position 5
Place both legs back, holding your body straight, supported only by your hands and toes. Continue to hold the breath taken at position 4.

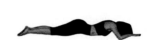

Position 6
Place your knees, chest, and forehead on the floor, but hold your abdomen up. Exhale.

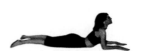

Position 7
Drop your hips to the floor and slowly raise your head and chest to arch the spine, supporting yourself on bent elbows. Point your chin to the ceiling while inhaling.

Position 8
Jacknife your hips toward the ceiling, keeping your legs straight and your heels on the floor. Exhale.

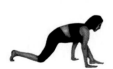

Position 9
Bring your left leg up between your hands while dropping the right knee to the floor. Raise your chin toward the ceiling and inhale.

Position 10
Bring your right foot forward so that both feet are together. Bend forward from the waist, keeping your legs straight and upper body relaxed. Try to touch your head to your knees. Exhale.

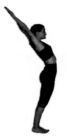

Position 11
Slowly straighten your body with arms extended over your head. When your arms are parallel to the floor, stretch toward the wall and slowly inhale. Straighten, then bend backward, arching your back.

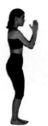

Position 12
Exhale while bringing your hands together in front of you. Close your eyes and relect on the sensations in your body.

FIGURE 7.1 The Sun Salute This Hatha yoga exercise is a series of twelve postures or asanas, intended to be done in one flowing routine. Each of the twelve postures is held three seconds. The entire routine should be done at least twice in succession, alternating the legs. The sun salute is an excellent way to stretch the body every morning or any time you may need to relax tense muscles and restore deep regular breathing.

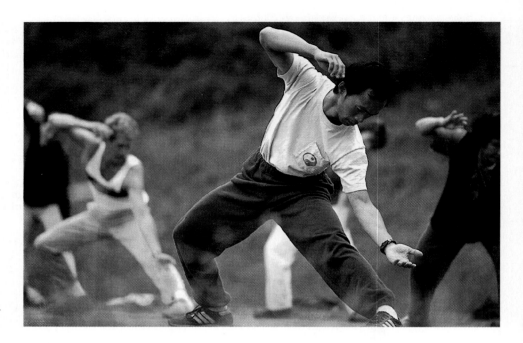

T'ai chi exercises help maintain physical fitness and mind-body harmony.

FITNESS AND CONDITIONING

A major outcome of regular physical activity is fitness. However, **fitness** is an elusive concept, not easily defined. For some, fitness means a lean, svelte, muscular body. For others, fitness means being in "top shape"— the capacity for strenuous exercise, such as hiking, swimming, running, or skiing long distances. But a lean,

muscular body or exceptional physical endurance probably represents the extreme of the concept of fitness. Most people do not have the time, physiological capacity, or desire to become models of fitness, however experts define it. Fortunately, nearly everyone can reach a level of fitness commensurate with good health, with life goals, and with individual capabilities. Sports physiologists usually define fitness as 1) adequate muscular strength and endurance to accomplish one's individual

Managing Stress

Stages of Exercise-Induced Relaxed Concentration

One means of managing everyday stress is through relaxed concentration. By following these stages you can help reduce such stress.

Stage 1: Paying Attention

At the beginning of an exercise session, you focus your mind on the activity and allow any thoughts that arise to pass out of your mind. When you notice them, simply say to yourself, "Oh, I have a thought," and bring yourself back to focusing on your activity.

Stage 2: Interested Attention

After a period of concentrating and letting go, you no longer have to concentrate on eliminating distractions and sense a flowing with the activity.

Stage 3: Absorbed Attention

Absorption with the activity is so great that it is very difficult for you to be distracted by what is going on around you. You may experience altered perceptions of space and time, and your mind may move through thoughts and images with-

out your direction. The experience can be dreamlike, except you are entirely awake and attentive.

Stage 4: Merger

You no longer are aware of any separation between you and what you are doing. The experience of union is complete: physical, mental, and spiritual. You attain a complete loss of self-consciousness, and even though you may be working your body very hard, mentally and spiritually you feel very calm.

Determine Your Fitness Index

The Harvard Step Test is a standardized measure of cardiorespiratory fitness. To carry out the Harvard Step Test, you need to be comfortably dressed (athletic clothes are best), you need a chair, stool, or bench 12–18 inches high, a stopwatch or clock with a second hand, a pencil and paper, and a metronome or some other method to produce a rhythmic 100–120 beats per minute, such as a recording of a march or some disco music. Once all this is assembled, you can begin.

1. Make a 15-second recording of your resting pulse and multiply by 4 to obtain your rate per minute.

2. Start the metronome or music; 120 beats per minute.

3. Step completely up on the bench with the left leg first, followed by your right leg, then step back down with the left leg first, followed by the right. The stepping should be done on a four-count: up-up-down-down; up-up-down-down . . .

4. Continue the exercise for 3 minutes unless you are over 30 years old and have been rather inactive for more than six months. In that case, do the test for only a minute or two, whichever you think you can do. If you are sure you cannot do the test for even a few seconds, don't.

5. When the 3 minutes of exercise are through, immediately take your pulse. Record the number of heartbeats between 15 and 30 seconds after exercising. Make another heart rate measurement between 60 and 75 seconds; another between 120 and 135 seconds; another between 180 and

195 seconds; another between 240 and 255 seconds; and a final measurement between 300 and 315 seconds.

6. Multiply each of the 15-second heart rates by 4 to give the beats per minute. Record your data on a graph.

7. Compute your Fitness Index: Add the per-minute heart rates for the first 3 minutes after exercise. Then divide that number into 30,000.

Fitness Index	Rating
Above 90	Excellent
80–89	Good
65–79	Average
55–64	Low Average
Below 55	Poor

Harvard Step Test Data Record

Time	Heartbeats per 15 seconds		Heartbeats per minute
At rest	‾‾‾	× 4 =	‾‾‾
15–30 sec.	‾‾‾	× 4 =	‾‾‾
60–75 sec.	‾‾‾	× 4 =	‾‾‾
120–135 sec.	‾‾‾	× 4 =	‾‾‾
180–195 sec.	‾‾‾	× 4 =	‾‾‾
240–255 sec.	‾‾‾	× 4 =	‾‾‾
300–315 sec.	‾‾‾	× 4 =	‾‾‾

goals, 2) reasonable joint flexibility, 3) an efficient cardiovascular system, and 4) body weight and percent body fat within the normal range.

Because modern life-styles do not require much physical movement, few adults in North America and northern Europe are naturally fit. Rather, achieving fitness requires a commitment of time and energy to regular activities other than school, work (particularly sedentary work), and family responsibilities. To be fit, one must engage in activities that challenge the mind and body beyond what is required by a sedentary life-style.

There are a wide variety of conditioning programs or training regimens to improve fitness, but they tend to fall into two major categories: **aerobic training**, which increases the body's ability to utilize oxygen and improves endurance, and **strength training**, which enhances the size and strength of particular muscles and body regions.

Aerobic Training

Aerobic exercise involves stimulating heart and lungs for a period sufficient to produce beneficial changes in the body. The main objective of aerobic exercise is to increase the amount of oxygen that the body can process within a given time (aerobic capacity). Changes in physiology resulting from aerobic exercise are collectively called the **training effect**. Inducing the training effect

> ### T E R M S
>
> *fitness:* the extent to which the body can respond to the demands of physical effort
>
> *aerobic training:* exercise that increases the body's capacity to utilize oxygen
>
> *strength training:* the use of resistance to increase one's ability to exert or resist force for the purpose of improving performance
>
> *training effect:* beneficial physiological changes as a result of exercise

involves exercising so that heart rate increases to between 60 and 80 percent of its theoretical maximum.

Three to four days of exercise per week is sufficient to produce a training effect. Two days per week may suffice for people already in good condition. One day a week does little to increase aerobic capacity and may increase the chances for injury. Exercise on more than five days a week does little to increase aerobic capacity. It may help expend calories, but it also makes one susceptible to injuries.

To obtain optimal training benefits you should exercise within your training heart rate zone. The simplest method of computing this is to subtract your age from 220 to determine your maximum heart rate (MHR) and then multiply by 60 percent and 80 percent. While you exercise, your heart rate per minute should fall between these two values. For a 21-year-old, the target heart rate range would be 149–174 (Table 7.2).

To measure your exercise heart rate, you should stop about five minutes into the aerobic part of your exercise to check your heart rate. Your heart rate should gradually increase during your warm-up, reach maximum level during your aerobic exercise, and gradually decrease during your cool-down exercises (Figure 7.2). Many activities can provide aerobic conditioning, including walking, running, bicycling, swimming, cross-country skiing, rowing, basketball, racquetball, and soccer.

Strength Training

Strength training involves repetitively moving muscles against resistance, commonly applied by weights such as

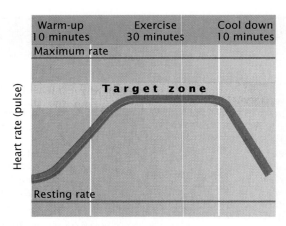

FIGURE 7.2 Heart Rate Pattern for a Typical Exercise Routine A diagram of your heart rate during warm-up, aerobic exercise, and cool-down.
Source: A. L. Thygerson, *Fitness and Health* (Boston: Jones and Bartlett, 1989), p. 38.

barbells, dumbbells, and exercise machines, but also by simple pushing against an immovable object (**isometric training**). A stronger body is better able to combat fatigue; in sports, strength can improve athletic performance and reduce the likelihood of injury. For some, "pumping iron" helps release stress-induced muscle tensions.

Many people are drawn to strength training for cosmetic reasons. In their desire to look good, individuals may not receive adequate instruction in strength-training methods and may injure themselves. It is essential to build strength gradually with proper techniques.

TABLE 7.2 Maximum and Target Heart Rates Predicted from Age By using the formula, 220 minus age, multiplied by .60 and by .80, you can determine your target heart rate range. Or by using this table take your pulse for 15 seconds immediately after exercising, and multiply by four. If your heart rate is in the target range, you have obtained optimal training benefits. If you are below this target range, you need to step up your activity. If you are above the maximum, you need to take it easier during your workouts and gradually increase intensity.

Age (in years)	Predicted maximum heart rate (in beats per minute)	Target heart rate range (in beats per minute)
20–24	200	149–174
25–29	200	129–174
30–34	194	145–170
35–39	188	142–165
40–44	182	138–160
45–49	176	134–155
50–54	171	131–151
55–59	165	128–146
60–64	159	124–142
60+	153	121–137

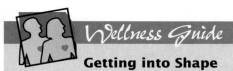

Getting into Shape

Undertake a program to increase aerobic conditioning by following these guidelines:

1. Frequency: you should exercise three to five times a week.
2. Intensity: you should exercise within 60–85 percent of your exercise heart rate.
3. Duration: you should exercise within your target zone for 20–60 minutes each time.
4. Type of exercise: appropriate exercises are rhythmic, are continuous, and utilize the large muscles of the legs and hips. Such exercises include walking, jogging, bicycling, swimming, cross-country skiing, and aerobic dancing.
5. Warm up and cool down. It is

The pattern of the preferred exercise session is shown in the following figure:

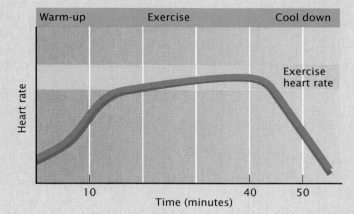

optimal to raise the body's core temperature about 1–3 degrees by doing the warm up and stretching activities before the aerobic workout. Following the aerobic workout you should slow your heart rate and cool down for 30–60 minutes. Optimal time to stretch is when the muscles are warmed (i.e., after aerobic exercise).

Compared to most aerobic exercise, strength training produces only a modest improvement in cardiovascular fitness. The time spent exercising is insufficient to increase the heart rate long enough to produce a training effect. The energy expended during strength training is about 4 calories per minute, about the same as for walking or swimming at a comfortable pace.

A common myth associated with strength training is that consuming high-protein foods and special vitamin supplements will increase muscle mass. This assumption is incorrect. Muscle tissue responds to the demands of work, not food. In a progressive strength-training regime, sufficient protein to build new muscle tissue will be obtained in a well-balanced diet. Excess protein and vitamins are simply excreted.

The current fashion of lean, muscular bodies has led some athletes and bodybuilders to take **anabolic steroids** (testosterone and testosterone-like substances) and growth hormones to increase muscle mass and stamina. Regular use of these drugs can, in both women and men, produce deepening of the voice, altered patterns of body hair growth, hair loss, liver damage, and infertility. Abuse of growth hormone can cause aberrations in metabolism and in bone structure. Sharing needles used to inject these drugs can also transmit the AIDS virus.

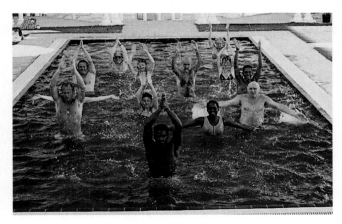

Water aerobics is a safe and enjoyable form of exercise for people of all shapes and ages.

MAKING PHYSICAL ACTIVITY A PRIORITY

For many people, the mere mention of physical activity conjures up unpleasant images of painfully boring exercises or rough competitive sports whose proposed beneficial effects on health and character development rarely seem to meet the promises made by enthusiastic players and coaches.

T E R M S

isometric training: another term for strength training
anabolic steroids: synthetic male hormones used to increase muscle size and strength

Twenty Nifty Facts about Your Muscles and Strength Training

1. The human body has more than 650 muscles.

2. Skeletal muscle is the body's largest tissue, accounting for about 45 percent of body weight in men and 36 percent in women.

3. Each muscle fiber is thinner than a human hair and can support up to 1000 times its own weight.

4. There are three distinct types of muscle: cardiac, smooth, and skeletal.

5. Cardiac muscle, found only in the heart, is responsible for the pumping action of the heart.

6. Smooth muscle surrounds nearly all of the body's organs.

7. Skeletal muscles are anchored to bones; when the muscle contracts and pulls on them, movement is initiated.

8. Proper training of a person's muscles has numerous health benefits, one of those being improving bone mineral density (reducing risk for osteoporosis).

9. The American College of Sports Medicine recommends a strength training program that includes a minimum of one set (8–12 reps) of eight to ten exercises that condition the major muscle groups, done at least two days per week.

10. By the age of 65, individuals who haven't engaged in exercise on a regular basis may incur a decrease in their muscular strength by as much as 80 percent.

11. Proper strength training poses little risk to a pregnant woman or her fetus, and it may be beneficial in helping to compensate for the postural adjustments that typically occur during pregnancy.

12. The level of strength of an individual is influenced by many factors, including genetics, type of training, hormone levels, body proportions, etc.

13. The optimal exercise program for controlling weight is one that combines aerobic conditioning and strength training.

14. Two types of sore muscles occur: acute and delayed. Acute soreness occurs during and immediately following exercise. Delayed soreness occurs well after the exercise is completed, often peaking in intensity within one to three days following unusually vigorous or unaccustomed exercise. Both can be prevented by proper training techniques.

15. Women can and should get strong: the benefits are just as important as for men, if not more so.

16. No pain . . . No gain . . . Nonsense! A sensible training program does not have to be painful. Uncomfortable perhaps, but not painful. Pain is your body telling you that you're doing too much.

17. Muscular dystrophy is a broad term applied to a group of nine disorders that literally robs a muscle of its power. They are characterized by weakness and wasting of skeletal muscles. Atrophy is a term used to describe a "shrinking" of muscle size, due to loss of use of the muscle.

18. Your muscles are attached to your bones by connective tissue called tendons. The tendons do not have as great a blood supply as muscles do, therefore, they take longer to heal if injured.

19. The basic methods of strength training can be grouped into three classifications: Isometric (you contract a muscle, but the involved joints don't move), Isotonic (contraction of a muscle with movement), and Isokinetic (a constant state of speed of contraction . . . this requires special equipment).

20. Extra protein will not enhance your effort to build larger muscles. Your body cannot store extra protein. If you consume more protein than your body needs the extra protein is excreted or converted to fat.

Source: Adapted from: "Nifty Facts about Your Muscles and Strength Training," *Fitness Management Magazine* (June, 1994).

Part of the idea of body work is to incorporate a playful or joyful activity into your life for its own sake. Americans are highly product-oriented; we tend to value what we do on the basis of outcome. With body work, the *process of doing* is itself the reward. So choose activities that you will enjoy. If you like to be around people, join an exercise class or organize some friends to work out with you. After you have accomplished a difficult task, reward yourself with praise. And remember, body work, even active sports, does not have to involve competition unless you want it to.

Choosing the Right Exercise

Once you have decided to begin exercising, it is tempting to do what others are doing (e.g., roller blading, jogging, racquetball, etc.). But before you go out and buy expensive running shoes and outfit or that new racquetball racquet, you must decide what exercise is right for you. First you may want to ask yourself what are your goals in an exercise program. Some goals may be: stress reduction; a healthy heart; weight control or weight reduction; greater strength; building muscles; greater stamina; or relaxation.

After you have determined your goals, you want to make sure that the activities you adopt go along with your goals. You may choose swimming as your main exercise. Swimming is good for weight maintenance, but not for body building. Other important factors when selecting your exercise of choice are: motivation; realistic expectations; comfort; convenience; and cost factors.

To be sure you are committed to an exercise class, take a trial class before signing up for several months. Make sure you enjoy the exercise. You should be able to enjoy working out and getting in shape at the same time. The more you enjoy what you are doing, the more likely you will stay motivated and continue to exercise and meet your fitness goals.

If you have never exercised or are not in good shape, do not expect to see results overnight. Achieving physical fitness takes time and commitment on your part. Changes will most likely be seen in the first month;

Wellness Guide

A Plan for Fitness

Some guidelines to keep in mind when incorporating any kind of physical activity into your life include:

1. **Have a plan.** Before beginning any body work program, you need to develop a plan and to commit yourself to it for a reasonable amount of time. To make a body work plan that will help you achieve your personal goals, you can consult a high school or college coach, attend a class at a YMCA or similar organization, or follow the plan in one of the "how to" books that have been written for almost every body work activity.

2. **Get a physical checkup.** If you have been inactive for many months or have concerns about your body's ability to perform at the level you would like, you may want to have a physician check you over.

3. **Accomplish goals.** The goal of any body work program is attainment of complete mind-body

harmony. This can be done by progressively attaining higher and higher goals. It is customary in our culture to measure progress by "how far" and "how fast." Such goals might be suitable for competitive athletes, but they are unsuitable for people who engage in body work activities for the purpose of receiving greater enjoyment from living. For most of us, personal goals based on such questions as "Does this level of activity make me feel good?" or "Does this help me toward my goal of losing weight?" make more sense than blind adherence to a stopwatch.

4. **Progress slowly.** Slow, deliberate progress give you the opportunity to integrate your body work activity into your normal life routine. Begin slowly; don't impulsively try to run a long distance the first day.

5. **Warm up and cool down.** All body work activity should be preceded by a brief period of

stretching, breathing, and relaxation to prepare your mind and body to receive the utmost benefit and pleasure from body work. This is a good time to focus attention on how your body feels. When you have finished your body work activity, it is a good idea to let your body cool down slowly. If you have been involved in strenuous aerobic exercise, slowly reduce the pace of your activity until your heart rate and breathing return to almost normal. By slowly reducing your activity level you also help prevent muscle cramps that sometimes occur when strenuous activity is suddenly stopped. You can prevent later muscle stiffness by doing a few stretching exercises to loosen the muscles that have worked hard during exercise. While cooling down, try to focus your attention on the sensations that your body work has brought you.

however, achieving total physical fitness will take months of constant exercise. Determine realistic expectations for yourself.

For some, a fitness club or recreation center can be intimidating if everyone else is in good shape. Some find more informal "shaping-up" classes better for them. However, for some people being surrounded by a lot of physically fit people in a fitness club is motivation. Some may wish to stay at home and exercise. You have to decide what environment you feel comfortable exercising in.

Make sure whatever activity you choose is convenient. Don't choose one that requires you to drive 30 minutes, because before you know it you will be saying "it's too far." Choose an activity within a convenient distance.

Decide how much money you can afford to spend. Remember to include the cost of equipment, proper clothing, and transportation. Look into exercise classes that allow you to pay as you go. Also, some fitness clubs will allow you to join for a one-month trial program. Both options are good if you are still unsure about which exercise program is right for you.

> *People through finding something beautiful think something else unbeautiful through finding one man fit judge another unfit.*
> Anonymous

Types of Beneficial Exercises

Different kinds of exercises provide different benefits. After you have determined goal(s) and which exercise is right for you, you must make sure the exercise provides the type of benefit you wish to achieve. There are exercises that help relieve stress, exercises for your heart, exercises for weight control, muscles, strength, and power and **endurance**, and exercises for **flexibility**. You may choose one or more of these exercises. You decide.

Exercising for Stress Reduction Exercise is a form of physical stress; one of its effects is to cancel the negative stresses that accumulate daily. Almost any exercise where you work out for at least one-half hour is effective. Pleasant surroundings also help in relieving stress. Swimming is soothing and relaxing for many people; others enjoy jogging.

Exercising for Your Heart Aerobic exercises are considered the most effective in terms of increasing heart capacity. Thirty minutes is what most studies believe is the magic number to produce maximum benefits from aerobics (this 30 minutes does not include the **warm-up** or **cool-down**).

Exercising to Maintain Weight When maintaining or trying to lose weight, you need to combine exercising with a balanced, nutritious diet. The net effect is to take in fewer calories and to use more calories through exercising (Wellness Guide, Energy Expenditures for Certain Activities, Chapter 6). To lose one pound you must expend 3500 calories. To expend 1350 calories you would need to walk for three hours at 5 mph. So when choosing an exercise for weight control, keep in mind the amount of time it takes to burn 3500 calories or lose one pound of fat.

Exercising for Strength Body building generally means weight training with light barbells, dumbbells, and weight machines. With strength training you use many of the same techniques as those for building muscles. The difference between muscle building and strength building is that less weight and more repetitions are used with strength building. In other words, instead of lifting 100 pounds ten times, you might lift 10-pound weights fifty times: the same amount of body work builds strength not bulk muscle.

Exercising for Endurance and Power Endurance is your body's ability to withstand stress over a period of time and power is your muscle's ability to perform over an extended period of time. Endurance is built by gradually increasing the length of time of high activity, whereas power is achieved by short bursts of high activity followed by rest periods. Sports not suitable for strength and endurance are softball or golf.

Exercising for Flexibility Calisthenics and yoga are great for flexibility. Keep in mind that flexibility should not be confused with fitness; flexibility is part of fitness, but flexibility exercises alone do not make a person physically fit. Almost all sports and exercises will increase flexibility.

T E R M S

endurance: the ability to work out over a period of time without fatigue

flexibility: the ability of a joint to move through its range of motion

warm-up: low-intensity exercise done before full-effort physical activity in order to improve muscle and joint performance, prevent injury, reinforce motor skills, and maximize blood flow to the muscles and heart

cool-down: the period in which an individual performs light or mild exercise immediately following competition or a training session; the primary purpose is to speed the removal of lactic acid from the muscles and allow the body to gradually return to a resting state

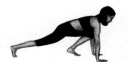

Ski stretch
Hold 30 seconds.

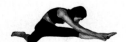

Hurdle stretch
Keep knee straight. Hold 30 seconds.

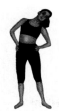

Trunk circling
Take 5 seconds to circle clockwise; relax. Repeat in counterclockwise direction. Do each direction at least twice.

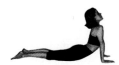

Cobra posture
Lie face down with hands under shoulders. With forehead on floor, slowly raise forehead, then nose, then chin, then shoulders, upper and middle back. Take 10 seconds to complete extension; hold extension 5 seconds. Relax.

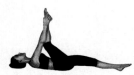

Hamstring stretch I
Slowly raise one leg to an angle of 90°, keeping the knee as straight as possible. Grasp the raised ankle with both hands and gently increase the stretch. Hold 5 seconds; relax. Repeat for other leg. Do each leg twice.

Hamstring stretch II
Bend at the waist holding onto toes or ankles. Attempt to place head on knees, hold 30 or 60 seconds.

Abdominal stretch I
Lie on back with arms in "T" position. Raise both legs to 90°. Lower legs to touch right hand, hold for 5 seconds. Raise legs to starting position, hold 5 seconds. Lower legs to touch left hand, hold 5 seconds. Raise legs, hold 5 seconds. Lower legs and relax. Repeat entire exercise.

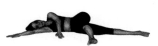

Abdominal stretch II
Lie on back with arms in "T" position. Raise left leg to 90°, keeping knee straight. Lower left leg across the body to touch right hand; hold 5 seconds. Raise leg to 90° position, then relax. Repeat for right leg, crossing over to touch left hand. Do exercise twice.

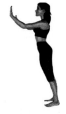

Gastrocnemius stretch
Lean against a wall at an angle of between 45° to 60°. Keeping heels on the floor, lean closer to the wall. Hold 15 seconds. Relax.

Groin stretch
Assume stretch position and pull ankles toward the body to increase the stretch on groin muscles.

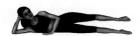

Abductor stretch
Lift leg to the point of resistance, hold 30 seconds; relax.

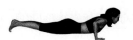

Push-ups
Do at least 30.

FIGURE 7.3 Flexibility Exercises That Can Be Used in Warming Up A good flexibility program for running is: 1) walk or run easily for one-quarter of a mile, 2) hamstring stretch I, 3) abdominal stretch I, 4) abductor stretch, 5) groin stretch, 6) hamstring stretch II, 7) push-ups, 8) hurdle stretch, 9) gastrocnemius stretch. A good flexibility program for tennis and other racket sports is: 1) trunk circling, 2) hamstring stretch II, 3) groin stretch, 4) abdominal stretch II, 5) push-ups, 6) gastrocnemius stretch, 7) ski stretch, 8) run in place for one minute, 9) jump in place for one minute, 10) practice strokes—ten each of forehand, backhand, and overhead.

Don't ask your muscles to do more than they can. Relishing the pain of overexertion—"going for the burn"—is dangerous. This pain is the body's message that something is wrong, not that the exerciser is lazy.

If you want to increase your performance, build muscle strength slowly, following a supervised regime. Also, pre- and postactivity stretching helps to prevent damage to muscles and joints. Injuries are more likely if equip-

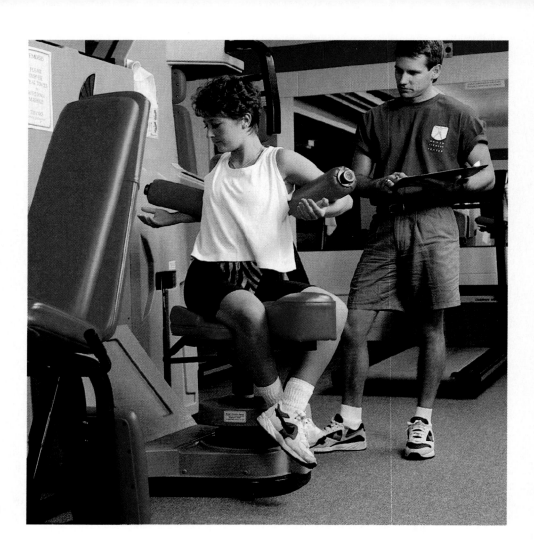

Weight-lifting machines build muscle strength.

Exploring Your Health

Determine Your Flexibility Index

Body flexibility is a fundamental aspect of feeling good and keeping your body young. Use this simple YMCA test to determine your degree of body flexibility, and continue to use it to determine your progress in becoming more limber. You can consult exercise and yoga books to find exercises that will help you improve your flexibility.

1. Warm up with some stretching before the test.
2. Sit on the floor with your legs extended and feet a few inches apart.
3. With a piece of adhesive tape, mark the place where your heels touch the floor. Your heels should touch the near edge of the tape.
4. Place a yardstick on the floor between your legs and parallel to them. The beginning of the yardstick should be closest to you and the 15-inch mark should align with the near edge of the tape.

5. Slowly reach with both hands as far forward as possible. Touch your fingers to the yardstick to determine the distance reached. Do not jerk to increase your distance—this may cause damage to your leg muscles.
6. Repeat the exercise two or three times and record your best score.

Inches reached		Rating
Men	Women	
22–23	24–27	Excellent
20–21	21–23	Good
14–19	16–20	Average
12–13	13–16	Fair
0–11	0–12	Poor

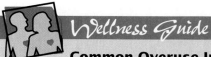

Common Overuse Injuries

Strain	Commonly referred to as "pulled muscles" or "pulled tendons." Caused by overstretching, tearing, or ripping of a muscle and/or its tendon	low-grade strain of a muscle-tendon unit	Sprain	Overstretching or tearing of ligaments
Tendonitis	Inflammation of a tendon caused by chronic,	Bursitis — Inflammation of the lubricating sac that surrounds a joint (*bursa*) caused by repeated low-grade strain of the joint's supporting tissues	Blisters	Fluid-filled swellings on the skin caused by undue friction from the rubbing of skin against shoes, clothing, and equipment

ment such as special shoes, weights, and various kinds of apparatus are improperly used or are in disrepair.

Most people participate in physical activity because 1) they want to have fun, 2) they want to gain a sense of accomplishment by doing something well, and 3) they want to feel physically and psychologically better. While pursuing these goals, no one wants to be hurt. It turns out that maximizing the have fun/do well/feel good aspects of exercise and minimizing the potential for injury go together. Physical activity is most satisfying when you are totally absorbed in it, when your body responds readily to your commands, when you run or play with confidence, and when your equipment and conditions are optimal. Take sports seriously enough to enjoy them, while minimizing the likelihood of injuries.

Walking and Health

If jogging, swimming, cycling, aerobic dancing, and other strenuous activities aren't for you, try walking. Regular walking contributes many of the health benefits of other activities. And walking has advantages that other activities do not: other than appropriate shoes, no special clothing or equipment is required and walking can be fit easily into a busy schedule.

Walking contributes the most to health when it is done regularly (about four times a week) for about an hour. How strenuous the walk should be depends on the desires and physical abilities of the walker. Most of the benefits can be derived by walking between two and four miles per hour. Aerobic capacity can be increased by walking briskly enough to increase the heart rate.

EXERCISE ABUSE

Although few would argue that being fashionably healthy and attractive are desirable goals, many people are so zealous in pursuing these goals that they harm themselves. For example, some individuals place higher priority on running or other fitness activities than they do on work, family, interpersonal relationships, and even their own health. Some are unwilling to stop exercising (even for a day!) to attend to other matters in life or to allow an exercise injury to heal properly. In their attempts to attain the "perfect body," a large number of women exercise and lose weight to such extremes that they stop menstruating **(athletic amenorrhea)** or develop anorexia or bulimia (Chapter 6).

The most common form of exercise abuse is exercising a body part or the entire body beyond its biological limit to the point of injury. Such injuries are referred to as *overuse syndromes*. It is estimated that between 25 and 50 percent of athletes visiting sports medicine clinics have sustained an overuse injury. Commonly, overuse injuries affect the muscles, tendons, ligaments, joints, and skin, which are constructed of fibrous bands of protein. These fibers can be torn if they are overloaded, as when lifting a heavy weight or running at top speed, or when forced to perform when fatigued. Damage can also occur by repeated small injuries that lead over time to a more serious problem. The common causes of overuse injuries are excessive exercising, faulty technique, and poor equipment.

All bodies are not anatomically capable of the same degree of physical exertion, especially the high performance exhibited by marathon runners or triathletes. The architecture of the body, the alignment of the legs, the capacity of the lungs, the size and strength of the bones and muscles, and other anatomical factors set limits on an individual's physical ability. Few people have the biological endowment to perform at championship levels. Physical activity can be much more enjoyable when you respect, accept, and appreciate your body's biological limits.

T E R M
athletic amenorrhea: irregular or cessation of menstruation due to excessive participation in athletics

HEALTH IN REVIEW

- Physical fitness is not a fad; it is a way of life. Being physically active helps us to be both physiologically and psychologically well.

- Physiological benefits from physical activity include increased efficiency and strength of heart, lungs, and muscles; more effective weight control; reduced fatigue and increased energy; higher level of immunity; lower blood cholesterol levels; improved sugar metabolism; more normal blood pressure; and improved posture.

- Psychological benefits from physical activity include: reduced fatigue and better sleep patterns; more positive mental outlook; less stress; release of tension and anxiety; and improved self-image and self-confidence.

- Fitness is the extent to which the body can respond to the demands of physical effort. Major fitness categories are aerobic training and strength training.

- Aerobic conditioning can be achieved through walking, running, bicycling, swimming, cross-country skiing, rowing, basketball, racquetball, and soccer.

- Aerobic exercise strengthens the heart. Strength training produces only a modest improvement in cardiovascular fitness, but builds muscle strength unlike aerobic conditioning.

- Goals for an exercise program include stress reduction; healthy heart; weight control or maintenance; greater strength; building muscles; greater stamina; or relaxation.

- The most common form of exercise abuse is exercising a body part or the entire body beyond its biological limit to the point of injury. Common injuries include strain, tendonitis, bursitis, sprain, and blisters.

REFERENCES

Blair, S. N., H. W. Kohl, R. S. Paffenbarger, D. G. Clark, K. H. Cooper, and L. W. Gibbons (1989). "Physical Fitness and All Cause Mortality: A Prospective Study of Healthy Men and Women." *Journal of the American Medical Association*, 262(17): 2395–2401.

Curfman, G. D. (1993). "The Health Benefits of Exercise: A Critical Appraisal." *The New England Journal of Medicine*, 528(8): 574–575.

Delza, S. (1961). *T'ai Chi Ch'uan*. New York: Cornerstone Library.

Lakka, T. A., J. M. Venalainen, R. Rauramaa, R. Salonen, J. Tuomilheto, and J. T. Salonen (1994). "Relation of Leisure-Time Physical Activity and Cardiorespiratory Fitness to the Risk of Acute Myocardial Infarction in Men." *The New England Journal of Medicine*, 330(22): 1549–1554.

Pate, R. R., et al. (1995). "Physical Activity and Public Health: A Recommendation from the Centers for Disease Control and Prevention and The American College of Sports Medicine." *Journal of the American Medical Association*, 273(5): 402–407.

SUGGESTED READINGS

Applewhite, M. P., G. R. Jansen, M. M. Marriot, and V. M. Breen (1994). "The Effects of Diet on Performance—An Initial Review." *Journal of the American Medical Association*, 271(2): 98–99. A review of the literature to determine the effects of diet on performance. The article discusses The Institute of Medicine's Food and Nutrition Board's review of diet and performance.

Jaret, P., and V. Fahey (1994). "The Old Advice: Work Out. The New Advice: Walk the Dog and Take the Stairs." *Health*, 8(5): 62. Article discusses how the definition of physical activity and exercise has changed. It includes anything from raking the leaves to roughhousing with the kids.

Roos, R. (1994). "Is Clinton's Plan Soft on Exercise?" *The Physician and Sportsmedicine*, 22(2): 31–33. A discussion on health-care reform and its relationship with physical fitness and disease prevention.

Tucker, S. H. (1994). "Getting Fit with a Personal Trainer." *Black Enterprise*, 24(8): 91–92. Personal trainers can assess personal fitness needs and prescribe a specific program for you.

The University of California, Berkeley Wellness Letter (1994). "Dynamic Yard Workout," 10(12): 6. Explains both the physical and psychological benefits of working in the yard.

Welty, E. (1994). "Fitness Through the Ages: Stay in Shape—in Your 20s, 30s, 40s, and Beyond." *American Health*, 13(6): 74. Describes how people can maintain a good level of fitness as they age.

PART three

Building Healthy Relationships

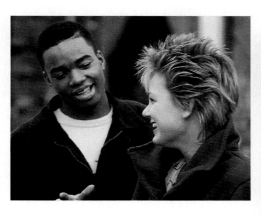

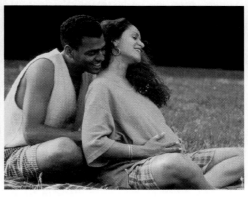

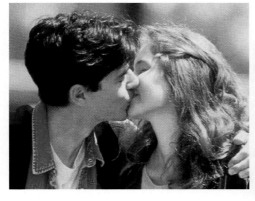

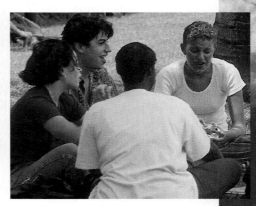

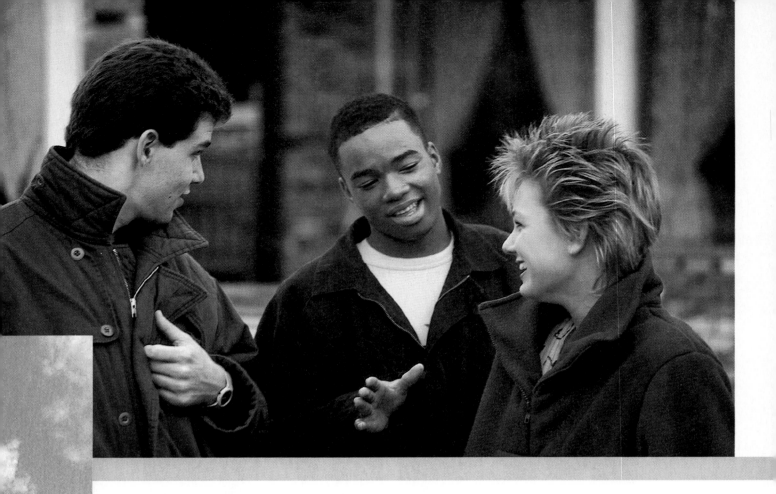

LEARNING OBJECTIVES

After reading this chapter you should be able to:

1. Define the terms sex, sexuality, sexual, menopause, masturbation, gender role, gender identity, sexual orientation, heterosexual, homosexual, bisexual.

2. Compare and contrast traditional gender roles for males and females.

3. Describe the male reproductive system.

4. Describe the female reproductive system.

5. Explain the menstrual cycle.

6. Explain the sexual response cycle.

7. Identify and discuss several different sexual difficulties.

8. Describe an intimate relationship.

9. Identify and describe the essential components of good communication.

8

Developing Healthy Intimate and Sexual Relationships

S exuality represents a truly holistic aspect of living, for it involves the simultaneous expression of mind, body, and spirit—the whole self. Although it is common to find sexuality represented in advertising and other media as having to do solely with physical gratification, most people are aware that sexuality involves much more than the stimulation of the body's sex organs. Sexuality involves thoughts, feelings, and identity. Sexuality is also a powerful form of communication between people.

From the standpoint of personal health, sexuality is an area over which you have considerable individual control. You choose when and with whom you wish to have sex, and which feelings you wish to express in sexual ways. With some fundamental knowledge of sexual biology, you can conduct your sexual life responsibly, thus avoiding unnecessary illness and exercising a choice of whether and when to have children. This chapter introduces the topic of sexuality and discusses the nature of the sexual self and of sexual expression.

DEFINING SEX AND SEXUALITY

Sex

Sex can refer to 1) an individual's classification as male or female as determined by the presence of certain anatomical and physiological characteristics, 2) a set of behaviors, and 3) the experience of erotic pleasure.

At the most fundamental biological level, **sex** refers to the mating of two anatomically distinct individuals, a male and a female, each of which manufactures specific cells, or **gametes**, which fuse to become the first cell of a new individual. To facilitate the fusion process (called **fertilization**), males and females of a species possess specific organs and display certain behaviors that are intended to bring about the union of gametes.

Often the word *sex* is used to denote aspects of an individual's personal characteristics that are thought to derive from her or his biological classification. Thus, the biological property of "femaleness" is associated with the social quality of "femininity," and the biological property of "maleness" is associated with the social quality of "masculinity." Although most modern dictionaries still define sex as having to do with personality characteristics, this concept is more accurately referred to as *gender* to distinguish its origins in culture rather than biology.

Besides biological classification, sex is also associated with certain behaviors that are defined as **sexual**. These activities usually involve touching in various ways certain anatomical regions of the body, such as the genitalia and breasts, and sexual intercourse.

Sex can also mean erotic pleasure, a certain kind of experience with unique and identifiable qualities that distinguish it from other kinds of pleasure, such as the satisfaction of hunger or the enjoyment of music. A variety of circumstances and events has the potential to activate the erotic pleasure centers, including certain kinds of tactile stimulation (e.g., touching, kissing) of certain body regions (e.g., mouth, breasts, genitals); certain kinds of visual, olfactory, and auditory stimulation; and fantasy. Potentially erotic stimuli become actual erotic stimuli when other centers in the brain interpret them as erotic. That is why not every touch, kiss, or potentially sexual situation is erotically arousing.

Identical behaviors may be erotically pleasurable in some instances but not in others. Kissing a child or a grandparent can be very different from kissing a spouse. The touching of the genitals in a medical examination is not the same as the touching of the genitals when expressing love and affection to a sexual partner.

Defining sex in terms of what is experienced makes no reference to any particular outcome other than the experience itself. Sex is not defined by certain genital responses, such as erection of the penis, nor is it defined in terms of a variety of changes in physiology, such as increased heart rate, blood pressure, and muscle tension. Nor is sex defined in terms of experiencing orgasm. Although it is true that sexual pleasure is usually associated with certain genital and physiological responses and sometimes orgasm, these outcomes are not sufficient to define sex because they can occur without the experience of erotic pleasure.

Defining sex in terms of the experience makes no reference to interaction with any particular person. Sexual

pleasure can be experienced by oneself through masturbation or fantasy. It can be experienced with someone of the same or the other sex. It can be experienced in a variety of social contexts.

Sexuality

Sexuality, as distinct from sex, consists of the aspects of a person's sense of self that are used to create sexual experiences. Another term for sexuality is the sexual self, which has several dimensions:

1. The *physical dimension* refers to any region of the body to which an individual gives sexual meaning, including the organs and organ systems that one employs to create erotic experiences (e.g., the skin, genitals). It also includes the physical features that define oneself to oneself and others as a sexual being.
2. The *psychological dimension* refers to one's emotions and one's conscious and unconscious beliefs that guide the interpretation of experience. This aspect of sexuality generates strategies for actions that are intended to satisfy one's wants and needs.
3. The *social dimension* refers to sexual attitudes and behaviors that affect an individual's interactions with members of the social groups to which she or he belongs.
4. The *orientation dimension* refers to the tendency to feel most "naturally" sexually attracted to, and the ability to emotionally bond with, members of a particular gender. About 85 to 90 percent of Americans are oriented to members of the opposite sex; the rest of the population orients to individuals of either sex (bisexuals) or, more often, exclusively to members of the same sex (homosexuals). Individuals do not choose their sexual orientation; it develops as a fundamental aspect of a person's personality. Scientific studies have failed to uncover genetic, hormonal, metabolic, or psychological mechanisms underlying sexual orientation.
5. The *development dimension* is the evolution of oneself throughout a lifetime. This evolution includes one's body, belief systems, and the ways sex is employed to create and maintain intimacy.
6. The *skill dimension* speaks to the physical and social skills that affect how well one meets one's sexual wants and needs.

GENDER IDENTITY AND GENDER ROLE

Although anatomy and physiology explain the biological bases of human sexuality, most people's sexual experiences also involve beliefs, thoughts, feelings, and social

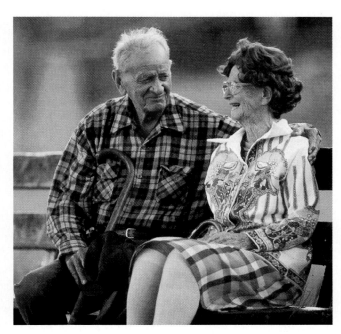

Intimacy is a basic human need at every age.

behaviors. How individuals come to think and behave sexually is almost entirely a product of what they learn as children about the kinds of behaviors that are expected of members of one sex or the other. Studies of psychosexual development indicate that the development of gender identity and the subsequent expression of sex-specific behaviors begins with the sex typing of newborn infants (Hampson and Hampson, 1961; Money and Ehrhardt, 1972). When a child is born, almost the first thing noticed is its biological sex as determined by the appearance of its external genitals. If the infant is born with a penis, those attending the birth will exclaim "It's a boy!" Similarly, "It's a girl!" follows the observation of a newborn's female external genitals.

Having been sex typed at birth, the infant is thereafter treated by adults in a manner they think is appropriate for a child of that sex, and eventually the infant incorporates into his or her self-image the awareness of being a male or a female. This awareness is called **gender identity,** and gender-specific behaviors are referred to as the **gender role.**

By about the age of two, a child's gender identity is fixed for life. How the child comes to act on the self-knowledge of its maleness or femaleness depends on the interrelationship of a variety of factors. Children learn attitudes and behaviors by modeling after adults such as parents, teachers, celebrities, and fictional characters, and they are also trained by reward and punishment. Whatever the sources of information and influence, children learn early which attitudes and behaviors are appropriate for males and which are appropriate for females. By the age of three, children are capable of cit-

ing a long list of behaviors that are expected of one sex and not the other.

Exactly which attitudes and behaviors are deemed appropriate for both sexes depends on the culture in which people live. In some societies, gender role behaviors are strictly defined, and little deviance from the stereotype is allowed. Our culture possesses a set of traditional stereotypic gender-role expectations that include economic role, dominance or submissiveness in social relationships, responsibilities for home and child care, mode of dress, personal appearance, and mode of expression of emotions.

DEFINING SEXUAL ORIENTATION

A person's **sexual orientation** is his or her attraction toward and interest in members of one or both genders. A **heterosexual** is a person who is attracted to someone of the opposite gender. A **homosexual** is attracted to people of the same gender. A **bisexual** is someone who is attracted to members of both genders. The terms heterosexual and homosexual do not imply normalcy or a type of sexual act; they simply describe a person's preference with regard to one gender or another. The concept of sexual orientation and identity has evolved over time, as views of masculinity and femininity have changed. Today we view masculinity and femininity as a

T E R M S

sex: has several definitions: 1) an individual's classification as male or female based on anatomical characteristics; 2) a set of behaviors; 3) the experience of erotic pleasure

gametes: sex cells, either sperm or ova, that fuse at fertilization; gametes carry a complete set of genetic information from each parent that is passed on to the child

fertilization: the fusion of a sperm cell and an ovum

sexual: characterized by or having sex; opposed to asexual

sexuality: a person's sense of self that is used to create sexual experiences

gender identity: awareness of being male or female

gender role: gender specific behaviors

sexual orientation: attraction toward and interest in members of one or both genders

heterosexual: someone who is attracted to people of the opposite gender

homosexual: someone who is attracted to people of the same gender

bisexual: someone who is attracted to members of both genders

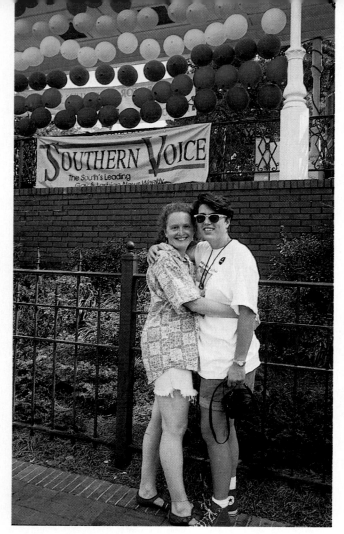

Intimate relationships between couples of the same sex are increasingly accepted in our society.

looked at behavior. Later research has shown the greater complexity of human sexuality.

A recent study of sexual practices in the United States tried to address the question, "how many people are homosexual?" (Lauman, Gagnon, Michael, and Michaels, 1994). Researchers asked a sample across the United States to self-report whether they considered themselves homosexual or heterosexual. About 1.4 percent of the women and 2.8 percent of the men reported same-gender sexuality. However, 6.2 percent of the heterosexual men reported being somewhat attracted to men, and 4.5 percent indicated the idea of sex with another man was appealing. Of the women 5.6 percent reported finding the idea of sex with a woman appealing, and 4.4 percent reported sexual attraction to women.

The researchers concluded: "Put simply, we contend there is no single answer to questions about the prevalence of homosexuality. Rather, homosexuality is a complex, multidimensional phenomenon whose salient features are related to one another in highly contingent and diverse ways."

SEXUAL BIOLOGY

One of the fundamental roles of sexuality is biological reproduction. The reproductive role of the male is to produce reproductively capable sperm and to deposit them in the female reproductive tract during sexual intercourse. The reproductive role of the female is to provide reproductively capable eggs, called **ova,** and to provide a safe, nutrient-filled environment in which the fetus develops for the nine months of pregnancy.

Male or female reproductive biology is genetically determined at conception. The fusion of an X-bearing egg with the X-bearing sperm produces a female (XX); fusion with the Y-bearing sperm produces a male (XY). Once the chromosome pattern is set, the development of the sexual anatomy follows from the precise instructions of the genes contained in the chromosomes. A particular

set of characteristics, which vary among both men and women.

Alfred Kinsey, a sex researcher in the mid-1900s, developed a seven-category sexual behavior rating scale to study the sexual behaviors of people (Figure 8.1). The scale ranges from 0 to 6, with 6 representing exclusively homosexual behavior, and 0 representing exclusively heterosexual behavior. Values 1 through 5 showed predominately heterosexual or homosexual behavior, respectively, but also indicate some of the other type of sexual behavior.

While this continuum represented the best approach at the time for classifying sexual behavior, it did not adequately reflect the sexual interests and needs of individuals. The scale indicated the type of sexual activity in which people participated, but it did not measure a person's degree of heterosexual or homosexual attractions. It did not take into account that some persons might be having heterosexual experiences, but really were attracted to others of the same gender. This scale only

$T \quad E \quad R \quad M \quad S$

ova: a term for female eggs (singular: ovum)

secondary sex characteristics: anatomical features appearing at puberty that distinguish males from females

ovaries: a pair of almond-shaped organs in the female abdomen that produces egg cells (ova) and female sex hormones

fallopian tubes: a pair of tube-like structures that transport ova from the ovaries to the uterus and that are the usual site of fertilization

uterus: the female organ in which a fetus develops

vagina: a woman's organ of copulation and the exit pathway for the fetus at birth

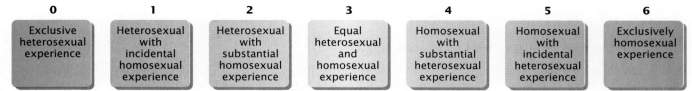

0	1	2	3	4	5	6
Exclusive heterosexual experience	Heterosexual with incidental homosexual experience	Heterosexual with substantial homosexual experience	Equal heterosexual and homosexual experience	Homosexual with substantial heterosexual experience	Homosexual with incidental heterosexual experience	Exclusively homosexual experience

FIGURE 8.1 Kinsey Scale of Sexual Behavior Kinsey believed that some people did not fit into strict same-gender or opposite-gender sexual behavior. His scale of sexual behavior reflects this belief.

chromosome set determines whether the as yet immature sex cells that appear at about the fifth week of development will eventually produce sperm or ova. The sex chromosomes determine whether the fetus will ultimately develop the male sex organs—testes, sperm ducts, semen-producing glands, and penis; or the female organs—ovaries, fallopian tubes, uterus, vagina, and external female genitals.

The genetic determination of sexual anatomy also specifies the pattern of male or female steroid hormone production, which in turn affects the **secondary sex characteristics** that distinguish adult males and females: the extent and distribution of facial and body hair; body build and stature; and appearance of breasts (Figure 8.2).

Female Sexual Anatomy

A woman's internal sexual organs consist of two **ovaries**, which lie on either side of the abdominal cavity, the **fallopian tubes**, the **uterus**, and the **vagina**; together these structures make up a specialized tube that goes from each ovary to the outside of the body (Figure 8.3). The function of the ovaries is to produce fertilizable ova as

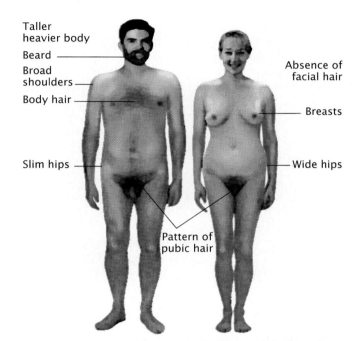

FIGURE 8.2 Secondary Sexual Characteristics of Men and Women

Health Update

Sex and the Brain

Simon LeVay, a neurobiologist at the Salk Institute in La Jolla, California, reported in 1991 that he found a minute but measurable difference in the brain between homosexual and heterosexual men. To be precise, a tiny cell cluster known as the third interstitial nucleus of the anterior hypothalamus, or INAH3, is "deeply involved in regulating male-typical sexual behavior."

Because you can't work on the brains of living humans, LeVay dissected and studied the brains of 41 people (19 homosexual men, 16 heterosexual men, and 6 heterosexual women) who had died. LeVay discovered that homosexual and heterosexual men did differ in a key area of the brain that controlled sexual behavior. Heterosexual men had INAH3 clusters almost twice as large as homosexual men.

Since LeVay published these data in *Science,* his personal and professional life have been dissected. LeVay is gay and like many other gays he lost his partner to AIDS. Does LeVay worry that his own research may be misused? His

response: "If scientists find a gay gene, and I think they will, it opens the possibility—even a probability—of misuse." If a gay gene is discovered, he foresees discriminatory employment tests and fetal tests followed by abortions of potentially gay children. Despite the possible misuse of research, LeVay believes the quest to understand the biology of sexual orientation should continue.

Source: D. Nimmons, "Sex and the Brain," *Discover* (March, 1994): 64.

Lifting the Gay Ban in the Military

The military is presumed to attract a relatively homogenous group of young men and women regarding cultural values and perspectives. The boundaries of acceptable behavior and values are more narrowly drawn in military compared to civilian life because of the more uniform social composition of the military.

Such views are reflected in the Department of Defense policy that bans homosexuals from military service. According to the current department directive, as revised on February 12, 1986:

Homosexuality is incompatible with military service . . . The

presence of such members adversely affects the ability of the Military Services to maintain discipline, good order, and morale; to foster mutual trust and confidence among service-members; to ensure the integrity of the system of rank and command; to facilitate assignment of worldwide deployment of service members who must frequently live and work under close conditions affording minimal privacy; to recruit and retain members of the Military Services; to maintain public acceptability of military services; and to prevent breaches of security.

Today, the military has instituted a "Don't ask, Don't tell" informal policy. This informal, unwritten policy basically implies that the military won't ask your sexual orientation and you won't tell them your sexual orientation. If you decide to tell the military that your orientation is homosexual, the military will take action to remove you from service. This policy continues to stigmatize the gay community and denies full rights to gays who serve in the military.

STUDENT REFLECTIONS

- Do you believe gays and lesbians should be allowed to join the military services? Why or why not?
- Should the Department of Defense's official policy be revised to protect the rights of gay military personnel? Why or why not?

well as sex hormones, which control the development of the female body type, maintain normal female sexual physiology, and help regulate the course of a normal pregnancy. The fallopian tubes gather and transport the ova that are released from the ovaries (about one each month). The two fallopian tubes connect to the uterus, an organ about the size of a woman's fist, which is situated just behind the pelvic bone and the bladder (Figure 8.4). The uterus is part of the passageway for sperm as they move from the vagina to the fallopian tubes to effect

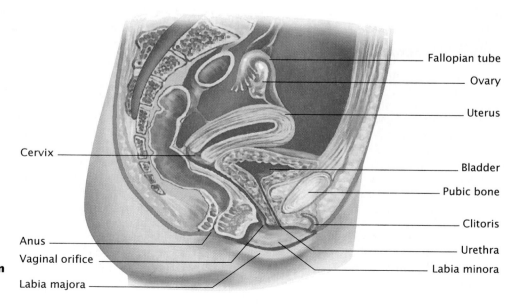

Fallopian tube
Ovary
Uterus
Bladder
Pubic bone
Clitoris
Urethra
Labia minora

Cervix
Anus
Vaginal orifice
Labia majora

FIGURE 8.3 A Cross-section of the Female Sexual-Reproductive System

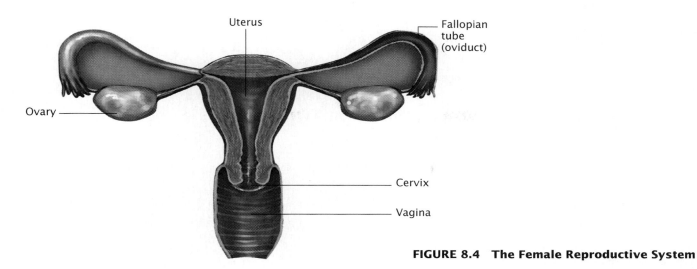

FIGURE 8.4   The Female Reproductive System

fertilization; after fertilization, it provides the environment in which the fetus grows. It is the inner lining of the uterus that is shed each month in menstruation.

The lower part of the uterus is the **cervix,** and the cavity of the uterus is connected to the vagina by means of a small opening called the cervical os. The cervix secretes mucus, which changes in consistency depending on the phase of the menstrual cycle. Some women learn to estimate the time of **ovulation** (ovum release) by examining their cervical mucus.

The vagina is a hollow tube that leads from the cervix to the outside of the body. Normally, the vaginal tube is rather narrow, but it can readily widen to accommodate the penis during intercourse, a tampon during menstruation, the passage of a baby during childbirth, or a pelvic examination. The vagina possesses a unique physiology that is maintained by the secretions that continually emanate from the vaginal walls. These secretions help control the growth of microorganisms that normally

inhabit the vagina, and they also help to cleanse the vagina. Because the vagina is a self-cleansing organ, it is usually unnecessary to employ any extraordinary cleansing measures, such as douching. Very often douching merely upsets the natural chemical balance of the vagina and increases the risk of developing vaginal infections, called **vaginitis.**

A woman's external genitals (Figure 8.5) consist of two pairs of fleshy folds that surround the opening of the vagina and the **clitoris.** The smaller, inner pair of folds are called the **labia minora,** and the larger, outer pair are called the **labia majora.** The clitoris, a highly sensitive sexual organ, is situated above the vaginal opening.

The opening of the **urethra,** which is the exit tube for urine, is located at the vaginal region just below the clitoris. The fact that the urethra is only about ½ inch long and located so close to the vagina makes it susceptible to irritation and infection, called **urethritis,** characterized by a burning sensation during urination and usually by the frequent urge to urinate. Occasionally, bacteria introduced into the urethra migrate the short distance to the bladder and produce a bladder infection called **cystitis.** The symptoms of cystitis are similar to those of urethritis.

The most frequent causes of urethritis and cystitis are irritation from sexual intercourse and the introduction of bacteria from the anal region into the vaginal region and into the urethra. To prevent urethritis and cystitis, care should be taken not to introduce anal bacteria into the vaginal region during sexual activity (manually or with the penis). It is recommended that a woman urinate immediately after having sex, wear absorbent cotton underpants or underpants with a cotton crotch, and wipe the urethra in the front-to-back direction after urinating.

A mild case of urethritis or cystitis can be helped by drinking a lot of fluids to wash the bacteria from the uri-

T E R M S

cervix: the lower and narrow end of the uterus

ovulation: release of an egg (ovum) from the ovary

vaginitis: an infection of the vagina

clitoris: small, sensitive organ located in front of the vaginal opening; center of sexual pleasuring

labia minora: a pair of fleshy folds that cover the vagina

labia majora: a pair of fleshy folds that cover the labia minora

urethra: a tube that carries urine from the bladder to the outside

urethritis: an irritation or infection of the urethra caused by bacteria

cystitis: inflammation of the bladder

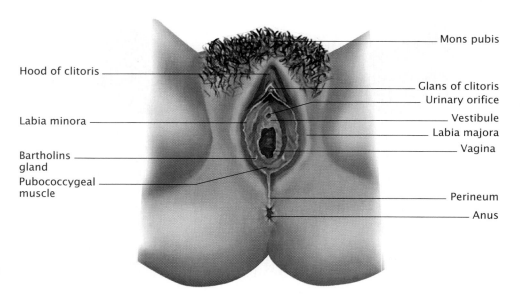

Mons pubis

Hood of clitoris

Glans of clitoris
Urinary orifice
Vestibule

Labia minora

Labia majora

Vagina

Bartholins
gland
Pubococcygeal
muscle

Perineum

Anus

FIGURE 8.5 The External Female Sexual-Reproductive Organs

nary tract and by making the urine more acidic, either by high doses of vitamin C or acidic fruit juices. It is also advisable not to drink alcohol and ingest caffeine or spices, for these substances may irritate an already inflamed urinary tract. If pain is severe or if there is blood in the urine, a physician should be consulted.

In addition to the primary sex organs, women have secondary sex characteristics including the **breasts.** The breasts consist of a network of milk glands and milk ducts embedded in fatty tissue. The variation in breast size among women is due to differing amounts of fatty tissue within the breasts. There is little variation among women in the amount of milk-producing tissue; thus, a woman's ability to breast feed is unrelated to the size of her breasts.

The breasts are supplied with numerous nerve endings, which are important in the delivery of milk to a nursing baby. These nerves also make the breast highly sensitive to touch, and many women find certain forms of tactile stimulation to be sexually pleasurable. Sexual arousal, tactile stimulation, and cold temperatures can cause small muscles in the nipples to contract, resulting in erection of the nipples.

The Menstrual Cycle

Each month or so women usually produce one ovum that is able to be fertilized. During each period of this ovum production—the menstrual cycle—a woman's body undergoes several hormonally induced changes that prepare her body for pregnancy if the ovum is fertilized. One of these changes involves the thickening of the lining of the uterus, the **endometrium,** in order to support the first stages of pregnancy. In addition, certain blood vessels in the uterus increase in size. Their role is to bring the maternal nutrients to the fetus via the placenta if pregnancy occurs. If the ovum is not fertilized,

the endometrium and the blood vessels within it are shed. This produces a loss of about 25 to 60 cc (about two or three tablespoons) of blood and tissue debris, which leaves the body through the vagina over the course of 3 to 6 days. This discharge is **menstruation.**

The length and regularity of the menstrual cycle vary from woman to woman. Most women experience cycles of approximately 28 days, with cycle lengths between 24 and 35 days being the most common. Shorter and longer cycles are possible, but they are regarded as irregular cycles. Irregular cycles can occur monthly, with the number of days between menstruations varying from cycle to cycle. Irregular cycles are common when females first begin to menstruate and also when they stop producing ova later in life.

The menstrual cycle is controlled by a number of hormones (Figure 8.6). Hormones from the hypothalamus in the brain, called **releasing factors,** are secreted and influence the release of other hormones from the pituitary gland. The pituitary hormones are called

T E R M S

breasts: secondary sex characteristics; a network of milk glands and ducts in fatty tissue

endometrium: the inner lining of the uterus

menstruation: the regular sloughing of the uterine lining via the vagina

releasing factors: hormones produced in the hypothalamus that control the release of hormones from the pituitary gland

gonadotropins: pituitary hormones; induce production of the hormones estrogen and progesterone in the ovary

menopause: the cessation of menstruation in mid-life

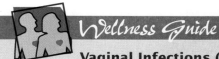

Vaginal Infections (Vaginitis)

Vaginitis is any irritation or inflammation of the vagina. Because one of the most common causes of vaginitis is infestation with the yeast *Candida albicans,* vaginitis is often referred to as a yeast infection. Other types of vaginitis are the result of infection with either *Trichomonas vaginalis,* a protozoan, or the bacterium *Hemophilus vaginalis,* or *Gardnerella vaginalis* as it is now called.

Regardless of the particular organism involved, the symptoms of vaginitis are usually a burning sensation, annoying itching in the vaginal region, and discharge from the vagina. This discharge is not to be confused with the normal vaginal discharge, *leukorrhea,* which is composed of sloughed-off vaginal cells and cervical mucus. The discharge of vaginitis is usually gray, yellow, or greenish in color. It may resemble cottage cheese or it may be foamy, and it may have an unpleasant smell.

Normally, the vagina is populated by bacteria and other microorganisms, including yeast. The relative proportion of these organisms is kept in check by the competition between them for nutrients and a suitable place to live. If something upsets the internal environment of the vagina, however, one or another of the organisms can take advantage of the change, their population can increase, and vaginitis results. Many factors can upset the vaginal environment and predispose a woman to vaginitis. Among them are antibiotics, which kill many of the bacteria in the vagina and therefore provide yeast and "Trich" a chance to thrive; pregnancy and birth control pills, which change the internal chemical composition of the vagina; tight clothing, hot and humid weather, and underwear made of synthetic fabrics, all of which increase the moisture in the vaginal region, thus improving the environment for the growth of microorganisms; obesity, diabetes, and other dietary metabolic problems; and having intercourse with someone carrying the infectious microorganisms.

Vaginitis can be treated by specific drugs after the infecting organism has been identified. Women can try to prevent vaginitis by

1. Wearing cotton underpants or at least pants with a cotton crotch.

2. Avoiding tight undergarments, girdles, and pantyhose, especially when wearing tight jeans or pants.

3. Avoiding routine douching, feminine hygiene sprays, and bath products that contain chemicals that irritate the vagina.

4. Avoiding oral contraceptives if vaginitis is a persistent problem and seeking medical advice.

5. Wiping from front to back after urinating to prevent spreading bacteria from the rectum to the vagina.

---

gonadotropins; their function is to induce the production of the hormones estrogen and progesterone in the ovary. These ovarian hormones circulate throughout the woman's bloodstream and induce changes necessary to support pregnancy. The preparation of the lining of the uterus for pregnancy is but one function of estrogen and progesterone (Table 8.1). The menstrual cycle is regulated so that if fertilization does not occur, the hormonal support of tissue growth in the uterus stops, and the uterine tissue is lost in a menstrual discharge.

Menopause

At some point in a woman's life she will stop menstruating altogether. This is **menopause,** otherwise known as "the change of life." It is a time when the ovaries stop producing ova and the ovaries' production of hormones wanes considerably. Therefore, the two principal biological consequences of menopause are that a woman no longer is capable of becoming pregnant and that her body may undergo some changes from the diminished production of ovarian hormones. The average age at which menopause occurs is about 50. The age at which menopause occurs may be affected by hereditary, social, and nutritional factors. There is no relation between the age at which menopause occurs and the age at which a woman first begins to menstruate.

Some people see menopause as a time of rapid degeneration of a woman's body and the onset of emotional instability. They also may have the mistaken idea that because menopause signifies the end of reproductive capacity that it necessarily means the end of a woman's sexual interest and abilities. None of these beliefs has a factual basis, but what is believed may have a powerful effect on changes in physiology. We have ample evidence all around us that age is no barrier to living a fulfilled and enjoyable life. Women who accept menopause as a natural part of their life process need not slow down. They can continue to be active and healthy and can continue to enjoy sex.

Male Sexual Anatomy

The principal reproductive role of male sexual organs is to make numerous viable sperm cells and to deliver them into the female reproductive tract during sexual

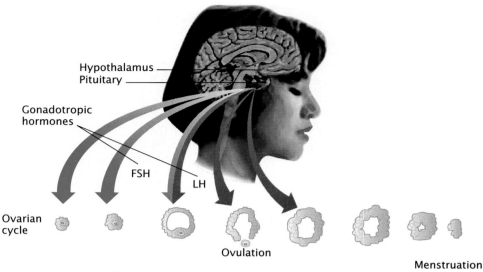

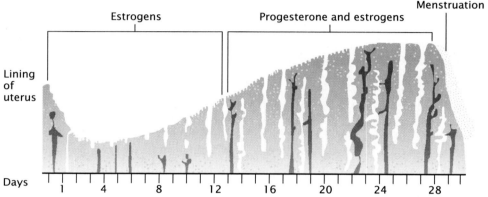

FIGURE 8.6 Hormonal Control of the Menstrual Cycle Hormones from the hypothalamus control the release of hormones from the pituitary gland, which in turn regulates the production of the ovum and sex hormones from the ovaries. Note how the rise and fall of the hormones is related to the building up and sloughing off of the uterine lining.

intercourse. The male sexual and reproductive system consists of two **testes**, the sites of sperm and sex hormone production; a series of connected sperm ducts that originate at the testes, course through the pelvis, and terminate at the urethra of the penis; glands that produce seminal fluid; and the **penis**, the organ of **copulation** (Figure 8.7).

The testes are located in a flesh-covered sac, the **scrotum**, that hangs outside the man's body. In the embryo, the testes develop inside the body, but just before birth they descend into the scrotum. Inside the scrotum the testes are kept at a temperature a few degrees cooler than the internal body temperature, a condition that is apparently necessary for the production of reproductively

TABLE 8.1 Functions of Estrogen and Progesterone

Organ	Effect of estrogen	Effect of progesterone
Ovary	Increases sensitivity to gonadotropins Stimulates growth in ovarian cells	
Fallopian tubes	Increases motility and secretion	Decreases motility
Uterus	Stimulates proliferation of blood vessels Increases size of muscle cells Stimulates production of cervical mucus	Increases secretory activity of endometrium Decreases contractions in uterine muscle Causes changes in viscosity of cervical mucus
Vagina	Stimulates growth and changes in vaginal cells Maintains vaginal secretions	Causes changes in cells of vagina
Breasts	Stimulates growth and development of nipple and milk ducts	
Secondary sex characteristics	Stimulates feminine pattern of hair growth Stimulates feminine pattern of fat distribution	

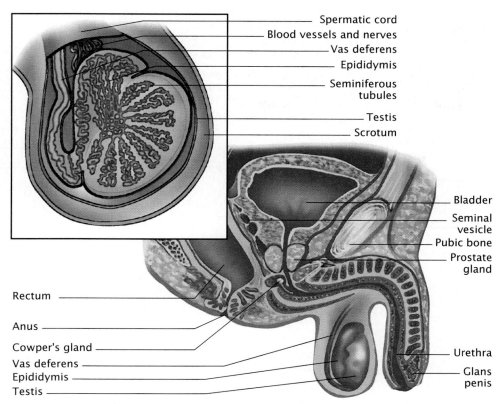

Spermatic cord
Blood vessels and nerves
Vas deferens
Epididymis
Seminiferous tubules
Testis
Scrotum

Bladder
Seminal vesicle
Pubic bone
Prostate gland

Rectum

Anus

Cowper's gland
Vas deferens
Epididymis
Testis

Urethra
Glans penis

FIGURE 8.7 The Male Reproductive Organs

capable sperm. One testis is usually a little higher than the other.

When a man ejaculates, sperm are propelled through the sperm ducts and out of the penis by contractions of the smooth muscles that line the ducts and the muscles of the pelvis. As they move out of the male body, the sperm mix with secretions of seminal fluid from the seminal vesicles, prostate gland, and Cowper's glands to form semen. The semen, which is the gelatinous milky fluid emitted at ejaculation, contains a mixture of about 300 million sperm cells and about 3 to 6 ml of seminal fluid. The seminal fluid contributes 95 percent or more of the entire volume of semen.

The penis is normally soft, but when a man becomes sexually aroused, its internal tissues fill with blood and the penis enlarges and becomes erect. All men are born with a fold of skin, the foreskin, that covers the end of the penis. For centuries, Jewish and Moslem families have surgically removed the foreskin from male children for religious reasons. This procedure is called circumcision. Although there is no clear medical indication that circumcision is beneficial, removal of the foreskin does eliminate the buildup of smegma, a white, cheesy substance that can accumulate under the foreskin. The belief that circumcision leads to an increase in sexual arousal because it exposes the glans, and the related belief that circumcision produces an inability to delay ejaculation are myths. For most men, circumcision has no effect on sexual arousal and sexual activity.

T E R M S

testes: a pair of male reproductive organs that produce sperm cells and male sex hormones

penis: the male's organ of copulation and urination

copulation: sexual intercourse

scrotum: the sac of skin that contains the testes

seminal vesicles: sac-like structures that secrete a fluid that activates the sperm

prostate gland: gland at the base of the bladder providing seminal fluid

Cowper's glands: small glands secreting drops of alkalinizing fluid into the urethra

semen: a whitish, creamy fluid containing sperm

foreskin: a fold of skin over the end of the penis

circumcision: a surgical procedure to remove the foreskin from the penis

smegma: a white, cheesy substance that accumulates under the foreskin of the penis

SEXUAL AROUSAL AND RESPONSE

Sexual arousal and response are often thought of in terms of genital stimulation, genital responses, and orgasm. But in reality, sexual experience is holistic

What Is Sexually Arousing to You?

What is sexually arousing to you? On the scale below indicate whether you are extremely aroused 5) by the activity or not aroused at all 1) by the activity. Numbers between 1 and 5 indicate sexual arousal between extremely aroused and not aroused at all.

There are no right or wrong answers. Share your responses with your partner. Did they know this about you? Have you ever communicated these desires?

	Extremely aroused		Neutral		Not aroused at all
	5	4	3	2	1
A shower with your partner	5	4	3	2	1
Fantasizing	5	4	3	2	1
French kissing	5	4	3	2	1
Oral sex	5	4	3	2	1
Petting	5	4	3	2	1
Partner undressing	5	4	3	2	1
Manual genital stimulation	5	4	3	2	1
Manual breast stimulation	5	4	3	2	1
Romantic music	5	4	3	2	1
Talking about sex	5	4	3	2	1
Talking dirty	5	4	3	2	1
Using a vibrator	5	4	3	2	1
Watching pornographic movie/video	5	4	3	2	1
When your partner is sexually assertive	5	4	3	2	1
Your partner's clothing					

involving one's body, mind, emotions, spirit, and relationship with the partner.

Sexual Arousal

Because sex is a whole-person experience, sexual interaction involves a change from a nonerotic to an erotic state of being, one in which erotic experience—for whatever reasons—is expected and sought. The change from a nonerotic to an erotic state usually involves these elements:

1. *Sexual interest:* openness to erotic arousal
2. *Desire or motivation:* energizing oneself toward creating an erotic experience
3. *Decision:* offering or accepting invitations for sex
4. *Participation:* engaging in behaviors that produce erotic arousal

Studies indicate that in both men and women sexual interest is influenced strongly and possibly maintained completely by androgens (principally testos-

terone), which are hormones manufactured in the testes, ovaries, and adrenal glands. For example, men with very low levels of androgen because of illness or disease usually report a loss of interest in sex. However, testosterone-replacement therapy in such men tends to restore sexual interest.

Similarly, women who have had their ovaries and adrenal glands surgically removed for treatment of cervical or breast cancer (to prevent production of hormones that might stimulate the growth of the cancer) often report a loss of interest in sex. Interest can be restored with replacement testosterone, but not estrogen or progesterone. Also, women's sexual interest does not change predictably when estrogen levels fall during the menstrual cycle or after menopause.

Although in our society people are expected to be highly and frequently interested in sex, in reality the desire for sexual activity varies among individuals and couples, changes over time, and is influenced by interpersonal and psychological factors. For example, many couples report a higher degree of sexual desire at the beginning of their relationship than after the relationship has matured. Alternatively, couples who have been together for many years may experience an increase in sexual interest when the childrearing phase of the family life cycle is completed. Various physical and psychological situations can affect sexual interest as well. For example, many women report a transient loss of sexual interest during the first few weeks after childbirth. And depression is almost always associated with loss of interest in sex.

Having sexual desire does not necessarily mean that a person will behave sexually. Human sexual behavior is not "reflexive"; activity does not occur automatically whenever one feels "horny" or one is presented with a sexual opportunity. Instead, sexual activity is the result of a decision (except in instances of sexual coercion and assault) that is based on desire to conform to social norms, personal values, and physical and psychological needs.

Creating a sexual experience involves two kinds of decision. The first concerns context, that is, the social situation in which sexual activity takes place. Societies have rules and norms that govern sexual activity. Individuals are not permitted to have sex with just anyone or in any social setting. For example, most people have sex only in the bedroom, not in the living room or kitchen or dining room.

The second type of decision concerns participation in a sexual episode. Even in a situation or relationship in which sexual activity is acceptable, and opportunities to have sex are present, a person can decide "yes," "no," "not yet," or "maybe" whenever a sexual opportunity occurs. The decision is made by evaluating how one feels physically and emotionally at the time, one's personal criteria for being sexual within the presenting situation, and one's expectation of how having sex at that time will affect one's self-esteem and the relationship.

There is no formula for creating sexual arousal. Everyone has preferences. In situations and circumstances that they deem appropriate for sex, most people respond sexually to being touched in certain ways. Certain regions of the body are highly sexually sensitive in nearly all people. These are the classic erogenous zones—the genitals, the breasts, the anus, the lips, the inner thighs, and the mouth.

The Sexual Response Cycle

When a person becomes sexually aroused, the brain and nervous system prepare the body for sexual activity. Impulses from the brain are transmitted by the spinal nerves to various parts of the body and cause physiolog-

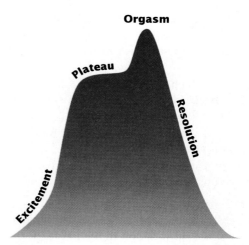

FIGURE 8.8   The Sexual Response Cycle as Identified by Masters and Johnson

ical changes. These changes include: the tightening of many skeletal muscles (**myotonia**); changes in the pattern of blood flow or **vasocongestion** (especially an increase in blood flow in the pelvis); increases in heart rate, blood pressure, and respiratory rate; increase in the general level of excitement; and increase in erotic feelings.

Increased pelvic blood flow in the male produces erection of the penis. The penis enlarges because the spongy tissues within it fill with blood. In the female, increased pelvic blood flow produces lubrication of the vagina and swelling of the clitoris and vaginal lips. Vaginal lubrication is produced by the release of fluids from the walls of the vagina. Swelling of the clitoris and vaginal lips is due to the filling with blood of spongy tissues within them. In some women the changes in blood flow due to sexual arousal also produces a swelling of the breasts.

Regardless of the type of sexual stimulation, the physiological response in both men and women is similar and follows a pattern called the **sexual response cycle**, which consists of four phases as identified by Masters and Johnson (Figure 8.8):

- *Phase 1:* Excitement in which the person experiences sexual arousal from any source and the body responds

> *The image of myself which I try to create in my own mind in order that I may love myself is very different from the image which I try to create in the minds of others in order that they may love me.*
>
> W. H. Auden,
> poet

T E R M S

myotonia: muscle tension

vasocongestion: the engorgement of blood vessels in particular body parts in response to sexual arousal

sexual response cycle: the physiological response in both men and women as described in four phases with specific changes: erection of the penis in males; vaginal lubrication and swelling of the clitoris and genitalia in females; and sex flush in both males and females.

- *Phase 2:* Plateau in which the physiological changes of the excitement phase level off, although subjective feelings of sexual arousal may increase.
- *Phase 3:* Orgasm in which the tensions that build up during excitement and plateau are released.
- *Phase 4:* Resolution in which the body returns to the physiologically nonstimulated state.

There is considerable variation in the extent and duration of the sexual response cycle among individuals of either sex. There is even variation in the nature of the response in the same person, for each sexual encounter is different. Masters and Johnson (1966) found more variation in the sexual response cycle for women than for men.

Orgasm

When sexual arousal builds to a certain point, the associated sexual tensions are released in an **orgasm.** The orgasmic response in both women and men frequently is associated with rhythmic contractions of the pelvic muscles; tightening of the muscles of the face, hands, and feet; and feelings of pleasure. Most commonly, men ejaculate during orgasm, although it is possible for males to experience orgasm without ejaculation and vice versa. The media have perpetuated the myth that during male or female orgasm, bells ring, the earth shakes, lights flash, and moans and groans are elicited. But often orgasms are quiet.

Orgasmic experiences vary greatly from person to person and from one encounter to another. For all persons there are "big orgasms" and "little orgasms" depending on the level of arousal. Sometimes, if a person is not sufficiently aroused, or too tired, tense or ill, there may be no orgasm.

Our society is oriented toward achievement, and it has become common to apply measures of success to sex, especially orgasm. For example, many people believe that "success" is determined by the number of orgasms a woman has during a sexual episode. By this standard, a successful male is someone who can delay ejaculation until his partner has experienced at least one

orgasm and preferably more, whereas a successful female is someone who can have several explosive orgasms in every sexual encounter. Men and women who cannot "manufacture" the appropriate number of orgasms may be erroneously labeled "inadequate" by themselves and others. When people become overly concerned with "succeeding" or "performing well," they can become psychologically detached from the activity. Rather than abandon themselves completely to sexual experience, they withdraw their attention and observe their actions. This is called **spectatoring.**

Couples are likely to enjoy sex more if they allow for different kinds of orgasm experience:

- Either partner may reach orgasm through manual, oral, or other means of sexual stimulation before or after intercourse.
- Sexual activity need not stop after one partner reaches orgasm. If a couple chooses, lovemaking can continue until both wish to stop.
- Neither individual may desire an orgasm during a particular sexual episode. Physically expressing love and caring does not require orgasm.

Masturbation

Masturbation is self-stimulation to produce erotic arousal, usually to the point of orgasm. While social and religious attitudes in many cultures consider it improper, immoral, or perverse, masturbation is nevertheless practiced widely throughout the world and even among other animals species.

Many people find masturbation a rewarding variation in their sex lives. People masturbate for many of the same reasons that they have partner sex: to experience erotic pleasure; to relieve physical tensions; to produce a sense of relaxation; to induce sleep; and when done with a partner, to create feelings of intimacy and bonding. Masturbation also helps people discover what pleases them sexually.

A number of personal harmful effects have long been rumored to result from masturbation. Among them are hair loss, insanity, pimples, warts, unhappy personal relations, and the inability to have children. There is no evidence that any of these claims are true. Physically, masturbation is harmless as long as it is not injurious to the stimulated organs.

Sexual Abstinence

Although for most people interest in and desire for sex is relatively constant, some people choose to abstain from sexual activity. For religious reasons certain people practice life-long sexual abstinence (sometimes called **celibacy**, which literally means remaining unmarried). Some individuals refrain from sexual intercourse until

> *T E R M S*
>
> *orgasm:* the climax of sexual responses and the release of physiological and sexual tensions
>
> *spectatoring:* observing one's own sexual experience rather than fully taking part in it
>
> *masturbation:* self-induced sexual stimulation
>
> *celibacy:* sexual abstinence

they marry. Still others avoid sexual interaction because they fear the closeness and intimacy implied by sex or they have strong negative feelings regarding sex.

Individuals not wishing to practice life-long sexual abstinence may nevertheless benefit from a sex "time out." For example, recovery from a physical or emotional illness may include sexual abstinence. No-sex is a sure way to avoid an unintended pregnancy or a sexually transmitted disease. Some people find abstaining helpful while recovering from the break-up of a love relationship. The healing of the emotional wound seems to proceed more smoothly without the emotional intensity that often accompanies sexual interaction.

Sexual abstinence can also provide an opportunity to develop a new set of personal and relational experiences. By avoiding the intimacy that accompanies a lot of sex, abstinence provides a way to discover new dimensions in interpersonal relationships. Without the diversion of sex (or the search for sex partners) an individual can focus on self-development, career, or school, and put energy into long-time friendships. New romantic relationships can develop without the pressure for sex early in the relationship, thus permitting the partners to develop trust and caring before becoming sexual.

For some, sexual abstinence seems like a hardship because their sexual needs and their needs for touching, physical contact, and emotional closeness may not be met. During a period of sexual abstinence, the need for touching and physical contact can be met through professional (nonsexual) massage, or hugging among friends and between parents and children. Masturbation can relieve sexual tensions. And intimacy needs can be met by deepening one's ongoing friendships, giving oneself to others through volunteer work, increasing one's level of self-awareness and self-development, or involving oneself in spiritual and/or religious activity.

Sexual Difficulties

Many individuals expect sex always to be exciting and satisfying; anything less is cause for concern. Life is full of changes, however, and the demands of career or parenting or occasional physical illness can sometimes produce a temporary loss in interest in sex and/or the ability to engage in sex (Table 8.2). Such changes in sexual interest and ability are normal and usually resolve themselves in time. Persistent difficulties with sex may signal that consulting a therapist would be helpful. Lack of interest in sex may be connected to many factors; failure to communicate likes and dislikes; boredom; stress, fatigue, and depression; alcohol and drugs; pregnancy and children; hostility and anger; change in physical appearance; and physical illness.

Lack of Interest   Therapists and counselors refer to the lack of interest in sex as hypoactive sexual desire or sexual aversion, and note that it can result from:

1. *Underlying sexual difficulty.* One or both partners may have some physical difficulty engaging in sex: a man

TABLE 8.2 Factors Contributing to Sexual Difficulties

Types of factors	Examples
Organic factors	Illness of any kind Hormonal, vascular, and neurological illness Fatigue and/or psychoendocrine stress Medications and recreational drugs

Values, beliefs, and attitudes	*Sex negative values:*
	    Sex is dirty; sex is sinful
	    Genitals (especially female) are dirty
	    Women are not supposed to enjoy sex
	    Men are supposed to always be interested in sex
	    Men are supposed to always be capable of sex
	Narrow definition of sex:
	    Sex = penis-in-vagina intercourse
	    Goal orientation (sex = orgasm)
	    Performance expectations

Personality and experiences	Low self-esteem Emotional difficulties (anxiety, depression, grief) Prior incidence of sexual abuse Poor body image
Relationship factors	Discomfort with intimacy Relationship problems Fear of pregnancy or sexually transmitted disease Sexual orientation

may be unable to gain or maintain an erection or a woman experiences pain during intercourse. Such problems can make sexual activity unpleasant for either or both partners, and they eventually lose sexual interest in each other.

2. *Failure to communicate likes and dislikes.* One partner may find some aspects of sex unsatisfying and not communicate this information to the partner. Resentment and displeasure may subsequently build up to the point that interest in sex is lost.

> There are two sides to every argument until you take one.
> Anonymous

3. *Boredom.* Like anything else that becomes predictable and routine, sex can become boring if it is always done in the same way and at the same time. As with other activities, the old cliché is true: "Variety is the spice of life."

4. *Stress, fatigue, and depression.* Being emotionally drained by work or other responsibilities or being "low" or "blue" can interfere with sexual desire.

5. *Alcohol and other drugs.* Frequent ingestion of alcohol and other drugs can lower sexual desire. Drug use can also turn off a partner who does not want to make love to someone who is drunk or on drugs. Some medications can also lessen interest in sex.

6. *Pregnancy and children.* During pregnancy and child raising the increase in responsibilities and the decrease in private time can lower interest in sex. Busy couples must make an effort to schedule time to be together (for sex and other activities).

7. *Hostility and anger.* Unresolved conflicts are a common cause of lost sexual interest. It may be difficult to feel intimate with someone with whom you are angry.

8. *Change in physical appearance.* Once they are in a relationship, some people stop caring about their appearance, which may lessen a partner's sexual interest.

9. *Physical illness.* Physical illnesses can cause some people to believe they shouldn't have sex. For example, the man who has a heart attack may be afraid to have sex because he fears another heart attack.

Erection Problems Difficulty in achieving or maintaining an erection can be the result of an injury or disease. It can also be due to alcohol, heroin, and other recreational drugs and some medications for high blood pressure. More often, however, erection problems are the result of fear of sexual performance (including anxiety about one's ability to get an erection) or the wish not to be sexual with a particular partner.

Ejaculation Control It is impossible to define "rapid" or "premature" ejaculation in terms of minutes; however, some therapists define it as absence of voluntary control of ejaculation. Ejaculation is a reflex activity that a man can learn to control just as he does bladder function. The key to controlling ejaculation is awareness of the bodily sensations that signal the onset of ejaculation, followed by modulating arousal according to one's desires.

Painful Intercourse In women, painful intercourse can be caused by vaginal infections, insufficient vaginal lubrication before intercourse (usually the result of not being sufficiently sexually aroused), and anxiety-produced spasms of the muscles surrounding the vagina, which makes vaginal penetration painful. Another source of pain associated with intercourse, which can affect both women and men, is a deep, aching sensation in the pelvis for women or scrotum ("blue balls") for men occurring during sex. This condition is caused by the congestion of blood in the pelvic region brought about by sexual arousal. Orgasm often reverses the congestion, but lack of orgasm can cause blood to remain and cause discomfort and pain.

Orgasm Difficulties Both men and women can have difficulty experiencing orgasm. Most often this difficulty is the result of insufficient sexual arousal, perhaps because of aversion to a particular partner, fear of pregnancy or sexually transmitted diseases, fear of letting go, lack of trust, or negative attitudes about sexual pleasure.

DEVELOPING POSITIVE SEXUAL RELATIONSHIPS

We all need intimacy—that feeling of closeness, trust, and openness with another person that tells us that our innermost self can be shared without fear of attack or emotional hurt and that we are understood in the deepest sense possible.

Intimate relationships can have an enormous impact on one's sense of vitality and well-being. When an intimate relationship is flowing smoothly, it can produce rich emotional satisfaction unparalleled by any other experience. Those who are involved in genuinely supportive and caring relationships tend to feel unswervingly confident about the potential of life to be harmonious and beautiful. On the other hand, when an intimate relationship is not going well, those involved can be overwhelmed by moroseness, unable to think of anything but their misery. They can be angry, depressed, anxious, or distraught, sometimes to the point of being unable to function at work or at school.

A lack of intimacy in life can adversely affect physical health as well as emotions and feelings. Studies indicate that married people are in better physical health than divorced, separated, and widowed people. The association of intimacy and physical health is suggested by the finding that recently widowed people suffer increased

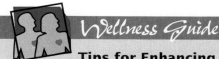

Wellness Guide

Tips for Enhancing Sexual Experience

- Create pleasure by stimulating the whole body, not just the genitals.
- Vary the manner and intensity of stimulation. Allow sensations to build and wane.
- Try not to make sex = work.
- Set aside time that is free of intrusions and distractions. Disconnect the phone, lock the door to ensure privacy.
- Make yourself an open, effective channel for sexual arousal before sexual activity begins. Satisfying

sex is not a mechanical activity involving only bodies, but a blending of mind-body energies. Remove sex-negative energies such as hunger, fatigue, and anger and focus your energy on sex through deep breathing or other relaxing activity.
- Be aware of differences between you and your partner in the state of readiness for sexual activity. Try to synchronize your and your partner's states of sexual arousal through talking, light touching,

dance, massage, and so on, before sexual activity begins.
- Address concerns about birth control and STDs.
- Take your time. Go slowly.
- Communicate likes and dislikes to your partner either verbally or nonverbally.
- Do not focus just on orgasms. Learn to appreciate the many sexual sensations from touching all parts of the body.

mortality during the first few months after the death of their spouse. Apparently these people do indeed die of a "broken heart." Such evidence demonstrates the substantial link between emotions and physical health that is so fundamental to the holistic health philosophy.

What Intimacy Is

Many people mistakenly equate genuine intimacy with sexual intercourse. That happens because love and affection are feelings associated with intimacy, and in our culture there is much confusion about love and sex. But intimacy is a feeling, not an act. It is the *quality* of a relationship between two people—a shared experiencing of their personal lives. People who have an intimate relationship may or may not choose to express their closeness with sex.

Many kinds of intimacies are possible. There are intimacies between other-sex peers, same-sex peers, children and parents, members of a family, neighbors, close friends, and even coworkers. Each intimacy has its unique and distinctive quality depending on the people involved, on the extent to which their personal histories are similar, and on the facets of themselves they choose to share with each other.

Yet intimacies possess certain common characteristics. They are relationships of mutual consent. One person cannot be intimate with another unless both agree that that is what they want. Intimacies tend to grow deeper and richer over time; partners need to share meaningful experiences in order to establish genuine trust and caring. Intimacies also carry the feeling that the personalities of the intimates are interconnected in some complex way. This is not the same as the feeling of hav-

ing their identities merge so they become "one," but rather that they feel both joined and separate at the same time in some way.

The Life Cycle of Intimate Relationships

Intimate relationships tend to develop through the stages of 1) selecting a partner, 2) developing intimacy, and 3) establishing commitment. Before an intimate relationship can develop, however, the partners have to be psychologically open to entering and maintaining it. Some individuals choose not to be involved in an intimate relationship, perhaps because they wish to devote energies to school, work, or self-development, or they find intimate relationships to be distracting or psychologically threatening. In some instances, previous life experiences can leave an individual fearful of emotional closeness, which can block the establishment of intimacy. In some

HEALTHY PEOPLE 2000

Increase to at least 85 percent the proportion of people aged 10 through 18 who have discussed human sexuality, including values surrounding their sexuality, with their parents and/or have received information through another parentally endorsed source such as youth, school, or religious programs.

Parents are the most important educators of their children in matters related to sexual behavior. From them, children receive their first lessons in sexual morality and appropriate sexual conduct.

of these instances, there are repeated attempts to form relationships; however, without the element of intimacy, these relationships often fail.

Factors that influence the choice of intimate partners include:

- *Proximity*. People are most likely to become intimate with someone with whom they are in physical proximity.
- *Similarity*. Similar age, religion, race, education, social background, attitudes, values, and interests affect the possibility for intimacy in two ways: 1) they influence proximity and 2) they reflect social norms for permissible peer intimacies. Note, for example, biases against interracial and older-younger intimacies. Colleges and universities provide students with relatively easy access to a "pool of eligibles" because they bring together individuals of similar age, religion, intelligence, expectations, and values.
- *Physical appearance*. Physical appearance provides cues that indicate who among the pool of eligibles is a desirable intimate partner. Those who are judged "attractive" tend to be thought of as kind, understanding, and affectionate ("what is beautiful is good"). Pairing with someone who is considered physically attractive enhances one's social status and self-esteem.

Developing Intimacy

Most people want their intimate relationships to develop feelings of closeness, positive regard, warmth, and familiarity with the other's innermost thoughts and feelings. This deep knowledge of each other comes from sharing the most important and often secret aspects of one's personality—one's goals, aspirations, strengths, weaknesses, and physical and sexual desires. The sharing of such private information is called **self-disclosure.**

When relationships begin, little intimate information is usually disclosed. People talk about the weather, the stock market, or politics. They gossip about professors, students, or other people they know. And they ask each other the classic leading questions: Where are you from? What do you do? What's your major? People face these questions so many times that they become adept at revealing as much or as little about themselves as feels comfortable. It is when they begin to talk about their personal history, current life problems, hopes and aspirations, and fears and personal failures that they begin to disclose important information—important because dis-

> *If I could tell you what it meant, there would be no point in dancing it.*
>
> Isadora Duncan,
> dancer

closing it makes them feel vulnerable. Most people discuss their deepest feelings only with those in whom they have developed considerable trust.

Intimacy develops through a progressive, mutual revealing of innermost thoughts. Psychologists compare people's personalities to onions—having many layers from an outer surface to an inner core. As acquaintances gain more and more knowledge about each other, they penetrate deeper and deeper through the layers of the other's personality, which establishes their intimacy. Another view compares intimate development to the peeling of an artichoke. Resistance and barriers to sharing information about oneself are like the leaves of the artichoke; as intimacy progresses, intimates peel away the leaves to get to the other's "heart."

Self-disclosure leads to the development of intimacy in two ways. First, you tend to be affected either positively or negatively by the information that is disclosed. If you make a positive judgment, you are likely to want to continue interacting with that person, for you believe that future interactions will be equally or even more positive. The same logic applies to negative assessments. If your reaction is unfavorable, you are likely to terminate the relationship, or perhaps maintain it on a lesser level of intimacy.

The second way that self-disclosure leads to intimacy is the *act* of self-disclosure, which, regardless of the information offered, often leads to reciprocal self-disclosure. By sharing important information, you communicate that you trust the other person, and usually that person accepts your trust and becomes more willing to disclose information. In this way intimacy progresses by a cycle of self-disclosure leading to trust, which brings about self-disclosure, which leads to more trust, and so on.

Establishing Commitment

After a period of self-disclosure, individuals may sense that their relationship has progressed to a state of "us-ness," that it has become a special friendship, a love relationship, or a marital-type dyad. This state of "us-ness" is one of commitment, which has three aspects.

- *An action, pledge, or promise.* One makes a promise and thus announces one's intention explicitly, even if it is only to the partner. Various social values and norms regarding keeping promises and the guilt and loss of self-esteem that come with breaking promises are among the "push" factors that keep a person committed. If the promise involves a social ritual (i.e., marriage ceremony, getting pinned), then family, friends, and the state become additional "push" factors.
- *A state of being obligated or emotionally compelled.* This state involves a cluster of emotions such as love, com-

T E R M

self-disclosure: sharing personal experiences and feelings with someone

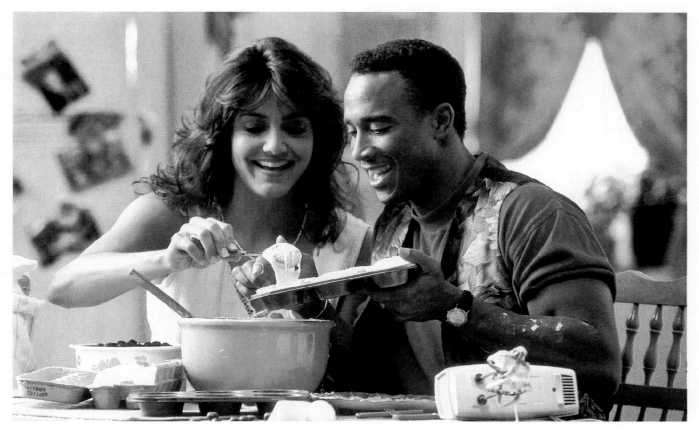

Intimacy begins by doing fun things together.

fort, caring, and relief from separation anxiety and loneliness.

- *An unwillingness to consider any partner other than the current one.* The rewards of the current relationship outweigh the costs of not exploring other opportunities for intimacy.

Endings

Everything in the universe (even the universe itself!) has a beginning and an end. Close relationships have a beginning and an end also. Sometimes a relationship lasts for only a few minutes; sometimes it lasts until one of the partners dies (and even then the relationship may still be "alive" in the imagination of the surviving partner). Sometimes the structure of a close relationship persists but the closeness and the dynamism wane, creating a "shell" relationship without vitality. Sometimes a relationship goes through cycles of birth and death within the structure of its ongoingness. When a close relationship ends, some or all of its structure, exchange of resources (love, caring, financial support, etc.), and feelings of attachment and emotional bondedness end also.

Endings occur for a variety of reasons. For example, partners' feelings of attachment and bondedness may be absent or weak. Life goals, values, and/or interests may no longer be shared. One or both partners may be unwilling or unable to invest personal resources such as greater time shared with the partner, or to commit to an exclusive relationship. Whether partners continue in a relationship also is affected by their assessment of other options such as another potential partner or singlehood. Without suitable alternatives, leaving a relationship may seem difficult, unwise, or impossible.

Another reason ongoingness stops is that the partners, either individually or as a dyadic unit, are unable to move the relationship into its next stage. For example, some couples cannot navigate the transition from being idealistic, passionate lovers to realistic, companionate lovers. In nonmarital close relationships, a partner may not be considered suitable as a potential marital partner, even in the presence of considerable love, attachment, and liking.

Another factor associated with endings is lack of support, or even hostility, from the partners' social network. Families may not accept a son's or daughter's choice of a dating or marital partner. Interracial, disabled, and same-sex relationships are still heavily stigmatized in our society.

Occasionally the seeds of an ending are sown into a relationship at its beginning. For example, partners may seek closeness as a way to cope with or avoid personal

How Intimate Are You?

Respond to the following statements. There are no right or wrong responses.

	Yes	No
1. Do you like to touch?	___	___
2. Do you like to be touched?	___	___
3. Do you often do things spontaneously or impulsively?	___	___
4. Can you put yourself in another's person's place?	___	___
5. Can you easily discuss sex in mixed company without feeling uncomfortable?	___	___
6. When you feel affection for someone, can you express it physically as well as verbally?	___	___
7. Do you like yourself?	___	___
8. Do you like others of your same gender?	___	___
9. Would you feel it a sign of weakness to seek help for a sexual problem?	___	___
10. Do you communicate with others through touch as well as words?	___	___
11. Do you fall in love at first sight?	___	___
12. Do you feel rejected if a person you love tries to preserve his or her independence?	___	___
13. Can you accept your loved one's anger and still believe in his or her love?	___	___
14. Can you express your innermost thoughts and feelings to the person you love?	___	___
15. Do you talk over disagreements with your partner rather than worry silently about them?	___	___
16. Can you accept the fact that your partner has loved others before you and not worry about how you compare with them?	___	___
17. Can you accept a partner's lack of interest in sex without feeling rejected?	___	___
18. Should fun and sensual please be the principal goals in a sexual relationship?	___	___
19. Do you feel pressure to "perform" all the time with your partner?	___	___
20. Is sexual intercourse for you an uninhibited romp rather than a demonstration of your love?	___	___

After completing this brief inventory of intimacy, if you find you are unable to openly communicate with your partner, unable to express your feelings emotionally and physically, and are frequently jealous of your partner, you may wish to seek advice from a counselor or health professional.

problems. They may feel rejected and lonely because of the break-up of a previous relationship. They may feel that they cannot take care of themselves. They may be afraid of leaving home or school. If, as often happens, a partner or relationship does not turn out to be the solution to a personal problem, a disappointed, angry, or frustrated partner may seek alternative ways of coping. These alternatives, such as drug or alcohol abuse, extra-relationship affairs, or physically or emotionally abusing the partner (or other family members) (Chapter 23), may very well be destructive to the relationship.

When a break-up does occur, individuals may feel tired, lethargic, lonely, sad, depressed, angry, resentful, and guilty. They may be unable to sleep or eat, may miss class, or be unable to work. They may withdraw from friends. They may find concentrating difficult, because they are continually thinking about the partner and what happened in the relationship. They may feel helpless ("what will become of me?") and hopeless ("I'll never find a true love") or skeptical and cynical ("love can never work out").

Some partners feel relaxed, hopeful, and relieved that what they identify as a bad or going-nowhere relationship has ended, and they are free to pursue personal goals or find a relationship partner who is better suited to them. Sometimes individuals feel euphoric and self-confident. They say that the separation was for the best, and they become more active and outgoing. This positive outlook may alternate with emotional distress.

When a person is emotionally (and sometimes physically) wracked with the pain of an ending, he or she may have difficulty seeing any good in that experience, but often endings mark the start of a new and better future. A study of remarried people showed that many had learned a lot about themselves and the nature of close relationships from a previous marriage(s) and found that their current marriage was much more satisfying.

COMMUNICATING IN INTIMATE RELATIONSHIPS

Communication is a symbolic process of creating and sharing meaning. At the heart of communication is an individual communication act, which involves imparting a message to another person to share information or feelings, to coordinate behavior with an individual or group of people, or to persuade someone to do something.

A communication act begins as a mental image; an idea, a wish, or a feeling (or some combination of all three). If humans were capable of mind reading, senders could impart mental images directly to receivers. Few people can read minds, *mind reading,* however, so communication requires that thoughts be transformed into symbols that can carry information. Those symbols make up the message. The most common symbols in communication are:

- *Words:* spoken or printed
- *Visual images:* paintings, sculpture
- *Posture or body language:* gaze, touch, smile, physical proximity
- *Objects:* flowers, gifts, food
- *Behaviors:* doing a favor, giving a kiss, ignoring an appointment

The sender's encoding of her or his mental images into the symbols that make up the message is only half of a communication act. The other half is the receiver's reactions: this involves taking in the symbols that make up the message and decoding them into her or his own mental images. Thus, a communication act requires two

transformations: in the sender, the transformation of mental images into symbols; in the receiver, the transformation of symbols into mental images.

Consider this example of a communication act between Beth and Ron one rainy morning. Beth doesn't want Ron to get wet in the rain, so she decides to use spoken words as the symbols to encode her thoughts. Beth says, "Ron, it's raining." Ron hears Beth's words, and decodes them into a mental image of the weather that day, and he picks up his umbrella.

In this communication act Beth accomplished her goal. But a different outcome could have occurred if one or more of the steps in the communication act had been distorted, weakened, or blocked completely. For example, if Beth had said "it's raining" in a tone of voice that Ron didn't appreciate, or if her words had been misunderstood, the communication process would have been distorted.

Every communication act carries two types of message or potential meaning. The first is the **literal message,** which is the message conveyed by the symbols themselves, as in the words "it's raining." The second is the **metamessage** ("meta" is the Greek word for "beyond," "additional," or "transcendent"), which carries implicit messages about the reason for the communication, how the message is to be interpreted, and the nature of the relationship of the sender and receiver. Most metacommunication occurs unconsciously.

When Beth said to Ron, "it's raining," not only did she send a literal message about the weather, but she also sent several metamessages, including "I care about you" and "an expectation in our relationship is that we help each other out."

After Beth had told Ron that it was raining, if Ron had kissed Beth and said, "Thanks, honey, for looking out for me," he would have been responding to one of the metamessages in the communication. If Ron had interpreted the metamessage as, "Ron, you're terribly childlike and I have to make decisions about you"—even though Beth didn't intend to impart that message—Ron might have responded angrily with something like, "Beth, I can look out for myself!" Her feelings may then have been hurt and possibly they would have had an argument. Acknowledging and responding to metamessages can sometimes be much more important than dealing with the literal ones.

Sending Clear Messages

A clear message is one in which the symbols represent as closely as possible the sender's intent. Clear messages are best delivered with **I-statements;** these are sentences that begin with (or have as the subject) the pronoun "I." I-statements clearly identify the sender as the source of a thought, emotion, desire, or act: I think . . . . I feel . . . . I want (need) . . . . I did (will do) . . . .

You-statements, which begin with (or have as the subject) the pronoun "you," as in "You always . . . ," "You never . . . ," "You are . . . ," or the interrogatives, "Why don't you . . . ?" or "How could you . . . ?" often are put-downs or character assassinations. They imply that the receiver is not-OK. Very often the not-OK message is explicit, as in "You're incompetent" or "You're stupid"—just about any negative adjective will do. People often respond to the metamessage in a you-statement, which is "I think you're no good," by feeling attacked, which can lead to hurt feelings and counterattacks or withdrawal.

Effective Listening

Effective communication requires both sending and receiving, both talking and listening. Effective listening is important because the receiver not only takes in the sender's message, but also helps establish the physical and emotional context for the communication. The lis-

tener also must communicate to the sender that the sender's message was received. This is called **feedback.** Some techniques for effective receiving are: giving the sender your full attention; making eye contact; listening; being empathic; being open for receiving the message; giving verbal feedback; acknowledging the sender's feelings; praising the sender's efforts; and being unconditional.

Give the Sender Your Full Attention Don't fake it. If you can't pay attention because you are tired, hungry, distracted, angry, or whatever, tell the sender how you feel and ask if it's OK to talk after you rest, or eat, or go to the bathroom, or just talk at another time. The sender is likely to grant your request if immediacy is not an issue because he or she wants your full attention.

Make Eye Contact Try to assume similar postures (i.e., both sitting or both standing) to create a sense of equal status. Making eye-to-eye contact allows the

Managing Stress

Pillow Talk

When problems arise among intimate couples, virtually every incident can be traced back to some misinterpretation in communication. "I thought you said this!" "I thought you meant that." Although not all communication styles are verbal, the amount of communication expressed through words lead to most of the difficulty in relationships. Poor communication in any relationship, and in particular sexual relationships, can lead to stress.

There are many issues involving sexual intercourse that can act as stressors. These include, but are not limited to, contraception, birth control, risk of pregnancy, infertility, venereal disease, vaginismis, molestation, celibacy, guilt, rape, self-respect, abortion, impotency, premature ejaculation, intimacy, ability to reach orgasm, homosexuality, and sexual satisfaction. This incomplete list is quite long and each item weighs heavy as a stressor for those who experience them. In addition, problems of this nature do not go away once a couple has

initiated sexual relations. To the contrary, if communications are poor at the start of a relationship, they tend to get worse as the relationship continues. Sex counselors advocate that *before* and *after* each and every act of sexual intimacy there should be a thorough conversation airing these and other issues. As any AIDS patient or women with an unwanted pregnancy will tell you, the short-term pleasures of sex are surely not worth risking your life, nor are they worth the days, months, and years of agony that may follow unresolved sex-related problems. The stakes of sexual encounters are high. Make it a point to include a healthy conversation as a requirement in all sexually intimate encounters.

Here are some suggestions for conversation with someone you become intimate with.

- Learn to become comfortable with words about sexual intimacy such as erection, penis, orgasm, and condom. The inability to articulate your feelings and preferences

creates additional stress in relationships.

- If you are anxious about explaining your feelings, rehearse a conversation in which you ask your partner how he or she feels about you, where he or she likes to be touched, or tell him or her that you wish to date him or her exclusively (specific aspects of this degree of intimacy).

- Learn to ask your partner what pleases him or her and what they don't like. Conversely, feel assertive enough to make known your preferences to your partner. Don't assume that he or she knows.

Open channels of communication are vital to the health of intimate relationships, whereas poor communication only adds to the stress of a relationship. In uncomfortable moments, your first reaction may be to avoid confronting issues of intimacy. At these times, rather than giving in to reactions of avoidance or silence, we must respond with an open heart.

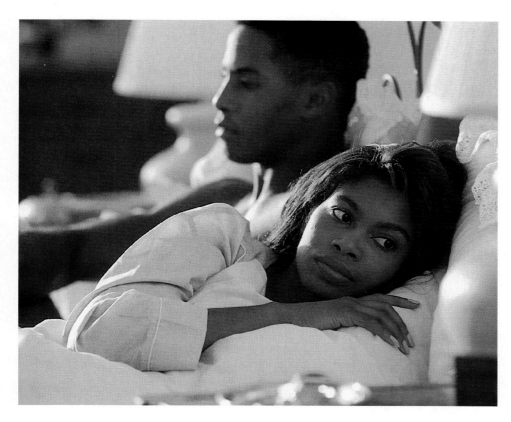

When communication breaks down, stress and tension ensue.

receiver to feel comfortable as well as conveying that you are listening to her and taking in the complete message.

Just Listen Don't interrupt until you have a signal that the sender is finished or until the sender has asked for a response, unless you don't understand what is being communicated. You can acknowledge that you are actively listening with gestures, nods, and vocalizations like "uh-huh," "yes," "go on," "I see," and so forth.

Be Empathic Try to "hear" the sender's feelings as well as the words. Be open to the sender's intentions and motivations as well as her or his ideas. Ask yourself, "What is this person feeling right now?"

Be an Open Channel for Receiving the Message Don't judge or evaluate the sender or the message while the sender is talking. Try not to correct the sender or, if the sender is being critical of you, to think of a defense.

Give Verbal Feedback Don't mind read. Summarize in your own words your understanding of the sender's thoughts and emotions. This way the sender can find out if the message that was intended was actually received. If so, then you can respond. If not, then the sender can try again. Ask for clarification if there's something you don't understand. You can say something like, "I don't think I understand everything you were saying about your mother. Can you tell me again, maybe in a different way?"

Acknowledge the Sender's Emotions "It seems to me that you're feeling . . ." and if you're not sure, add "do I have that right?" By acknowledging or providing feedback, you are sharing what you believe are the sender's emotions. If you are incorrect, the sender can relay that to you.

Praise the Sender's Effort Acknowledge the sender's efforts for investing the time, energy, and care to communicate with you, especially if the communication was a difficult one.

Be Unconditional Let the sender know that you respect him or her even if you are uncomfortable with the messages that are being communicated. Assure the sender that even though things may be difficult, you are willing to continue talking and working through difficult feelings.

Expressing Anger Constructively

Disagreements and conflicts are inevitable in any close relationship. The notion that people in intimate relationships shouldn't have to fight because love makes them see eye to eye on everything or the idea that you can't possibly be angry with someone you love are romantic myths. By expressing anger constructively, intimates fight for the success of their relationship as well as for their individual needs.

In constructive fighting, there should be no "winner" and no "loser." Good fights are efforts of individuals to be heard and to improve the relationship. The best fights occur when the people involved feel that they have gained something.

Here are some suggestions for expressing anger constructively:

- Try not to let anger and resentment build up over time. Express feelings when you become aware of them.
- Agree on a time, a place, and the content for fights. It is certainly acceptable to get mad spontaneously if that is how you feel, but it is better to set aside a specific time for the resolution of an issue rather than trying to deal with it when you or your partner may not be psychologically or physically ready to argue. Be sure that the person you are angry with knows what the issue is before the fight.
- Be specific as to what you are angry about and stick to the issue. Don't bring up old hurts. Try not to discuss second and third topics, especially as a means of retaliation.
- Attack the problem, not each other. Don't denigrate the other's personal qualities. Use I-statements to communicate resentments. I-statements tell how you feel. You-statements are often received as personal attacks.
- Try to resolve the issue with an air of compromise and respect. Try to understand the other's point of view.
- Know when it is time to stop. Sometimes you can sense that the argument isn't getting resolved. It is okay to acknowledge that and to take a few hours or days to reconsider things and to discuss the issue again. Sometimes emotions are too high and it is not possible to think clearly. That may be the time to stop the fight until tempers cool.
- Engaging in sex or any other affectionate behavior before an issue is resolved should not be taken as a sign that everything is forgotten. Such behavior shows that the fight fits into what is believed to be healthy relationship.
- Don't hold grudges.

HEALTH IN REVIEW

- Sex refers to one's biological classification as male or female and to the experience of creating erotic pleasure.
- Sexuality consists of the aspects of oneself that affect sexual experience: the physical, psychological, social, orientational, developmental, and sexual skill dimensions of the whole self.
- One's sexual biology is determined by genetic make-up, which in turn determines the nature of sex organs: the testes, sperm ducts, semen-producing glands, and penis in the male; the ovaries, fallopian tubes, uterus, vagina, and external genitalia in the female.
- One's sexual psychology is rooted in gender identity, which guides gender role behaviors.
- Sexual arousal and response involves four phases: excitement, plateau, orgasm, and resolution.
- Sexual difficulties include lack of interest in sex, lack of erection, lack of ejaculatory control, painful intercourse, and difficulties with orgasm.
- Intimate relationships involve sharing one's innermost self. They develop through three stages: selecting a partner, developing intimacy through self-disclosure, and commitment.
- Effective communication is crucial for developing and maintaining relationships.

REFERENCES

Hampson, J. L., and I. G. Hampson (1961). "The Ontogenesis of Sexual Behavior in Men." In W. C. Young (ed.), Sex and Internal Secretions, 3rd ed. Baltimore: Williams and Wilkins.

Laumann, E. O., J. H. Gagnon, R. T. Michael, and S. Michaels (1994). The Social Organization of Sexuality: Sexual Practices in the United States. Chicago: The University of Chicago Press.

Masters, W., and V. Johnson (1966). *Human Sexual Response.* Boston: Little, Brown.

Money, J., and A. Ehrhardt (1972). *A Man and Woman: Boy and Girl.* Baltimore: Johns Hopkins University Press.

Nimmons, D. (1994). "Sex and the Brain." *Discover,* March: 64.

SUGGESTED READINGS

Henry, W. A. (1993). "Born Gay?" *Time,* July 26: 36–39. This article discusses what it would mean if homosexuality was genetic.

Michael, R. T., J. H. Gagnon, E. O. Laumann, and G. Kolata (1994). *Sex in America.* Boston: Little, Brown. Findings from a national study of adult sexual behavior. Book is intended for the general audience.

"The Power and the Pride" (1993). *Newsweek,* June 21: 54–60. Lesbians are no longer considered invisible homosexuals. This article discusses how as a group they are struggling to define themselves socially and politically.

Tannen, D. (1990). *You Just Don't Understand: Women and Men in Conversation.* New York: Ballantine Books. Looks at the gender differences in conversation. Provides an easy way to understand the differences between men and women, and how we can learn from each other's conversation styles.

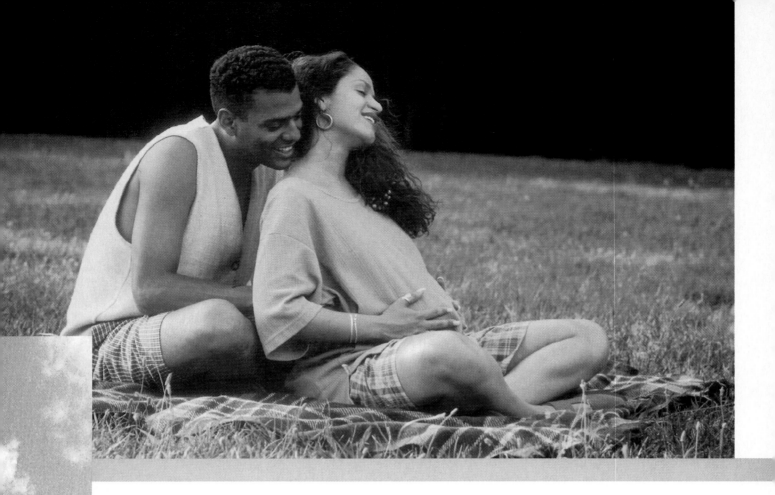

LEARNING OBJECTIVES

After reading this chapter you should be able to:

1. Discuss reasons for becoming pregnant and reasons for not becoming pregnant.
2. Explain what takes place during pregnancy, beginning with fertilization.
3. Discuss childbirth preparation.
4. Describe the birthing process.
5. Identify the pros and cons of breast-feeding.
6. Identify and briefly describe four important health habits during pregnancy.
7. Identify several reasons for infertility and options for infertile couples.

Understanding Pregnancy and Parenthood

*T*his chapter is about one of the most profound of life's experiences: creating a child. Many people are awed by the idea that the union of one of their body's cells with a cell from their mate can bring forth a unique human being whose well-being is highly dependent on the physical and emotional foundations they provide. There is a tremendous responsibility in being the best kind of parent so that both the child and society benefit.

People want children for a variety of reasons. A couple may believe that a child is an expression of their love, and having children adds to their sense of bonding. Some see a child as a way to leave a legacy to the world or to carry on the family name. Some couples may feel pressured by their families or by societal or religious expectations to have children, and others may hope that having children will improve their marriage. Being a parent can make some people feel important, needed, or proud. Parenthood may reinforce the ideals of feminine and masculine roles (Chapter 8). Prospective parents may also see children as adding fun, excitement, love, and companionship to their lives.

CHOOSING WHETHER OR NOT TO BE A PARENT

Not everyone chooses to become a parent. About 5 percent of fertile American married couples do not become parents. Some see parenthood as infringing on their career goals or as an unnecessary or unwanted addition to their intimate partnership. Some may have doubts about their psychological or economic abilities to nurture or support children. Others may know or suspect that their children might inherit a genetic disease. Still others may feel that they do not want to contribute more children to an already overpopulated world.

Giving birth to and raising a child requires major adjustments in the parents' lives. The career plans of one or both parents and the distribution of family resources—time, energy, physical space, and money—may change. First-time parents may feel overwhelmed by their responsibilities. The decision to parent should not be taken lightly. The years of parenting are often intense. However, you will never experience such responsibility, hard work, and intimacy as that involved in the growth and development of another human being.

Children do not ask to be born. Parents make that decision. Therefore, before committing to this decision, potential parents must be as certain as they can that their decision is appropriate for their life goals and that they have the means for caring for their children.

BECOMING PREGNANT

For most people, becoming a parent involves pregnancy—a 40-week period during which a fetus grows inside the mother's uterus and the mother's body undergoes important changes to nurture the developing child. Every pregnancy begins with **fertilization**, which is the fusion of a father's sperm cell with a mother's ovum to form the first cell of their child, called the fertilized egg or **zygote**. When a man ejaculates during sexual intercourse, hundreds of millions of sperm cells are released into the vagina. Propelled by the swimming motion of their long tails, these tadpole-like cells make their way through the uterus and into the fallopian tubes, the usual site of fertilization (Figure 9.1). Only one of the many sperm cells actually fertilizes the egg. After fertilization, the zygote moves to the uterus, where it implants in the inner lining and proceeds to develop as an **embryo.**

During each of a woman's menstrual cycles usually one ovum, but sometimes two or more, are able to be fertilized. Once freed from the ovary at ovulation, these eggs can survive for about 24 hours. After ovulation, the lining of the uterus thickens, its glands become filled with nutrients, and small blood vessels enlarge to bring maternal nutrients to the embryo should pregnancy occur.

Sperm are produced in the testes in narrow, highly coiled, tube-like structures called **seminiferous tubules** (Chapter 8). It takes about 70 days for an immature sperm cell to develop into a mature sperm. Once in the vagina, sperm must travel about 30 cm to the site of fertilization in the fallopian tube, which, on a comparative basis, is equivalent to a person traveling nearly six miles.

The cervix is the gateway for passage from the vagina to the uterus (Chapter 8). For most of the month, fluid produced by glands in the cervix is dense. This thick cervical mucus keeps sperm from penetrating as readily as they do at the woman's most fertile time. It also prevents some microorganisms from entering the uterus. Near the time of ovulation, the cervical mucus becomes more fluid and has the consistency of egg white, and becomes organized into channels that orient sperm movement toward the uterus. A woman can learn to "read" her cervical mucus to determine the days on

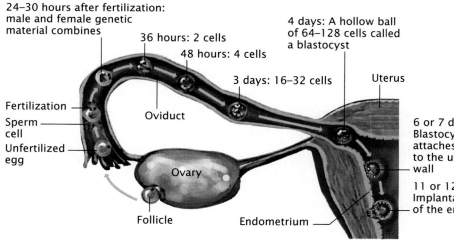

FIGURE 9.1 Fertilization and Early Development of the Embryo The joining of sperm and egg in fertilization. After fertilization, the zygote travels down the fallopian tube to the uterus. Implantation of the zygote begins approximately six days after fertilization.

24–30 hours after fertilization: male and female genetic material combines

36 hours: 2 cells

48 hours: 4 cells

3 days: 16–32 cells

4 days: A hollow ball of 64–128 cells called a blastocyst

Uterus

Fertilization

Sperm cell

Unfertilized egg

Oviduct

Ovary

Follicle

Endometrium

6 or 7 days: Blastocyst attaches itself to the uterine wall

11 or 12 days: Implantation of the embryo

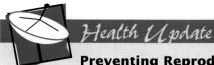
Preventing Reproductive Problems

Many infertile couples wonder why something so easy for most people is so hard for them. Although science cannot fully answer that question, it does know that some reproductive problems are preventable.

Heading the list is damage to the structures that allow sperm and egg to meet, caused by gonorrhea, chlamydia, and other sexually transmitted diseases (STDs). This damage accounts for about 20 percent of all infertility in men and women alike. Use of barrier methods of contraception—condoms for men, or diaphragms (with spermicide) for women—can stop many of these infections before they start.

Both women and men who are sexually active should be regularly checked for the possible presence of STDs as these infections often have no symptoms. The longer the delay before antibiotic treatment is started, the greater the risk of impaired fer-

tility. This risk rises the more sexual partners a person has and with the number of times he or she has these infections.

Tobacco, alcohol, and the use of illicit drugs can also diminish the reproductive potential of both sexes, as can the use of steroid drugs for bodybuilding purposes and for enhancing sports performance. So can poor nutrition, rapid weight loss, and either too much or too little body fat. The same goes for excessive rigorous exercise, meaning more than an hour a day. While too much exercise is more likely to impair female than male fertility, neither sex can count on escaping its reproductive effects.

Childhood immunizations also have a bearing on future fertility. Immunization against mumps and rubella (German measles) is particularly important because the male who gets mumps in adolescence or later runs a high risk of becoming

permanently sterile, and the female who gets rubella while pregnant— particularly early in pregnancy—is at high risk of miscarriage or having a baby with birth defects.

In addition, boys who are born with an undescended testicle, which is fairly common, are more likely than other boys to later have reproductive problems. They are also at a somewhat higher risk for later developing testicular cancer. Undescended testicles can be surgically corrected during childhood.

Girls who don't menstruate by age 16 or are plagued with menstrual problems need to be evaluated by a physician. Neither condition is necessarily an indication of impaired fertility, but it is also true that delaying needed treatment can sometimes make the situation worse.

Source: J. Randal, "Trying to Outsmart Infertility," *FDA Consumer* (May 1991): 22–29.

---

which she is fertile, either as a way to increase the probability of conception or as a form of birth control (Chapter 10).

Within seconds following ejaculation in the vagina, some sperm move through the cervix and uterus and into the fallopian tubes. The majority of sperm, however, become trapped in coagulated semen in the upper portion of the vagina. After about 20 minutes, the coagulated semen liquefies and sperm move into microscopic folds in the cervix. Weak or abnormal sperm are unlikely to move beyond the cervix. Healthy, motile sperm tend to be released into the uterus continuously throughout the ensuing 48 hours. Several hundred sperm capable of fertilization approach an ovum, but only one succeeds in penetrating the ovum's outer membrane.

During the first three days after fertilization, the cells of the embryo replicate at about daily intervals, and the embryo moves along the fallopian tube toward the uterus. By about the fourth day after fertilization, the embryo, now comprised of between 50 and 100 cells arranged as a fluid-filled sphere, enters the uterus. On about the sixth day after fertilization the embryo attaches to the lining of the uterus; shortly thereafter it implants in the uterus by eroding the uterine lining.

PREGNANCY

Soon after the embryo implants in the uterus, it secretes a hormone unique to pregnancy, called **Human Chorionic Gonadotropin**, or **HCG**, into the maternal bloodstream (Figure 9.2). Under the influence of HCG the mother's ovaries are stimulated to increase the production of estrogen and progesterone, which in turn forestalls the next menstrual period and permits the preg-

T E R M S

fertilization: the fusion of a sperm cell and an ovum

zygote: the first cell of a new person, formed at fertilization

embryo: the developing infant during the first two months of conception

seminiferous tubules: convoluted tubules in the testicles that produce sperm

Human Chorionic Gonadotropin (HCG): a hormone produced furing the first stages of pregnancy; it is used as a basis for pregnancy tests

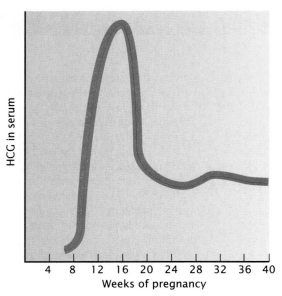

HCG in serum

4 8 12 16 20 24 28 32 36 40
Weeks of pregnancy

FIGURE 9.2 The Pattern of Human Chorionic Gonadotropin (HCG) Secretion during Pregnancy

nancy to continue. Increases in the levels of estrogen and progesterone bring about the first noticeable signs of pregnancy: absence of the next menstrual period, occasional nausea and vomiting referred to as "morning sickness," enlarged and tender breasts, increased frequency

of urination, and enlargement of the uterus. Both clinical and home pregnancy tests are based on analyzing a woman's urine for the presence of HCG. Such tests are about 75 percent accurate. Their most frequent inaccuracy is a false negative—reporting no pregnancy when one actually exists.

On rare occasion, the fertilized egg implants outside the uterus, usually in a fallopian tube where its passage is blocked by tubal malformation or scarring or twisting from an earlier infection, often gonorrhea or chlamydia. A pregnancy in which the fertilized egg implants somewhere other than in the uterus is called an **ectopic pregnancy.** Ectopic implantation in a fallopian tube also is called a tubal pregnancy. If the ectopic nature of a tubal pregnancy remains undiscovered, the embryo will become too large for the fallopian tube sometime between the eighth and twelfth weeks of pregnancy and the tube will burst, creating internal bleeding and a critical situation that requires immediate medical intervention.

The Developing Fetus

Fetal development occurs in two major phases. In the first phase, which takes about 10 weeks, nearly all of the fetal body forms. By the tenth week of development, the fetal body appears to have a human form and weighs

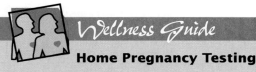

Home Pregnancy Testing

When a woman wants to know if she is pregnant, she can consult a physician or go to a family planning or public health clinic. Or, she can administer a pregnancy test herself. Several home pregnancy testing kits are now available without prescription at low cost, and they are relatively easy to use.

Virtually all chemical tests for pregnancy—those carried out in clinics and the self-test kind—analyze a woman's blood or urine for the hormone of pregnancy, Human Chorionic Gonadotropin, HCG. In some home pregnancy tests, a woman puts a few drops of her first morning urine (it contains the highest concentration of HCG) into a test tube, adds the test chemicals, and within seconds receives results. A brown ring appearing at the bottom of the test tube indicates that she is pregnant. In other tests a

chemically coated test stick is used to detect HCG in urine. A change in the test stick's color signals the presence of HCG.

The home pregnancy tests are not 100 percent accurate. Only rarely (about 3 times in 100) does the test indicate pregnancy when the woman is not pregnant. A "false positive" is likely to be discovered when the woman seeks prenatal care.

The home test for pregnancy is wrong about 20 percent of the time when it indicates that a woman is not pregnant when in fact she is. About half of these "false negatives" occur because the test has been administered too early in the pregnancy. About half of the "false negatives" are corrected if the test is re-administered in about a week. However, about 10 percent of women who are pregnant still get the inaccurate test result that they

are not pregnant. This is one of the most serious drawbacks of home pregnancy tests, for the risk of complications in pregnancy and abortion rise the longer in pregnancy a woman waits to obtain professional care.

In spite of the possibility of inaccuracy, many physicians and family planning consultants believe home pregnancy testing to be useful. It enables women to take a more active part in their own health care, and it may help women who "would rather not think about it" confront the possibility that they are pregnant. Home pregnancy testing may protect the privacy of women who may not want it known that they are sexually active. And it may help women with irregular menstrual periods relieve anxiety about the possibility of being pregnant.

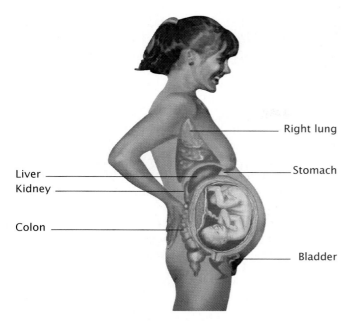

Liver

Kidney

Colon

Right lung

Stomach

Bladder

FIGURE 9.3 The Woman and Fetus during Last Months of Pregnancy Note the positioning of the fetus.

about 1 gram. During the second phase of development, which normally takes another 28 weeks, the fetal body grows and many of the organs become functional. Healthy **fetuses** born after the normal 266-day **gestation period** weigh between 5 and 10 pounds.

Fetal development and growth take place with the fetus enclosed in a fluid-filled membranous sac called the **amnion**, which forms during the second week of development. As it develops in the **amniotic fluid**, the fetus is able to grow unimpeded by the mother's internal organs. The amniotic fluid also protects the fetus from potentially damaging jolts when the mother changes her body position. The amnion ruptures just before birth, sometimes called "breaking of the bag of waters."

The growth and development of the fetus are supported by the **placenta**, an organ unique to pregnancy. The placenta manufactures many hormones needed to sustain pregnancy and is responsible for transporting oxygen and nutrients from the mother to the fetus and waste products from the fetus to the mother.

A number of changes occur in a pregnant woman's physiology (Figure 9.3). For example, the blood plasma increases in volume as much as 50 percent over her non-pregnant levels; the heart beats 10 percent faster and with 20 to 30 percent greater output per minute; the number of red blood cells increases; and breathing becomes deeper and slightly faster. One of the most striking changes during pregnancy is the growth of the uterus. The nonpregnant uterus is approximately 7–8 cm long (2.75–3.5 inches) and weighs about 60–100 grams. By the end of pregnancy the uterus is approximately 30 cm long (12 inches) and weighs nearly 1,000 grams (2.2 pounds).

CHILDBIRTH

For the parents, the moment of childbirth can bring a mixture of feelings that might include great joy, relief that the nine months of waiting are over, and surprise at the baby's appearance. All in attendance may experience concern for the condition of the mother and baby and awe and wonder at the miracle of new life.

Learning about Childbirth

In some cultures, childbirth is highly ritualized and participants follow long-established customs. But in our culture childbirth is accompanied by a variety of choices. These choices offer prospective parents opportunities to make childbirth experiences meaningful and rewarding. Decisions include where the baby will be born; the philosophy that will guide the birth; who will be present at the birth; how pain and intense sensations will be dealt with; and how much access the new parent(s) will have to the baby immediately after the birth.

It is important to know that in many cases doctors and others who assist in childbirth do not make decisions in accordance with individual and couple needs, but perform procedures they have learned and that have become routine. There are times when medical procedures are needed for the safety of the mother and/or baby, but many interventions routine in some birth settings are unnecessary and may even be harmful (Smith et al., 1991). Medications for relief of pain, **cesarean section, episiotomy,** and fetal monitors often are taken for granted as beneficial rather than being thought of as choices that may have no positive impact on the birth of the child or the experience of the parents.

T E R M S

ectopic pregnancy: a pregnancy occurring outside the uterus, usually in the fallopian tubes

fetus: the developing infant during the second and third trimesters of pregnancy

gestation period: 266 days of fetal development

amnion: the inner membrane which forms a fluid-filled sac surrounding and protecting the embryo and fetus

amniotic fluid: fluid from the amnion

placenta: the flat circular vascular structure within the pregnant uterus that provides nourishment to and eliminates wastes from the developing embryo and fetus and is passed as afterbirth after the baby is born

cesarean section: delivery of the fetus through a surgical opening in the abdomen and uterus

episiotomy: an incision in the perineum to facilitate passage of the baby's head during childbirth while minimizing injury to the woman

Prospective parents should learn the policies of a birthing center and discuss their preferences with those who will assist with the birth. Some prospective parents develop a written birth plan clearly stating their preferences. This plan is given to doctors or others who will assist the birth so all will know what is expected.

Prospective parents can learn about their options by taking childbirth preparation classes, talking with other parents about their experiences, interviewing doctors and midwives, and reading. Obtaining a variety of opinions, while sometimes frustrating and confusing to sort out, nevertheless offers the chance to make the most informed choices.

> When I was born I was so surprised I
> didn't talk for a year and a half.
> *Gracie Allen*

Childbirth Preparation

A variety of programs and organizations provide education for parents-to-be in preparation for the childbirth experience and parenthood. These are usually six-to-eight week courses, sometimes called "natural childbirth," "Lamaze," or simply childbirth preparation. Childbirth preparation classes can enhance the intimate relationship of the expectant couple and increase their confidence and self-esteem. In addition, women who participate in childbirth preparation are likely to have less pain and discomfort in childbirth, to require less medication, and to have fewer complications. Prepared women are also more likely to have positive attitudes toward childbirth and parenting. Fathers who attend childbirth preparation classes tend to feel more comfortable about sharing the birth experience with their partners and about helping them during it. They are also more likely to be interested and involved in parenting after the baby is born.

Almost all childbirth preparation courses teach prospective parents the basic biology of pregnancy and childbirth. They also teach breathing and relaxation exercises, and some teach imagery and affirmations, all intended to make the delivery of the baby proceed more smoothly and comfortably. While attending these courses, parents-to-be meet other expectant couples with whom they can share their feelings and experiences. The classes also address birthing options. Since childbirth preparation courses reflect the biases of those who teach them, prospective parents are likely to gain more complete information about birthing options by consulting additional sources (books, other parents, etc.).

Studies have shown that continuous emotional support during labor can shorten labor time, give the woman in labor greater perception of control, decrease her need for pain medication, and, overall, lead to fewer complications that affect the baby (Kennell et al., 1991). On the other hand, labor can be slowed or stopped if the woman feels uncomfortable, anxious, frightened, or experiences performance pressure due to others' expectations about how the labor should be proceeding.

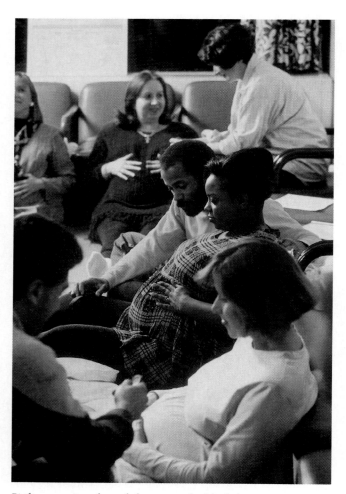

Birth preparation classes help ensure a healthy baby.

Options for Controlling Discomfort

Intense discomfort or pain can be associated with labor, especially in the later phases of the first stage and the early stages of the second. The intensity of feeling is caused by stretches and strains on the uterine muscle tissue, effacement of the cervix, and stretching of the perineum. Pain relief methods include relaxation techniques, deep breathing, acupuncture, hypnosis, massaging and supporting of the perineum by the birth attendant, medications that block pain awareness (analgesia), and medications that block the pain sensations (anesthesia). The most common anesthesia used during labor is a regional anesthetic to diminish sensation only in the pelvic region. This leaves the mother conscious during labor so that she can actively "bear down" to help push the baby out. General anesthesia (complete unconsciousness) is used only in cases of difficult births and interventions, such as cesarean sections.

Occasionally the course of labor may slow to the degree that may be harmful to both mother and fetus. Because the hormone oxytocin stimulates uterine contractions, modern obstetric practice often calls for administering oxytocin during difficult childbirth. For centuries, midwives and birth attendants in many countries have stimulated the breasts of laboring mothers to augment labor, as breast stimulation causes the natural release of oxytocin from the mother's posterior pituitary gland.

 Managing Stress

Pregnancy and Childbirth: Belly Breathing Exercise

In Lamaze classes expectant mothers (and fathers) are taught to place the emphasis of their breathing on the lower stomach, or diaphragm. During the several hours of labor and the actual delivery, this breathing skill is employed to ease the pain of childbirth. What is taught and practiced in the stressful event of childbirth is now taught and practiced in several other stressful situations as well.

Each breathing cycle is said to be comprised of four distinct phases:

Phase I: Inspiration, taking the air into your lungs through the passage of your nose or mouth

Phase II: A very slight pause before exhaling the air out of your lungs

Phase III: Exhalation, releasing the air from your lungs and though the passage it entered

Phase IV: A very slight pause after exhalation before the next inhalation is initiated.

These phases can be enhanced when the breathing cycle is exaggerated by taking a very slow and comfortable deep breath. When trying this technique, try to isolate and recognize these four phases by identifying them as they occur. It is important to remember not to hold your breath at any one time during each phase. Rather, learn to regulate your breathing by controlling the pace of each phase in the breathing cycle. Remember that diaphragmatic breathing is not the same as hyperventilation: this style of breathing is slow, relaxed, and as deep as feels comfortable. It is commonly agreed that the most relaxing phase of breathing is the third phase, exhalation. In this phase the chest and abdominal areas relax, producing a relaxing effect throughout the body. When focusing on your breathing, feel how relaxed your whole body becomes during this phase of exhalation, especially your chest, shoulders, and abdominal region.

An Energy Breathing Exercise

There are three phases to this exercise and you can use this technique either sitting or lying down.

1. First get comfortable, allowing your shoulders to relax. If you choose to sit, try to keep your legs straight. As you breathe in, imagine that there is a circular hole at the top of your head. As the air enters your lungs, visualize energy in the form of a beam of light, entering the top of your head. Bring the energy down, from the crown of your head to your abdomen as you inhale. As you exhale, allow the energy to leave through the top of your head. Repeat this 5 to 10 times, trying to coordinate your breathing with the visual flow of energy. As you continue to bring the energy down to your stomach area, allow the light to reach all the inner parts of your upper body. When you feel comfortable with this first phase, you are ready to move on to the second phase.

2. Now, imagine that in the center of each foot, there is a circular hole through which energy can flow in and out. Again think of energy as a beam of light. Concentrating on only your lower extremities, allow the flow of energy to move up from your feet into your abdomen as you inhale from your diaphragm. Repeat this 5 to 10 times, trying to coordinate your breathing with the flow of energy. As you continue to bring the energy up into your stomach area, allow the light to reach all the inner parts of your lower body.

3. Once you have coordinated your breathing with the visual flow of energy through your lower extremities, begin to combine the movement of energy from the top of your head and your feet, bringing the energy to the center of your body as you inhale air from your diaphragm. Then, as you exhale, allow the flow of energy to reverse from the direction of which it came. Repeat this 10 to 20 times. Each time you move the energy through your body feel each body region—each muscle, organ, and cell—become energized. At first it may be difficult to visually coordinate the movement of energy coming from opposite ends of your body, but this will become very easy with practice.

Giving Birth

A few weeks before the onset of childbirth, or **labor**, the fetus becomes positioned for birth by descending in the uterus, a process called **lightening**. When this happens the pressure on some of the mother's internal organs is relieved and she may find it easier to breathe, stand, and digest food. In about 95 percent of all births the fetus is in a head-down position. When not head-down, the fetus may be head-up, referred to as a breech position. In nearly all instances the fetus' legs are tucked up against its abdomen in the "fetal position."

> *When my kids become wild and unruly, I use a nice, safe playpen. When they're finished, I climb out.*
> Erma Bombeck,
> columnist

Throughout much of pregnancy, the uterus contracts intermittently, tightening in waves that sometimes are so gentle that the woman is unaware of them. During the last half of pregnancy, a woman may at times feel her abdomen becoming hard or otherwise perceive the uterine contractions as they prepare her body for the true labor. Health professionals refer to these as **Braxton-Hicks contractions**. They can be distinguished by their occurrence at irregular intervals and rather short duration.

Although childbirth is one continuous process, it is often described as occurring in three stages. During the first stage the mother's cervix dilates to allow the baby to pass from the uterus. The second stage is the actual emergence of the baby from the mother's body. The third stage, called the **afterbirth**, is the expulsion of the placenta and membranes. Childbirth usually lasts 2 to 24 hours; the overall length and the length of each stage varies tremendously among women, and for each woman from baby to baby. Labor tends to be longer for first-time mothers, but this may not always be so.

The onset of labor is marked by the appearance of strong, rhythmic, and eventually frequent uterine contractions. These initially dilate the cervix and later change in character to move the baby out of the mother's body. The contractions of labor usually begin as roughly minute-long contractions coming at approximately 10- to 20-minute intervals. As labor progresses, these regular contractions usually become more intense, frequent, and of longer duration, perhaps up to 90 seconds.

During the first stage of labor, the cervical opening enlarges or effaces from about 1 centimeter to about 10 centimeters to allow passage of the baby from the mother's body. In the first stage the birth attendants will likely encourage the mother to relax her body around her uterus and baby so that her uterine muscles can work efficiently, unimpeded by other bodily tensions. She is told to avoid pushing, which could interfere with the work of her contractions in dilating the cervix.

The second stage begins when the cervix is fully dilated and the baby's head moves into the birth canal. During this stage the baby passes through the

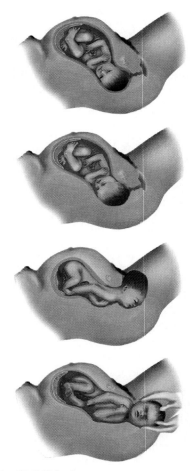

FIGURE 9.4 Childbirth

T E R M S

labor: the process of childbirth

lightening: the positioning of the fetus for birth by descent in the uterus

Braxton-Hicks contractions: normal uterine contractions that occur periodically throughout pregnancy

afterbirth: the third stage of labor, in which the placenta is discharged

puerperium: the six weeks after childbirth, also called postpartum period

colostrum: yellowish liquid secreted from the breasts; contains antibodies and protein

prolactin: a hormone produced by the anterior lobe of the pituitary gland that stimulates milk secretion

vaginal canal and out of the mother's body (Figure 9.4). The mother's role shifts and she actively assists during contractions by bearing down to push the baby out; indeed, she may feel an almost irresistible urge to push. To allow her perineum to stretch gradually, it can be useful for the mother to replace the image of "pushing" with a mental image of "opening up" or "expanding" for her baby's passage.

THE POSTPARTUM TRANSITION

After the child is born, the mother goes through a several-week period of postpartum transition called the **puerperium.** During this time, the physiological changes of pregnancy slowly reverse and the vagina and the surrounding structures recuperate from labor. Uterine tissue that is no longer needed is discharged for the first month or so after childbirth. The discharge, called lochia, at first resembles a heavy menstrual flow, then typically tapers off after a week or two. Following delivery, estrogen and progesterone levels, which were high during pregnancy, drop rapidly, reaching almost zero about 72 hours after birth.

During this period the mother and her partner begin to adjust to their often demanding new life situation. For example, childbirth and infant care are exhausting. Many women experience the "baby blues," transitory mood changes involving tiredness, depression, loneliness, and/or fear. These feelings usually abate in the weeks following childbirth, but a minority of women experience postpartum depression severe enough to be disabling and require professional help. Postpartum mood changes are so common that experts suggest they may be related to the massive changes in hormone levels that accompany childbirth. Others, while not denying the effects of hormonal changes, point out that childbirth is a life transition that brings many changes and psychological adjustments for the woman, her partner, and other family and household members.

Breast-Feeding

The preparation of the breasts for nursing begins in the early weeks of pregnancy with an increase in the number of milk ducts and the deposit of fat in the breast tissue. This growth causes breast tenderness early in pregnancy. In addition to the increase in breast size, the nipples enlarge and often deepen in color. About midway into pregnancy, the breasts begin to manufacture **colostrum,** a yellowish precursor to actual mother's milk. For the first few days after birth, colostrum is the major substance emitted from the breasts. As the newborn nurses, colostrum is drained from the breasts and is replaced by mother's milk. Colostrum contains nutrients and is especially high in antibodies that protect the infant against

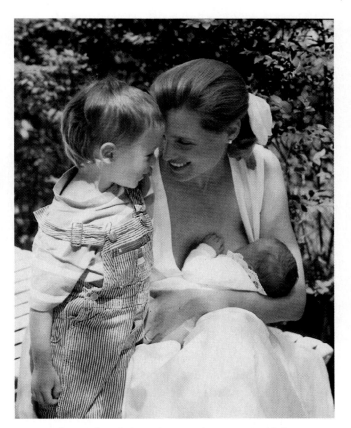

Breast milk provides a baby with essential nutrients and helps prevent infections.

infection. Mother's milk contains specific milk proteins, antibodies, lactose, fat, and water. The synthesis of milk is controlled by the pituitary hormone **prolactin,** the levels of which rise tremendously during pregnancy and are maintained as long as the mother continues to nurse.

HEALTHY PEOPLE 2000

Increase to at least 75 percent the proportion of mothers who breast-feed their babies in the early postpartum period and to at least 50 percent the proportion who continue breast-feeding until their babies are 5 to 6 months old.

Breast-feeding is the optimal way of nurturing full-term infants while simultaneously benefiting the lactating mother. The advantages of breast-feeding range from biochemical, immunologic, enzymatic, and endocrinologic to psychosocial, developmental, hygienic, and economic. Human milk contains the ideal balance of nutrients, enzymes, immunoglobulin, anti-infective and anti-inflammatory substances, hormones, and growth factors.

Milk is delivered from the breast through the coordinated activity of the mother and infant. Inserting the nipple into the baby's mouth activates the baby's sucking reflex. When the baby sucks, nerve impulses are transmitted from the breast to the mother's brain, which stimulate the release of the hormone oxytocin. Oxytocin circulates through the mother's bloodstream to the breasts, where it causes the muscle cells that line the milk ducts to contract and eject milk from the nipple. Oxytocin also stimulates contractions of the uterus, so breast-feeding helps return the uterus to its prepregnant size.

A mother can nurse for many months. As long as the baby is sucking and the breasts are regularly drained of milk, the hormonal stimulation of milk production will continue. Without such stimuli, milk production stops. The many advantages of breast-feeding include:

- It is economical, readily available, and eliminates the effort involved in purchasing, preparing, and heating bottles and formula.
- It transfers immunity (protection against infections) from the mother to the infant, and breast milk itself and the act of nursing stimulate the development of the infant's own immune defenses.
- Breast milk promotes development of the infant's digestive system.
- Breast-fed babies have fewer allergies, less diarrhea, fewer dental problems, and less colic (stomachache).
- Breast milk is nutritionally balanced for human infants; formulas containing cow's milk are not nutritionally identical to human milk, although they are nutritionally adequate.
- Breast-feeding may increase the psychological attachment between mother and infant.
- The hormones involved in the production and release of milk cause uterine contractions, which help the uterus return to its normal size. During the first week or so after childbirth these contractions may be intense and even painful. Thereafter some women describe them as pleasurable, sensual, or erotic.

Many women find that breast-feeding offers them a relaxing, pleasurable experience with their babies. Often the pleasurable feelings of breast-feeding will have an erotic tone, possibly producing genital sensations and even occasionally orgasm. These feelings and responses are normal and natural, and a women need not feel guilty or distressed by them.

The many advantages of breast-feeding do not mean that bottle feeding is not wholesome. Many healthy, well-

T E R M

weaned: to discontinue breast-feeding, using other means to provide nutrients

Reduce the incidence of fetal alcohol syndrome to no more than 0.12 per 1,000 live births.

Heavy alcohol consumption during pregnancy is known to cause alcohol-related defects among infants and fetal alcohol syndrome, which is characterized by growth retardation, facial malformations, and central nervous system dysfunctions including mental retardation. Although the lower limit of safe alcohol consumption during pregnancy has not been documented, it is clear that most known adverse effects in infants are associated with heavy maternal alcohol use.

adjusted people were bottle-fed infants. Some women are physically unable to breast-feed. Some mothers choose not to breast-feed because work, family, and other responsibilities make it inconvenient. Breast-feeding in public or at work is still not acceptable in many communities or places of employment. Some women choose not to breast-feed because they fear that changes in the shape of their breasts will decrease their sexual attractiveness.

Some women breast-feed their infants for several weeks or months and then gradually substitute bottle-feedings for breast-feedings until the child is completely **weaned,** that is, has stopped nursing altogether. More important than whether the milk comes from the breast or a bottle is the physical contact and loving the infant receives while being fed.

HEALTH HABITS DURING PREGNANCY

Every child deserves to be born as healthy as possible. It is only fair to the unborn child—who did not ask to be conceived—that all the genetic potential to develop a healthy body and mind be given the opportunity to be fully expressed. Few of us are as careful about maintaining proper health habits as we could be. Most people live with whatever risk might be associated with nonhealthy behaviors and are presumably willing to accept the consequences of those behaviors. But when a woman is pregnant, disregarding fundamental health practices endangers her child as well as herself, and perhaps more so, because the developing baby's body and mind are extremely vulnerable to damage. It is extremely important that a mother-to-be make every effort to practice good health habits. If her developing baby could talk, he or she might say, "Mom, my life-long health and well-being are in your hands now. I know nine months is a long time to have to be concerned about what you eat and drink, but it's important to me that you do the right

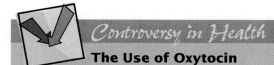

The Use of Oxytocin

There is controversy about the use of oxytocin to augment labor. Critics charge that some hospital staff administer oxytocin to force the birth to occur when the staff is most available rather than letting the mother deliver on her own schedule. Also, there is no consensus regarding what conditions should signal the use of oxytocin. Labor augmentation is needed when uterine contractions are weak or absent or when the fetus is in distress (not breathing). To determine the state of the fetus during childbirth, an electric heart-rate monitor is applied to the baby's body, and sometimes the oxygen content of the blood is monitored by taking blood samples from the scalp. If the fetal heart rate and blood samples indicate fetal distress, then oxytocin may be given. Studies fail to show, however, that in the majority of normal births, fetal monitoring, scalp blood monitoring, and oxytocin are required (Smith et al., 1991).

STUDENT REFLECTIONS
- Would you request that no oxytocin be used during the birth of your child?
- Under what circumstances would you request oxytocin?

things for both of us. Not only will that give me the chance to become the best person I can be, but will also keep you healthy so we can share a lot of good times after I'm born." The factors that deserve a pregnant woman's attention to ensure her own health and that of her baby are proper nutrition, obtaining professional prenatal care, getting enough exercise, refraining from smoking and consuming alcohol or other drugs while pregnant, and accepting and dealing with emotional and sexual feelings that may be different from those experienced when not pregnant.

Nutrition

Throughout pregnancy, the fetus' cells and physiological capacities are developing. Perhaps more than at any other time of life, an ample supply of nutrients is required so that the making of new cells and the devel-

oping of organs proceeds optimally. All of the fetus' nutrients come from the mother via the placenta. Therefore, a pregnant woman directly influences the nutritional status of her baby, and she must be aware that she must "eat for two," meaning that she must be sure her diet contains adequate nutrients for herself and for her baby. Mothers-to-be who eat highly nutritious diets during pregnancy are more likely to give birth to healthy babies than are mothers whose diets are nutritionally poor. It is recommended that pregnant women increase their intake of essential nutrients and calories (Table 9.1). Some women are advised to supplement a generally well-balanced diet with extra iron and folic acid.

Many pregnant women are concerned with the amount of weight they gain. Not long ago, most doctors severely restricted weight gain by pregnant women in their care because they felt that gaining too much weight caused a serious high blood pressure disease of preg-

TABLE 9.1 Recommended Daily Dietary Allowances for Nonpregnant, Pregnant, and Lactating Women, Ages 25–50

	Nonpregnant	Pregnant	Lactating		Nonpregnant	Pregnant	Lactating
Protein (g)	50	60	64	Folacin (mg)	180	400	280
Vitamin A (mcg)	800	800	1300	Vitamin B_{12} (mcg)	2	2.2	2.6
Vitamin D (mcg)	5	10	10	Calcium (mg)	800	1200	1200
Vitamin E (mg)	8	10	12	Phosphorus (mg)	800	1200	1200
Vitamin C (mg)	60	70	95	Magnesium (mg)	280	320	355
Thiamine (mg)	1.1	1.5	1.6	Iron (mg)	10	15	15
Riboflavin (mg)	1.2	1.6	1.8	Zinc (mg)	12	19	16
Niacin (mg)	13	20	20	Iodine (mcg)	150	200	200
Vitamin B_6 (mg)	1.6	2.2	2.1				

Source: Food and Nutrition Board, *Recommended Dietary Allowances* (Washington, D.C.: National Academy of Sciences National Research Council, 1989).

nancy, **toxemia.** While it is never good to weigh too much, current obstetric practice allows a mother-to-be to gain a reasonable amount of weight, about 28 to 30 pounds by the end of pregnancy, most of which comes in the last two-thirds of pregnancy. About 7 of these pounds are contributed by the fetus. The enlarged uterus accounts for another 2 pounds and the placenta and amniotic fluid contribute 1 pound each. About 4 to 8 pounds of fluid are added to the maternal system as extra blood and extracellular fluid. And the mother may gain about 4 pounds of body fat. It was once considered good obstetric practice to prescribe diuretic drugs (to reduce water in the body) and appetite suppressants (amphetamines) to control a mother's body weight and thereby to try to prevent certain diseases that are characteristic of pregnancy. This is no longer recommended.

Prenatal Care

Pregnancy involves several profound biological changes. Not only does the fetus develop from a single cell to a 7- or 8-pound newborn infant composed of many millions of cells, but also the mother's body undergoes a number of anatomical and physiological changes in order to support fetal development. Moreover, the fetal-maternal relationship is maintained by the placenta, an organ that develops only during pregnancy and is expelled from the mother's uterus after the baby is born. Any rapidly changing system is vulnerable to errors and problems, and so it is with pregnancy and fetal development. That is why it is recommended that mothers-to-be receive professional prenatal care. A number of studies have shown that the more prenatal care a woman receives, the fewer will be her problems during pregnancy and childbirth and the more likely that her infant will be born healthy. Professional prenatal care can help a mother-to-be avoid the consequences of a number of pregnancy-specific illnesses, such as toxemia, pregnancy-induced diabetes, and infection. These illnesses can threaten both the mother's health and the proper development and delivery of her baby. Professional prenatal care can also help manage problems resulting from a malfunctioning placenta and

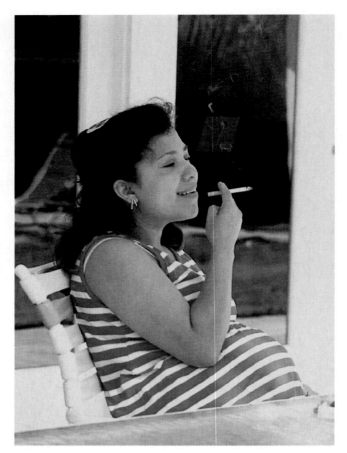

Chemicals in cigarette smoke can damage the developing fetus.

can educate a mother about proper nutrition and advise her on how smoking at any time during pregnancy can adversely affect her baby's development, as can consumption of alcohol. Maternal infections that are harmful to the fetus, such as rubella (German measles), syphilis, gonorrhea, toxoplasmosis, herpes, and the HIV virus, can be detected and managed. Another reason for prenatal care is to be sure the maternal and fetal blood cells are immunologically (Rh factor) compatible.

Physical Activity and Exercise

There are special benefits to being physically active during pregnancy. Some women feel lethargic during pregnancy. In just a few weeks their bodies take on unfamiliar proportions and they have to carry up to 20 percent more weight than when they are not pregnant. They may feel uncomfortable, unattractive, and clumsy. Through

T E R M S

toxemia: an infrequent complication of pregnancy characterized by high blood pressure, swelling, and possible convulsions

infertile: unable to become pregnant or to impregnate

movement and exercise, a pregnant woman can become accustomed to the temporary changes in her body and can accept pregnancy as a positive and fulfilling time of her life. Physical activity also helps prepare the mother's body for childbirth, which is often physically demanding. By keeping active, a pregnant woman can improve her circulation and thereby reduce swelling and formation of varicose veins in the lower legs, which can be common in pregnancy. Perhaps the greatest benefit from physical activity during pregnancy is maintaining the habit of being active. That way, after the baby is born, the mother can lose body fat gained during pregnancy and return her body to a firm nonpregnant state.

The degree of physical activity a pregnant woman engages in depends on her desires and abilities. Some athletic women engage in sports almost to the day of delivery. Women who are not routinely athletic are wise to begin a program early in pregnancy that involves exercises to maintain correct posture, strengthen abdominal muscles, and improve breathing and ability to relax (Figure 9.5).

Emotional Well-Being

Pregnancy can be a time of intense feelings, not only for the mother-to-be but also for her partner and others who are close to her. Enthusiasm, excitement, anticipation, fear about the baby's condition, uncertainties about one's suitability as a parent, a desire for more (or less) love, affection, and sex are all natural. Recognizing that intense feelings are normal in pregnancy and accepting them with patience and understanding are the keys to a rewarding pregnancy experience.

Perhaps the best way to deal with intense feelings at any time in life, including pregnancy, is to take time each day to quiet the mind and body with meditation, yoga, or other relaxation methods. Massage is also beneficial, and it fulfills some of the desires of those who feel more sensual during pregnancy. Some couples feel increased desire for sexual intercourse during pregnancy, which is all right unless the woman has a medical problem that would be worsened by sex. In that event couples can engage in the many forms of pleasuring that do not involve sexual intercourse.

INFERTILITY

Approximately 14 percent of all American married couples of childbearing age are **infertile**, which means that they are unable to become pregnant after a year of trying. Male factors are responsible for infertility in about 40 percent of infertile couples; female factors in another 40 to 50 percent. In about 10 percent of infertile couples, no cause can be determined. With professional help, about half of all infertile couples can eventually

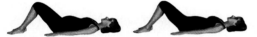

Pelvic tilt
Lie on back with both knees bent and feet on the floor, 18 inches apart. Press small of back to the floor for a count of four, then relax. Repeat ten times.

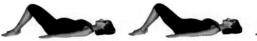

Universal toner
Same position as pelvic tilt. Press small of back to floor and lift head and stretch right arm to left knee, hold a few seconds, then relax. Repeat stretching left arm to right knee.

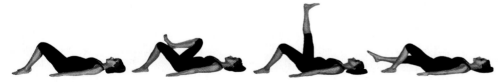

Hip-knee-ankle toner
Lie on back or on side. Upon exhalation, bend right leg, bringing knee to chest. Then stretch leg straight, trying to touch ceiling with heel. Slowly lower leg to floor. Repeat twice for both legs.

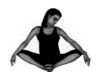

Neck and shoulder toner
Sit with back straight. Slowly drop chin to chest and gently circle to left in a large arc, making a complete circle. Repeat in other direction.

FIGURE 9.5 Some Recommended Exercises during Pregnancy
Source: P. Shrock, Clinical Obstetrics, Vol. 2.

Infertility Tests for Women

Women-only tests, more varied and extensive [than those for men], generally begin with a determination of if and when the woman is ovulating. One of the most popular techniques for pinpointing ovulation relies on the typically slight rise in resting body temperature midway in the menstrual cycle, signaling that ovulation has recently occurred.

A woman's body temperature fluctuates throughout her menstrual cycle, and she is instructed to record these fluctuations on a chart after taking her temperature each morning before getting out of bed. If the chart—called a basal body temperature, or BBT, chart—indicates that the woman has been ovulating, it can often be used to predict when ovulation will happen during subsequent menstrual cycles. The couple can then use the information to attempt to time conception. Several urine test kits, approved by the Food and Drug Administration for sale over the counter, can be used by consumers to supplement the temperature chart.

Still other methods widely used to predict ovulation rely on examinations of the cervical mucus, which undergoes a series of hormone-induced changes at various times in the menstrual cycle. Some versions of these tests require a health professional's expertise. There are, however, versions of them that some women—with a physician's guidance—can learn to do themselves.

Other methods widely used to diagnose female infertility and to monitor therapy include:

- *Endometrial Biopsy:* A long, hollow tube is passed into the patient's uterus late in her menstrual cycle, and a little of the lining is scraped off and examined with a microscope. The examination helps the physician tell whether the development of the egg and of the lining are in proper phase with each other. In most cases, the scraping is done in a physician's office and because it is only very briefly painful no anesthetic is used.

- *Ultrasound:* This technology relies on sound waves to produce images of internal structures. It is used, often in combination with one or more of the tests already discussed, to find the presence or absence of follicles that contain and release the eggs. Ultrasound is also sometimes used to detect abnormalities in the ovaries or uterus.

- *Hysterosalpingogram:* This is an X-ray study of the uterus and fallopian tubes. It is done just after a woman's menstrual period so there is no danger of her being pregnant and thereby exposing the fertilized egg or embryo to radiation.

  A dye containing iodine—technically called a contrast medium—is injected through the cervix. It spreads into the uterus and the fallopian tubes, allowing them to be visualized. Among other things, this study often enables the physician to determine if the fallopian tubes are open. It is usu-

ally done without an anesthetic in the X-ray department of a hospital or clinic.

- *Hysteroscopy:* The patient's uterus is filled with a liquid or gas, instilled through the cervix. A thin, lighted tube called a hysteroscope that works like a telescope is then inserted into the uterus through the cervix, enabling the surgeon or physician to look directly inside. Many hysteroscopes have a separate channel through which instruments can be passed, often making it possible to immediately correct any abnormalities. Patients undergoing hysteroscopy are usually given an anesthetic, which may be local or general.

- *Laparoscopy:* A laparoscope, like a hysteroscope, is an instrument with a light that works like a telescope. It is slipped into the abdominal cavity through a small incision in or near the navel. For a clearer view of the woman's reproductive tract, the cavity is filled with gas during the procedure, and a colored solution—usually blue—is injected into the uterus and fallopian tubes. A general anesthetic is required. Advanced operative techniques may allow the repair of defects in the reproductive tract to be made at the same time as the examination.

Source: J. Randal, "Trying to Outsmart Infertility," *FDA Consumer* (May 1991): 22–29.

---

have children. A significant percentage of couples medically diagnosed as infertile eventually have children without medical interventions.

In both sexes, infertility can be caused by a variety of conditions that adversely affect the functioning of an otherwise normal reproductive system. For example, ill health, cigarette smoking, chronic alcohol use, marijuana and other drug abuse, exposure to radiation or toxic chemicals, malnutrition, anxiety, stress, and fatigue can lessen a person's reproductive capabilities. Medical treatments and/or changes in life-style can often restore fertility.

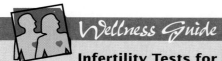
Infertility Tests for Men

A semen analysis is almost always the first test done on men and is usually repeated several times. After abstaining from intercourse for about 48 hours, the man collects a sperm sample in a container.

The sample is microscopically examined to determine the number, activity and shape of individual spermatozoa (sperm cells) and the characteristics of the fluid part of the semen.

A healthy, potent ejaculate typically contains 1.5 to 5 cubic centimeters (5 cc = 1 teaspoon) of semen and each cc will contain an average of 70 million sperm that look to be of normal size, shape, and behavior. If the specimen markedly differs on any of these factors, further tests may be done to determine whether infection, hormonal imbalance, or another problem could be the culprit.

Among these tests may be a testicular biopsy, a minor operation—performed with a local or general anesthetic—in which a small amount of tissue from the testes is removed for laboratory studies. Since even men with sperm counts well below 70 million per cubic centimeter sometimes father children, this test is ordinarily done only when the count is zero.

If damage to one or both of the vas deferens, is known or suspected, an X-ray examination may also be ordered. As an iodine-containing solution has to be injected into the tubes to make them visible on X-rays, the patient is first given local or general anesthesia. If the examination discloses damage, surgical repairs are often attempted at the same time the diagnosis is made.

Other special tests may be ordered if none of the tests already mentioned seems to explain the man's infertility. The most common of these tests are the bovine mucus test and the hamster-oocyte penetration test.

In the first, bovine (cow) mucus (from the cervix, or neck of the uterus where it opens into the vagina) is placed in a special glass column. Samples of the man's semen are applied to the column, and measurements are made of how well the sperm are able to enter and swim through the mucus, giving some indication of their ability to swim through human cervical mucus.

In the hamster-oocyte penetration test, some of the man's semen is mixed with hamster egg cells that have had their outer shells (membranes) removed. If the sperm are functioning normally, they will penetrate the hamster eggs, an indication that they are also capable of fertilizing human eggs. However, failure of the sperm to penetrate the hamster eggs does not always mean that they are incapable of fertilizing human eggs.

Source: J. Randal, "Trying to Outsmart Infertility," *FDA Consumer* (May 1991): 22–29.

Obstacles to Fertility

Because sperm and ovum production and the functions of the male and female reproductive tracts are absolutely dependent on adequate hormone production, hormonal problems are a common cause of infertility in both men and women. Infertility can also be caused by anatomical abnormalities or damage to the male or female reproductive systems (Chapter 8). A common cause of damage is scarring and subsequent blocking of the fallopian tubes and, less frequently, the epididymis, by gonorrhea and chlamydia infections. The scar tissue from such diseases blocks the tubes and prevents the passage of sperm and ova. Growths and tumors in the reproductive tract can also block the passage of sperm and ova. Sometimes surgical repair of blocked or damaged tubes can restore fertility.

Problems with **insemination** and sperm transport can also cause infertility. For example, a man may have difficulty getting and maintaining an erection or ejaculating into the vagina. A woman may produce very thick or voluminous cervical mucus, which can block entry of sperm into the uterus. Sometimes a couple has trouble conceiving because they are not having intercourse near the time of ovulation.

Enhancing Fertility Options

A variety of medical interventions are available to help infertile couples become pregnant. For example, if a male partner produces too few sperm but those he does produce are healthy, conception is unlikely to occur. For conception to occur, more than 20 million healthy

T E R M S

insemination: introduction of semen into the uterus or oviduct

artificial insemination: introduction of semen into the uterus or oviduct by other than natural means

in vitro *fertilization* **(IVF):** a procedure in which an egg is removed from a ripe follicle and fertilized by a sperm cell outside the human body; the fertilized egg is allowed to divide in a protected environment for about two days and then is inserted back into the uterus

sperm need to be deposited in the vagina. Fertilization can be facilitated by introducing semen obtained from the man directly into the cervix with a syringe. This is called **artificial insemination.** If the male partner cannot produce sufficient numbers of healthy sperm even for artificial insemination, the couple may become pregnant by artificial insemination with semen from a donor.

Another way to overcome infertility is *in vitro* **fertilization (IVF),** which involves obtaining several ova from the ovaries and fertilizing them in a laboratory dish. The resultant embryo is placed into the woman's uterus. *In vitro* fertilization is employed when a woman's fallopian tubes do not function correctly. GIFT (gamete intrafallopian transfer) and ZIFT (zygote intrafallopian transfer) are similar to *in vitro* fertilization. With GIFT, the ova are placed in equal numbers in each of the fallopian tubes and semen is introduced directly into the tubes. With ZIFT, eggs are fertilized *in vitro* and an embryo is placed in the fallopian tube. These procedures are successful between 10 and 20 percent of the time.

For some couples, the prospect of not being able to have a child is devastating (Stanton, Tennen, Affleck, and Mendola 1991). Many of these couples embark on lengthy efforts to become pregnant and have a healthy baby, which may cost thousands of dollars and consume much of their emotional energy. Such couples may be asked to keep careful records of the woman's fertility cycle and to time intercourse for maximum likelihood of conception. They may be counseled to have intercourse at certain times after hormone treatments. They may make repeated visits to fertility clinics to undergo IVF or other medical interventions.

About 40,000 infertile couples in the United States attempt to have a child using IVF techniques each year. However, for most of these couples repeated attempts to conceive end in failure. For women under age 35 the success rate is approximately 20 percent; for women over age 40 the success rate is under 10 percent (Begley, 1995). In addition to the poor success rate, couples pay approximately $10,000 for each attempt to become pregnant and health insurance generally does not cover any IVF costs.

HEALTH IN REVIEW

- Conception, pregnancy, and childbirth are important and meaningful life experiences. The decision to become a parent requires psychological and physical preparation so every child can have parents prepared to meet its needs.
- Children are produced by the fusion of an ovum and a sperm. Ova are produced in the ovaries at near-monthly intervals and released into the fallopian tubes, where fertilization usually takes place.
- Sperm are produced in the testes and transported outside the body through the penis.
- Fertilization is followed by cleavages of the embryo as it moves into the uterus. About the sixth day after fertilization the embryo implants in the lining of the

uterus, and for the next 266 days or so the fetus develops. After 38 weeks of pregnancy a baby is born.
- Optimal childbirth can be achieved by attending childbirth preparation classes, assuring emotional support for the mother during childbirth, and making wise choices about medical interventions such as episiotomy and pain management.
- The period after childbirth may involve breast-feeding and resumption of sexual activities.
- Approximately 14 percent of American couples are infertile. Some of these couples can be medically assisted to become pregnant; pregnancy also may occur with *in vitro* fertilization or artificial insemination.

REFERENCES

Begley, S. (1995). "The Baby Myth." *Newsweek*, September 4.

Kennell, J., M. Klaus, S. McGrath, S. Robertson, and C. Hinkley (1991). "Continuous Emotional Support during Labor in a U.S. Hospital." *Journal of the American Medical Society*, 265: 2197–2201.

Smith, M. A., L. S. Acheson, J. E. Byrd, P. Curtis, T. W. Day,

S. H. Frank, et al. (1991). "A Critical Review of Labor and Birth Care." *Journal of Family Practice*, 33: 281–292.

Stanton, A. L., H. Tennen, G. Affleck, and R. Mendola (1991). "Cognitive Appraisal and Adjustment to Infertility." *Women and Health*, 17: 1–16.

SUGGESTED READINGS

Nilsson, L., and L. Hamberger (1990). *A Child Is Born*. New York: Delacorte/Lawrence. The story of birth from the beginning, with excellent photographs.

Randal, J. (1993). "Trying to Outsmart Infertility." *FDA Consumer*, May: 22–29. A complete review of fertility drugs, surgery, artificial insemination, *in vitro* fertilization, and fertility tests.

Rosenberg, J. (1995). "How Pregnancy Affects Your Sex Life." *Parents*, March: 66–68. Discusses the physical changes that occur during pregnancy and their influence on sexual response, who should not have sex, creative lovemaking, and the importance of communication.

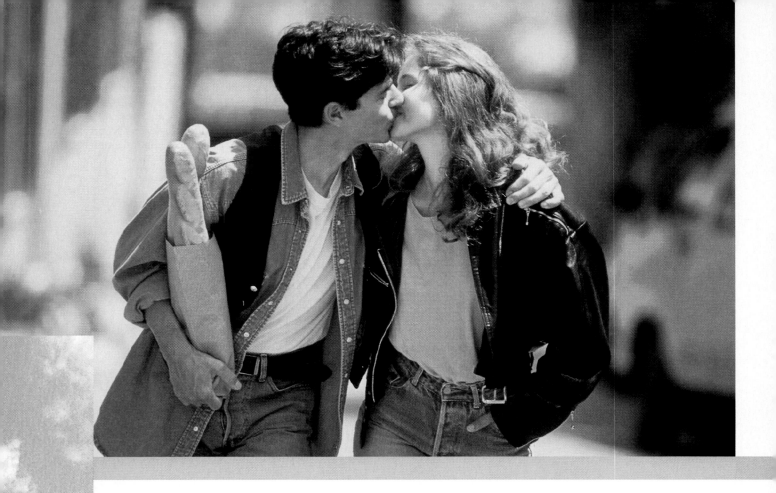

LEARNING OBJECTIVES

After reading this chapter you should be able to:

1. Identify the advantages and disadvantages for the following birth control methods: male condom, female condom, spermicides, diaphragm, cervical cap, hormonal contraceptives, Norplant, Depo-Provera, IUD, abstinence, sterilization, withdrawal, and postcoital methods.

2. Identify several different types of fertility awareness methods.

3. Identify the most effective and least effective birth control method.

4. Determine the best birth control method for your sexual life-style.

5. Discuss the importance of communication when determining the right birth control method to use with your partner.

6. Explain why some sexually active people do not use birth control.

7. Define abortion and describe the different types of abortion procedures.

Choosing a Fertility Control Method

To be aware of the many facets of human sexuality—sexual values, the structure of sexual anatomy, aspects of sexual identity and sexual behavior, and sexual responsiveness—is the first step toward attaining a healthy and fulfilling sex life. Because sexual activities nearly always involve others, our sexual decisions must also involve concern for the health and well-being of the partner. In this chapter, we discuss responsible sexual decision making as it pertains to the avoidance or termination of unintended pregnancy and the prevention of sexually transmitted (venereal) diseases.

FERTILITY CONTROL

Approximately 70 million Americans engage in between 1 and 6 billion acts of sexual intercourse each year for reasons other than to produce children. Instead of procreation, people often have sex because it is pleasurable and a way to express love and affection. Given the choice, most persons would prefer to separate nearly all of their sexual experiences from conception. People have many reasons for practicing birth control (Table 10.1) and, fortunately, modern biotechnology has produced highly effective aids for preventing unintended pregnancies.

TABLE 10.1 Some Common Reasons for Birth Control

Reason	Explanation
Enhancing sexual pleasure	Anxiety about the possibility of pregnancy can divert a person's attention from the sexual experience and interfere with the flow of sexual feelings. Also, worry during intercourse can cause difficulties with erection and ejaculation in men, and with vaginal lubrication and orgasm in women.
Family planning	Safe, reliable birth control affords couples the opportunity to plan the size of their family and the timing of their children's births. Couples can have children when the family's financial resources are sound and the parents' relationship is ready for raising a child or children.
Increasing women's life choices	Birth control allows women to choose when to devote time and energy to various life pursuits, including parenthood. In the not-too-distant past, when birth control methods were unreliable, it was difficult for a woman to integrate her personal goals with parenthood because she had little control over the timing of the births of her children.
Health considerations	Birth control helps couples reduce the risk of passing a hereditary disease to children. Birth control also is advantageous for women for whom pregnancy and childbirth may be a significant health risk. Birth control can prevent pregnancy in teenagers, who experience more pregnancy-related problems than older women.
World overpopulation	Some couples keep their families small because they want to take some responsibility for limiting the growth of the human population. At the current rate of growth, the world's population is doubling about every 30 years, which means that by the end of this century it will total almost 8 billion. Some people fear that overpopulation will create pressures for food, water, living space, energy, and other resources.

Throughout history hundreds of methods of birth control have been advocated, including potions, elixirs, vaginal inserts (pessaries), and douches made of assorted plant and animal substances; having the woman jump or sneeze after intercourse to try to dispel semen from the vagina; and will power. However, at no time in the past have people had available to them as many safe, reliable methods of birth control as they have today. Unlike the ancient methods, which were rooted in superstition and folklore, today's birth control methods are based on scientific knowledge of human reproductive biology. Some of the modern birth control techniques are preconcep-

tion methods (contraceptives). They work by preventing the development or union of sperm and ova. Other techniques are postconception methods. They inhibit in various ways the development of the fertilized ovum or embryo.

When you consider the several methods of fertility control, keep in mind that sex without intercourse is a highly effective way to prevent pregnancy. Genital (penis-in-vagina) intercourse is not the only way to give and receive sexual pleasure. Touching, kissing, and stroking can bring intense sexual enjoyment and even orgasm to both partners.

There is no fertility control method that is perfect for everyone. Except for abstinence from sexual intercourse, no single method is 100 percent effective, 100 percent free of side effects, absolutely safe, financially available to everyone, and 100 percent reversible. Without a perfect contraceptive, avoiding an unintended pregnancy requires weighing the benefits and drawbacks of the various methods and choosing the one(s) that both partners are comfortable using and that they will use properly each time sexual intercourse takes place. Even the most technologically perfect contraceptive would fail if it were not used properly and consistently.

T E R M S

failure rate: likelihood of becoming pregnant if using a birth control method for one year

lowest observed failure rate: likelihood of becoming pregnant if using a birth control method consistently and as intended

typical failure rate: likelihood of becoming pregnant considering all the potential problems associated with a birth control method

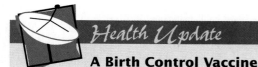

A Birth Control Vaccine

For decades, researchers have been trying to develop a vaccine that would "trick" the immune system into preventing pregnancy. This hard work is finally beginning to pay off. The ideal contraceptive vaccine would:

- prevent pregnancies for 6 to 12 months with a single dose
- have none of the side effects associated with other contraceptives

- be more reliable than mechanical methods
- restore male or female fertility by administering a counteractive drug

Researchers at Northwestern University are talking with the Food and Drug Administration about testing a vaccine that would induce a woman's immune system to attack sperm. Testing of a contraceptive vaccine in men and women is currently underway in India, Sweden, and the United States.

The challenge to scientists is the requirement that the contraceptive vaccine must past rigorous scientific standards for effectiveness and safety and also be acceptable to people.

Source: Adapted from D. L. Wheeler, "A Birth Control Vaccine," *The Chronicle of Higher Education* (April 7, 1995).

A birth control method's effectiveness is measured in terms of its **failure rate**, which is the percentage of women who, on average, are likely to become pregnant using a particular method for one year (Table 10.2). Each method has two failure rates: the **lowest observed failure rate**, a measure of how a method performs when used consistently and as intended, and the **typical fail-**ure rate, a measure of how a method performs allowing for all of the errors and problems typically associated with a method. In the United States, the most popular contraceptive methods are oral contraceptive pills (10.7 million), female sterilization (9.6 million), condoms (5.1 million), and male sterilization (4.1 million) (Hatcher et al., 1994).

TABLE 10.2 Effectiveness of Modern Contraceptives (reported as failure rates)

Method	Typical failure rate (percentage)	Lowest rate observed failure (percentage)
Abstinence	?	0
Tubal ligation	0.4	0.4
Vasectomy	0.1	0.1
Pill (combination)	3	0.1
Progestin-only pill	3	0.5
Depo-Provera	0.3	0.3
Norplant	0.1	0.1
IUD (Copper T-380)	0.8	0.6
Male condom	12	3
Female condom	21	5
Diaphragm	18	6
Cervical cap	18	9
Sponge	18	9
Spermicides	21	6
Penile withdrawal	19	4
Calendar rhythm	20	9
Chance	89	89

Sources: R. A. Hatcher et al., *Contraceptive Technology, 1994–1995,* 15th edition (Atlanta: Printed Matter, Inc.). and J. Tussell and K. Kost (1994), "Contraceptive Failure in the United States," *Studies in Family Planning,* 18 (September/October): 237–283.

WITHDRAWAL

The withdrawal method of birth control (**coitus interruptus**) requires that the man withdraw his penis from the vagina before ejaculation. In theory, withdrawal prevents sperm from being deposited in the vagina and subsequently fertilizing an ovum. Contrary to what many believe, withdrawal provides protection similar to that of vaginal barrier methods. Among typical users, there is about a 19 percent fail rate during the first year of use, compared to a 12 percent fail rate for condoms (Hatcher et al., 1994). The male must exercise great control and restraint in order to withdraw the penis in time. Withdrawal is risky because a small emission may occur prior to ejaculation (pre-ejaculate), which may contain HIV or other STD bacteria or viruses. Even if no sperm are actually deposited in the vagina, pregnancy is possible if sperm are released near the vagina and enter later, perhaps inadvertently, through body-to-body contact.

Withdrawal can diminish a couple's sexual pleasure. When the man must concentrate on withdrawing and the women is concerned about whether he will withdraw in time, neither is free to fully experience the pleasure of sexual intercourse.

Liberty means responsibility. That's why most men dread it.
George Bernard Shaw

HORMONAL CONTRACEPTION: THE PILL

In 1960, the U.S. Food and Drug Administration (FDA) approved the use of oral hormonal contraceptive agents for women. Today millions of women in the United States are "on the pill." Worldwide, the number of users is thought to exceed 150 million.

The reasons for the pill's popularity include its convenience, low cost, reversibility, tolerable side effects (for most users), and, most significantly, effectiveness. The pill is 98–99 percent effective in preventing conception when used correctly.

Combination Birth Control Pills

The most common hormonal contraceptives contain a combination of two synthetic hormones that in many ways mimic the actions of a woman's natural ovarian hormones. One of the synthetic hormones is similar to the natural hormone estrogen, and the other is similar to the natural hormone progesterone. The progesterone-like compound is called a progestogen or progestin. In addition to combination oral contraceptives, a progestin-only pill (minipill) is available. The mechanisms by which the synthetic hormones are thought to prevent pregnancy are shown in Table 10.3.

Over forty brands of birth control pills are available. Many have similar ingredients in identical dosages, but are produced by different manufacturers. Combination pills generally contain between 20 and 35 micrograms of estrogen and 0.5 and 1.5 milligrams of progestin. Progestin-only minipills contain 0.35 milligrams of progestin or less. Some combination pills also have an iron supplement to help prevent iron-deficiency anemia. Combination pills vary from one brand to the next in the potency of estrogen and progestin (Hatcher et al., 1994).

Regardless of brand or dose of synthetic hormones, the method of taking the combination oral contraceptives is the same. The pills come in packages of 21 or 28 pills. In the 21-pill packets, all the pills contain a prescribed mixture of the two synthetic hormones. In the 28-pill packets, 21 of the pills contain hormones; the other seven pills are inert or contain iron and serve as a

TABLE 10.3   Mechanisms of Action of Estrogens and Progestogens Used in Oral Contraceptives

Hormone	Mechanisms of action
Estrogens	1. Inhibition of ovulation by suppressing the release of pituitary hormones FSH and LH 2. Inhibition of implantation of the fertilized egg 3. Acceleration of transport of the ovum in the fallopian tube 4. Accelerated degeneration of the corpus luteum, which secretes progesterone, and consequent prevention of normal implantation of the fertilized ovum
Progestogens	1. Production of thick cervical mucus, which blocks sperm transport from the vagina to the uterus 2. Change in the character of cervical mucus such that sperm are less able to effect fertilization 3. Deceleration of ovum transport in the fallopian tubes 4. Inhibition of implantation 5. Interruption of the hormonal regulation of ovulation

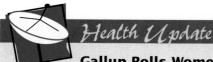

Health Update

Gallup Polls Women about Birth Control Pills

Most American women don't believe birth control pills are safe enough to buy without a doctor's prescription, according to a Gallup Poll released January 1994. However, the proportion of women who believe substantial health risks are associated with the pills has declined significantly since 1985.

The American College of Obstetricians and Gynecologists commissioned the poll to compare women's views with a similar poll in 1985. Based on telephone interviews nationwide with 997 women 18 and over, the results show that:

- 86 percent of women overall, and 91 percent of women on birth control pills, don't believe the pills are safe enough to buy without first seeing a doctor.
- 54 percent of women believe there are substantial risks associated with use of the pills, down from 76 percent who held such views in 1985; of these women, 29 percent cite cancer as the chief risk, as did 31 percent in 1985.
- 41 percent believe the pills provide no health benefits other than preventing pregnancy, and only 6 percent are aware of the pills' protection against cancer, such as ovarian and endometrial cancer.
- 65 percent believe using birth control pills is more risky or as risky as childbirth, as did 64 percent in 1985; in fact, childbearing carries twice the risk of death as use of birth control pills.

Source: FDA Consumer (May 1994).

way to keep track of the days that no hormone is to be taken. The pills with the hormones are usually a different color from the inert or iron-containing tablets. The first pill in a packet is taken on a predetermined day, and one pill is taken each day. Approximately two days after the last active pill is taken, a menstrual period should occur. Minipills come in 28-day packets; each pill contains active hormone. One pill is taken each day for an entire cycle, even during menstruation.

Those using pills are encouraged to take their daily pill with some routine activity, such as eating a meal, brushing their teeth, or going to bed. Taking the pill at the same time each day increases its effectiveness and decreases the likelihood of forgetting to take it. The hormones in today's birth control pills only prevent ovulation for approximately 24 hours. This is why the timing of taking the pill is important.

If you forget to take one pill, take it as soon as you remember. Take the next pill at your regular time. This means that you take two pills in one day. You do not need to use a back-up birth control method if you have sex. If you forget to take two pills in a row during week one or week two, you need to take two pills on the day you remember and two pills the next day. Then take one pill a day until you finish your package of pills. You may become pregnant if you have sex in the seven days after you miss your pills. You must use another birth control method (such as condoms, foam) as a back-up for those seven days. If you forget to take two pills in a row during the third week, throw out the rest of the pill pack and start a new pack that same day, unless you start your pills on a Sunday. Then you should keep taking one pill a day until Sunday and on Sunday throw out the rest of the pack and start a new pack of pills that same day. As before, you may become pregnant if you have sex in the seven days after you miss your pills. You must use a back-up birth control method for those seven days.

TERM

coitus interruptus: removing the penis from the vagina just prior to ejaculation; also called withdrawal or pulling out

HEALTHY PEOPLE 2000

Increase to at least 90 percent the proportion of sexually active, unmarried people aged 19 and younger who use contraception, especially combined method contraception that both effectively prevents pregnancy and provides barrier protection against disease.

The only certain way to prevent pregnancy is through abstinence from sexual intercourse. Abstinence also provides protection from sexually transmitted diseases, including AIDS. Mutually faithful monogamy with an uninfected partner will also protect people from STDs. However, for sexually active teenagers and young adults who chose not to postpone sexual activity and who do not wish to become pregnant or infected with an STD, consistent use of dual methods of contraception is the most effective means of reducing rates of pregnancy and STDs.

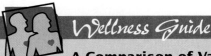
A Comparison of Various Contraceptive Methods

Method	How it works	Effectiveness	Advantages	Disadvantages
Withdrawal	Man withdraws penis from vagina before ejaculation	Low	Causes no health problems	Requires considerable control on the part of the male; may decrease sexual satisfaction
Fertility awareness	Intercourse only on a woman's "safe" days	Moderate if used consistently and conscientiously	Causes no health problems Little if any religious objection	Sometimes difficult to predict "safe" days May require long periods of abstention from sexual intercourse
Hormonal contraceptives	Prevents the release of eggs from the ovaries	High	Easy to use Does not interfere with sexual activity	May cause unintended physiological effects (weight gain, breast tenderness) May cause serious health problems
IUD	Prevents implantation and first stages of pregnancy	High	Always available when needed Does not interfere with sexual activity	May cause heavy menstrual bleeding and cramps May increase the chance of pelvic infection
Diaphragm	Blocks sperm from reaching egg; kills sperm	High if used consistently and correctly	Causes no health problems	Must be used with each incidence of intercourse Must be fitted by a clinician

The effectiveness of birth control pills may be lessened when they are taken simultaneously with certain other medications, such as antibiotics, anticonvulsants, and a variety of pain relievers and anti-inflammatory drugs. Pill users should continue birth control pill use and consult their health professional about this possibility when taking other medications.

Approximately half the women using oral contraceptives experience unwanted and unintended side effects. Most of the time the side effects present little long-term risk to health, and often they disappear after several cycles on the pill. The more common of the less serious side effects are nausea, weight gain, breast tenderness, mild headaches, spotty bleeding between periods, decreased menstrual flow, increased frequency of vaginitis, increased depression, and lowering of the sex drive. Some other frequent side effects of the pill are considered beneficial by many women. Among these are diminution and even absence of menstrual cramps, decreased number of menstrual bleeding days, and absolute regulation of the menstrual cycle, which can be important for travelers and athletes.

Studies indicate that pill use may help prevent certain diseases. Women who take combination birth control pills have about one-third the chance of developing pelvic inflammatory disease, one-half the chance of developing benign (noncancerous) breast disease and ovarian cysts, nearly complete protection against ectopic pregnancy, and one-half the risk of developing iron-deficiency anemia (Baird and Glasier, 1993). Data also indicate that combination birth control pills may protect against rheumatoid arthritis, endometrial cancer, and ovarian cancer.

There is no evidence that fertility is affected by taking the pill even after many years of use. Some women, however, experience menstrual irregularities after discontinuing the pill. Despite the myth, after discontinuing the pill, women can become pregnant immediately. Studies indicate that there is no association between pill usage and the possibility of birth defects in children born to pill users.

For a small percentage of women, oral contraceptives present a severe health risk. Several studies have shown that the risk of fatal blood clots and heart attack is greater for some women who take oral contraceptives than for those who do not. Women most at risk are those who are over 35 years old and who smoke cigarettes. These women should consider using a birth control method other than the pill. Any pill user who experiences severe abdominal pain, chest pain, headaches, unusual eye problems (blurred vision, flashing lights, temporary blindness), or severe calf and thigh pain should consult a physician or family planning agency immediately. The risk of developing liver disease, gallbladder disease, high blood pressure, and stroke is also slightly greater for pill users. Recent studies show that pill usage carries no increased risk of developing breast cancer.

Method	How it works	Effectiveness	Advantages	Disadvantages
Cervical cap	Blocks sperm from reaching egg; kills sperm	Moderate	Can remain in place for up to 24 hours	Must be fitted by a clinician May cause cervical irritation
Vaginal foam or creams	Kills sperm	Moderate if used consistently and correctly	Causes no health problems Can be obtained without a doctor's prescription Protects against sexually transmitted diseases	Must be used before each incidence of intercourse Found messy by some couples
Condom	Prevents sperm from entering vagina	High if used consistently and correctly	Causes no health problems Can be obtained without a doctor's prescription Helps prevent spread of sexually transmitted diseases	May detract from sexual pleasure May break or tear
Vaginal foam and condom together	Prevents sperm from entering vagina and kills any sperm that accidentally enter	High	Causes no health problems Can be obtained without a doctor's prescription Helps prevent spread of sexually transmitted diseases	Same as for condom alone and foam alone

Progestin-Only Contraceptives

Progestin-only contraceptives are available as pills, injections, and implants. Progestin-only contraceptives work by inhibiting ovulation and thickening the cervical mucus, making it more difficult for sperm to reach the egg. Side effects may include menstrual irregularities, weight gain, depression, fatigue, decreased sex drive, acne or oily skin, and headaches. Progestin-only contraceptives are completely reversible. A woman returns to her previous level of fertility when she stops using any of the methods.

Depo-Provera Depo-Provera is a 12-week supply of progestin that is injected intramuscularly by a health care provider. The hormone is released at a steady rate. At the end of the 12 weeks, a replacement injection or another contraceptive must be obtained.

T E R M S

progestin-only contraceptives: work by inhibiting ovulation and thickening of the cervical mucus; completely reversible

Depo-Provera: injectable form of medroxyprogesterone acetate

Norplant: hormone-containing capsule inserted under the skin

Depo-Provera's active ingredient is a chemical similar to (but not the same as) the natural hormone progesterone that is produced by women's ovaries during the second half of the menstrual cycle. Depo-Provera acts by preventing the egg cells from ripening. If an egg is not released from the ovaries during the menstrual cycle, it cannot become fertilized by sperm and result in pregnancy. Depo-Provera also causes changes in the lining of the uterus that make it less likely for pregnancy to occur. Depo-Provera is over 99 percent effective.

Depo-Provera is reversible. To stop using Depo-Provera, the woman simply does not get the next injection. Most women who get pregnant do so within 12 to 18 months of the last injection. The most common side effects include: irregular menstrual bleeding, amenorrhea, weight gain, headache, nervousness, stomach pain or cramps, dizziness, weakness or fatigue, and decreased sex drive. Depo-Provera is intended to prevent pregnancy only, and does not protect against the transmission of sexually transmitted diseases. Therefore, another method needs to be used in conjunction with Depo-Provera to prevent STD transmission.

Norplant Norplant consists of six thin, hormone-containing capsules made of soft flexible material, which are placed in a fan-like pattern under the skin on

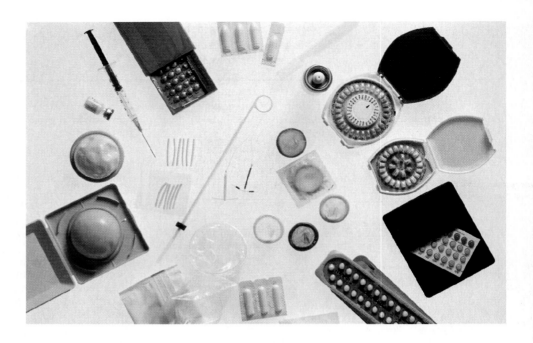

An assortment of fertility control options available today.

the inside surface of the upper arm. After insertion, the hormone is released into the body continuously. One insertion is effective for up to 5 years. Norplant is inserted by a trained medical professional in an office or clinic; the procedure takes about 10 to 15 minutes. Once under the skin, the capsules are invisible, but the outline of the capsules can be felt and sometimes seen. For some women, discoloration over the placement site occurs, which usually reverses when the capsules are removed, as well as irregular menstrual bleeding and weight gain. The removal procedure (or replacement with fresh hormone-filled capsules) is supposed to be simple. In some women, however, fibrous scar tissue builds up around the capsules, making their removal difficult and painful.

THE INTRAUTERINE DEVICE

The **intrauterine device**, or **IUD**, is a small plastic object that is placed inside the uterus. The possible mechanisms by which IUDs work include: 1) killing or weakening sperm; 2) altering the timing of the ovum's or embryo's movement through the fallopian tube; and/or 3) inhibiting implantation of the embryo in the uterine lining. Although IUDs have been available for many years, the exact mechanism of action of IUDs is not completely understood (Hatcher et al., 1994).

During the 1960s and 1970s, several kinds of IUD were available. Early in 1986, however, all but one of the major types of IUD had been withdrawn from the U.S. market because hundreds of IUD current and former

users claimed that they were harmed by the device. These users sued the manufacturers of IUDs and manufacturers chose to withdraw the devices from the U.S. market rather than face the enormous costs of both legal defense and large financial settlements. So costly were the damages assessed against one IUD, the Dalkon Shield—the use of which was associated with pelvic infections, ectopic pregnancies, and several deaths—that its manufacturer declared bankruptcy.

Currently, three types of IUD are available in the United States; the Progestasert, the Copper T-380A, and the LNg 20. The Progestasert and the Copper T-380A are plastic devices shaped like a "T." The Progestasert is filled with progesterone, which diffuses slowly from the device. The Copper-T is wrapped with copper metal. The plastic IUD without progesterone or copper is itself an effective contraceptive, but with the addition of either substance the failure rate drops to about one pregnancy per year per 100 women. The LNg 20 (Levonorgestrel IUD) has the active ingredient levonorgestrel released directly into the uterus at a constant rate of 20 milligrams per day. The LNg 20 is the single most effective method of reversible contraception available in the world today, followed closely by the Copper T-380A (Hatcher et al., 1994).

Research indicates that IUD use increases the risk for pelvic inflammatory diseases, uterine perforations, and increased risk of **ectopic pregnancy** should a pregnancy occur with the device in place. **Pelvic inflammatory disease (PID)** can damage the fallopian tubes sufficiently to make a woman infertile or to increase the likelihood of ectopic pregnancy.

BARRIER METHODS

Barrier methods of birth control are devices that physically block the path of sperm movement in the female reproductive tract and usually bring sperm in contact with a sperm-killing (spermicidal) chemical, most often nonoxynol-9. Several contraceptive methods work on this principle, including the diaphragm; the cervical cap; spermicidal foams, jellies, and creams; and the condom.

The Diaphragm

The **diaphragm** is a dome-shaped latex cup, which is placed in the vagina to cover the cervix (Figure 10.1). A metal spring in the rim of the diaphragm holds the device snugly in place between the back wall of the vagina and the pubic bone in the front of the pelvis. In this position the diaphragm blocks the movement of sperm from the vagina to the uterus, although it does not fit snugly enough to keep all of the sperm out. Its primary purpose is to hold a spermicide in place next to the cervix. Correct usage requires that the rim and cup of the diaphragm be coated with a tablespoon or two of a spermicidal jelly or cream. The diaphragm should be left in place for at least six hours after intercourse. The spermicides used with the diaphragm also help prevent the transmission of some microorganisms responsible for genital infections.

The diaphragm can be highly effective if used correctly every time a woman has intercourse. The typical failure rate is about thirteen pregnancies per 100 women per year.

One major advantage of the diaphragm is the absence of major medical problems associated with its use. A very few women or their partners may be allergic to the latex or the spermicide and some contract urinary tract infections. Some women may experience discomfort with the diaphragm in place. Changing brands or

getting a better fitting diaphragm often solves these problems.

Another advantage is that the diaphragm can be inserted up to six hours before intercourse, so a couple does not have to interrupt sexual pleasuring to insert the device. If a diaphragm is inserted several hours before sexual activity, however, it is advisable to put an additional amount of spermicidal jelly or cream into the vagina before intercourse. The diaphragm must be left in place at least 6 hours after intercourse, but should not be used longer than 24 hours because of possible risk of toxic shock syndrome.

Each woman must be fitted (by a family planning professional or a physician) with a diaphragm that is the correct size for her. The need for proper fitting is one reason that diaphragms are available only by prescription. Any change in a woman's body size from a gain or loss of several pounds, pregnancy, or pelvic surgery is reason to check the diaphragm and get a new diaphragm prescribed if necessary. A woman should not use another woman's diaphragm because the fit might be wrong, lowering the device's effectiveness.

After each use the diaphram should be washed with mild soap and water, rinsed thoroughly, and dried in the air or with a towel. Perfumed talcum powders, petroleum jelly, or scented creams should not be used with the diaphragm. Occasionally the rubber darkens, but this generally does not impair effectiveness.

One disadvantage of the diaphragm is the possibility of dislodgement during intercourse. Only rarely will a man feel the diaphragm during sexual intercourse if the device is inserted properly. If either the man or the woman experiences unusual sensations or discomfort during intercourse, then the diaphragm may not be inserted correctly, it may have become dislodged during intercourse, or it may be the wrong size.

Periodically the diaphragm should be held against a light to check for tiny holes and weak spots (where the rubber buckles). With proper care a diaphragm will last a year or two.

The Cervical Cap

The **cervical cap** is a cup-shaped rubber device that snugly covers the cervix similar to the way a thimble fits on a finger (Figure 10.2). Like a diaphragm, a cervical cap needs to be coated with spermicide to be as effective as possible, but unlike a diaphragm, a cervical cap remains in place for up to 24 hours. Cervical caps come in several sizes and must be fitted for each woman. The typical failure rate is about seventeen pregnancies per 100 users per year.

The principal advantages of the cervical cap are:

- low cost and convenience.
- can be inserted any time of the day intercourse is anticipated.

T E R M S

intrauterine device (IUD): a flexible, usually plastic device inserted into the uterus to prevent pregnancy

etopic pregnancy: implanting of the embryo outside the uterus, usually in the fallopian tubes

pelvic inflammatory disease (PID): inflammation of the pelvic structures, especially the uterus and fallopian tubes; often caused by a sexually transmitted disease

diaphragm: a soft, rubber, dome-shaped contraceptive device worn over the cervix and used with spermicidal jelly or cream

cervical cap: small latex cap that covers the cervix, used with spermicidal jelly or cream inside the cap

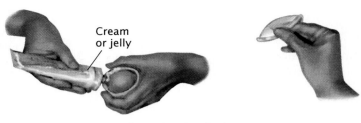

Cream
or jelly

Preparing the diaphragm

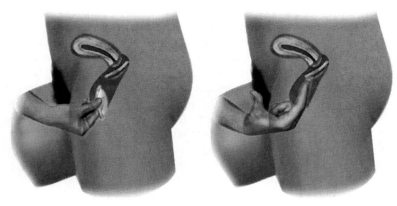

Inserting the diaphragm

Checking the diaphragm

FIGURE 10.1 Procedure for Inserting a Diaphragm

• sexual activity can take place spontaneously during the ensuing 24 hours without having to be concerned with birth control.

The major disadvantages of the cervical cap are difficulty with insertion and removal, occasional discomfort during intercourse, dislodgment during intercourse, and possibly irritation of the cervix. Like the diaphram, the cervical cap should not be left in place for more than 24 hours at a time.

> ### T E R M S
>
> *contraceptive sponge:* a polyurethane sponge that contains one gram of the spermicide nonoxynol-9
>
> *toxic shock syndrome:* a severe bacterial illness characterized by a sudden high fever, vomiting, diarrhea, aches, and a sunburn-like rash; it usually occurs in menstruating females using superabsorbant tampons
>
> *spermicide:* a chemical that kills sperm; particularly foams, creams, jellies, and suppositories used for contraception
>
> *suppositories:* a medicine placed in a body orifice to dissolve and sometimes to be absorbed; birth control suppositories contain spermicidal chemicals
>
> *condom:* a latex or polyurethane sheath worn over the penis (male condom) or inside the vagina (female condom); can be both a barrier method and act as a prophylactic against sexually transmitted diseases

The Contraceptive Sponge

Currently, the **contraceptive sponge** is no longer being manufactured or distributed in the United States (Health Update, page 201). The contraceptive sponge is made of a compressible spongy synthetic material in the shape of a mushroom cap. The sponge fits in the vagina with the concave side against the cervix. The sponge is impregnated with spermicide and works in three ways: 1) by destroying sperm, 2) by absorbing ejaculate, and 3) by blocking sperm entry into the uterus.

As with other barrier methods, allergies to the device or the spermicide can cause vaginal and/or penile irritation. A few cases of **toxic shock syndrome** have been associated with sponge usage, especially if the device is left in the vagina for over 24 hours. Information about

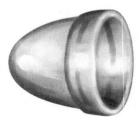

FIGURE 10.2 Cervical Cap

toxic shock syndrome was included in the package inserts.

Vaginal Spermicides

A variety of birth control methods consist solely of a spermicidal chemical (usually nonoxynol-9) and an inert substance that transports and retains the **spermicide** in the vagina. These agents include foams, gels, creams, and vaginal **suppositories**. Although often displayed in stores with other feminine hygiene products, vaginal spermicides should not be confused with douches, deodorant products, or lubricants, none of which are effective birth control methods.

The effectiveness of all of the vaginal spermicides depends on a sufficient quantity of sperm-killing chemical bathing the cervix at the time of ejaculation. Among typical users, however, the failure rate is about eighteen pregnancies per 100 women per year. Using vaginal spermicides requires dedication and competence. Users must put the spermicide in the vagina immediately before every act of intercourse and before each subsequent intercourse in the same sexual encounter.

Users of foam should be sure that the foam is frothy and bubbly, which is achieved by shaking the container about twenty times before filling the applicator. Because there is no way to know how much foam remains in a container, a spare container should be kept on hand.

Suppositories should be placed as far back in the vagina as possible so that the dissolved spermicide covers the cervix. It is important to allow enough time (from 10 to 30 minutes, depending on the product) for the suppository to dissolve completely before each act of intercourse. Vaginal suppositories have the disadvantage of having to wait the prescribed time to allow the tablet to melt.

Major advantages of vaginal spermicides are:

- They are available without a doctor's prescription.
- They can be purchased in pharmacies and many supermarkets.
- The spermicidal chemicals give some added protection against STDs.
- The effectiveness of spermicidal agents increases to nearly 100 percent when they are used simultaneously with a condom.

> Whenever I hear people discussing birth control, I always remember that I was the fifth.
>
> Clarence Darrow,
> lawyer

Vaginal spermicides tend to be slippery, which occasionally can be a nuisance, but the moisture can augment a woman's natural vaginal lubrication and enhance sensation. These methods may also be a hindrance to oral-genital stimulation. In rare instances someone may be allergic to a particular product. Changing brands may alleviate this problem. Some women experience irritation if the tablet has not dissolved completely before intercourse takes place. Some erroneously believe that spermicides cause birth defects; this belief is a myth.

Male and Female Condoms

The male **condom**, or rubber, is a membranous sheath that covers the erect penis and catches semen before it enters the vagina. About 99 percent of male condoms

Health Update

Today Sponge Discontinued

The manufacturer of the Today Sponge, a nonprescription contraceptive for women, will no longer make the product.

Whitehall-Robins Healthcare, the only manufacturer of contraceptive sponges, decided to discontinue the sponge after determining that correcting problems found during an FDA inspection would be too costly.

FDA's March 1994 inspection of the firm's plant in Hammonton, N.J.,

disclosed bacterial contamination of the water used to make the Today Sponge and other products, including nasal sprays, ointments, and suppositories.

FDA investigators also established that the firm had neglected to validate its microbiological test methods, thereby raising questions about the reliability of the tests. Other problems were found in the firm's equipment sanitization.

Longstanding public health standards do not allow the marketing of contaminated products that have the potential to transmit disease. However, had the problems been corrected, FDA would not have objected to continued production of the Today Sponge.

Source: FDA Consumer (April 1995): 4.

are made of latex; the rest, so-called "skin" condoms, are manufactured from lamb intestines. The female condom (Figure 10.3) is a polyurethane sheath with plastic rings at each end to hold the device in place inside the vagina. The female condom covers the external genitals to offer protection against the transmission of sexual infections.

Condoms can be obtained in pharmacies, supermarkets, vending machines, and through mail order advertisements in newspapers, magazines, and catalogs. When stored in a cool, dry place, condoms retain their effectiveness for up to five years. Kept in a warm environment, such as in a wallet in the back pocket of one's pants or in the glove compartment of a car, the latex will deteriorate. To be effective, condoms must be used with water-based lubricants, as petroleum-based lubricants will cause the latex to deteriorate.

There are many advantages to using condoms. Condoms are:

- easy to obtain.
- inexpensive.
- free of medical risk (on rare occasions a man or a woman may be allergic to the latex, lubricant, or spermicide).
- reliable.
- effective.

The typical failure rate is about twelve pregnancies per 100 women per year. This first-year failure rate among typical users of condoms is lower than the rates

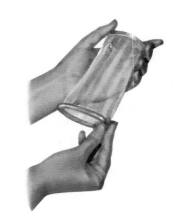

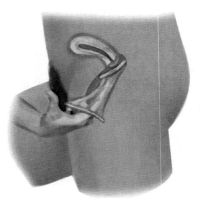

FIGURE 10.3   Reality Female Condom

Health Update

Challenges in Marketing the Female Condom

The first female condom came on the market in early fall 1994, and the advertising industry was challenged with promoting an unknown product to a skeptical public. Advertisers admit that it won't be easy to market because sales for over-the-counter female contraceptives have been steadily declining.

The maker of the Reality female condom conceded that it faces a major challenge and decided to focus the first phase of advertising on educating consumers about the female condom. The company believes consumers need to know how to use the product before buying it so that they do not become discouraged from using it due to lack of knowledge.

Ads for the female condom began appearing in November 1994 in magazines that cater to women ages 18 to 24, such as *Cosmopolitan, Essence,* and *Mademoiselle.*

The contraceptive is not inexpensive, costing $2.70 to $3.00 per Reality condom, compared to about $1.00 per male condom. The Reality package answers three questions: "Will it protect me?"; "How do I insert Reality?"; and "What does it feel like during sex?" The package also includes information indicating that the female condom has a failure rate of 26 percent which is considerably higher than for other contraceptives.

Reality is manufactured in London, by a company which markets female condoms in twelve countries under the name *Femy* and *Femidom.* The company says that about half of the women who bought the product once, purchased it again.

Source: Adapted from K. Goldman, *Wall Street Journal* (July 27, 1994), B4.

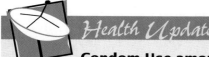

Condom Use among College Students

A recent study of undergraduate students enrolled in health sciences and engineering classes at a California university found that females were more comfortable talking about condoms with a partner, that males had more negative attitudes about condoms but reported higher usage, and that relationship status was a significant factor for females in determining condom usage. Specific survey results include:

- 51 percent of males and 33 percent of females used a "condom more than half the time" during the past year

- 71 percent of the males and 54 percent of the females intended to use a condom the "next time" they have sexual intercourse
- when asked "Do Condoms make it easy to have sex on the spur of the moment," 46 percent of the females said yes, while 28 percent of the males said yes
- when asked "Do Condoms decrease my sexual pleasure," 51 percent of the males said yes and 37 percent of the females also said yes
- In answering the statement "Condoms are difficult to use," 21 per-

cent of the males agreed, and 6 percent of the females agreed
- 98 percent of the females and 88 percent of the males had previously talked with a partner about condoms
- 21 percent of the males and 13 percent of the females were embarassed to talk about condoms

Source: J. B. Bontempi, "Gender Differences in Condom Use among Sexually Active Undergraduate College Students." Paper delivered at the American Alliance for Health Physical Education, Recreation, and Dance National Convention, March 31, 1995.

---

for typical users of other barrier methods. A primary reason for condoms to fail in preventing pregnancy is error in condom use. Used in conjunction with another barrier method, such as a diaphragm or spermicidal foam, condoms are nearly 100 percent effective. Another advantage is that condoms help prevent the transmission of chlamydia, gonorrhea, herpes, HIV, and other kinds of infections.

Some people complain that the condom diminishes pleasurable sensations, but the device does not totally block genital feeling, which, in any event, is only one of many factors that contribute to sexual arousal and pleasure. A negative attitude about condoms may diminish pleasure far more than a thin layer of latex ever could. Instead of thinking about how condoms block sensations, it might enhance lovemaking to think of them as a fun way to help make lovemaking more pleasurable because of the protection they provide.

When using a condom, consider ways to incorporate putting on the device without interrupting lovemaking. For example, having a condom available before sexual activity begins makes breaking off contact to obtain one unnecessary. Before intercourse begins, either partner can put the condom on the erect penis while the couple continues to fondle, talk, or play.

FERTILITY AWARENESS METHODS

Fertility awareness methods of birth control (sometimes called natural family planning, the rhythm method, or periodic abstinence) attempt to determine a woman's most fertile period; that is, when an ovum has been released from the ovary and is capable of being fertilized. Fertility awareness methods of birth control either estimate when ovulation is most likely to occur or indicate when ovulation has already taken place, thereby telling a couple the days in the menstrual cycle not to have unprotected intercourse. Those are referred to as "unsafe days." The days when a woman is not likely to be fertile are referred to as "safe days." On unsafe days, a couple should use an alternative method of birth control, such as condoms, a diaphragm, or spermicidal foam. Other options include enjoying ways of sexual pleasuring other than genital intercourse or complete sexual abstinence.

Couples using fertility awareness methods should realize that even on safe days fertilization is still possible because of natural variations in a woman's reproductive processes. Therefore, safe days are really *relatively* safe days.

> **T E R M**
>
> **fertility awareness methods:** methods of birth control in which a couple charts the cyclic signs of the woman's fertility and ovulation, using basal body temperature, mucus changes, and other signs to determine fertile periods

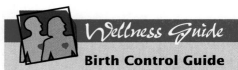

Birth Control Guide

Birth control efficacy rates in this chart are yearly estimates. The percent effectiveness depends on conscientious and correct use. Human error and other factors result in reduced effectiveness. For comparison, 60 to 85 percent of sexually active women using no contraception would be expected to become pregnant in a year.

	Male condom	Female condom	Spermicides used alone	Diaphragm with spermicide	Cervical cap with spermicide
Estimated effectiveness	About 85%	An estimated 74–79%	70–80%	82–94%	At least 82%
Risks	Rarely, irritation and allergic reactions	Rarely, irritation and allergic reactions	Rarely, irritation and allergic reactions	Rarely, irritation and allergic reactions; bladder infection; very rarely, toxic shock syndrome	Abnormal Pap test; vaginal or cervical infections; very rarely, toxic shock syndrome
STD protection	Latex condoms help protect against sexually transmitted diseases, including herpes and AIDS	May give some protection against sexually transmitted diseases, including herpes and AIDS; not as effective as male latex condom	Unknown	None	None
Convenience	Applied immediately before intercourse; used only once and discarded	Applied immediately before intercourse; used only once and discarded	Applied no more than one hour before intercourse	Inserted before intercourse; can be left in place 24 hours, but additional spermicide must be inserted if intercourse is repeated	Can remain in place for 24 hours, not necessary to reapply spermicide upon repeated intercourse; may be difficult to insert
Availability	Nonprescription	Nonprescription	Nonprescription	Rx	Rx

Pills	Implant (Norplant)	Injection (Depo-Provera)	IUD	Periodic abstinence (NFP)	Surgical sterilization
97%–99%	99%	99%	95–96%	Very variable, perhaps 53–86%	Over 99%
Blood clots, heart attacks and strokes, gallbladder disease, liver tumors, water retention, hypertension, mood changes, dizziness and nausea; not for smokers	Menstrual cycle irregularity; headaches, nervousness, depression, nausea, dizziness, change of appetite, breast tenderness, weight gain, enlargement of ovaries and/or fallopian tubes, excessive growth of body and facial hair; may subside after first year	Amenorrhea, weight gain, and other side effects similar to those with Norplant	Cramps, bleeding, pelvic inflammatory disease, infertility; rarely, perforation of the uterus	None	Pain, infection, and, for female tubal ligation, possible surgical complications
None	None	None	None	None	None
Pill must be taken on daily schedule, regardless of the frequency of intercourse	Effective 24 hours after implantation for approximately 5 years; can be removed by physician at any time	One injection every three months	After insertion, stays in place until physician removes it	Requires frequent monitoring of body functions and periods of abstinence	Vasectomy is a one-time procedure usually performed in a doctor's office; tubal ligation is a one-time procedure performed in an operating room
Rx	Rx; minor outpatient surgical procedure	Rx	Rx	Instructions from physician or clinic	Surgery

Source: M. S. Goldberg, "Choosing a Contraceptive," *FDA Consumer* (1993): 18–25.

Fertility awareness offers the advantages of being safe and inexpensive; furthermore, some peoples' religious convictions make fertility awareness the only acceptable method of birth control for many. The effectiveness of fertility awareness is among the lowest of the common methods, about twenty pregnancies per 100 women per year. Failures occur because people do not keep careful records, they find the intervals of abstinence during the unsafe days too long, and they find having to plan sex only for the safe days a hindrance to spontaneous love-making.

Calendar Rhythm

Calendar rhythm is a way to estimate the most likely fertile, or unsafe, days in a woman's menstrual cycle by assuming that:

1. Ovulation usually takes place 14 days (plus or minus 2 days) prior to the onset of the next menstrual flow.
2. An ovum is capable of being fertilized for 24 hours.
3. Sperm deposited in the vagina remain capable of fertilization for up to 3 days.

Using calendar rhythm effectively requires knowledge of the female fertility cycle and instruction in doing the calculations correctly. Family planning agencies, women's health clinics, and books on fertility awareness methods can be helpful in learning the method.

The Temperature Method

The **basal body temperature (BBT)** is the lowest temperature in a healthy person during waking hours. In 70–90 percent of women the BBT rises approximately one degree after ovulation, presumably because of changes in hormone levels. By keeping a daily record of the BBT, a woman can determine when ovulation has occurred and therefore the unsafe and safe days between ovulation and the beginning of the next menstrual cycle. Because the BBT method cannot predict when ovulation will occur, a woman must still estimate with another fertility awareness method (calendar method, mucus method) the safe and unsafe days before ovulation.

Temperature measurements should take at least five minutes. Daily temperature measurements should be taken at the same time each day, and a record should be kept on a graph (Figure 10.4). Once the BBT has risen for three consecutive days, a woman can assume that ovulation has taken place and that the rest of the days in that menstrual cycle are safe for unprotected intercourse.

The Mucus Method

Certain hormone-sensitive glands in the cervix produce mucus that changes in amount, color, and consistency during different phases of the menstrual cycle. Learning to recognize the changes in cervical mucus can help determine when ovulation occurs, and safe and unsafe days for intercourse can be planned accordingly.

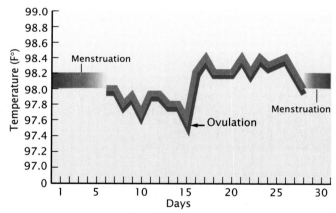

FIGURE 10.4 The Basal Body Temperature Method of Contraception A woman's body temperature rises about one degree during the days following ovulation. Once the BBT has risen for three consecutive days, it can be assumed that ovulation has taken place and that the rest of the days in that menstrual cycle are safe for unprotected intercourse. To use the BBT method, a woman must record her basal body temperature each morning before engaging in *any* activity. Thus, it is advisable to record the body temperature before going to sleep. Temperature measurement should last at least 5 minutes.

The mucus method requires that cervical mucus be examined frequently during the cycle. Samples of mucus can be obtained with a finger, on toilet tissue, or observing discharge on underpants. Collection with a finger is best because it permits direct determination of the amount and consistency of mucus.

Because douching, vaginal infections, semen, contraceptive foams and jellies, vaginal lubricants, medications, and vaginal lubrication from sexual arousal can interfere with the recognition of mucus patterns, women wishing to use the mucus method should obtain instructions from an experienced user, a family planning clinic, or a health center. A woman should plan on charting her cervical mucus for at least one month to learn her individual pattern of mucus changes before relying on the method for birth control.

The **sympto-thermal method** involves using the temperature and mucus methods simultaneously.

Chemical Methods

Chemical methods of fertility awareness measure the amount of **lutenizing hormone** in a woman's urine, which peaks at the time of ovulation. Ovulation predictor kits to measure the levels of LH can be purchased in pharmacies. Manufacturers claim that the kits are 85 percent accurate.

Douching

Douching (rinsing of the vagina with fluid) after sexual intercourse is a method of birth control that is almost totally ineffective. After ejaculation in the vagina, thousands of sperm move through the cervix and enter the uterus within a few seconds. There simply isn't time to flush out sperm from the vagina before a significant number enter the uterus. Furthermore, the force from the spray of the douche may propel sperm into the uterus, aiding conception rather than preventing it. Douching is unnecessary for most women as the vagina is constantly cleansing itself.

STERILIZATION

Sterility is being permanently unable to have children. For people who are certain that they do not want children, or, as is more often the case, no more children, surgical methods that render a person sterile but have no effect on sexual arousal or activities may be the most desirable form of birth control. Indeed, for married couples over 30 years old, "permanent birth control" (sterilization of either the male or female partner) has become the most frequently chosen method of birth control. The popularity of sterilization as a method of birth control stems from its nearly 100 percent effectiveness, the relative safety of the procedure, and its relatively low one-time cost.

Male Sterilization

The sterilization of a man is called **vasectomy**. This procedure involves the cutting and tying of each of the two vas deferens, the tubes that connect the testes (where sperm are made) to the penis (Figure 10.5). When these tubes are cut, sperm are no longer emitted upon ejaculation because their passage is blocked. Because the cut is made upstream from the organs that produce seminal fluid, a man still ejaculates, but the semen contains no sperm cells. And because the sperm cells make up only a small percentage of the total volume of the semen, neither a man nor his partner is aware of any change in their sex life, except that no other form of contraception is needed.

Although vasectomy should be considered a permanent form of contraception, it is sometimes possible to reverse the condition by rejoining the cut ends of the vas deferens. The success of vasectomy reversal as measured by the ability to have children again is about 50 percent, although some surgeons claim much higher reversal rates.

One of the reasons vasectomy is such a popular method of contraception is that it is uncomplicated and causes few problems. The procedure is usually carried out in a doctor's office with a local anesthetic in about 15 to 30 minutes. The incidence of postoperative complications is very low, and within a week most men can return to regular activities, including sex. About one-

T E R M S

calendar rhythm: an estimate of fertile or unsafe days to have intercourse

basal body temperature (BBT): a method of contraception that uses daily temperature readings immediately after wakening to identify the time of ovulation; approximately 24 hours after ovulation the BBT increases

sympto-thermal method: using both the BBT and the mucus methods at the same time

lutenizing hormone: anterior pituitary hormone that causes a follicle to release a ripened ovum and become a corpus luteum; in the male it stimulates testosterone production and the production of sperm cells

douching: rinsing the vaginal canal with a liquid; not an effective means of birth control or STD prevention

sterility: not being able to be impregnated or impregnate

vasectomy: a surgical procedure in men in which segments of the vas deferens are removed and the ends tied to prevent the passage of sperm

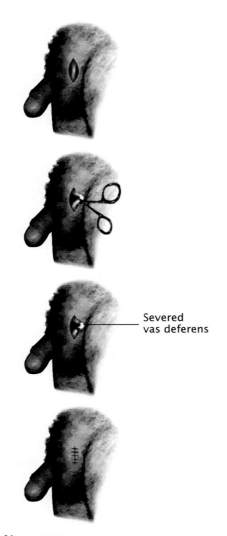

FIGURE 10.5 Vasectomy

Severed
vas deferens

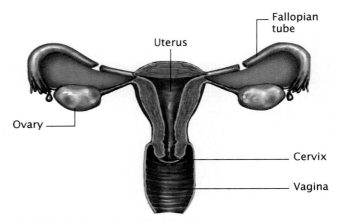

FIGURE 10.6 Tubal Ligation

half to two-thirds of vasectomized men develop anti-bodies to sperm, but there is no evidence to suggest that this is harmful. A man can be fertile for several weeks, because the sperm pathway contains sperm present before the vasectomy. Once these are ejaculated the man is sterile.

Female Sterilization

The principal sterilization procedure for women is **tubal ligation,** which is the blocking of the fallopian tubes (Figure 10.6). Blocking can be accomplished by cutting and tying the tubes, by sealing the tubes (cautery), or by closing them with clips, bands, or rings. Most tubal ligations can be performed under local anesthesia in about 20 minutes in a clinic or a doctor's office, and the woman can usually go home the same day or the day after. The incidence of postoperative complications is very low.

Most tubal ligations are "band-aid" surgeries, so-called because the operation requires only one or two inch-long incisions to be made. The incisions allow the surgeon to enter the abdominal cavity and locate and block the fallopian tubes. Entry to the abdominal cavity is generally through an incision just below the embilicus. Vaginal tubal ligation is called **culpotomy.** There are two types of abdominal tubal ligations, **minilaparotomy** and **laparoscopy.** The main difference between the two is the way the fallopian tubes are visualized. With minilaparotomy, the doctor exposes the tubes to direct view, whereas in laparoscopy the tubes are visualized with a cylindrical viewing device (the laparoscope), which is placed in the abdominal cavity through a small surgical incision.

Although tubal ligation is intended to be a permanent form of birth control, accidental pregnancies occur because a blocked tube spontaneously reopens. Surgical reversal of tubal blocking may be possible if a woman later decides that she wants to have children, with a success rate of 50 to 70 percent.

Another female sterilization technique is **hysterectomy,** the surgical removal of the uterus. Most experts do not recommend hysterectomy solely for sterilization purposes because, when compared to tubal ligation, the chances for postoperative complications are 10 to 100 times greater, the operation is more expensive, and the negative psychological impact may be greater.

CHOOSING THE RIGHT BIRTH CONTROL METHOD

Most users of birth control are principally concerned with two questions: How well does the method work, and is it safe? The efficacy of a birth control method can be evaluated in terms of both theoretical effectiveness and actual effectiveness. The **theoretical effectiveness** is how well the method performs if it is used consistently and as intended. The **actual effectiveness** is a measure of how well a method performs in actual use in a population. Measures of actual effectiveness take into account improper, inconsistent, and careless usage.

Considerations of the safety of birth control methods must take into account the health risks of a particular method, such as serious illness, the possibility of infection and its consequences, the risk of death, the risk of being unable to have children in the future, any effects on unborn children, and undesirable and unhealthful changes in the body.

Evaluation of a birth control method's safety should also assess the physical and psychological consequences of an unintended pregnancy. These include the risks associated with terminating the pregnancy with an abortion and the risks associated with carrying the pregnancy to term. Factors such as a woman's age, her physical health, whether she has had previous children, and her capacity to care for another child also need to be evaluated. Of course, the most serious risk associated with the use of any contraceptive is the risk of death, which is rare except for older pill users who smoke heavily.

RESPONSIBILITY FOR BIRTH CONTROL

Most people engage in sexual activity because they want a joyous, rewarding experience. Because an unintended pregnancy can cause enormous hardship, birth control is an important part of every sexual relationship. Denying the possibility of pregnancy by assuming "it can't happen to me" is just gambling against the odds.

T E R M S

tubal ligation: a surgical procedure in women in which the fallopian tubes are cut, tied, or cauterized to prevent pregnancy; a form of sterilization

culpotomy: a female sterilization procedure

minilaparotomy: female sterilization procedure in which the fallopian tubes are ligated or cauterized through a small abdominal incision

laparoscopy: a surgical incision into the abdomen used to visualize internal organs

hysterectomy: surgical removal of the uterus

theoretical effectiveness: how well a birth control method performs if it is used as intended and consistently

actual effectiveness: how well a birth control method performs in actual use in a population

The responsibility for birth control has two components. First, a birth control method must be chosen, taking into consideration the nature of an individual's sexual activities or a couple's sexual relationship, the frequency of intercourse, future plans regarding children, and personal and religious values. Second, the chosen method must be used consistently and correctly.

For both technological and sociological reasons, there has been a tendency to associate the responsibility for birth control with the partner for whose body a particular method is designed. For example, in the late nineteenth century, when withdrawal and the condom were the principal methods of birth control, and women were not supposed to be interested in sex, men were considered to be the ones responsible for birth control (when it was used at all). In the late 1960s when the pill and IUD were heralded as "perfect" contraceptives and women began to assert themselves socially and politically, the responsibility for birth control shifted almost totally to women.

Today a large percentage of sexually active people believe that both partners in a sexual relationship should share the responsibility for birth control. Yet, because so many methods are intended for use by the woman, in actual practice many women are left to manage birth control on their own. Having to take total responsibility for birth control can create resentment that blocks the feelings that many people wish to express with sex.

The responsibility for birth control can be shared in a number of ways. The most important is to discuss it. In an ongoing relationship there are many opportunities to talk about birth control. Couples can go to birth control clinics together, they can read and discuss information about the advantages and disadvantages of the different methods, and they can try out various methods to find out which are best suited for them. They can share the time and the financial costs of their chosen method, or they can divide responsibilities. For example, if a woman has to take time to go to a clinic or doctor, her partner could pay for the clinic visit and the contraceptives.

Partners can also share in using their chosen method. They can discuss any difficulties or concerns they have with their method of birth control. A man can learn how a diaphragm is used, a woman can learn about the condom, and they can incorporate into their lovemaking preparing to use these and other barrier methods. If a woman is using fertility awareness methods, a man can share the responsibility by helping to determine the safe and unsafe days and by sharing the responsibility for abstaining from sexual intercourse.

Partners who share the responsibility for birth control are more likely to use their chosen method(s) properly, which makes birth control more effective. And

Choosing the Best Contraceptive for You

Which contraceptive options do you think are best for your sexual practices? Identify the contraceptives below as "very suitable," "suitable," or "not suitable" and then list the reasons for your decisions. There are no right or wrong decisions.

Method	Very suitable	Suitable	Not suitable	Reasons
Male condom	☐	☐	☐	_____
Female condom	☐	☐	☐	_____
Spermicides used alone	☐	☐	☐	_____
Diaphragm	☐	☐	☐	_____
Diaphragm with spermicide	☐	☐	☐	_____
Cervical cap with spermicide	☐	☐	☐	_____
Pill	☐	☐	☐	_____
Implant (Norplant)	☐	☐	☐	_____
Injection (Depo-Provera)	☐	☐	☐	_____
IUD	☐	☐	☐	_____
Periodic abstinence	☐	☐	☐	_____
Vasectomy	☐	☐	☐	_____
Tubal ligation	☐	☐	☐	_____
Withdrawal	☐	☐	☐	_____
Postcoital methods	☐	☐	☐	_____

reducing the fear of pregnancy makes sex more enjoyable. Another benefit of sharing this responsibility is that it tends to enhance intimacy in a relationship. The discussion of birth control and the mutual decision making involved in choosing and using a method lead to better communication.

It is always a good idea for you to have some method of birth control with you if you anticipate that sexual intercourse might occur. For example, both men and women can carry a condom and/or spermicides with them on dates or to parties if they think that sexual activity is a possibility.

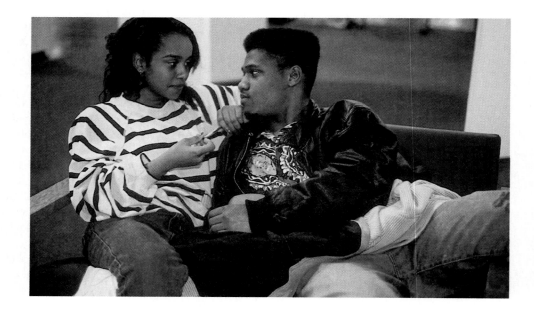

Choosing a fertility control method should be a decision made by both sexual partners.

DISCUSSING BIRTH CONTROL RESPONSIBILITY

A couple shares the responsibility for birth control because both partners are responsible if an unintended pregnancy occurs. This fact alone is the most important reason for discussing birth control. Although it is important to discuss birth control before having sex, many individuals are embarrassed to do so. Talking about contraception implies that sex is going to take place, which may force an individual to face internal conflicts about engaging in sex. Many individuals subscribe to the myth that good sex should be spontaneous rather than planned. Therefore, sex and birth control remain undiscussed. First-time partners may not discuss birth control before sex because they fear spoiling a romantic mood.

Still, the best time to discuss birth control is *before* sexual intercourse. A partner might say, "I would really like to make love (have sex) with you, and I want to be sure we're protected." That kind of introduction can be followed by a statement of preference and personal responsibility, such as, "I prefer to use condoms" or "I'm

on the pill" or, using a question, such as, "What birth control method do you prefer?" or "What are we going to do about birth control?"

In some cases, even if a man is concerned about an unintended pregnancy and sexual diseases, he may not feel comfortable bringing up the topic of birth control, fearing embarrassment or appearing ignorant or weak. Many women, however, welcome a man who initiates a discussion of birth control. Communication about birth control and other sexual matters, such as the role of sex in a relationship, likes and dislikes, and preventing sexually transmitted diseases is vital to a healthy sexual relationship.

WHY SEXUALLY ACTIVE PEOPLE DO NOT USE BIRTH CONTROL

Despite a presumed and sometimes stated desire not to become pregnant, approximately 5 percent of married individuals and 15 percent of unmarried sexually active individuals use no birth control. Some of the major reasons that people do not use birth control, even if they wish to avoid pregnancy, include:

Wellness Guide

Your Health Matters: Talking with Your Health Care Provider about Sexual Health

Taking personal responsibility for your sexual health is essential in maintaining a healthy life-style. Many women have a reproductive tract infection (RTI), but are unaware they do. On average, one in every five women has an RTI, and some women are at a greater risk for contracting an RTI than others. Because RTI's symptoms are not always noticeble, a woman can have an infection but not know it. Diseases like chlamydia and gonorrhea can go undetected for years and may cause a serious threat to a woman's health. Fortunately, diagnosis and treatment is available for many infections. **Don't wait any longer, talk to your health care provider.**

Often women, and sometimes even the health care providers, are embarrassed to talk about sexual health. Discussing your sexual prac-

tices may be awkward; however, it is critical in assessing your risk level for having an RTI. Here are some helpful tips to keep in mind when discussing your sexual health with your provider:

- **Be completely honest.** Your health care provider is sworn to privacy, so give as many facts as possible.
- **Tell your provider how old you were when you first had intercourse.** Women who have sex at an early age have a greater risk for infection.
- **Tell your provider how many sexual partners you have had.** The more sexual partners a woman has, the greater her risk of infection.
- **Discuss your sexual practices.** A woman can get an infection through vaginal, anal, oral sex,

and non-insertive sexual contact.

- **Tell your provider if you regularly use condoms.** Regular condom use reduces your risk of RTI infection.
- **Discuss any symptoms you or your partner(s) may be experiencing.** Genital itching, burning, redness, swelling, blisters, or warts may indicate infection.

After talking with you about your sexual health, your provider may decide to test you for infection. Testing is easy and no more uncomfortable than a routine gynecological exam. Early diagnosis and treatment is critical for maintaining health.

Source: Tami Kaszuba, "Wellness Watch," Illinois State University Health Promotion Office (Spring, 1995).

- *Low motivation.* People who have mixed feelings about avoiding pregnancy are less motivated to use birth control. For example, a couple that has decided that they want to have a child "sometime in the near future" is less likely to be motivated to use birth control than is a couple that is absolutely certain it does not want a child until some specified time, or at all.

- *Lack of knowledge.* Lack of knowledge about the process of conception and how to use birth control effectively can lead to an incorrect perception of risk of becoming pregnant. For example, some people believe the myths that pregnancy is not possible if a woman has an orgasm, if she urinates after intercourse, or if she is having sexual intercourse for the first time. Sometimes a method is believed to be more effective than it really is, or the chosen method is used incorrectly. For example, some people erroneously believe that a woman is most fertile during the bleeding days of the menstrual cycle and thus practice fertility awareness at the wrong time. Some couples lose, misplace, or run out of their primary method and do not have a back-up method available.

- *Negative attitudes about birth control.* Some people believe that birth control is immoral, a hassle, unromantic, or harmful. One's own negative attitudes or the perceived negative attitudes of others, such as peers or parents, can inhibit one from obtaining contraceptives. People use these as excuses not to visit doctors or clinics, or they may shy away from obtaining over-the-counter contraceptives.

- *Relationship issues.* Individuals in committed relationships are better contraceptors than individuals who are not in such relationships. Involvement with a committed partner tends to lessen guilt associated with sexual activity, and hence improves attitudes about contraceptive practice. People in a committed

> *It goes without saying that you should never have more children than you have car windows.*
> Erma Bombeck,
> humorist

relationship tend to have sexual intercourse more often and regularly, which gives the couple opportunities to talk about contraception and to become adept at using method(s). Individuals with irregular sexual contact, either because of geographical separation or relationship problems, may have difficulties in establishing a birth control regime. In new or casual sexual relationships there is a tendency to use no method or a poor method at first.

EMERGENCY CONTRACEPTION

An early acting method of contraception is the post-coital or **morning-after pill**. With this method, a woman who suspects that she may have conceived after a particular episode of intercourse can receive (preferably within 12, but up to 72, hours after intercourse) from a clinic or a doctor a large dose of synthetic estrogen and progesterone, which renders the reproductive tract incapable of supporting a pregnancy. This method is meant to be used as an emergency method only. It is not meant to be used as a regular means of birth control.

Because the morning-after pill works before implantation, a woman will not know for sure that she was pregnant. Morning-after pill treatment has a failure rate of approximately 1.5 percent. Side effects are infrequent. Nausea and vomiting are the most common, along with breast tenderness, irregular bleeding, and headache.

ABORTION

Abortion, in the form of the intentional, premature termination of pregnancy, is one of the oldest and most widely practiced methods of birth control. Chinese medical writings from 2700 B.C. recommended abortion. A cross-cultural study found that all but one of 300 societies has used abortion to control the size of families (Devereaux, 1995). Currently in the United States approximately 1.5 million abortions are performed annually. This number represents about one-fourth of all pregnancies and about one-half of all unintended pregnancies.

Women undergoing abortions tend to be young, white, and unmarried (Hatcher et al., 1994). Women in their teens account for only one in four abortions performed in the United States, while older teenagers and young adults have higher abortion rates (National Abortion Federation, 1990). Ninety percent of women obtain abortions in the first trimester (first 12 weeks) of pregnancy, and over 80 percent are not married at the time of the abortion (National Abortion Federation, 1990).

HEALTHY PEOPLE 2000

Increase to at least 85 percent the proportion of people aged 10 through 18 who have discussed human sexuality, including values surrounding sexuality, with their parents and/or have received information through another parentally endorsed source, such as youth, school, or religious programs.

Parents are the first and most important educators of their children in matters related to sexual behavior. From them, children receive their first lessons in sexual morality and appropriate sexual conduct, including lessons about the meaning of mutual respect, love, and marital fidelity.

Surgical Methods of Abortion

Vacuum or **suction curettage** is the safest and most commonly used abortion method; about 90 percent of all abortions are vacuum aspiration. Vacuum curettage is a two-part procedure. First, the woman is given general or (more often) local anesthesia and the cervix is gradually widened, either with a series of progressively tapered cylinders called dilators, or by insertion of slim rolls of **laminaria,** a seaweed product that expands when exposed to the liquid in cervical secretions. In the second part of the procedure, a narrow wand, called a **cannula,** is connected to a suction device, which is used to empty the uterus. Vacuum curettage is usually performed within the first 12 weeks of pregnancy.

An alternative to vacuum curettage is **dilatation and curettage** or "D and C." In a "D and C," the cervix is dilated as in the vacuum method, but instead of suction, the uterus is emptied by cleaning the inner lining with a spoon-shaped scraping-instrument (the curette).

If abortion is performed between the thirteenth and twentieth weeks of pregnancy, a procedure combining vacuum and surgical curettage, called **dilatation and extraction,** or "D and E," is usually performed.

Surgical methods of abortion are relatively simple and safe. If done before the third month of pregnancy, they can be carried out in 30 minutes or less. The cost usually ranges from $150 to $750. The rate of major complications, such as excess bleeding, damage to the uterus, or infection, is very low.

T E R M S

morning-after pill: a hormonal drug which, if taken within 72 hours after unprotected intercourse, temporarily disrupts the uterine environment to prevent implantation of the fertilized egg; morning-after pills also prevent ovulation

abortion: the expulsion or extraction of the products of conception from the uterus before the embryo or fetus is capable of independent life; abortions may be spontaneous or induced

vacuum (suction) curettage: removal of fetal tissue by suctioning off contents of the uterus

laminaria: a plug of sterile dried kelp (seaweed) which expands when in contact with water and can thus be placed in the cervical canal to dilate the cervix

cannula: a hollow tube for insertion into the body cavity

dilation and curettage (D and C): dilation of the cervix with use of a wand or laminaria and scraping the uterine lining; this procedure is often used during abortion

dilation and evacuation (D and E): dilation of the cervix and evacuation of the uterine contents using vacuum techniques

mifepristone or *RU 486:* a drug that blocks the natural hormone progesterone; used to prevent or abort an early pregnancy

Chemical Methods of Abortion

Chemical methods of abortion act very early in pregnancy or after the thirteenth week. An early acting chemical method of abortion is administration of **mifepristone,** also called **RU 486,** which blocks the action of the naturally occurring hormone progesterone. Because progesterone is absolutely essential for successful implantation and pregnancy, blocking the hormone's actions with mifepristone interrupts the early phases of pregnancy and causes the pregnancy to end, as in a miscarriage.

Mifepristone is given within 50 days of a woman's last menstrual period, usually in conjunction with prostaglandin, a hormone that induces uterine contractions. The drug is given by trained medical personnel in a clinic over the course of a week, after which a menstrual period occurs, which ends the pregnancy. Mifepristone plus prostaglandin is 95 percent effective, and side effects and other complications are minor (Peyron et al., 1993).

Late-acting (post-thirteen weeks of pregnancy) chemical methods of abortion are usually used as alternatives to D and E. These methods involve infusing saline, urea, or prostaglandin (a hormone) into the uterus. Saline and urea kill the fetus, and uterine contractions that follow empty the uterus. Prostaglandin induces uterine contractions directly, which result in expulsion of the uterine contents.

The Legality and Morality of Abortion

The propriety of abortion as a socially sanctioned method of birth control has been debated in Western societies for centuries. Over 2,000 years ago the Greek philosophers Aristotle and Plato recommended abortion, whereas Hippocrates, the founder of modern medicine, forbade it. Throughout the Middle Ages and the Renaissance, abortion was common, although various religious leaders objected to the practice on ethical grounds.

When the U.S. Constitution was ratified, and for several decades after, abortion was legal if it took place before the time of "quickening"—when a woman could feel fetal movements. Quickening usually occurs near the sixteenth week of pregnancy. The first statutes regulating abortion were enacted in the 1820s in Connecticut and New York. These laws prohibited abortion before the time of quickening, principally to protect women from what by modern standards were primitive and dangerous surgical techniques. By the end of the Civil War, more states had enacted restrictive abortion legislation, not only to preserve the health and life of a pregnant woman, but also to encourage American-born women to have children and to discourage nonreproductive sex. By 1900, abortion was illegal in all U.S. jurisdictions, and it remained so for over 60 years.

Restrictive abortion laws did not stop women from having abortions, however. In the first decades of the twentieth century, millions of women obtained illegal

Discovering Your Feelings about Abortion

There are no right or wrong responses.

Statement	I strongly agree	I tend to agree but have some reservations	I am undecided	I tend to disagree but have some reservations	I strongly disagree
Abortion penalizes the unborn for the mother's sake.					
Abortion places human life at a very low point on the scale of values.	___	___	___	___	___
A woman's desire to have an abortion should be considered sufficient reason to do so.	___	___	___	___	___
I approve of legal abortions so a woman can obtain one with proper medical attention.	___	___	___	___	___
Abortion ought to be prohibited because it is an unnatural act.	___	___	___	___	___
Having an abortion is not something that one should be ashamed of.	___	___	___	___	___
Abortion is a threat to society.	___	___	___	___	___
Abortion is the destruction of one life to serve the convenience of another.	___	___	___	___	___
A woman should have no regrets if she eliminates the burden of an unwanted child with an abortion.	___	___	___	___	___
The unborn [fetus] should be legally protected against abortion since [it] cannot protect itself.	___	___	___	___	___
Abortion should be an alternative when there is contraceptive failure.	___	___	___	___	___
Abortions should be allowed since the unborn is only a potential human being and not an actual human being.	___	___	___	___	___
Any person who has an abortion is probably selfish and unconcerned about others.	___	___	___	___	___
Abortion should be available as a method of improving community socioeconomic conditions.	___	___	___	___	___
Many more people would favor abortion if they knew more about it.	___	___	___	___	___

Statement	I strongly agree	I tend to agree but have some reservations	I am undecided	I tend to disagree but have some reservations	I strongly disagree
A woman should have an illegitimate child rather than have an abortion.	___	___	___	___	___
Liberalization of abortion laws should be viewed as a positive step.	___	___	___	___	___
Abortion should be illegal, for the 14th amendment to the Constitution holds that no state shall "deprive any person of life, liberty, and/or property without due process of the law."	___	___	___	___	___
The unborn should never be aborted no matter how detrimental the possible effects on the family.	___	___	___	___	___
The social evils involved in forcing a pregnant women to have a child are worse than any evils in destroying the unborn.	___	___	___	___	___
Decency forbids having an abortion.	___	___	___	___	___
A pregnancy that is not wanted and planned for should not be considered a pregnancy but merely a condition for which there is a medical cure.	___	___	___	___	___
Abortion is the equivalent of murder.	___	___	___	___	___
Easily accessible abortions probably cause people to become unconcerned and careless with their contraceptive choices.	___	___	___	___	___
Abortion ought to be considered a legitimate health measure.	___	___	___	___	___
The unborn ought to have the same rights as the potential mother.	___	___	___	___	___
Any outlawing of abortion is oppressive to women.	___	___	___	___	___
Abortion should be accepted as a method of population control.	___	___	___	___	___
Abortion violates the fundamental right to life.	___	___	___	___	___
If a woman feels that a child might ruin her life, she should have an abortion.	___	___	___	___	___

abortions. Those with money could travel to other countries where abortion was legal and performed in a hospital with trained personnel, or they could obtain a clandestine abortion performed by an American physician who accepted the risk of prosecution in return for a high fee. Most women, however, had to obtain abortions from nonmedical people who often performed the procedure using coathangers, spoons, disinfectant, or lye. Many women were maimed or killed by such procedures. The psychological trauma even of successful procedures was enormous. By the 1950s, an estimated 200,000 to one million women were getting illegal abortions annually.

By the 1960s, people began to take into account the social and psychological costs of illegal abortion, and on January 22, 1973 the U.S. Supreme Court declared that states could not make laws prohibiting abortion on the ground that they violated a woman's right to privacy, in this case, the right to decide about the outcome of a pregnancy. This decision, known as *Roe* v. *Wade*, declared 1) that the decision to have an abortion during the first trimester (12 weeks) of pregnancy should be left entirely to the woman and her physician, and 2) during the second trimester, individual states could regulate the abortion procedure for only one purpose—to protect the woman's health.

Many people have mixed feelings about abortion. Because there is no universally accepted scientific definition of when a life begins, some individuals view abortion as murder. Some opponents of abortion believe that its availability encourages irresponsible sexual behavior or haphazard use of birth control. Some see abortion as a threat to family life. Even the staunchest proponents of abortion rights would prefer that abortions never occur, but they argue that women must have the right to control their bodies. They believe that abortion is a necessary last resort if contraception fails, if a woman becomes

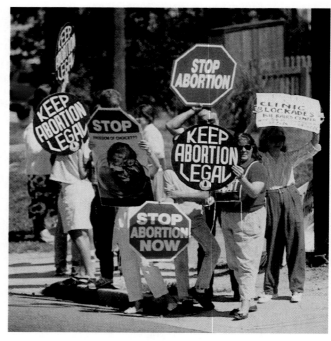

The option for abortion is a very controversial subject in our society.

pregnant because of rape or incest, if the child may suffer a birth defect, or if the woman's life and health are jeopardized by pregnancy or childbirth.

Whether pro-choice or pro-life, both positions agree on the value and dignity of human life, but are divided on when life begins, how conflicts such as religion, morals, and philosophy are to be balanced, and how human life is best preserved and enhanced. Several factors ensure that the abortion debate will continue. These factors include: 1) advances in neonatal medicine; 2) political aspects of abortion; and 3) ethical issues regarding when life begins.

Controversy in Health

Mrs. Martinez's Dilemma

Mrs. Martinez grew up in Mexico and emigrated to the United States as a young girl. She was educated by nuns and is a devout Catholic. Her first husband died and at age 40, she married Charles Perkins, who had no religious preferences. When Mrs. Martinez became pregnant, her doctor insisted that she undergo amniocentesis because of her age. The test showed that she was carrying a fetus with Down syndrome. The doctor recommended an abortion. The father wanted to abort the pregnancy. Mrs. Martinez refused an abortion because of her religious convictions.

STUDENT REFLECTIONS
- What should the doctor do in light of his patient's convictions?
- What should the father do?
- What would you do?

HEALTH IN REVIEW

- A variety of safe, reliable, and effective birth control methods are available today. These include hormonal contraceptive (the birth control pill and progestin-only contraceptives), barrier methods (condom, diaphragm, cervical cap, and spermicides), fertility awareness methods, the IUD, sterilization, and withdrawal.
- A contraceptive's effectiveness is measured in terms of lowest observed and typical failure rates.
- Although most birth control methods are designed for use in the woman's body, both partners share the responsibility for birth control. Communication and cooperation are keys to shared responsibility.

- People who say they do not want to have a baby yet do not use birth control methods tend to have low motivation, lack of knowledge of human reproduction and birth control methods, have negative attitudes toward birth control, or are in relationships that hinder correct birth control practice.
- The most common type of abortion is vacuum aspiration. Abortion became legal in the U.S. in 1973 with the Supreme Court's *Roe* v. *Wade* decision.

REFERENCES

Baird, D. T., and A. F. Glasier (1993). "Hormonal Contraception." *New England Journal of Medicine,* 328: 1543–1549.

Devereaux, G. (1995). *A Study of Abortion in Primitive Societies.* New York: Julian Press.

Goldberg, M. S. (1993). "Choosing a Contraceptive." *FDA Consumer,* December: 18–25.

Hatcher, R. A., J. Trussell, F. Stewart, G. K. Stewart, D. Kowal, F. Guest, W. Cates, and M. S. Policar (1994). *Contraceptive Technology,* 16th edition. New York: Irvington Publishers.

Peyron, R., E. Aubery, V. Targosz, L. Silvestre, M. Renault, F. Elkik, P. Leclerc, et al. (1993). "Early Termination of Pregnancy with Mifepristone (RU 486)." *New England Journal of Medicine,* 328: 1509–1513.

"Women Who Have Abortions" (fact sheet) (1990). Washington, D.C.: National Abortion Federation.

SUGGESTED READINGS

Baker, B. (1993). "The Female Condom." *MS.* magazine, March/April: 80–81. Describes the two kinds of female condoms available for women.

Goldberg, M. S. (1993). "Choosing a Contraceptive." *FDA Consumer,* December: 18–25. Discusses all the birth control options.

Hatcher, R. A., J. Trussell, F. Stewart, G. K. Stewart, D. Kowal, F. Guest, W. Cates, and M. S. Policar (1994). *Contraceptive Technology,* 16th edition. New York: Irvington Publishers. A comprehensive, up-to-date book on contraceptive technology and sexual reproduction.

Stehlin, D. (1993). "Depo-Provera: The Quarterly Contraceptive." *FDA Consumer,* July. Discusses the pros and cons of Depo-Provera use.

Stewart, F., F. Guest, G. Stewart, and R. Hatcher (1987). *Understanding Your Body: Every Woman's Guide to Gynecology and Health.* New York: Bantam Books. A complete guide to women's health issues.

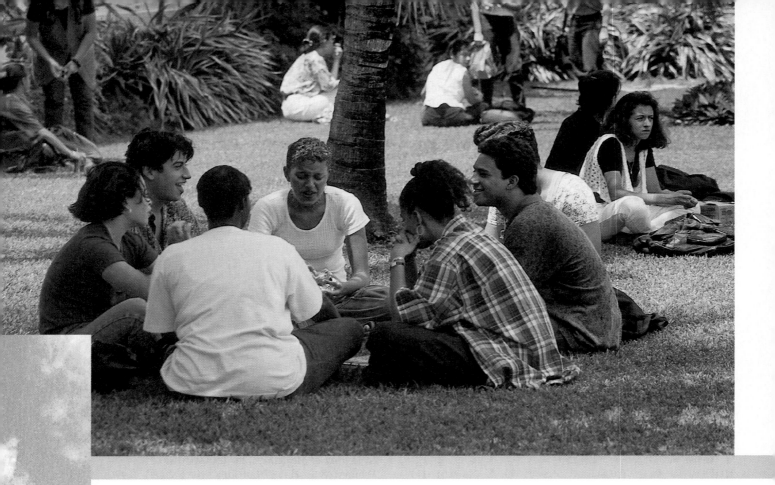

LEARNING OBJECTIVES

After reading this chapter you should be able to:

1. Describe the impact of STDs on society.
2. Explain how different sexual behaviors increase your risk of contracting an STD.
3. Identify the causative agent, symptoms, and treatment for the following: trichomonas vaginalis and gardnerella vaginalis, chlamydia trachomatis, gonorrhea, syphilis, genital herpes, genital warts, pubic lice, scabies, and AIDS.
4. Understand the importance of testing for HIV and the proper testing procedures.
5. Identify several "safer sex" practices.
6. Describe the importance of effective communication in reducing the risk of STDs and HIV/AIDS.

Protecting against Sexually Transmitted Diseases and AIDS

*A*bout twenty-five kinds of infections can be passed from person to person through sexual contact (Table 11.1). Traditionally, these infections have been called venereal diseases or "VD"—the word *venereal* being derived from Venus, the mythical Roman goddess of love. To identify more clearly their origins, these diseases are now called **sexually transmitted diseases,** or **STDs.**

Sexually transmitted diseases have been afflicting humans for thousands of years. Ancient Chinese medical writings describe diseases of the genitalia that were probably syphilis. The ancient Egyptians described genital diseases that were probably gonorrhea. Old Testament and Talmudic writings describe a condition called "ziba," which was associated with the emission of fluid, referred to then as "issue," from the nonerect penis or the vagina. "Ziba" was probably gonorrhea, and "issue" was probably the discharge associated with gonorrhea. A number of famous historical figures are thought to have been afflicted with sexually transmitted diseases (Table 11.2).

The number of people infected with STDs is a major concern for our society. Approximately thirteen million Americans may have a symptomatic STD. The economic costs of STDs are enormous, especially when one includes treatment for infertility (often due to STDs), treatment for pelvic inflammatory dis-

TABLE 11.1   Agents Causing Common Sexually Transmitted Diseases

Disease	Infectious agent
	Bacteria
Chlamydia	*Chlamydia trachomatis*
Gonorrhea	*Neisseria gonorrhea*
Syphilis	*Treponema pallidum*
Vaginitis	*Gardnerella vaginalis*
	Viruses
Genital herpes	Herpes virus 1 and 2
Anogenital warts	Papilloma virus
AIDS	Human immunodeficiency Virus
Hepatitis	Hepatitis viruses A, B, C, D
Molluscum contagiosum	Molluscum contagiosum virus
	Protozoa
Vaginitis	*Trichomonas vaginalis*
	Insects
Lice ("crabs")	*Phthirus pubis*
Mites ("scabies")	*Sarcoptes scabiei*

TABLE 11.2   Famous People Afflicted with an STD
No one knows for sure, but historians say these famous people were infected with an STD.

Abraham	Job
Sarah	King David
Julius Caesar	Cleopatra
Charlemagne	Napoleon
Henry VIII	Columbus
The Greats: Peter and Catherine	Goya
Dürer	Gauguin
Schubert	Boswell
Molière	Goethe
Van Gogh	Oscar Wilde
Nietzsche	

ease, and STD treatment. There are also the serious human costs of lost work and study, as well as physical suffering due to STDs.

In the United States today, the total number of reported cases of STDs exceeds that of all other infectious diseases except the common cold (Figure 11.1). Individuals under age 25 make up the majority of STD cases. Two-thirds of gonorrhea and chlamydia cases occur in young adults 24 years old or younger.

UNDERSTANDING SEXUAL BEHAVIOR

Everyone accepts different levels of risk in life. Certain sexual behaviors increase your risk of contracting an STD and it is important to know what they are. Understanding your sexual behaviors will allow you to make the appropriate decision to decrease your risk of contracting an STD, becoming pregnant, or impregnating someone.

Multiple Sexual Partners

There is a large pool of unmarried sexually active people, because many individuals become active in late adolescence. This group consists of those who delay marriage until their mid-to-late 20s and early 30s, and those who become divorced and have sexual partners before remarriage. One-third of unmarried sexually active people report having more than one sexual partner in the previous year (Kost and Forrest, 1992).

False Sense of Safety

Using birth control pills tends to decrease the use of condoms and spermicides, which help prevent transmission of STDs. The availability of antibiotics makes many people less afraid of sexually transmitted diseases. They believe that as long as there is a cure for syphilis and gonorrhea there is nothing to worry about.

Absence of Signs and Symptoms

Some STDs have very mild or no symptoms, which permit a worsening of the infection and unknowingly passing it to others. One study showed that approximately 8 percent of college students were infected with chlamydia and did not know it. Another 1.5 percent were infected with gonorrhea and did not know it. People infected with HIV can have mild or no symptoms for years, yet still be infectious.

Untreated Conditions

Some individuals lack sufficient knowledge of the signs and symptoms of STDs to know that they are infected. Those who are not accustomed to seeking health care, or who financially cannot afford it, are less likely to seek treatment for an infection. Furthermore, many individuals with STDs do not comply with treatment regimes. When medications are not taken for the required length of time, an infection may not be completely eradicated even though symptoms may disappear. People who do not complete treatment may still be infectious.

T E R M
sexually transmitted diseases (STDs): infections passed from person to person by sexual contact

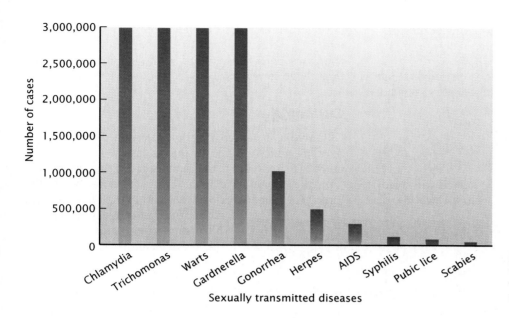

FIGURE 11.1 Estimated Yearly Number of Sexually Transmitted Diseases in the United States

Impaired Judgment

The use of drugs, including alcohol, can increase the risk of transmitting STDs because people with impaired judgment do not stop to think about using condoms. Also, people in this state may be more likely to have sex with someone they do not know; they may know nothing of their partner's past sexual and drug history.

Lack of Immunity

Some STD-causing organisms, especially viruses, can escape the body's immune defenses, causing individuals to remain infected and transmit the infection. This may permit reinfection and also makes the development of vaccinations difficult or impossible (Sparling et al., 1994) (Chapter 10).

REACTIONS TO STDs

Many people who contract a sexually transmitted disease are often embarrassed or ashamed to discuss this with their health care provider or partner. There are usually two reactions to a sexually transmitted disease: 1) it is sinful to have one and 2) "it won't happen to me."

Value Judgments

Unlike nearly all other kinds of infections, STDs are associated with sinfulness, dirtiness, condemnation, shame, guilt, and disgust. These negative attitudes keep people from getting check-ups, contacting partners when an STD has been diagnosed, and talking to new partners about previous exposures. In the nineteenth century, when syphilis was a scourge of Europe, rather than trying to prevent its spread (effective treatments had not yet been invented), countries blamed the disease on the weak character or immorality of their neighbors: the English referred to syphilis as the "French disease," and the French called it the "Spanish disease." Prejudice and scapegoating helped spread the disease.

Denial

With respect to contracting an STD, many people think, "It can't happen to me," or "He/she is too nice to have an STD" or "He/she isn't the type of person who would have an STD." Because there are no vaccinations against infectious agents that cause sexually transmitted diseases, the only way to prevent them is for sexually active individuals, who are not in life-long single-partner ("monogamous") sexual relationships, to assume responsibility for protecting themselves and their partners. This means

HEALTHY PEOPLE 2000

Provide HIV education for students and staff in at least 90 percent of colleges and universities.

High rates of STDs among students using college and university student health centers suggest that students are not practicing safer sex. For example, 40 percent of women seeking pregnancy tests at the University of Maryland student health center in 1987 tested positive for an STD other than HIV. Colleges and universities can help prevent the spread of HIV infection by assuring that their students and staff are educated about how HIV is and is not transmitted, how to prevent transmission, and how to assess their own risk of infection accurately.

becoming aware of the signs and symptoms of the common STDs and seeking treatment when such signs occur. It means that sexually active people who have more than one partner within a year should obtain periodic (about every six months) STD check-ups. It also means knowing about and practicing "safer sex."

COMMON STDs

Although many nonviral STDs can be treated with medications, the epidemic of STDs persists worldwide (Holmes, 1994). There are no vaccinations for either the bacterial or viral infections that cause the most common sexually transmitted diseases. Dealing directly and responsibly with STDs is not easy. However, we owe it to the people we care about to do so. Table 11.3 outlines the major STDs, including their symptoms and treatment.

> *Prejudice, not being founded on reason, cannot be removed by argument.*
> Samuel Johnson

Trichomonas and Gardnerella

Although not often regarded as sexually transmitted diseases, vaginal infections caused by the protozoan *Trichomonas vaginalis* and the bacterium *Gardnerella vaginalis* are transmitted during intercourse. Symptoms tend to occur only in women (vaginal itching and a cheesy, odorous discharge from the vagina), but the organisms can survive in the urethra of the penis and under the penile foreskin. A man who harbors these organisms can infect other partners or even reinfect the partner who transmitted the organisms to him. Medications can eliminate these infections and it is essential for both partners to undergo treatment.

Chlamydia

Chlamydia is caused by the bacterium *Chlamydia trachomatis,* which specifically infects certain cells lining the mucous membranes of the genitals, mouth, anus, and rectum, the conjunctiva of the eyes, and occasionally the lungs. The chlamydial bacteria bind to their surfaces and induce the host cells to engulf them. After gaining entrance to the cell, these organisms resist a host cell's defenses and eventually "steal" from the host cell the biochemical compounds required for their own survival. The chlamydial organisms use the stolen nutrients to reproduce and multiply, and ultimately the host cells die.

In the United States and other Western countries, chlamydia is the most prevalent sexually transmitted disease. Each year approximately three million Americans are reported to contract chlamydia, which public health experts estimate represents only one-third of all actual cases. In as many as half of all cases, chlamydia occurs simultaneously with gonorrhea. Newborns also are susceptible to chlamydial infection if their mothers are infected at the time of delivery. The most common complications of chlamydial infection in newborns are conjunctivitis (eye infection) and pneumonia.

Health Update

New Lab Test for Chlamydia

A new laboratory test offers improved reliability and speed in detecting chlamydia, a sexually transmitted genital tract infection common in sexually active teenagers and young adults.

The new Amplicor Chlamydia Trachomatis Test can catch chlamydia cases that might be missed by current cell culture methods. The test can be performed on a man's urine or on a swab sample from a woman's cervix or urethra. It is quick— about four hours, compared to three to seven days for current procedures.

Studies show the new test to be superior to culture techniques in detecting the disease in both sexes, but it is particularly effective in males. Traditionally, chlamydia in men has been difficult to diagnose. Current urine tests are undependable, and swab methods are uncomfortable.

Men are primary carriers of chlamydia but often don't show symptoms. Left untreated, the disease can cause disorders such as pelvic inflammatory disease and ectopic pregnancy in women, as well as respiratory and eye infections in babies of infected mothers.

Four million people contract chlamydia annually in the United States.

On male urine, the new test showed 95 percent sensitivity in detecting infection compared with 68 percent for culture methods. On urethral samples, the new test had 91 percent sensitivity versus 83 percent for culture methods. Cervical specimens from women showed 94 percent for the new test compared with 86 percent for culture methods. In a few instances, the new test missed cases detected by the culture methods.
Source: FDA Consumer (September 1993).

TABLE 11.3 Common Sexually Transmitted Diseases (STDs)

STD	Symptoms	Treatment
AIDS	Flu-like symptoms followed by any of a number of diseases characteristic of immunodeficiency	AZT may retard viral reproduction temporarily. Opportunistic infections can be treated to some degree.
Chlamydia	Usually within 3 weeks: infected men have a discharge from the penis and painful urination, women may have a vaginal discharge, but often are asymptomatic	Antibiotics
Gardnerella	Yellow-green vaginal discharge with an unpleasant odor; painful urination; vaginal itching	Metronidizole
Genital warts	Usually within 1 to 3 months: small, dry growths on the genitals, anus, cervix, and possibly mouth	Podophyllin
Gonorrhea	Usually within 2 weeks: discharge from the penis, vagina, or anus; pain on urination or defecation or during sexual intercourse; pain and swelling in the pelvic region; genital and oral infections may be asymptomatic	Antibiotics
Hepatitis	Low-grade fever, fatigue, headaches, loss of appetite, nausea, dark urine, jaundice	Rest, proper nutrition
Herpes genitalis	Usually within 2 weeks: painful blisters appear on site(s) of infection: genitals, anus, cervix; occasionally itching, painful urination, and fever	None; acyclovir relieves symptoms
Pubic lice	Usually within 5 weeks: intense itching in the genital region; lice may be visible in pubic hair; small white eggs may be visible on pubic hair	Gamma benzene hexachloride
Syphilis	Usually within 3 weeks: a chancre (painless sore) appears on the genitals, anus, or mouth; secondary stage—skin rash—appears if left untreated; tertiary stage includes diseases of several body organs	Antibiotics
Trichomoniasis	Yellowish green vaginal discharge with an unpleasant odor; vaginal itching; occasionally painful intercourse	Metronidizole

One reason that chlamydial infections are so prevalent is that infected individuals often have extremely mild or no symptoms. Thus infected individuals can unknowingly transmit the infection to new sex partners. When symptoms do occur, they include pain during urination in both men and women (dysuria) and a whitish discharge from the penis or vagina. Symptoms generally appear within 7 to 21 days after infection.

Chlamydia can be treated with antibiotics. Left untreated, the chlamydial bacteria can multiply and cause inflammation and damage of the reproductive organs in both sexes. In men, untreated chlamydia can result in inflammation of the epididymis (**epididymitis**), characterized by pain, swelling, and tenderness in the scrotum, and sometimes by a mild fever. Damage to the tissues in the epididymis can eventually lead to sterility. In women, chlamydial infections affect the cervix, uterus, fallopian tubes, and peritoneum. Often chlamydial infections of the reproductive tract produce no symptoms until the infection is advanced. A woman may then experience chronic pelvic pain, vaginal discharge, intermittent vaginal bleeding, and pain during intercourse. Infection of the fallopian tubes can produce scar tissue

> T   E   R   M   S
>
> *chlamydia:* a sexually transmitted disease caused by the bacterium *Chlamydia trachomatis*
>
> *epididymitis:* inflammation of the epididymis (a structure that connects the vas deferens and the testes)

that damages the tubes' lining and partially or completely blocks the tubes. These effects may increase the risk of ectopic pregnancy or render a woman infertile; in fact, about 10,000 cases of female infertility per year result from fallopian tube damage from chlamydia (Grodstein and Rothman, 1994).

Chlamydial infections induce an immune response in the host, but for unknown reasons infected individuals do not gain immunity to future chlamydial infections. This means that treated individuals can be reinfected upon exposure to the bacteria.

Gonorrhea

Gonorrhea, also known as "the clap," is caused by the bacterium *Neisseria gonorrheae.* Gonorrheal organisms specifically infect the mucous membranes of the body, most often the genitals, reproductive organs, mouth and throat, anus, and eyes. Neisseria cannot survive on toilet seats, doorknobs, bedsheets, clothes, or towels. Transmission in adults almost always occurs by genital, oral, or anal sexual contact; infection of the eyes occurs by hand (often through self-infection). Each year, about one million American adults are infected with gonorrhea.

Newborn babies exposed to gonorrheal organisms in the mother's birth canal may develop gonorrhea of the eyes. Most states require that antibiotics or a few drops of silver nitrate be put into the eyes of babies immediately after birth to kill the gonorrhea bacteria and prevent possible blindness.

Although the bacteria causing them are quite different, the symptoms of gonorrheal and chlamydial infections are very similar. Like chlamydia, many people infected with gonorrheal organisms do not develop symptoms and their infections go unnoticed. If the infection progresses, men may develop epididymitis and woman may develop infections of the uterus, fallopian tubes, and pelvic region. Such infections may cause sterility. When symptoms appear they include painful urination in both sexes and a yellowish discharge from the penis or vagina. Occasionally there is pain in the groin, testes, or lower abdomen. The first symptoms of gonorrhea usually appear within a week to ten days after exposure.

Gonorrhea can be treated with antibiotics. However, new antibiotic-resistant strains of the organism are constantly evolving. In nearly half of all cases of gonorrhea, chlamydia also is present. Individuals undergoing diagnosis for gonorrhea should also be tested for chlamydia.

Syphilis

Syphilis is caused by a spiral-shaped bacterium called *Treponema pallidum.* These organisms are transmitted from person to person through genital, oral, and anal contact, as well as being acquired from blood. Syphilis can also be transmitted from a mother to her unborn fetus, perhaps as early as the ninth week of pregnancy.

The first noticeable sign of syphilis is a painless open sore called a **chancre** ("shanker"), which can appear any time between the first week and third month after infection. If the infection is not treated within that period, the chancre will heal and the disease will enter a secondary stage, characterized by a skin rash, hair loss, and the appearance of round, flat-topped growths on most areas of the body. Left untreated, the signs of the secondary stage also disappear, and the infection enters a symptomless (latency) period during which the syphilis organisms multiply in many other regions of the body. In the final, tertiary stage, the disease eventually damages vital organs, such as the heart or brain, and can cause severe symptoms or death. Syphilis can be treated with antibiotics at any stage of the infection.

Herpes

Herpes is caused by the virus *Herpes simplex,* or HSV. Various strains of HSV can cause cold sores on the mouth ("fever blisters"), skin rashes, mononucleosis, and lesions on the penis, vagina, or rectum. Herpes viruses can infect the eyes, leading to impaired vision and even blindness. If the virus is present in the birth canal, newborn babies can be infected, often resulting in brain damage and abnormal

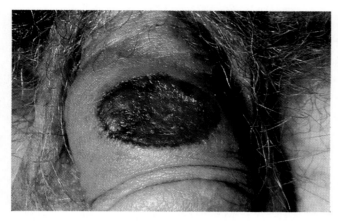

The first physical sign of a syphilis infection is an open lesion called a chancre.

development. About 500 babies are born each year with herpes and two-thirds of infected babies who are not treated die. Pregnant women who have had herpes should tell their physicians of the previous infection in order to prevent transmission of HSV to their babies.

Each year up to one million adults acquire a genital herpes infection. As many as thirty million American adults have already been infected with genital herpes. Oral herpes infections occur in many children and by age 50 more than three-fourths of the adult population has experienced an oral herpes infection.

Genital herpes infections are caused most frequently by the viral strain HSV-2. Oral herpes is caused most frequently by HSV-1. However, both HSV-2 and HSV-1 can cause genital and oral infections with virtually identical symptoms. Thus people with oral herpes can transmit the infection to partners via oral sex. They can also transmit it to themselves through masturbation. Once a person has been infected, oral HSV-1 infections tend to recur much more frequently than do oral HSV-2 infections. Conversely, genital HSV-2 infections tend to recur more frequently than genital HSV-1 infections. Oral herpes can occur without sexual contact; however, genital herpes cannot occur without some form of sexual contact, either vaginal, anal, oral, or through masturbation.

A herpes lesion on the genitals usually appears within 2 to 20 days after contact with the virus. Trans-mission of the virus via bed linen, clothing, towels, toilet seats, and hot tubs is highly unlikely. The major symptoms of a genital herpes infection are the presence of one or more blisters, which eventually break to become wet, painful sores that last about two or three weeks; fever; and occasionally pain in the lower abdomen. Eventually these initial symptoms disappear, but the herpes virus remains dormant in certain of the body's nerve cells, permitting periodic recurrences of the symptoms, called "flare-ups," at or near the site(s) of the initial infection. Stress, anxiety, improper nutrition, sunlight, and skin irritation can bring on flare-ups.

There is no cure for herpes. Infected individuals remain so for life. The drug acyclovir can minimize the duration and severity of the symptoms of an initial infection or a flare-up.

Herpes is extremely contagious when a sore is present. People with open lesions should avoid sex with others until the lesions disappear. Even if no sore is present, transmission is possible, although much less likely, through the "shedding" of virus particles from the skin.

Because the herpes virus remains in the body, and because flare-ups are a persistent possibility, some people believe that infected persons can never be sexually active. This is not true. People with herpes can learn to manage the condition. In many instances, after one or two episodes, additional flare-ups never occur. Some people can anticipate a flare-up because they get a tingling sensation, itching, pain, or numbness at the site of the initial infection. This can be a signal to refrain from sexual contact. If used appropriately, condoms and spermicides can protect against the spread of herpes.

Because genital herpes is associated with a risk of cervical cancer, women with herpes are advised to have annual Pap smears to ascertain the condition of the vagina and cervix.

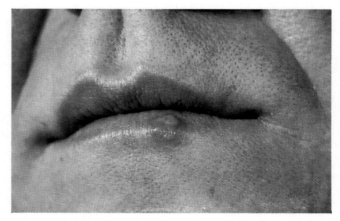

"Cold sores" on the lip or inside the mouth are a common occurrence in people who are infected by the herpes simplex virus. The sores usually heal in a week or so but can flare up again, because the viral infection is permanent.

Sexually Transmitted Warts

Sexually transmitted warts (*Condylomata acuminata*), also known as genital or venereal warts, are hard, cauliflower-like growths that appear in men on the penis, in women on the external genitals and cervix, and in both sexes in the anal region. Warts are caused by several of the approximately fifty varieties of **human papillomavirus, HPV.** When HPV infects skin cells and cells of the genital tract, it causes them to multiply, thus forming the wart. Infection with many varieties of HPV is often more of a nuisance than it is dangerous. However, two varieties of HPV, HPV-16 and HPV-18, may cause or facilitate uncontrolled multiplication of cells of the cervix and eventually cancer of the cervix (Lowry et al., 1994).

Sexually transmitted warts usually appear about three months after contact with an infected person. They can be removed by coating the wart with a liquid containing podophyllin, which dries the wart. In severe cases, wart removal is accomplished by freezing the warts with liquid nitrogen or removing them with laser surgery (Table 11.4).

Pubic Lice

Pubic lice (*Phthirus pubis*), also known as "crabs," are barely visible insects that live on hair shafts primarily in the genital-rectal region and occasionally on hair in the armpits, beard, and eyelashes. The organisms' claws are specifically adapted for grasping hairs with the diameter of pubic and axillary hair, which differs in diameter from the shafts of scalp hair. Thus pubic lice are not usually found on the head. (Scalp hair is the ecological niche of the head louse, *Pediculus humanus capitis*.)

Lice feed on blood taken from tiny blood vessels in the skin, which they pierce with their mouth. Some people are sensitive to the bites and may experience itching, which is often the main symptom of infestation. The lice can also been seen; they look like small freckles. The eggs of lice are enclosed in small white pods (called "nits"), which attach to hair shafts. The presence of nits is also a sign of infestation.

Transfer of lice is via physical—usually sexual—contact. They can also be transmitted via contact with objects on which eggs might have been laid, such as towels, bed linens, and clothes. An infestation of pubic lice can be eliminated by washing the pubic hair with liquids or shampoos containing agents that specifically kill lice (e.g., pyrethrins, piperonyl butoxide, and gamma benzene hydrochloride). All of an infected person's clothes, towels, and bed linens should also be washed with cleaning agents made specifically for killing lice.

Scabies

Scabies is an infestation of certain regions of the skin by extremely small (invisible to the naked eye) mites, *Sarcoptes scabiei*. The mites burrow into the skin where they live and lay eggs. The tiny lesions produced by the mites often cause intense itching, which is the major sign of a scabies infection. The mites produce tiny burrows across skin lines, which often go unnoticed. Occasionally, an infestation will produce small round nodules. The mites tend to live in the webs between the fingers, on the sides of fingers, and on the wrists, elbows, breasts, abdomen, penis, and buttocks. Rarely do mites live on the face, neck, upper back, palms and soles.

Scabies can be transmitted both sexually and nonsexually. All that is required is close personal contact. The itching and physical symptoms often take several weeks

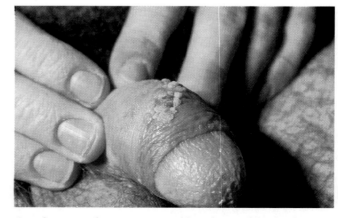

Genital warts on the penis are caused by infection of the skin by papilloma viruses. Genital warts can be removed by a variety of treatments but sometimes recur.

TABLE 11.4 Genital Wart Treatments

Treatment	Efficacy	Recurrence*
Cryotherapy	63–88%	21–39%
Interferon	44%	0% (recombinant alone)
Interferon + podophyllin	61%	67%
Laser vaporization	23–40%	Not known
Podofilox	45–88%	33–60%
Podophyllin	32–79%	27–65%
Surgical excision	93%	29%
Trichloroacetic acid or bichloroacetic acid	81%	36%

*Up to 1 year, depending on the study.

Source: R. Lewis, "New Choices for Coping with Genital Herpes," *FDA Consumer* (1995): 17–21.

to appear. Scabies can be treated with topical agents that kill the mites and their eggs.

Acquired Immune Deficiency Syndrome (AIDS)

Cause of AIDS AIDS is caused by **human immunodeficiency virus,** or **HIV** (Chapter 12). HIV infection causes disease by destroying immune system cells and weakening the body's immune system, and also damages certain cells in the brain. Destruction of the body's immune system makes HIV-infected individuals susceptible to a variety of bacterial, viral, and fungal infections that a person with an intact immune system could readily ward off. Individuals who are HIV-positive are also susceptible to cancer because the immune system protects the body against cancer. AIDS patients tend to develop cancer of the immune system (lymphoma) and a skin cancer called **Kaposi's sarcoma.** HIV infection

T   E   R   M   S

sexually transmitted warts: hard growths caused by an infection with human papilloma virus, HPV, that appears on the skin of the genitals or anus

human papillomavirus (HPV): a genus of viruses including those causing papillomas (small nipple-like protrusions of the skin or mucous membrane) and warts

pubic lice: small insects that live in hair in the genital-rectal region

scabies: infestation of the skin by microscopic mites (insects)

human immunodeficiency virus (HIV): the virus that causes AIDS; it causes a defect in the body's immune system by invading and then multiplying within the white blood cells

Kaposi's sarcoma: skin cancer that occurs with (and without) HIV infection

in the brain leads to loss of mental faculties (AIDS dementia).

AIDS, like cancer, is not a single disease. AIDS is defined by the U.S. Centers for Disease Control and Prevention (CDC) as having one or more of twenty-seven specific infectious diseases plus 200 or fewer CD4 T-cells in the blood. (A normal CD4 T-cell level is 800–1200 cells per ml of blood.)

Incidence of AIDS Trends of HIV infection in the United States indicate that as many as one million persons may be infected. Although the infection has occurred primarily in men, women are becoming increasingly infected. HIV is a public health problem not only in the United States but around the world. About 80 percent of reported new cases now arise in developing countries where no funds are available for AIDS education and prevention programs. Some researchers estimate that as many as 100 million people worldwide will be infected by the year 2000.

In the United States during the past decade, AIDS accounted for a tremendous increase in the death rate of men ages 25–44 (Figure 11.2). What is now alarming public health officials is the number of HIV infections in young people ages 13–24 (Figure 11.3). In 1993 alone almost 25 percent of the total number of HIV cases were contracted, suggesting more teenagers and young adults are becoming HIV infected and eventually will develop AIDS.

The Centers for Disease Control and Prevention estimate that about one million people, or one in 250, in the United States are infected with HIV. Currently, AIDS is the sixth and seventh leading cause of death in men and women, respectively, ages 15–24 (Chapter 1).

According to data through 1993, the majority of males become HIV infected through sex with men (62 percent) and intravenous drug use (21 percent). While 49 percent of the women contracted HIV through intra-

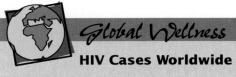
HIV Cases Worldwide

Worldwide, approximately 4.5 million people have developed AIDS since the beginning of the epidemic. The greatest number of HIV infection has occurred in Africa. According to Dr. Michael Merson of the World Health Organization, HIV infections are increasing most rapidly in Asia. (Floyd et al., 1995, p. 150). At right is a breakdown of HIV cases worldwide. Many believe the number of people with HIV is only the tip of the iceberg. As more men and women of different sexual orientations, age, race, and geographic locations become affected by HIV, the numbers of HIV-infected people worldwide will increase dramatically. All experts believe that education is key to stopping this worldwide epidemic.

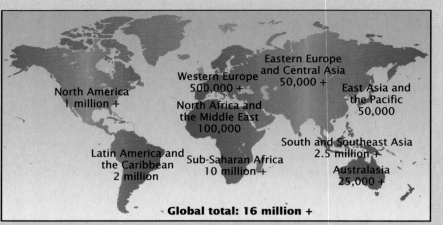

Source: World Health Organization.

venous drug use, about one-third (35 percent) became HIV infected through heterosexual contact (Figure 11.4). The increase in the number of heterosexual individuals infected with HIV is beginning to dispel the myth that AIDS is a homosexual disease. All sexually active people

need to take the necessary precautions to decrease their risk of contracting HIV/AIDS.

A recent survey by the National Opinion Research Center (1995) indicated that 30 percent of adults say they have changed their sexual behaviors because of

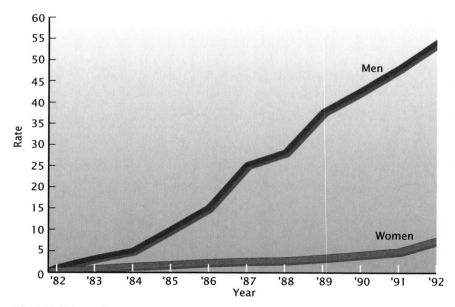

FIGURE 11.2 HIV/AIDS Death Rates* among Men and Women Ages 25–44: U.S. 1982–1992**
Source: Centers for Disease Control HIV/AIDS Prevention 1994 Fact Book, pp. 8 and 9.

*Per 100,000 population.

**National vital statistics based on underlying cause of death, using final data for 1982-1991 and provisional data for 1992. Data for liver disease in 1992 were unavailable.

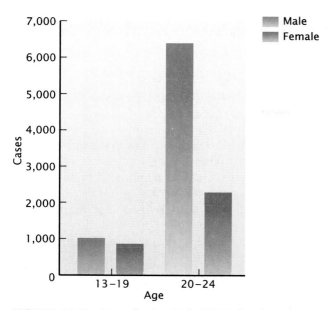

FIGURE 11.3 Cumulative U.S. HIV Infection Cases (not AIDS) among Young People Ages 13–24 (from States with Confidential HIV Infection Reporting*) through 1993

*Includes data from 25 states.

Source: Centers for Disease Control/U.S. Public Health Service, HIV/AIDS Surveillance Report (July 1994): 14.

AIDS. Of these, 29 percent used condoms more often, 26 percent have limited their sexual activity to one partner, 25 percent are more selective in partners, 11 percent abstain from sexual intercourse, and 11 percent have reduced their number of sexual partners. Clearly, these behaviors will help reduce the risk of contracting HIV; however, everyone needs to practice safe sex behaviors.

Methods of Transmission HIV is transmitted exclusively via blood, semen (which contains small amounts of blood), and vaginal fluids. HIV is not transmitted by touching the skin or clothes of an infected person, from saliva, from shared toilets or from air, food, or water that has been touched by an infected person. Indeed, hardly any HIV transmission has been found among family members who live in intimate contact with HIV-infected hemophiliacs who received the virus from HIV-contaminated blood products used to treat their hereditary bleeding disorder.

HIV is a **retrovirus,** which means that once it gains entry to a cell it incorporates itself into the host cell's DNA. This allows HIV to manufacture many copies of itself, which eventually infect neighboring cells. Because HIV incorporates itself into host cells, it cannot be eliminated from an infected person's body. HIV infections are life-long (Chapter 12).

When individuals become infected with HIV, within a few weeks they usually experience flu-like symptoms from which they eventually recover. Their immune systems are still intact and they produce copious antibodies to HIV. The mounting of an immune response in the early phases of an HIV infection provides the basis for HIV testing. Nearly all of the tests for HIV infection detect antibodies to HIV. A positive result ("seropositive") indicates that a person has been exposed to sufficient quantities of HIV particles to mount an immune response.

An HIV-infected individual may not manifest symptoms of AIDS for as many as 15 or 20 years after the initial infection. During this latency period the infected person is contagious and can spread the infection to oth-

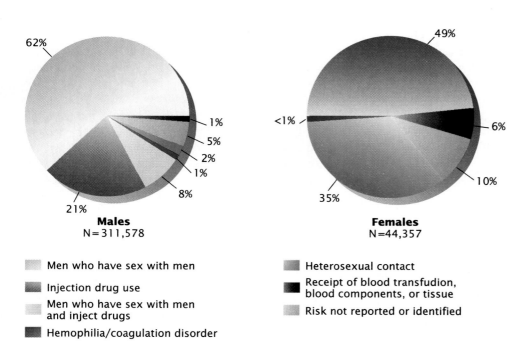

Males
N=311,578

Men who have sex with men

Injection drug use

Men who have sex with men and inject drugs

Hemophilia/coagulation disorder

Females
N=44,357

Heterosexual contact

Receipt of blood transfudion, blood components, or tissue

Risk not reported or identified

FIGURE 11.4 AIDS Cases among Adults and Adolescents, by Sex and Exposure Category, Reported through December 1993

Source: Centers for Disease Control HIV/AIDS Prevention 1994 Fact Book, p. 12.

ers, even though she or he is symptomless. The first signs of AIDS are usually mononucleosis-like symptoms (e.g., swollen lymph glands, fever, night-sweats) and possibly headaches and impaired mental functioning caused by HIV infection of the brain. As the disease progresses, individuals most often suffer weight loss, infections on the skin (shingles) or in the throat ("thrush"), and one or more opportunistic infections and/or cancer.

Because there is now no way to rid the body of HIV and hence cure AIDS, the best treatment available to infected individuals is medications and care for the opportunistic infections that result from immune suppression. In addition, there have been attempts to slow the replication of the virus. The drug *zidovudine,* or AZT, was given to HIV-infected individuals to slow replication of the virus. Initial hopes that AZT would be effective in prolonging the lives of HIV-infected individuals have not been fulfilled. Also, because HIV mutates rapidly, people taking AZT usually develop drug-resistant strains of the virus.

Because many viral diseases have been conquered by vaccination, much effort has gone into developing vaccines against HIV, but without success so far. The only effective way to control the spread of AIDS is to prevent the transfer of HIV from person to person. This is accomplished by using condoms and spermicides (which destroy the virus), reducing exposure to infected individuals, and avoiding casual sex.

Reducing the Risk of HIV/AIDS   Because the first reported cases of AIDS in the United States were among male homosexuals, and because many thousands of men in that group have died from AIDS, some people mistakenly believe that only homosexual men can get AIDS. This is not so. Anyone can get AIDS. The reasons that so many male homosexual males acquired AIDS include:

- Without knowledge of the infectious agent HIV, it was impossible to take precautions.
- In the late 1970s and early 1980s, sexual mores among young people, including male homosexuals, permitted multiple sexual partners affording HIV rapid access to a large population.
- Anal intercourse provides HIV a highly efficient route of infection because microscopic tears in the rectum give the virus access to the recipient's blood. Microscopic tears in the penis also allow blood transmission as well as blood in semen.

After it was determined that HIV caused AIDS and once strategies were developed to stop its transmission, the frequency of new HIV infections among homosexual males declined dramatically. This decline demonstrated that educational efforts and motivation can prevent the transmission of HIV/AIDS and other STDs. Although AIDS is still a threat to male homosexuals, the majority of new cases of AIDS are among intravenous drug users who share their drug paraphernalia (needles and

T E R M S

retrovirus: a type of virus (such as the one that causes AIDS) that can invade cells and integrate its own genetic information into chromosomes

hemophilia: a hereditary disease (primarily in men) caused by a lack of an essential blood clotting factor; results in excessive bleeding in response to any scratch or injury

syringes) with others, and persons who engage in sexual intercourse with these individuals. AIDS is increasing among heterosexuals around the world.

Before HIV tests became available, thousands of people were inadvertently infected with HIV as a result of receiving HIV-tainted products derived from blood or blood transfusions (for example, tennis star Arthur Ashe). In the 1980s thousands of people with **hemophilia** (a hereditary blood disease) received clotting factor derived from pooled blood that was contaminated with HIV, and many have since been stricken with AIDS. In France, a national scandal erupted when it was learned that French health officials knowingly continued to allow hemophiliacs to receive contaminated blood products. All clotting factor products used today are manufactured by biotechnology companies and are free of viral contamination. In addition, all blood donations in the United States today are tested for HIV and other viral contamination. However, new strains of HIV continually arise, and tests are not available for all of them. For any elective surgery, patients often are advised to donate their own blood beforehand should a transfusion be required.

There are many unresolved questions about HIV and its role in AIDS. Some scientists have suggested that infectious agents other than HIV may be involved in the development of AIDS. Others have argued that extensive use of cocaine and other drugs is the cause of AIDS and that infection by HIV is not the primary cause of AIDS (Duesberg, 1991). Much more needs to be learned to reach a complete scientific understanding of HIV and its role in AIDS. In the meantime, everyone should avoid high-risk sexual behaviors, and support AIDS research and prevention programs to stop the spread of this fatal disease.

PREVENTING SEXUALLY TRANSMITTED DISEASES

Preventing STDs requires that societies provide continuous, widespread public health programs and services for STD education and treatment. It is also crucial that infected individuals seek prompt treatment, take responsibility for not infecting other individuals, and practice safer sex to lower their risk of infection.

 Controversy in Health

Should Students Be Tested for HIV?

Health officials do not advocate that all sexually active individuals be tested for HIV. But certainly those who suspect that they have been exposed to the virus are candidates for testing.

There are two AIDS tests: ELISA (enzyme-linked immunosorbent assay) and the Western blot. ELISA is technically easier and less expensive than Western blot, so it is used first to test for HIV infection. If ELISA is positive, usually a second ELISA is carried out. If that test is positive, then the more sensitive Western blot is carried out. A positive result is called "seropositivity" or "seropositive."

ELISA and Western blot work on the principle that an individual exposed to HIV produces antibodies to the virus, usually within four to

twelve weeks, but sometimes much longer. This "latency" is one reason that the tests can produce a false negative. A person could be infected with HIV but may not have produced any detectable quantity of anti-HIV antibodies. This is why some individuals, to be absolutely certain, obtain two tests, each six months apart.

The tests can also produce false positives, that is, the test indicates the presence of anti-HIV antibodies even though the individual has not been exposed. False positives occur in about four per 1000 samples taken from the general population.

HIV tests can be obtained from private physicians and a variety of health agencies. Blood banks ask that people not use blood donation as a way to obtain HIV test results.

Confidentiality

There are two types of AIDS-testing centers: anonymous and confidential. In an anonymous system, individuals receiving the test are identified only by a number and so their true identity is never recorded. In a confidential system, one's name is part of the record, although the record is kept confidential and the information regarding the results is supposed to be controlled by the tested individual.

For most people, getting tested is frightening. People fear a positive result and all of the emotional, social, and health ramifications. These are serious considerations, and testing for HIV is often facilitated with HIV counseling.

STUDENT REFLECTIONS
- Would you be willing to have an HIV blood test if your partner requested it of you?
- Under what circumstances would you ask your partner to take an HIV antibodies test?

Testing Blood

One of the cornerstones of maintaining a safe blood supply is testing. FDA requires that all blood establishments test each unit of blood for a variety of blood-borne diseases. Furthermore, FDA reviews and approves all assay test kits used to detect infectious and transmittable diseases in donated blood. Each unit of blood must be tested for:

- hepatitis B, using hBsAg (an indicator of the virus) and hB core antibody (an indicator of the antibody) tests
- hepatitis C, using a hepatitis C antibody test
- HIV-1 (AIDS virus), using an HIV-1 antibody test

- HIV-2 (also causes AIDS, but it is far less prevalent in the United States than HIV-1), using an HIV-2 antibody test
- HTLV-1 for evidence of a rare leukemia virus found mainly outside the United States
- syphilis for evidence of this sexually transmitted disease.

In the early 1970s, the risk of contracting some form of hepatitis from a unit of blood was as high as 6 to 8 percent. Now the risk of contracting hepatitis B per unit of blood is approximately 1 in 250,000, and the risk for contracting hepatitis C is less than 1 in 3,300.

For HIV, the risk of infection has decreased from 1 in 2,500 in 1985

to around 1 in 225,000 today. In 1985, FDA licensed the first test, HIV-1 enzyme immunoassay, capable of detecting HIV antibodies in blood. In 1987, the agency licensed the more precise Western blot test, which is used as a confirmatory test.

Screening tests are continually being improved. The test for hepatitis C detects the antibody in about 90 percent of chronic non-A, non-B hepatitis cases. However, more sensitive tests are being developed. The screening test for HIV is among the most sensitive, detecting evidence of infection in more than 99 percent of infectious samples.

Source: FDA Consumer (April 1995):24.

The stigma associated with STDs is a great hindrance to prevention efforts. Thinking about STDs in moral terms, that is, associating them with dirtiness and immorality makes people reluctant to think and talk about them. It also makes society want to ignore STD epidemics. During World Wars I and II, American society supported massive gonorrhea and syphilis control programs; as a result, the incidence of these infections dropped tremendously. When the threat of a postwar STD epidemic seemed to wane, moralistic concerns thwarted the continuation of control efforts, and the incidence of STDs increased. Public health officials realize that ongoing efforts are the only way to control STDs.

Judgmental attitudes also make talking about STDs difficult. To have to tell a partner that you have an STD, or even to say that you once had an infection and are now perfectly OK, can bring feelings of guilt and shame, which can lead to the avoidance of discussion altogether. Similarly, to ask about a partner's previous STDs may be interpreted as an accusation that the person is "loose" or immoral. To avoid feeling embarrassed or risk offending a sexual partner, people are likely to avoid the topic of STDs. Prevention would be enhanced if sexually active individuals developed an open attitude about talking about STDs (and other aspects of sex) and acquired the necessary communication skills.

> The way I see it, if you want the rainbow, you gotta put up with the rain.
>
> Dolly Parton,
> singer

Practicing Safer Sex

The surest way to reduce the risk of acquiring a sexually transmitted disease is to abstain from sexual intercourse. This does not mean that one has to give up sexual interaction. There are many ways of giving and receiving sexual pleasure without engaging in sexual intercourse: touching, kissing, exchanging a massage, even sleeping together without intercourse.

Another way to reduce risk is to know a partner's sexual history, including all high-risk activities in which a partner may have engaged. Often this kind of information is difficult to gain early in a relationship, because exchanging information about sexual histories requires a certain level of trust, which takes some time to develop.

Until you have this knowledge, it is essential to protect yourself by using condoms and spermicides when having sex, even if some other form of birth control is employed. Birth control pills offer no protection against STDs. Women and men who are sexually active should come to accept as standard practice with new partners the use of condoms and spermicides, even if the pill is used for birth control. Sexually active women and men should carry condoms and spermicides whenever the possibility of sex exists and use them. This requires overcoming the gender-role stereotypes that women who admit to being sexual are "sluts" and men who behave the same way are "studs."

An HIV Ethical Dilemma

You are a young male hemophiliac (person with a hereditary bleeding disorder) who became infected with the AIDS virus from HIV-contaminated blood that was given to you periodically to control bleeding. You have met a beautiful young woman; both of you are in love with each other and are eager to make love to one another.

STUDENT REFLECTIONS

- Should you tell her about your HIV status and risk losing her?
- Should you have protected sexual intercourse (with a condom) and tell her about the HIV later?
- Should you not tell her about the HIV unless you both decide to marry and have children?
- What would you do?

Some barriers to safer sex include:

- **Denying that there is a risk.** Many people assume that STDs happen only to "dirty," "promiscuous," and "immoral" people, and since they have sex only with people who are "clean" and "nice," getting an STD is impossible. Another form of denial is to tell oneself, "I eat right. I exercise. I can't get an STD."

- **Believing that the campus community is somehow insulated from STDs.** The truth is that about half of college students are sexually active before they enter college. As a result, students can arrive on campus with an infection. Also, on many campuses, students in the same living groups and student organizations have sex with one another. One infected person could lead to a whole chain of infections.

- **Feeling guilty and uncomfortable about being sexual.** This prevents individuals from planning sex and carrying condoms and spermicides, and talking about possible risks with new partners.

- **Succumbing to social and peer pressure to be sexual.** These pressures encourage people to be sexual in

situations that are potentially risky, such as one-night stands and brief relationships that are sexual virtually from the beginning. The risk of infection is lessened when individuals resist peer pressure to have sex with a relative stranger, and ask themselves instead, "Is this the right relationship?," "Is this the right partner?," "Am I going to feel OK about this afterwards?"

Effective Communication Skills

The pressure to be sexual early in a relationship, before the partners know each other well enough to talk about their past sexual experiences, may force partners to deny there may be a risk. A less risky strategy would be to postpone sexual interaction by saying, "I'd like to be close to you, but I'm not ready to have sex until we get to know each other better." "Not yet" and "maybe" are options when weighing an invitation to be sexual.

Even if a person is ready to talk about the sexual aspects of a new relationship, including birth control and possible exposure to STDs, it can be difficult because of fear of being rejected, offending the partner,

Wellness Guide

Guidelines for "Safer Sex"

- Abstain from sexual intercourse or be sexual only in long-term, monogamous relationships.
- Know a partner's sexual history, including any possible previous STDs.
- Limit the number of sexual partners. Sexually active individuals with more than one partner should be tested for STDs every six months.

- Use condoms and devices that incorporate spermicide (diaphragm, sponge, foams, creams, gels) with new sexual partners, even if the pill is used for birth control.
- With a new partner look for sores, unusual discharges, lice, or warts on the skin.
- Learn the signs and symptoms of the common STDs and be aware

of any changes in your body's normal functions.
- Tell partners if you learn that you've become infected.
- Tell new partners of your actual or possible exposure to STDs. Ask new partners about their actual or possible exposure.
- Comply with STD treatment regimes. Always follow treatment with a "test of cure" examination.

Condom Sense

Researchers and public health officials agree that latex condoms and the spermicidal chemical nonoxynol-9 are usually effective in preventing the transfer of the organisms that cause AIDS and other STDs. Some brands of condoms already come with nonoxynol-9. Natural or skin condoms, while effective as contraceptives, are somewhat porous and do not block the transmission of infectious agents.

The STD-preventing effectiveness of condoms depends on both quality and proper use. The Food and Drug Administration tests the quality of both domestic and foreign-made condoms. FDA officials sample condoms at random (in factories or at ports of entry) for cracks and other defects in the rubber, and they test for resistance to leaks and breakage by filling condoms with 10 ounces of water. If more than four condoms out of a thousand are defective or leak, the entire lot from which the samples were obtained cannot be distributed. Another test is the "airburst test": condoms are inflated under controlled conditions until they break. The minimum standard of acceptable quality is inflation to a volume of 15 liters (about the size of a watermelon) and 0.13 pounds per square inch of pressure. These values have been proposed as an international standard of condom quality.

Laboratory testing for leaks can help improve the structural quality of condoms, but there's more to condom efficacy than manufacturing quality. People have to use them properly. When condoms fail, it is often because users inadvertently damage the condom.

Using Condoms Correctly

- Use fresh condoms to lessen the possibility of leakage or breakage. Condoms that have been in a wallet or a purse for several weeks may have small punctures or may have been weakened by exposure to heat. Store condoms in a dark, cool, dry place. Condoms that are brittle, sticky, discolored, or from damaged packages should not be used.
- To prevent the transfer of STD-causing organisms, condoms should be used from the very beginning of a sexual episode and not put on just before the man ejaculates. This prevents contact with all genital and rectal regions.
- Open the package carefully, being careful not to puncture the condom with fingernails or teeth.

- The condom should be unrolled onto the erect penis. While unrolling, pinch the tip of the condom to push out the air. This leaves space for the ejaculate and prevents breakage. Some condoms come with reservoir tips.
- Adequate lubrication should be present to prevent breakage due to friction. If additional, nonbody lubricant is desired, it should be water-based and not oil-based, as oil-based materials weaken the latex. Water-based lubricants include vaginal lubricants (e.g., K-Y Jelly) and contraceptive foams, creams, and jellies. Oil-based lubricants include Vaseline, baby oil, cooking oils, butter, margarine, skin creams, and suntan lotions.
- After ejaculation, one of the partners should hold the condom on the penis as the penis is withdrawn. This prevents semen from spilling out of the condom. If the condom breaks before ejaculation, another condom should be put on immediately. If the condom breaks, leaks, or slips off after ejaculation, vaginal spermicide should be employed (always have some available). Discard the condom after use. *Never* reuse a condom.

or just spoiling the mood. Disclosing one's discomfort about talking about the subject is one way to relieve anxiety about it. A conversation could begin with one partner saying, "There's something I want us to talk about and I feel sort of uncomfortable about it, but I think it's important to both of us, so here goes."

After that introduction, the individual can offer information by saying something like, "We don't know each other very well; I'm concerned about sexual diseases. I want you to know this about me." That person should offer all of the information that he or she would like to be told. After

> The time is always right to do what is right.
> Martin Luther King

hearing the disclosure, the other person is more likely to respond in kind. And if more information is desired, one could say something like, "Thanks for telling me all of that. I'd feel more comfortable if I knew a little more about . . . " whatever it is.

What if the other person gets offended or won't talk about this subject? Or what if the other person can't be trusted? If partners cannot discuss something as serious as STDs, it is prudent to postpone sexual interaction until the relationship has progressed to a greater level of trust. Potential sexual partners should remember that being under the influ-

Preventing STDs and AIDS: Confidence Building

Pressure from a friend to be sexually intimate when it is not your first choice to do so can result in some serious consequences. Thoughts of disease, illness, and death are almost nonexistent in the mind of a young college student. Rather, feelings of immortality and invincibility are the norm. However, in today's society where the risk of AIDS and sexually transmitted diseases are ever so prevalent, no one can be afford to be naive. Having the world at your feet ready to explore is a wonderful prospect, yet it can be cut short without taking precautions. Precautions don't begin with condoms. They begin with attitudes, beliefs, and values.

One attitude that is essential to dealing with the stress of sexual intimacy is confidence. Confidence is a feeling at your gut level that guides your sense of willpower to make choices that make you feel comfortable, not guilty. While we all have access to confidence, most people let it atrophy like an unexercised muscle. Yet it is confidence, a belief in yourself, a feeling of security, a feeling of groundedness that guides you through times of peer pressure or undesired sexual impositions. With confidence, there is a responsibility to honor your integrity, not jeopardize it with feelings of arrogance.

When confidence is coupled with a sense of intuition and humbleness, they prove to be powerful inner resources that can help steer you clear of the unnecessary dangers like AIDS and STDs. When confidence acts alone, the result is often cockiness. Rather than helping you avoid potentially dangerous or unhealthy situations, this arrogance leads you straight into them.

So what are some ways to increase your sense of confidence? You can begin by telling yourself that you feel comfortable and responsible about your sexual behavior. Try it. Say to yourself, *"I feel comfortable and responsible with my sexual behavior."* When you say it to yourself, don't only think it to yourself, feel it in your stomach, at the gut level. Once you have said this, say it again. Say it to yourself enough that you feel comfortable with saying it and understand the message you are giving yourself. Then make a habit of saying this or a similar phrase to yourself every day, enough so that it becomes second nature to you, part of your own being. And when you find yourself preparing for a moment of sexual intimacy, repeat the phrase to yourself again, so that it guides you through each experience, feeling good about yourself and your partner.

It is impossible to live life without regrets, for regret teaches many of life's lessons. Yet we can also learn from others. Those who have encountered AIDS and STDs firsthand will tell you that this is one lesson you don't have to experience firsthand to grasp fully. Let your confidence and balanced solid intuition be your guides.

ence of alcohol or other drugs can affect one's judgment in making decisions about what is and is not safe. Also, being drunk or stoned can impair using condoms effectively—or using them at all!

Safer sex does not mean no sex. It does not mean that sex is dangerous. It does not mean that sex cannot be fun. It does mean that sex is cooperative. It means that partners are making choices together.

HEALTH IN REVIEW

- Sexually transmitted diseases (formerly called venereal disease, or VD) are infections passed from person to person most frequently by sexual contact.
- About 30 million sexual infections occur each year in the United States.
- STDs are epidemic in the United States because people are uninformed about them, because they engage in high-risk behaviors, and because vaccines and cures (for several) are unavailable.

- The most common STDs in the United States are: trichomonas, gardnerella, chlamydia, gonorrhea, syphilis, herpes, genital warts, pubic lice, and AIDS.
- Preventing STDs involves supporting public health efforts to inform the populace about STDs, their prevention and treatment. It also requires individuals to practice "safer sex" and to comply with treatment when they are infected.
- PREVENTION is the key!

REFERENCES

Duesberg, P. H. (1991). "AIDS Epidemiology: Inconsistencies with Human Immunodeficiency Virus and with Infectious Disease." *Proceedings of the National Academy of Sciences,* 88: 1575–1579.

Floyd, P. A., S. E. Minus, and C. Yelding-Howard, *Personal Health: A Multicultural Approach* (Englewood, Col.: Morton Publishing Co., 1995), p. 150.

Grodstein, F., and K. J. Rothman (1994). "Epidemiology of Pelvic Inflammatory Disease." *Epidemiology,* 5: 234–242.

Holmes, K. K. (1994). "Human Ecology and Behavior and Sexually Transmitted Bacterial Infections." *Proceedings of the National Academy of Sciences,* 91: 2448–2455.

Kost, K., and J. D. Forrest (1992). "American Women's Sexual Behavior and Exposure to Risk of Sexually Transmitted Diseases." *Family Planning Perspectives,* 24: 244–246.

Lowry, R., D. Holtzman, B. I. Truman, L. Kann, J. L. Collins, and L. J. Kolbe (1994). "Substance Use and HIV-Related Sexual Behaviors among U.S. High School Students." *American Journal of Public Health,* 84: 1116–1120.

National Opinion Center Research (1995). *USA Today* Snapshots, "Behavior Changed by AIDS." April 10.

SUGGESTED READINGS

Ashe, A. (1993). *Days of Grace: A Memoir.* New York: Alfred A. Knopf. Arthur Ashe discussing his life and AIDS.

Keeling, R. P. (1993). "Campuses Confront AIDS: Tapping the Vitality of Caring and Community." *Educational Record,* Winter: 30–36. As college campuses are confronted with the issue of AIDS, they need policies to reduce occupational risk, as well as educational programs focused on prevention and behavior.

Kurtzweil, P. (1995). "Warding Off HIV Wasting Syndrome." *FDA Consumer,* April: 16–20. Describes the wasting syndrome and the problems associated with it.

Morbidity and Mortality Weekly Report (1995). "Update: AIDS among Women—United States, 1994." February 10: 81–84. Atlanta: Centers for Disease Control and Prevention.

Revelle, M. (1995) "Progress in Blood Supply Safety." *FDA Consumer,* April: 21–24. Discusses the importance of a safe blood supply and the safeguards taken to prevent contaminated blood.

Shilts, R. (1988). *And the Band Played On: Politics, People, and the AIDS Epidemic.* New York: Penguin Books. An account of the AIDS epidemic and how politics affected the lives of people.

Centers for Disease Control and Prevention AIDS Hotline 1-800-342-AIDS (24 hours daily). 1-800-344-7432 (In Spanish, 8:00 A.M.–2:00 P.M., 7 days a week)

four

Understanding and Preventing Disease

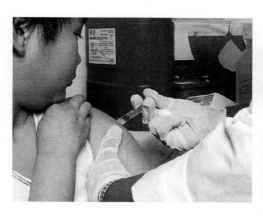

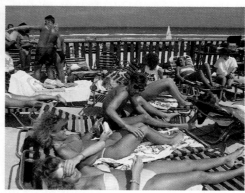

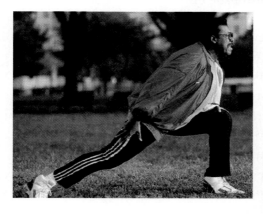

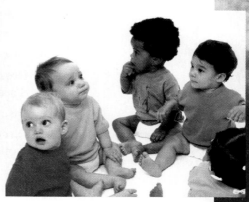

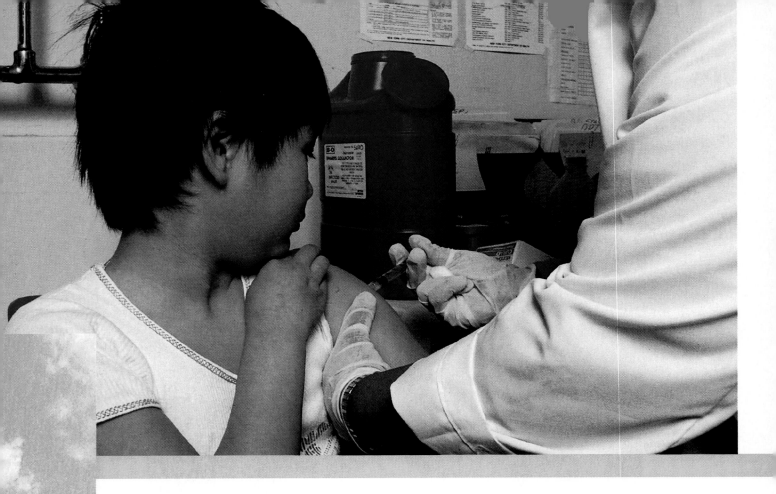

LEARNING OBJECTIVES

After reading this chapter you should be able to:

1. Define pathogen, communicable disease, vector, immunizations, opportunistic infections, nosocomial disease, immune system, antibodies, antigens, and autoimmune diseases.

2. Review the historical perspective of infectious diseases, including plague, yellow fever, smallpox, and typhus.

3. Identify and explain how infectious diseases are fought.

4. Discuss the importance of antibiotics with regard to infectious diseases.

5. Describe the implications of antibiotic-resistant strains of infectious diseases.

6. Discuss the importance of immunizations.

7. Discuss the following infectious diseases: cold and flu, Lyme disease, mononucleosis, and ulcers.

8. Describe the infectious implications of HIV and AIDS.

9. Explain how the immune system works.

10. Describe how reactions of the immune system cause allergies.

11. Discuss organ transplants, blood transfusions, and the Rh factor.

12. Explain how understanding communicable diseases will help you in protecting yourself from sexually transmitted diseases.

Reducing the Risk of Infectious Disease

Knowledge Encourages Prevention

Until very recently, human beings have succumbed by the hundreds of millions to diseases caused by bacteria, viruses, protozoa, and other infectious organisms that cause sickness and death. Improvements in public sanitation, personal hygiene, nutrition, and immunization have drastically reduced the deaths from infectious diseases in the United States. In many poor countries of the world, however, infectious diseases such as cholera and malaria still cause millions of deaths each year. In both developed and underdeveloped countries, poverty creates conditions that lead to disease, particularly infectious diseases (McKeown, 1988).

For most people in the United States, life consists of long periods of being well. However, even though we try to stay well, it would be foolish to pretend that we never will become sick or that we will not contract an infectious disease. Health is achieved not only by preventing diseases, but by having the necessary information and attitudes during times of sickness to help in the healing process. Catching a cold that seems to linger on and on may be your body's way of telling you that you have been pushing too hard in your studies or job—maybe you need to slow down and rest.

Periods of sickness often can be used to reflect on the stresses and habits that may be contributing to susceptibility to frequent infections. Serious sickness often can be used in a positive way to refocus your needs and goals (Price, 1994;

Selzer, 1993). In any event, understanding how infections occur and how they affect the body is essential to their prevention and to recovery.

RECOGNIZING AGENTS OF INFECTIOUS DISEASE

A remarkable variety of microorganisms including bacteria, viruses, protozoa, yeast, and small worms can infect cells in the human body and cause disease and sickness (Figure 12.1). Viruses are the smallest agents of disease, but are not alive in the same sense that a bacterium is; all microorganisms except viruses are cells that can grow and reproduce on their own. Viruses only grow and reproduce after they infect a cell and usurp the cellular machinery to make more viruses. Some common human diseases caused by viruses are colds, flu, polio, hepatitis, chicken pox, mumps, measles, and herpes sores. Each of these viruses is different and infects a specific tissue or organ in the body where a disease is produced. While most bacteria that grow in and on the body are beneficial, if they grow in the wrong places they can cause disease. Other bacteria are not present to any significant degree. When these **pathogens** (disease-causing organisms) infect the body, they cause infectious diseases.

Many infectious diseases such as pneumonia, tuberculosis, cholera, plague, typhoid fever, and gonorrhea are caused by infections of specific kinds of pathogenic bacteria. Often pathogenic bacteria cause disease only if the individual is already in a weakened state, particularly if the immune system is not functioning optimally. Many people carry tuberculosis (TB) bacteria in their lungs without any infection as long as they are in general good

health. However, malnutrition or stress can trigger an outbreak of the TB bacteria and disease.

If an infectious disease is shown to be caused by a specific organism, that cause is called its **etiology**. For example, tuberculosis usually is caused by a specific bacterium called *Mycobacterium tuberculosis;* infectious mononucleosis is caused by the *Epstein-Barr virus;* and giardiasis (an infection of the small intestine) is caused by the protozoan *Giardia lambia.*

Infectious agents enter the body in a variety of ways. If the infectious organism is usually passed from person to person, the disease is called a **communicable disease.** Colds, measles, chicken pox, and gonorrhea are all communicable diseases. Infectious organisms also can be transferred to people from other animals, especially insects. In these instances the animal or insect is said to be the **vector,** or carrier, of the disease-causing microor-

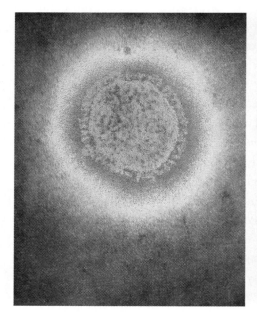
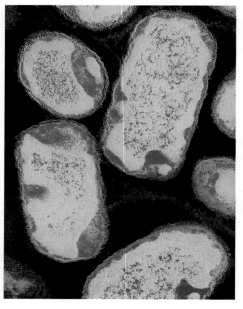

FIGURE 12.1 Infectious Organisms Electron micrographs of (left) an influenza virus that causes flu and (right) *Salmonella* bacteria that cause food poisoning. Both the "flu" virus and the bacteria are easily passed from person to person and cause widespread epidemics.

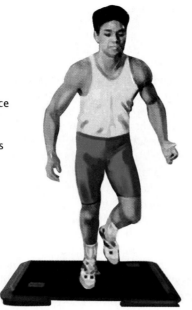

Internal

Age
Sex
Immunological competence
Previous infections
Hormonal status
Presence of other diseases
Nutritional state
Emotional stress
Heredity

External

Infections in the community
Season of the year
Hygiene and sanitation
Drugs and medications
being used
Environmental pollution

FIGURE 12.2 Various internal and external factors determine if disease results from infections by viruses, bacteria, and other kinds of infectious agents.

ganism. For example, **malaria** is usually caused by microscopic protozoa called *Plasmodium falciparum.* When a person with malaria is bitten by a mosquito, blood (and the parasite) is taken up by the mosquito and injected into another person bitten by the mosquito. Thus, mosquitoes are the vectors for malaria. (Only a few species of mosquitoes carry the malarial parasite.) Rabies is a disease of the nervous system caused by the rabies virus present in infected dogs, cats, bats, skunks, and other animals. The infected animals are the vectors for rabies and the virus is transmitted in the saliva of the rabid animal.

While infectious diseases are usually ascribed to a specific etiologic agent as described above, in reality most infectious diseases do not have a single cause. Whether or not a person gets an infectious disease depends on a wide range of factors, including the competence of the immune system, nutritional status, the presence of other diseases, and environmental conditions (Figure 12.2). For example, many people are exposed to bacteria that can cause pneumonia. However, pneumo-

nia usually develops in very old people whose immune systems are weak or in younger people who are susceptible to infections for a variety of reasons. Some people are more resistant to infectious organisms than others. Resistance to infection is increased by previous exposure to a similar virus; for example, a person generally is not infected by the same strain of cold virus in succession. Resistance to infection can be reduced by stress, poor nutrition, or by infection by HIV, the virus that causes AIDS (discussed in a later section and in Chapter 11).

Tuberculosis is not simply caused by infection with the bacterium *Mycobacterium tuberculosis.* Robert Koch, a famous nineteenth-century microbiologist, called TB the "disease of poverty" because it was associated with squalor, overcrowding, poor nutrition, and poor sanitation. Today many people have small tubercular lesions in

---

T E R M S

pathogens: disease-causing organisms

etiology: specific cause of disease

communicable disease: an infectious disease that is usually transmitted from person to person

vector: the carrier of infectious organisms from animals to people or from person to person

malaria: a disease of red blood cells that produces fever, anemia, and death

---

H E A L T H Y   P E O P L E   2 0 0 0

Reduce tuberculosis to an incidence of no more than 3.5 cases per 100,000 people.

Over the ten-year period 1975–1984, the percentage decline in TB case rates was essentially the same for whites and nonwhites. However, the incidence of TB in 1988 was seven times higher among blacks than among non-Hispanic whites, nine times higher among Asians and Pacific Islanders, four times higher among American Indians, and four times higher among Hispanics. Minorities account for nearly two-thirds of reported cases; among children, minority groups members constitute 83 percent of cases.

their lungs, but have no symptoms of disease because they enjoy good nutrition, good living conditions, and are in good general health. Today, in some urban areas where people live in squalor and poverty, TB is once again emerging as a communicable infectious disease.

REVIEWING THE HISTORY OF INFECTIOUS DISEASES

Throughout human history, infectious diseases have killed hundreds of millions. To appreciate how human health has benefited from the eradication of many infectious diseases, it is worth reviewing some of that history. Keep in mind that while specific diseases are causally associated with a particular organism, the epidemics, deaths, and human suffering of the past also were the result of ignorance, poor sanitation, absence of sterile techniques, lack of antibiotics, malnutrition, and other factors.

Plague

During the Middle Ages, **plague** repeatedly decimated Europe. Plague is estimated to have killed more than 130 million persons in past centuries. Caused by the bacterium *Pasteurella pestis,* plague is primarily a disease of rats and is transmitted to people by fleas that bite both rats and people. If rat populations are controlled, there is no reservoir of the bacteria and people do not become infected. This is why rodent control measures are critical in controlling plague. Occasional, small outbreaks of plague still occur in the United States, but deaths are rare because of antibiotic treatments.

In 1994 the world was alarmed by a plague epidemic that broke out in India. Many flights to and from India were curtailed and people leaving India were examined to ensure they were not infected. In these days of rapid travel, an epidemic in one part of the world can quickly spread.

Yellow Fever

In 1703 in Philadelphia, 5000 people died from yellow fever. At that time no one even suspected that the disease was caused by a virus transmitted to people by mosquitoes. Now, with mosquito control measures, yellow fever has virtually disappeared from most areas of the United States, although it is still common in many tropical areas of the world. Travelers can protect themselves by being vaccinated for yellow fever before traveling to areas that still have the disease.

We learn from history that we learn nothing from history.
George Bernard Shaw

Smallpox

In the sixteenth century, Spanish explorers brought smallpox to the Americas. It is estimated that *half* of the entire North and South American Indian population was killed by this deadly viral disease. The spread of smallpox greatly facilitated the Spanish conquests and later also played a major role in destroying native populations in Hawaii and throughout the Pacific.

Smallpox is the first, and as yet the only, infectious human disease to be eradicated from the world. As a result of a worldwide vaccination program carried out by the World Health Organization (WHO), not a single person in the world is infected with the smallpox virus and vaccination for smallpox is no longer necessary. Three factors led WHO to attempt total eradication of the disease: 1) no animal carriers of smallpox exist, 2) there is no chronic human carrier condition in which the virus could survive in a person without causing the disease, and 3) a safe, effective vaccine is available.

In 1967 smallpox was still a serious disease in more than thirty-three countries and an estimated ten to fifteen million cases occurred worldwide. By October 1977 the last known naturally occurring case of smallpox was reported from Somalia. Since then not a single case of smallpox has been detected anywhere. The only places the smallpox virus exists today are two national laboratories, one in Russia and the other in the United States. Many scientists believe that these smallpox stocks should be destroyed to completely eliminate the virus from earth. Others think they should be preserved in case the genetic information carried in the viral DNA could be useful in the future.

Other Epidemics

Following the Russian Revolution in 1917, three million Russians died of typhus, a disease caused by a bacteria-like organism called *Rickettsia prowazekii.* Typhus is transmitted from person to person by body lice; in this epidemic poor sanitation and personal hygiene were responsible for spreading the disease. In 1918 a worldwide influenza epidemic killed more than twenty million people, including millions in the United States. Every few years new strains of the flu virus develop and these are carried from country to country by travelers. This results in the annual flu epidemic, which is more severe in some years than others depending on the particular strain of virus.

T E R M

plague: a bacterial infectious disease that killed hundreds of millions of people in the past before antibiotics were discovered

TABLE 12.1 Estimated Deaths Worldwide from Infectious Diseases in 1990

Cause of death	Estimated number
Acute respiratory infections	6,900,000
Diarrheal diseases	4,200,000
Tuberculosis	3,300,000
Malaria	1,000,000–2,000,000
Hepatitis	1,000,000–2,000,000
Measles alone	220,000
Meningitis, bacterial	200,000
Schistosomiasis (parasitic tropical disease)	200,000
Pertussis alone (whooping cough)	100,000
Amoebiasis (parasitic infection)	40,000–60,000
Hookworm (parasitic infection)	50,000–60,000
Rabies	35,000
Yellow fever (epidemic)	30,000
African trypanosomiasis (sleeping sickness)	20,000 or more

Source: World Health Organization.

In many areas of the globe, hundreds of millions of people still suffer and die from infectious diseases (Table 12.1). Various kinds of worms (roundworm, pinworm, hookworm, and tapeworm) infect at least a billion people worldwide. Another 200 million people are debilitated by the water-borne parasite that causes the disease schistosomiasis. Malarial parasites still infect as many as 300 million people each year and cause at least a million deaths annually in Africa. Surveys show that about a billion children in Asia, Africa, and Latin America suffer from severe diarrhea caused by infectious organisms, and about five million children die from diarrhea each year in these areas. Many countries lack the resources to ensure safe water supplies, public sanitation, safe waste disposal, and adequate health care—factors that can control the spread most infectious diseases.

In the United States public health measures have largely eliminated infectious diseases that are still prevalent in many other countries. However, serious infectious diseases still break out in the United States, some of which are caused by new strains of viruses and bacteria (Table 12.2). The frequency of these outbreaks has aroused concern that many infectious diseases, even TB

TABLE 12.2 Emerging Infectious Diseases and Recent Epidemics in the United States

Disease: symptoms	Cause	Cases
Bloody diarrhea: kidney failure	*Escherichia coli* strain (0157:H7) in contaminated meat, especially hamburger	Estimated 20,000 cases annually
Cryptosporidiosis: diarrhea	*Cryptosporidium,* a parasite in water supplies	Estimated 400,000 people became ill in Milwaukee in 1993; 44,000 were treated
Pulmonary disease: impaired lung functions	Hantavirus, a new virus spread in rodent urine and feces	A serious outbreak in the Southwest in 1993
Lyme disease: neurological symptoms	*Borrelia burgdorferi,* a tick-borne spirochete (form of bacteria)	More than 15,000 cases since 1980
Otitis media: ear infection in children	Various species of bacteria; some are antibiotic-resistant	An estimated one-third of all children will have 3 serious ear infections by age 5
AIDS: susceptibility to many infectious diseases	Human immunodeficiency virus (HIV)	Estimated 200,000 deaths since 1982
Hepatitis B: symptoms range from none, to mild, to death	Hepatitis B virus	Estimated 300,000 cases annually
Chronic fatigue syndrome: persistent fatigue plus other symptoms	Unknown	Nonreportable
Tuberculosis: impaired lung functions; also affects bones	*Mycobacterium tuberculosis*	Estimated 30,000 cases annually; many strains antibiotic-resistant

that was believed to be virtually eliminated, are again on the rise in the United States.

Another new source of infectious diseases in the United States comes from immigrants from underdeveloped countries who may arrive with untreated infections that spread to others. In addition, many poor people in this country still do not have access to medical services and drugs that could cure them of their infectious diseases. And when poor patients are treated, they often sell the medicines to obtain money. Treatment for TB requires taking drugs for six to eighteen months, but patients often stop taking the drugs as soon as they feel a little better.

Fighting Infectious Diseases

Infectious diseases are fought in four ways: sanitation, treatment with antibiotics and other drugs, vaccinations, and healthful living. Stopping the spread of infectious organisms requires that they be destroyed in infected people, in the environment, or in both.

Scientific understanding of the causes of infectious diseases first began in the late nineteenth century with the research of the French scientist Louis Pasteur, who established the "germ" theory of disease by showing that microscopic organisms could cause infections and disease. Pasteur discovered that these microorganisms could be rendered harmless by heat or by treatment with antiseptic chemicals. Like many radically new scientific ideas, Pasteur's admonitions were ignored at first.

Pasteur aroused the anger of many doctors when, in 1874, he advocated the use of sterile surgical techniques. At the time more than half of patients who underwent surgery died from infections. Pasteur wrote:

> If I had the honor of being a surgeon, I would never introduce into the human body an instrument without having passed it through boiling water or, better still, through a flame and rapidly cooled right before the operation.

—Bender, 1966

The use of antiseptic (sterile) techniques to reduce infections and deaths following surgery was adopted slowly in the United States, despite the fact that a famous American physician, Joseph Lister, had successfully implemented Pasteur's advice in his hospital. (The antiseptic mouthwash Listerine is named in his honor.) Before antiseptic techniques were introduced in hospitals, surgery or giving childbirth in a hospital often led to death from subsequent infection. Sanitation, sterile techniques, and public health programs were not actively implemented in the United States until the beginning of the twentieth century. Only then did the incidence of many infectious diseases such as tuberculosis, plague, pneumonia, and diphtheria begin to decline dramatically.

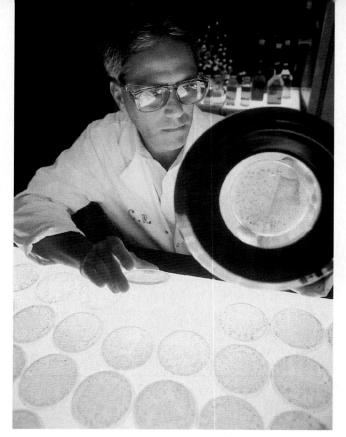

Medical research often involves the use of sophisticated instruments.

Many medical historians argue that sanitation is the most significant medical advance of all time because it contributed to preventing many millions of cases of infectious diseases caused by contaminated water and food.

UNDERSTANDING ANTIBIOTICS

In the late 1940s another highly effective tool was discovered for combatting infectious diseases caused by bacteria. The antibiotic **penicillin**, which is produced by a species of mold, was able to cure many kinds of bacterial infections. Today hundreds of antibiotics are available for treating infectious diseases caused by bacteria, yeast, worms, and other microorganisms except viruses.

T E R M S

penicillin: an antibiotic produced by mold and capable of curing many bacterial infections

acyclovir: an antiviral drug that is used to treat herpes virus infections

DNA (deoxyribonucleic acid): a chemical substance in chromosomes that carries genetic information

Antibiotics block essential biochemical reactions in microorganisms, thereby preventing them from growing in the body. The most useful antibiotics selectively interfere with the growth of the infectious organisms without affecting the functions of body cells. Antibiotics kill both harmful and helpful bacteria; however, once the harmful bacteria have been killed, the helpful bacteria quickly repopulate their normal sites.

Antibiotics do not prevent the growth of viruses that infect body cells because viruses are not living cells. Viruses infect and take over the cellular functions of body cells, thus ensuring their own growth and propagation. Finding a drug that will specifically kill a virus but not also kill body cells is very difficult. The few antiviral drugs that have been developed, such as **acyclovir** used to treat herpes virus infections, are only partially effective. The drug slows down the reproduction of the viruses but does not actually destroy them.

Some viruses, once they infect certain cells hide in them for life and can never be eliminated (Table 12.3) The most common of these, herpes simplex I, causes cold sores around the lips and mouth, and is carried by a majority of people in the United States. In most people these viruses remain dormant for life, and if they do erupt, cause only mild temporary symptoms (Chapter 11). Herpes viruses can be activated by a number of factors such as physical or emotional stress, poor nutrition, or lowered immunity. Viruses may have learned to coexist with people because killing their hosts would also lead to their own extinction.

Antibiotics Are Becoming Less Effective

When antibiotics were first discovered they were greeted as wonder drugs capable of curing some of the most deadly infectious diseases, such as plague, tuberculosis, pneumonia, syphilis, and a slew of less serious diseases. Indeed, antibiotics have been exceptionally useful drugs over the past fifty years, but we are now witnessing a decline in their general effectiveness. One of the primary reasons is many pathogenic bacteria have acquired new genes that make them resistant to one or several of the most common antibiotics (Begley, 1994).

Within a few years of the discovery of penicillin, penicillin-resistant bacteria began appearing in patients treated for bacterial infections. Bacteria also acquired resistance to later antibiotics, such as tetracycline, erythromycin, and chloramphenicol. Antibiotic resistance can be transferred among bacteria in nature in a small piece of genetic material (**DNA**) that carries antibiotic-resistant genes. Harmless bacteria of one species can transfer antibiotic-resistance genes to many other species of bacteria, including ones that cause disease. In this way bacteria that cause gonorrhea, pneumonia, and tuberculosis have become resistant to many previously effective antibiotics.

TABLE 12.3 Some Types of Viruses Remain in the Body for Life Once Individuals Are Infected

Virus	Symptoms	Spread by	Remains in
Herpes simplex I	Cold sores on lips or in mouth	Direct contact; most infectious when lesions are present	Nerve cells
Herpes simplex II	Painful blisters on genital organs	Direct contact; oral-genital sex can transmit type I or II to mouth or genital area	Nerve cells
Cytomegalovirus (CMV)	No symptoms in most children and adults; CMV can cause stillbirth and mental retardation in fetuses	Body fluids: blood, urine, saliva	White blood cells
Varicella-Zoster virus	Chicken pox in children; shingles in adults	Person to person	Nerve cells
Epstein-Barr virus (EBV)	Mononucleosis	Saliva (kissing)	Lymph glands
Human immunodeficiency virus (HIV)	None to full symptoms of AIDS	Sexual intercourse (homosexual or heterosexual), blood transfusions, contaminated needles of IV-drug users	T-cells of the immune system and other body cells

For example, vancomycin is the only effective antibiotic for treating deadly infections of the circulatory system and surgical wounds caused by a species of bacteria called *enterococci*. Since 1988, vancomycin-resistant bacteria have been increasing in patients with these diseases; consequently, some of these patients die because the antibiotic is no longer effective. The antibiotics rifampin and isoniazid had been very effective in treating TB, but now these drugs are sometimes ineffective because the TB bacteria have acquired multiple antibiotic resistance. New antibiotics are constantly being developed but nature is never far behind in the selection of resistant strains of bacteria. For example, millions of tons of antibiotics have been released into the environment as a result of their use in animal feed. The antibiotics in soil and water encourage the selection of resistant strains of bacteria that normally grow in soil and water. Only increased caution in the use of antibiotics will permit them to remain "wonder drugs" (Cohen, 1992).

IMMUNIZATIONS

One of the great achievements of modern medicine has been the development of **immunizations** (vaccinations) to prevent a variety of serious infectious diseases caused by bacteria and, more importantly, by viruses (Beardsley, 1995). Viral diseases that have been eliminated or markedly reduced include smallpox, whooping cough (pertussis), poliomyelitis, measles, mumps, and hepatitis B. Vaccination is the administration, usually by injection (hence, the name "shots"), of substances called vaccines. When you are vaccinated, specific proteins from inactivated viruses, bacteria, or toxins are injected into the body. The body's immune system responds by producing other unique proteins and cells that can inactivate the infectious organisms. If you later encounter the active, disease-causing viruses, you are protected by the vaccination.

For example, the crippling disease poliomyelitis has been virtually eradicated in the United States as a result of the widespread use of the polio virus vaccine. The first polio vaccine was developed in 1954 by Jonas Salk using chemically inactivated viruses. The polio vaccine now used is derived from a genetically inactivated virus developed in 1957 by Albert Sabin. Both methods of viral inactivation prevent the dead virus from causing disease and confer long-lasting immunity.

In general, vaccination is safe and effective in pre-

T E R M

immunizations: vaccinations to prevent a variety of serious diseases caused by both bacteria and viruses

---

venting a number of infectious diseases. Vaccinations are recommended for both children and adults, but the majority of shots are administered to young children. Other vaccinations are only recommended for people at particular risk of exposure to a certain disease. For example, travelers to a country where cholera, typhoid fever, or polio is prevalent should be vaccinated for these diseases.

Health-care workers who may be exposed to the hepatitis virus present in blood should be vaccinated for that particular disease. Vaccination for a disease such as influenza usually is recommended for people susceptible to lung infections, such as the elderly or asthmatics. Since the flu shot is only partially effective, and in some years not effective at all, it is not recommended for healthy persons.

The most recent addition to the list of effective vaccines is one for the hepatitis B virus. About 200,000 cases of hepatitis B (HBV) are diagnosed in the United States annually. HBV is a serious viral disease that can lead to death from cirrhosis or liver cancer. Some people experience only mild symptoms after being infected, but others develop a chronic infection that gradually destroys the liver. Because HBV causes such a serious disease, vac-

---

H E A L T H Y   P E O P L E   2 0 0 0

Increase immunization levels as follows:

- **Basic immunization series among children under age 2 to at least 90 percent.**
- **Basic immunization series among children in licensed child-care facilities and kindergarten through postsecondary education institutions to at least 95 percent.**
- **Hepatitis B immunization among high-risk populations, including infants of surface antigen mothers to at least 90 percent; occupationally exposed workers to at least 90 percent; IV-drug users in drug treatment programs to at least 50 percent; and homosexual men to at least 50 percent.**

A goal of the National Childhood Immunization Initiative is to establish a system for effective delivery of vaccines to the preschool population, that is, adequately immunizing at least 90 percent of all children by 2 years of age. The current immunization level is believed to be about 70 to 80 percent; blacks and Hispanics appear to have a substantially lower immunization level than the general population. Lifetime risk for hepatitis B varies from almost 100 percent in high-risk groups to 3 to 5 percent for the general population, yet only about 30 percent of people in high-risk groups have been immunized.

Exploring Your Health

Your Vaccination Record

Make a record of your vaccinations using a chart like this one:

Vaccine	Year initial series completed	Years revaccinated					
Diphtheria							
Influenza							
Measles							
Mumps							
Pertussis (whooping cough)							
Polio							
German measles (rubella)							
Tetanus							
Tuberculosis							
Other							

cination of infants also is now recommended (Fendrick, 1994).

Two other forms of viral hepatitis are caused by viral strains A and C. Hepatitis A is commonly acquired from fecal contamination of food or water and usually does not cause serious long-term sickness. Hepatitis C is primarily acquired from blood transfusions or by people who are intravenous (IV) drug abusers. No vaccinations are currently available for these forms of hepatitis, but vaccines are in development.

RECOGNIZING SPECIFIC INFECTIOUS DISEASES

Some infectious diseases such as AIDS and Lyme disease have captured more-than-average public attention and press coverage recently. Colds and flu are so common that almost everyone gets one or more infections each year. While infectious diseases are not necessarily more dangerous nor even more prevalent than chronic dis-

Wellness Guide

The Newly Revised Schedule for Childhood Vaccinations

In 1995 the Centers for Disease Control and Prevention issued a schedule for childhood vaccinations. Almost one-third of children in the United States under 3 years of age have not had all of the recommended shots.

Age	Vaccine
Birth to 2 months	Hepatitis B
2 months	Polio, diphtheria, tetanus, pertussis (DTP); *Haemophilis B* (Hib)
2–4 months	Hepatitis B
4 months	Polio, DTP, Hib
6–18 months	Polio, Hepatitis B
6 months	DTP, Hib
12–15 months	Hib, measles, mumps, rubella (MMR)
12–18 months	DTP
4–6 years	Polio, DTP, MMR (MMR can be given alternatively at 11–12 years)
11–12 years	Diphtheria, tetanus

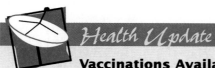

Vaccinations Available in the United States

Disease	Vaccination effectiveness; recommendations
Cholera	Only partial immunity; recommended renewal every 6 months for duration of exposure in foreign country
Diphtheria, tetanus, pertussis (DTP)	Highly effective; recommended renewal every 10 years
German measles (rubella)	Highly effective; recommended for women of childbearing age
Hepatitis B	Effective; recommended for individuals at risk
Influenza	Renew every year (because viral strains change) if in high-risk group; recommended for people ages 65 and over
Measles	Highly effective; usually produces lifelong immunity
Mumps	Lifetime immunity if immunized as a child
Plague	Incomplete protection; boosters necessary every 3 to 6 months
Pneumonia	Renew every six years; recommended for people age 65 and over
Polio	No longer required in the United States
Rabies	A vaccination each day for 14 to 21 days beginning soon after the bite
Tetanus	Very effective; renew every 10 years or when treated for a contaminated wound if more than 5 years have elapsed since last booster
Tuberculosis	Bacille Calmette-Guerin (BCG) vaccine; recommended for immunocompromised persons and others at risk for TB
Typhoid fever	About 80 percent effective
Yellow fever	Highly effective; provides long-lasting immunity

eases, they do present special public health problems and personal concerns for many people. To better understand common infectious diseases, we'll review: 1) colds and flu; 2) Lyme disease; 3) mononucleosis; and 4) ulcers. AIDs and HIV are discussed later in this chapter and also in Chapter 11.

Colds and Flu

Most people contract one or more colds and a flu every year. Both diseases are caused by viruses that infect cells of the respiratory tract. Colds are caused by more than 200 different species and strains of viruses. A cold caused by one virus does not protect a person from catching a cold caused by a different one, explaining why colds can occur one after another or several times a year.

While cold symptoms may be quite discomforting, colds generally do not result in long-term illness or death. Billions of dollars are spent by Americans every year on medications that are supposed to alleviate cold symptoms, such as sore throat, cough, congestion, runny nose, and pain. Physicians joke that a cold will go away in about a week with rest and medications or in about seven days if nothing is done. It takes the immune system of the body about a week to produce the specific proteins that inactivate the viruses and for all the tissues to heal.

High-tech modern medicine has nothing to offer that can prevent a cold, although enormous research efforts have been expended to find a cold remedy that would reduce the risk of catching a cold. While many of the "discoveries" of cold research were announced with great fanfare, none have worked.

Influenza, or flu, is caused by a different kind of virus than the ones that cause colds. Flu is a much more serious disease. The symptoms of flu are body aches, high fever, loss of appetite, and other complications that may result from the infection. Infections of the respiratory system by a flu virus can so weaken people that they contract pneumonia, a bacterial infection, and die.

As described earlier, flu epidemics have killed millions of people over the past century, especially before the development of vaccines and modern medical care. There are many different strains of flu virus and new strains arise continually. Because flu is so debilitating and serious, vaccines are prepared each year that are supposed to be specific to the expected yearly epidemic. The problem is that scientists have to guess which flu strain will be the cause of the next epidemic because it takes about a year to prepare and distribute the vaccine.

T E R M

Lyme disease: a serious, difficult to diagnose infectious disease caused by disease-carrying ticks

In some years flu vaccine is quite effective, but in others it is not effective at all if it was prepared with the wrong strains of the virus. People with respiratory problems such as asthma, people with immune system deficiencies, or the elderly who are most susceptible to pneumonia are advised to get a flu shot each year to help prevent infection.

Never catching a cold or flu is probably impossible in modern society. However, certain precautions can help reduce the risk. During seasons when colds and the flu are present, try to stay away from crowds as much as possible. The viruses are easily transmitted in droplets from people who are coughing or sneezing. Being in a classroom, theater, bus, or any crowded place increases the risk of being infected. The viruses also are easily transmitted by bodily contact, such as shaking hands with someone with a cold who has recently wiped his or her nose or mouth.

Lyme Disease

People in some parts of the United States live in fear of being bitten by a disease-carrying tick with the exotic name *Ixodes dammini* (Figure 12.3). This species of tick transmits a bacterium (*Borrelia burgdorferi*) that causes a serious disease with long-lasting effects on joints and the

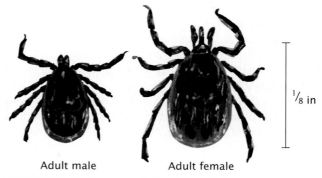

Adult male   Adult female

FIGURE 12.3 Forms of the Deer Tick

nervous system in some patients. **Lyme disease** first gained notoriety in the 1970s when numerous cases broke out in Lyme, Connecticut. In 1991, almost 10,000 cases were reported mainly from eight states: California, Connecticut, Massachusetts, Minnesota, New Jersey, New York, Rhode Island, and Wisconsin. However, cases have been reported from all states except Alaska and Hawaii. Next to AIDS, Lyme disease is what people worry about most in terms of becoming infected (Barbour and Fish, 1993).

Lyme disease is difficult to diagnose because the symptoms are similar to those caused by other diseases

Health Update

Conquering the Common Cold: A Brief History

Virtually everybody catches a cold sometime or other. Schoolchildren may contract as many as a dozen different colds a year. It is estimated that 100 million serious colds occur each year in the United States, causing 30 million days lost at school and work.

In 1914 a German scientist, W. Von Kause, first proposed that colds are caused by viruses. However, an actual cold virus (adenovirus R-167) wasn't isolated until 1953. Finally, in 1985, a detailed x-ray picture of a cold virus was obtained. Six major classes of cold viruses—rhinoviruses, coronaviruses, adenoviruses, myxoviruses, paramyxoviruses, and coxsackieviruses—have been identified. And within the rhinovirus class alone more than 120 different types have been observed. Scientists hope to find some common feature shared by the different cold viruses so that

a single vaccine can be developed. Such a boon to health is still just a remote possibility, even with modern medical expertise.

Here is a brief history of the evolution of research on the common cold. It shows how little our understanding has progressed.

- **1930s:** Scientists announce that colds are contagious and are caught by shaking hands. Recommended treatment is aspirin, fluids, and rest.

- **1940s:** Scientists announce that taking hot baths followed by cold showers, eliminating wheat from the diet, and eating fruits and vegetables help develop immunity to colds.

- **1950s:** Scientists announce that a low-sugar, low-starch diet prevents colds. Bioflavenoids are the

rage as cold remedies. Vitamin C is declared worthless. Development of a cold vaccine is predicted within two years.

- **1960s:** Scientists declare war on the common cold. They announce that a salt-free diet prevents colds. They also discover that more women than men catch colds.

- **1970s:** Linus Pauling, a Nobel prize winner, declares that massive doses of vitamin C prevent colds. The National Institutes of Health announce they have given up hope of finding a cure for the common cold.

- **1980s:** Scientists announce that colds are spread by hand contact. They recommend aspirin, fluids, and rest if you catch a cold.

- **1990s:** Gesundheit! Scientists recommend chicken soup.

and because there is no reliable test for the infecting bacterium. Most people get bitten in the spring or summer when the ticks are prevalent in lawns and woods. Wearing protective clothing and boots when walking in areas known to be tick infested helps to prevent getting tick bites and Lyme disease.

Until a definitive test for *B. burgdorferi* becomes available, Lyme disease can only be diagnosed based on clinical patterns of symptoms. Fortunately, most cases of Lyme disease respond to antibiotic therapy if treatment is begun soon after infection.

Mononucleosis

Mononucleosis (mono) is an infectious disease common in young adults, especially those in college or living in crowded, unsanitary conditions. The disease is caused by infection by the Epstein-Barr virus (EBV) that is ubiquitous in human populations. About half of all children in the United States become infected with EBV by age five; in most of these children the infection goes unnoticed since it causes few or no symptoms. Once a person has been infected with EBV, it remains in the body for life without necessarily causing any disease symptoms. Periodically, infected people shed the virus, primarily in secretions of the nose and mouth. The virus is very contagious and if saliva is shared between an infected and uninfected person, transmission of EBV occurs. This is why mononucleosis is described as the "kissing disease."

Infection by EBV as a child provides protection against infection as an adult because of the immunity that develops. However, infection by EBV as a young adult usually produces mononucleosis, a disease characterized by fatigue, fever, and swollen lymph nodes. There is no specific treatment for mononucleosis except rest, and most symptoms usually disappear within one to two weeks. Persons recovering from mononucleosis, however, should refrain from sports activities and weightlifting for at least two months because of the risk of rupturing the spleen. In a very few cases (less than 1 percent) mononucleosis can precipitate more serious diseases. Once people have had mononucleosis, they are immune to subsequent infections by EBV.

Ulcers

For most of this century medical dogma held that **stomach ulcers** were caused by behavioral or environmental factors such as stress, anxiety, smoking, or alcohol. Ulcers are open sores that can arise anywhere on or in the body. An ulcer develops in the stomach or small intestine of some susceptible persons for reasons that are largely unknown. The ulcer gradually eats a hole in the stomach, causing pain, soreness, burning, and other symptoms. The acid normally secreted in the stomach to help digestion also contributes to the enlargement of the ulcer.

Treatment for ulcers includes antacid drugs such as cimetidine (trade name Tagamet) or ranitidine (trade name Zantac). Together, these drugs account for more than $4 billion in annual sales in the United States, which attests to the frequency of stomach and intestinal ulcers.

In 1983, two physicians in Australia shocked the medical world with the announcement that a new bacterium, later named *Helicobacter pylori,* was the cause of ulcers. Much skepticism followed, but the evidence is now very convincing that most stomach ulcers can be classified as an infectious disease. This does not mean that stress or smoking or alcohol have nothing to do with developing ulcers. What it does mean is that without the presence of the *H. pylori* bacteria in the stomach, one is unlikely to develop an ulcer.

The real voyage of discovery consists not in seeking new landscapes but in having new eyes.
Marcel Proust

As a result of this new information, stomach ulcers are now treated with antibiotics as well as with antacids. The antibiotics kill the bacteria and the antacids help heal the ulcer. Despite extensive research showing the involvement of bacteria in ulcers, some physicians remain unaware or unconvinced by the findings and still recommend only antacids as therapy. However, persons who undergo antacid treatment only usually find that their ulcers return, whereas persons who receive antibiotics can be permanently cured (Graham, 1993). The ultimate goal now is to develop a vaccine that could be administered to children before they become infected by *H. pylori.*

T E R M S

mononucleosis: an infectious disease caused by the Epstein-Barr virus, common among college-age adults

stomach ulcers: open sores that occur in the stomach or small intestine for reasons largely unknown

nosocomial diseases: an infectious disease contracted while in the hospital for an unrelated disease or problem

immune system: an interacting system of organs and cells that protect the body from infectious organisms and harmful substances

antibodies: proteins that recognize and inactivate viruses, bacteria, and other organisms and toxic substances that enter the body

HOSPITAL-ACQUIRED INFECTIONS

We usually regard the hospital as a safe, sterile environment. Unfortunately, the modern hospital has become a place that sometimes endangers the health of patients because it is a source of serious infectious diseases. About 5 percent of all hospital patients in this country contract an infectious disease while hospitalized for an unrelated problem. These infections are called **nosocomial diseases.** Each year, approximately 7.5 million Americans undergo bladder catheterization in hospitals because they are immobilized. About a half million of these patients develop serious bacterial urinary tract infections and some patients die from the hospital-acquired infections. Nosocomial diseases also prolong the patient's stay in the hospital and require extra treatment.

The two bacteria mainly responsible for nosocomial diseases are *Escherichia coli* and *Staphylococus aureus.* These bacteria normally are present in healthy individuals and usually do not cause disease. In hospital patients, however, these bacteria may invade other tissues and cause an infectious disease. Since hospitals use large quantities of antibiotics, bacteria that grow in hospitals are often resistant to the antibiotics. Thus, nosocomial diseases are difficult to treat.

Because of the problem of nosocomial diseases, the U.S. Centers for Disease Control and Prevention established a program that monitors their frequency in hospitals across the country. Hospitals are supposed to keep records of nosocomial diseases. It has been found that rates vary considerably among hospitals. If you need to be admitted to a hospital, you might want to find out its rate of nosocomial diseases and how the rate compares to other hospitals in your area.

PREVENTING INFECTIONS

Infections to some degree are unavoidable. However, the elements of healthy living that we have been emphasizing can both reduce the risk of contracting an infectious disease and also hasten recovery. Foremost is maintaining health by proper nutrition and a reasonable amount of exercise. These factors, as well as sufficient rest and sleep, increase the ability of the immune system to fight infectious organisms.

Vaccinations against certain infections can provide almost complete protection in most cases. Check your record of immunizations with your family physician and update any that have not been received on schedule or that you are not sure that you received as a child. Many infections, such as mumps or measles, that are usually mild in childhood, can be serious if acquired as an adult.

Never forget that the mind interacts with the immune system and also contributes to the body's propensity to ward off or to succumb to infections. Stressful situations and emotional disturbances lower the body's defenses and make it more vulnerable to infectious microorganisms. Finally, use common sense and stay away from people and situations that are known to carry a high risk of infection. For example, do not travel to an area that is having a cholera epidemic. Do not become sexually intimate with someone who is HIV positive. Do not expose yourself unnecessarily to people with colds, flu, or other highly contagious diseases. With reasonable precautions many infectious diseases are preventable. And by maintaining good health, the body will quickly and completely recover from most infections when they do occur.

UNDERSTANDING THE IMMUNE SYSTEM

The world teems with infectious viruses, bacteria, and other microorganisms that can cause disease if they invade the body. Most people stay well most of the time because the body contains a remarkable array of defense mechanisms that help keep disease-causing microorganisms out or that can destroy them if they should invade the body. We suffer only occasionally from an infectious disease because the **immune system** acts to protect the body from infectious organisms and foreign substances.

The immune system takes time to develop. At birth, a baby is protected from infectious diseases by antibodies that were present in the mother's blood and passed on to the fetus. **Antibodies** are proteins that recognize and inactivate viruses, bacteria, and harmful substances that can cause disease. Babies also receive antibodies in breast milk, which help to protect them while their own

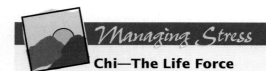
Chi—The Life Force

In the Western culture, there are several classifications of diseases: the two most predominant are infectious diseases and life-style diseases. In Chinese culture, diseases are grouped into one category; energy disease. Unlike Westerners, who view health as the absence of diseases and illness, the Chinese view health as an unrestricted current of subtle energy throughout the body.

According to the Chinese philosophy, there is a life force of subtle energy that surrounds and permeates us all. The Chinese call this force "Chi." To harmonize with the universe, to move in unison with this energy, to move as freely as running water, is to be at peace with the universe. This harmony promotes tranquillity and inner peace. It also appears to support the integrity of the immune system.

Scientists are beginning to explore and study the connection of the mind to infectious diseases. Perhaps these explorations will help to explain why some people exposed to disease microbes show no symptoms and contract no disease while others become very ill. The study of mind-body-spirit medicine already indicates that the practices of stress management techniques are influential in maintaining optimal health and, indeed, these techniques may work to create a sense of harmony between the subtle and gross anatomies of our being, thereby strengthening our immune systems and inhibiting the predisposition of infectious diseases.

The following relaxation technique may help you to calm yourself and possibly strengthen your immune system.

Breathing Clouds

Breathing Clouds is a meditation that serves as a cleansing process for the mind and body. To begin, close your eyes and focus all your attention on your breathing. Visualize the air you breathe as being clean, pure, and full of vitalizing energy. As you breathe in this clean, pure air, visualize and feel air enter your nose (or mouth) and travel down your spine and circulate throughout your entire body. Now, as you exhale, visualize the air leaving your body carrying with it all the body's stress and frustrations in the form of a cloud of smoke. With each breath, allow the clean, pure air to clear your mind and rejuvenate your body. Repeat this breathing cycle for five to ten minutes. As you repeat this cycle of breathing in pure air and breathing out cloudy, smoky air filled with undesired feelings and toxins from the body, you should notice your body and mind becoming more relaxed and comfortable.

---

immune systems mature during the first year or so of life.

Many factors can adversely affect the development and functioning of the immune system. Perhaps the most important factor is poor nutrition, especially early in life. Without a healthy diet, a child is extremely susceptible to infections that a weak immune system cannot fight. Inadequate nutrition and starvation are the principal reasons that children die in many underdeveloped and impoverished countries of the world. Other factors that affect the development or functions of the immune system are hereditary disorders, viral infections, stress, and many drugs and chemicals including alcohol and tobacco.

The Lymphatic System

The immune system, which is part of a larger and more complex system called the **lymphatic system,** has many organs and cells that must act in concert to protect people from infectious diseases (Figure 12.4). The lymphatic vessels contain fluid called lymph. At various intervals along the lymphatic vessels are nodules called **lymph nodes.** The "swollen glands" that people experience in the neck, under the arms, in the groin, or in other areas of the body are due to enlarged lymph nodes that are

T E R M S

lymphatic system: a system of vessels in the body that trap foreign organisms and particles; the immune system is part of the lymphatic system

lymph nodes: nodules spaced along the lymphatic vessels that trap infectious organisms or foreign particles

T-cells: cells of the immune system that attack foreign organisms that infect the body

cell-mediated immunity: the response of T-cells to infections

macrophages: special cells of the immune system that engulf and destroy foreign cells and particles

B-cells: cells of the immune system that produce antibodies

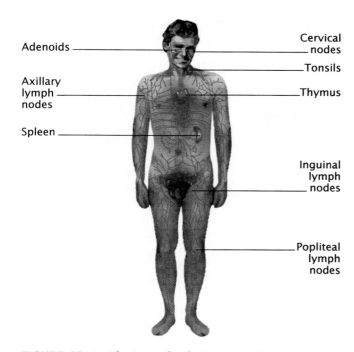

Adenoids

Axillary lymph nodes

Spleen

Cervical nodes

Tonsils

Thymus

Inguinal lymph nodes

Popliteal lymph nodes

FIGURE 12.4 The Lymphatic System Bone marrow, lymph nodes, and other organs of the immune system are shown. The lymphatic system performs many functions in protecting the body from infectious diseases.

engaged in filtering out infectious organisms or foreign particles capable of causing disease. Thus, swollen and sore lymph nodes are a sign that the body is fighting an infection.

Bone marrow, tonsils, adenoids, spleen, and thymus are all organs of the immune system that produce the various cells that allow the body to mount an immune response against infectious organisms. When bacteria or viruses infect the body, the immune system produces diverse kinds of white blood cells that function in different ways to destroy infectious organisms (Figure 12.5).

The **T-cells** (also called T-lymphocytes) circulating in the blood are ready to attack infectious organisms immediately because T-cells recognize the "foreignness" of specific proteins on the surface of bacteria, viruses, and other pathogens. The response of the T-cells is called **cell-mediated immunity** because the T-cells attach directly to the infectious organisms and inactivate them. Once cells have been identified as foreign by the T-cells, the **macrophages** and other immune system cells complete the process of their destruction and elimination from the body.

The **B-cells** (also called B-lymphocytes) comprise the final and most effective immune system defense; the

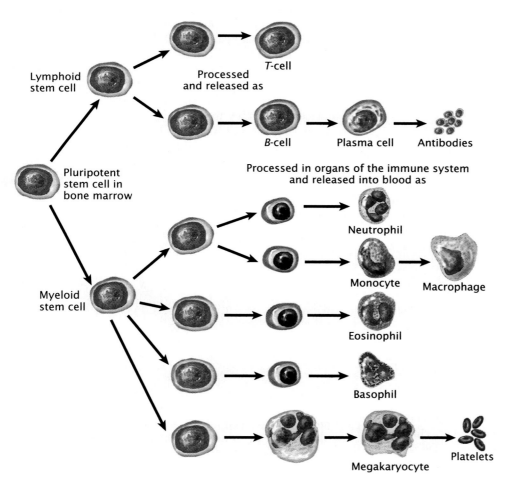

Lymphoid stem cell

Processed and released as

T-cell

B-cell   Plasma cell   Antibodies

Pluripotent stem cell in bone marrow

Processed in organs of the immune system and released into blood as

Neutrophil

Monocyte   Macrophage

Myeloid stem cell

Eosinophil

Basophil

Megakaryocyte   Platelets

FIGURE 12.5 Specialized White Blood Cells Specialized white blood cells originate in bone marrow. These cells carry out different functions of the immune system. The B-cells and T-cells recognize foreign proteins on infectious bacteria, viruses, and other organisms and substances. B-cells are converted to plasma cells that manufacture antibodies.

response of the B-cells is called **humoral immunity.** The B-cells function by producing antibodies, which recognize all proteins that are foreign and potentially harmful to the human body.

All mammals have similar immune systems and manufacture antibodies; these immune systems evolved with the earliest animals on earth. Without a functional immune system, people and animals would quickly succumb to the countless infectious microorganisms in the environment. Because the immune systems of all mammals are quite similar, rats, mice, and other small animals are used to study how cells of the immune system are synthesized and how they function.

The foreign proteins on viruses, bacteria, and other infectious organisms are called **antigens** (*anti*body *gen*erators). Every person has a collection of B-cells circulating in the blood that can recognize any foreign protein on any infectious organism in the world that may be encountered during a person's lifetime. How this collection of many millions of different B-cells develops in the human body is a fascinating but complex story, much of which is now well understood.

A particular B-cell can recognize a particular foreign antigen on a virus or bacterium and begin to make more B-cells just like itself. Eventually these B-cells (now called plasma cells) synthesize vast amounts of one specific kind of antibody that attaches to all of the infectious bacteria or viruses in the body. Once the antibodies have recognized and inactivated an invader, other white blood cells finish the job of destruction. To produce the correct antibodies in large amounts takes about a week after an infection, which is why other quicker acting immune system defense mechanisms are also needed.

The B-cells and T-cells interact among themselves in complex ways to produce a full-fledged immune response. Small molecules called **cytokines** coordinate the activities of the B-cells and T-cells. Many of the cytokines that regulate the functions of the immune system have been identified and are manufactured by biotechnology companies. Some of these products are being tested as potential drugs in the treatment of cancer and other diseases in which the functions of the immune system are impaired.

T-cells are also divided into different classes according to their specific functions. Helper T-cells increase the proliferation of B-cells, killer T-cells destroy cancer cells and other pathogenic organisms, and suppressor T-cells retard the growth of other immune system cells. A special class of T-cells called CD4 cells are important in the diagnosis and development of AIDS. When the level of CD4 cells in the blood falls to a low level, a person becomes extremely susceptible to infection by many different microorganisms causing one of the more than twenty different infectious diseases that characterize AIDS. How the immune system and CD4 cells are affected by HIV infection is discussed in a later section.

How the Body Protects Itself

The best way to avoid infectious diseases caused by pathogenic microorganisms is to keep them out of the body. The skin and mucous membranes prevent the entry of most microorganisms into the body by functioning as physical barriers. That is why a wound often exposes the body to infection (Figure 12.6). The skin is mildly acidic and provides a poor habitat for most harmful microorganisms, although the skin is covered with beneficial bacteria.

The eyes, nose, throat, and breathing passages are protected by mucous membranes that continuously produce secretions that flush away harmful organisms and particles. Mucous membranes also secrete enzymes that can destroy toxic substances. The mouth, digestive system, and excretory organs also are protected by membranes that guard the internal organs.

Tears keep the surface of the eyes moist and serve to wash away foreign particles. Wax secreted from the ears protects the delicate hearing apparatus. The mucus coating of the respiratory tract is sticky and provides a trap for irritating particles and microorganisms in the air; microscopic hairs called **cilia** keep the mucus moving out of the bronchial tubes. Coughing and spitting are mechanisms that remove foreign material from the breathing passages. Sneezing and blowing the nose eliminate irritating particles that are inhaled.

Cells and enzymes in the blood quickly form clots that seal off any break in the skin, thereby preventing the entry of harmful substances and infectious organisms. If some bacteria do enter the wound before it is sealed off, other special cells that are part of the immune system attack and destroy the invaders.

If microorganisms or foreign particles should penetrate the skin and enter the blood, they soon encounter specialized cells called **leukocytes,** the colorless white

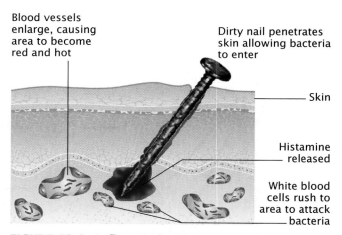

Blood vessels enlarge, causing area to become red and hot

Dirty nail penetrates skin allowing bacteria to enter

Skin

Histamine released

White blood cells rush to area to attack bacteria

FIGURE 12.6 Inflammation Response Penetration of the skin by any unsterile sharp object often produces an inflammation response, the regular response of the body to injury or infection.

CASE STUDY

Five-year-old Billy is brought to the hospital emergency room suffering from severe stomach pain. His parents want an X-ray because they think he has swallowed something. The doctor takes a blood sample and finds a high white blood cell count. He determines that Billy has acute appendicitis and wants to operate immediately. The parents refuse because they are Christian Scientists and do not believe in medical treatment. They want to take the child home and have God heal him. The doctor says Billy may die unless operated on.

STUDENT REFLECTIONS

- What should the doctor do?
- What should the parents do?
- Does Billy have any right to choose?

blood cells that can be distinguished from the red blood cells that transport oxygen. Only about 1 in 700 cells in the blood is a leukocyte, but their number can increase dramatically if an acute infection occurs. That is why blood is tested for the number of white blood cells when an infection is suspected. For example, **appendicitis**, an infection of the appendix, will cause the white blood cell count to rise appreciably.

Specialized white blood cells called macrophages are associated with specific organs and are vital to the body's internal defense mechanisms. Macrophages are able to engulf and digest foreign cells and particles that invade the body. Organ-specific macrophages protect the lungs, stomach, and other organs from damage by foreign substances (Figure 12.7).

UNDERSTANDING ALLERGIES

Allergies are the immune system's response to foreign substances called **allergens** that the body thinks are harmful, but which usually are not. Pollens, molds, house dust, animal hair, foods, drugs, chemicals, and many other substances can act as allergens. The body responds by synthesizing a particular class of antibodies (immunoglobulin E or IgE) that triggers the allergic reaction (Figure 12.8). No one knows why allergic responses evolved or what benefit they might have provided, but millions of people today can attest to the misery caused by allergic responses.

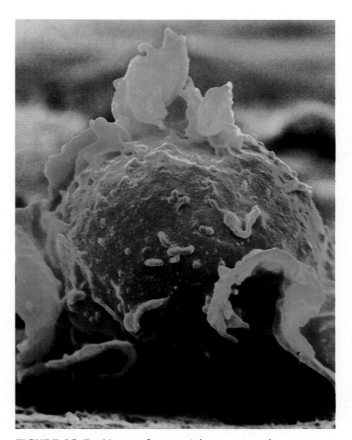

FIGURE 12.7 Macrophage A lung macrophage as seen in the electron microscope. These cells "eat and destroy" foreign particles and microorganisms that are breathed into the lungs.

T E R M S

humoral immunity: the response of B-cells to infections

antigens: foreign proteins on infectious organisms that stimulate an antibody response

cytokines: small molecules that coordinate the activities of B-cells and T-cells

cilia: microscopic hairs in the lining of the bronchial tubes

leukocytes: white blood cells that fight infections

appendicitis: an infection of the appendix

allergens: foreign substances that trigger an allergic response by the immune system

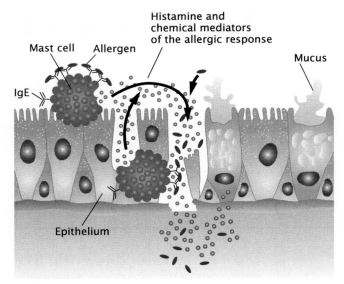

FIGURE 12.8 **The Chemistry of an Allergic Response** An allergen (a substance from a plant, insect, or other organism) binds to antibody proteins (IgE) on mast cells. This triggers the release of histamines and other inflammatory substances that characterize the allergic response. These reactions occur mainly in the nose, lungs, skin, and digestive tract.

The allergic reaction is usually accompanied by the secretion of mucus and the release of **histamine**, an inflammatory chemical that is abundant in cells of the skin, respiratory passages, and digestive tract. That is why most allergic reactions are associated with the skin (eczema, hives, contact dermatitis), the respiratory passages (asthma, hay fever), and the digestive tract (swelling, vomiting, diarrhea).

Contact dermatitis affects millions of people because of the things we touch (Table 12.4). Walking in the woods can bring on ugly rashes if poison ivy or poison oak touches the skin. Peeling a mango can also cause people to break out, although they usually can eat the fruit without a reaction. Allergic reactions of doctors and nurses to rubber gloves and other rubber products have been increasing with the increased use of rubber gloves, and has become a particular problem for some surgeons and others who use them daily (Gonzalez, 1992).

Millions of people with allergies receive shots that are supposed to desensitize them to the substances to which their immune systems react in allergy tests. Some people do benefit from a program of shots that are given over months or years. However, it is now recognized that only a small number of people actually benefit from the allergy shots. When asthma, hay fever, or other allergy can be shown to be caused by an elevated level of a particular antibody, then shots are appropriate and can lessen a person's sensitivity to the allergen. Other people who benefit from allergy shots are probably being helped by the placebo effect (Norman, 1990).

TABLE 12.4 Some chemicals that can cause atopic (contact) dermatitis, usually manifested as skin rashes. These chemicals are found in many everyday materials. Contact dermatitis can also result from touching plants such as poison ivy or the skin of mangos.

Chemical	Source
Ethylenediamine hydrochloride	Antifungal cream Aminophylline Hydroxyzine Antihistamines
p-Phenylenediamine	Hair dye Fur dye Black, blue, or brown clothing
Thiuram	Rubber compounds Fungicides Wood preservatives
Formalin, formaldehyde	Cosmetics Insecticides Wearing apparel (drip-dry, wrinkle-resistant, water-repellent)
Potassium dichromate	Leather (chrome tanned) Yellow paints
Paraben	Cosmetics Pharmaceuticals
Epoxy resin	Adhesives
Sodium hypochlorite	Bleach Cleansing agents
Carba mix	Rubber Lawn and garden fungicides
Imidazolidinyl urea	Cosmetics (preservatives)
p-ß-Naphthylamine, p-tert-Butylphenol	Rubber compounds Plastics Adhesives
Mercury, nickel, copper	Topical ointments, coins, jewelry, Insecticides

Asthma

Although allergies are caused by physiological and immunological responses in the body, they can also arise or be made worse by a person's emotional and psychic state. Some asthmatic children often improve dramatically when separated from family situations that are stressful and emotionally upsetting. Adult asthmatics

> T E R M S
>
> **histamine:** a chemical released by cells in an allergic response; causes inflammation
>
> **contact dermatitis:** an allergic reaction of the skin to something that is touched
>
> **food allergies:** allergic responses to something that is eaten
>
> **anaphylactic shock:** a severe allergic reaction involving the whole body that can cause death

often notice that their attacks occur more frequently or become worse when they are upset or under stress that cannot be managed. Thus, asthmatics have an immunological make-up that makes them sensitive to allergens, but also respond to emotions and stress in ways that other people do not.

For example, an asthmatic who gets into a violent argument with a husband, wife, or parent may begin to experience breathing difficulties whereas an equally angry, nonasthmatic person would not. For these reasons asthma is classified as a psychosomatic disease, meaning that both the body and the mind contribute to the symptoms (Chapter 2).

Many medicines are now available to relieve, control, and prevent asthmatic attacks. Although a small number (a few thousand) of people die from asthmatic attacks each year in the United States, the rate has been increasing. Anyone who is diagnosed with asthma should take medications prescribed to prevent serious attacks. It is also important to know that the severity or frequency of asthmatic attacks can be reduced by reducing stress and emotional upsets.

Food Allergies

Food allergies, also called food intolerance, are allergic responses to a particular food. The reaction can be local (such as a stomach upset or swelling in the mouth) or it can involve the whole body. For example, an allergic reaction to a food or to an insect bite can cause hives to break out all over the body. Food allergies are most common in children but can occur in anyone at any age.

When people are tested for food allergies, six substances account for 90 percent of the allergic reactions—eggs, peanuts, milk, fish, soy, and wheat (Sampson, 1987). Severe allergic reactions produce **anaphylactic shock,** a systemic reaction that can quickly cause death. Anaphylactic shock can be brought on by an immediate, strong allergic reaction to food, a bee sting, or a drug.

About 20 percent of people report food intolerance of one sort or another at some time in their lives, yet studies show that the actual number of people who are physiologically sensitive to foods is more like 2 percent or less (Young et al., 1994). The discrepancy between what people report as an allergic reaction and what is demonstrated by allergy tests is probably due to the power of suggestion. If someone reads or is told that many people are allergic to eggs, he or she may begin to experience an allergic reaction when eggs are eaten. Also, throwing up after eating a particular food can produce a subsequent aversion or allergic reaction to that food.

The power of suggestion in causing food allergies has been demonstrated by experiment (Jewitt, 1990). In this study, patients who reported that they had a food allergy were given a series of injections to desensitize them to the food causing the allergy. One group was desensitized with a placebo (saline) injection; another group was desensitized with an injection of the allergen. Neither the patients nor the doctors knew which injections contained saline and which contained the allergen. Seven of eighteen patients reported that their food allergies were prevented by the placebo shots. Others reported that their symptoms worsened when they received the saline placebo. Thus, placebo effects can cure food allergies or they can cause them to become worse as in this experiment. How we view food in our minds has a powerful effect on how it is received by the body (Chapter 2).

Food allergies (as well as other forms of allergy) should not be regarded as the result of imagination and, therefore, in some sense "unreal." Whether the allergic reaction is brought on specifically by the interaction of an allergen with IgE antibodies or by a state of mind, is largely irrelevant. In both instances the physiological responses are real and need to be treated. For centuries, allergies have been successfully treated by eliminating the cause of the allergic reaction, by the power of suggestion, or both.

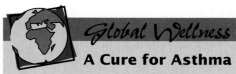

Global Wellness

A Cure for Asthma

One of the first successful treatments for an allergy dates from the sixteenth century. An Italian physician, Girolamo Gardano, was asked to come to Scotland to treat John Hamilton, Archbishop of St. Andrews, who suffered from asthma. After watching his patient for several days, Gardano asked the archbishop to give up his swan-feather pillows. This was almost heresy because only the upper classes were allowed to use such pillows. However, the archbishop did give them up and was cured.

Today avoidance of allergy-causing foods and environmental substances that cause allergic reactions is still the best therapy. In many patients with allergies, mental imagery, hypnosis, or suggestion are also effective in reducing or eliminating allergic reactions.

RECOGNITION OF "SELF"

The immune system is able to recognize and destroy virtually any foreign cell, which is how it protects the body from infectious diseases. What prevents the immune system from recognizing and attacking the body's own cells and organs? By mechanisms that are not yet completely understood, the immune system can distinguish cells of the body that are recognized as "self" from all other cells (even those of another person) that are "nonself."

During fetal development, as the body's tissues are being formed, all of the antibody-producing cells that could attack the body's own cells are destroyed. It is not yet known how these particular antibody-producing cells are selected out of the millions of different cells and destroyed, but such a mechanism is vital to protect the organs and tissues of the body from destruction.

Also during development, the fetus receives antibodies from the mother's blood that protect it from infections. These antibodies last for several months after birth and continue to protect the baby from infections. And, as noted earlier, the mother's antibodies are present in breast milk which will continue to protect the child as long as it is breast-fed. Eventually the child's own immune system develops and is able to manufacture the cells and antibodies that afford protection from infections.

Autoimmune Diseases

The immune system must function without mistakes in order to distinguish "self" from "nonself" because any mistake that caused antibodies to attack the body's own cells could result in serious disease or death. Unfortu-

nately, mistakes in the functioning of the immune system do occur and produce **autoimmune diseases** (Figure 12.9). Some inherited disorders, fortunately quite rare, can result in the loss of the immune system's ability to distinguish "self" from "nonself." Environmental factors such as viral infections, nutritional problems, and other unknown agents may also cause the immune system to make mistakes that lead to autoimmune diseases.

Lupus erythematosus is an autoimmune disease that most frequently affects women between the ages of 18 to 35. In this disease, for reasons still unknown, antibodies are synthesized that attack the genetic information in cells (DNA), especially in cells of the blood vessels, skin, and kidneys. Many organs of the body are affected, and the symptoms—rashes, pain, and anemia—flare up and wane throughout life, which usually is shortened.

Another autoimmune disease that affects millions of people is **rheumatoid arthritis.** In this disease antibodies are synthesized that attack cells of the joints, causing inflammation, pain, and loss of movement. No cause for arthritis has been found and it occurs in many forms both in children and, more often, in adults. Some people have found that the symptoms of arthritis can be controlled through nutritional changes or by the use of meditation, imagery, or other mental relaxation techniques.

An autoimmune disease that affects the central nervous system is **multiple sclerosis** or **MS**. Recent research suggests that MS may be initiated by a viral infection that somehow causes the immune system to produce antibodies that attack **myelin,** a substance that sheaths and insulates nerve fibers in the brain and spinal cord.

Although drugs can help reduce the symptoms of autoimmune diseases, these diseases cannot be cured since they are caused by complex malfunctions of the immune system that are not understood. Because the mind also affects the functions of the immune system, many people who suffer from autoimmune diseases find relief in alternative therapies, mental relaxation techniques, and nutritional changes.

Organ Transplants

Like blood cells, all body cells have antigens on their surfaces that are different for everyone except identical twins. If tissue or organs from one person are grafted onto another, the immune system produces antibodies to the foreign cell antigens, causing destruction of the cells and rejection of the transplanted organ.

The more alike two persons are genetically, the more likely it is that proteins are the same and that the transplanted tissue will be accepted by the body. Identical twins are genetically identical; this is why tissue transplants between identical twins have the greatest chance of being accepted. To minimize the risk of rejection of

---

T E R M S

autoimmune diseases: mistakes in the functioning of the immune system that cause it to attack tissues in the body

lupus erythematosus: an autoimmune disease that mostly affects women

rheumatoid arthritis: an autoimmune disease that affects joints

multiple sclerosis (MS): an autoimmune disease that affects the central nervous system

myelin: a substance that sheaths and insulates nerve fibers in the brain and spinal cord

histocompatibility: the degree to which the antigens on cells of different persons are similar

HLA (human leukocyte antigens): antigens that are measured to determine the suitability of an organ for transplantation from donor to recipient

immunosuppressive drugs: drugs to suppress the functions of the immune system, for example, following organ transplants

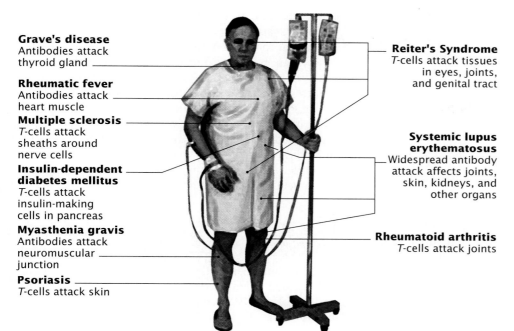

Grave's disease
Antibodies attack thyroid gland

Rheumatic fever
Antibodies attack heart muscle

Multiple sclerosis
T-cells attack sheaths around nerve cells

Insulin-dependent diabetes mellitus
T-cells attack insulin-making cells in pancreas

Myasthenia gravis
Antibodies attack neuromuscular junction

Psoriasis
T-cells attack skin

Reiter's Syndrome
T-cells attack tissues in eyes, joints, and genital tract

Systemic lupus erythematosus
Widespread antibody attack affects joints, skin, kidneys, and other organs

Rheumatoid arthritis
T-cells attack joints

FIGURE 12.9 Various Autoimmune Diseases
These occur when the body's immune system goes awry and cells of the immune system begin attacking the body's own cells because they are mistakenly recognized as foreign.

transplanted organs, the **histocompatibility** (similarity of cell surface antigens) between the donor and recipient is determined by immunological tests. Just as red blood cells have particular groups of strongly antigenic proteins on their cell surfaces, other cells in the body have antigenic proteins called **HLA (human leukocyte antigens)** that are crucial in determining whether a transplanted organ will be accepted or rejected (Figure 12.10). The greater the similarity in HLA antigens between donor and recipient, the greater the chance that the tissue will be accepted and function normally in its new host. From the number of HLA antigens already determined, calculations show that there are so many different HLA antigen combinations that each unrelated person is immunologically unique.

A few years ago the first successful heart transplants made headlines. Today the transplantation of hearts, kidneys, livers, and other organs has become a relatively common procedure in many hospitals. However, organ transplants are extremely costly, complicated procedures and are not always successful. Many more people are waiting for suitable organs than can be supplied from living donors or accident victims. Patients whose survival depends on the availability of a suitably matched organ often wait months to receive one. And often no organ becomes available before the patient dies.

The organ transplanted most often is the kidney. Since people have two kidneys, relatives sometimes donate one of their healthy kidneys to another close relative if their HLA genes are well matched. If the match is perfect for HLA antigens and ABO blood type, the success rate is 90 percent survival at one year. Brothers and sisters have one chance in four of inheriting the same

HLA genes from their parents, which is why close relatives are examined first as possible donors. Bone marrow transplants also are used as a last resort in cases of aplastic anemia, acute leukemia, and radiation sickness.

The rejection of transplanted organs can be controlled to some degree with **immunosuppressive drugs** (corticosteroids, cyclosporin); however, treatment with these drugs lessens resistance to infections and sometimes enhances development of other diseases. The long-term use of immunosuppressive drug therapy itself results in increased susceptibility to cancer. It makes more sense to seek ways to prevent kidney and heart diseases, so that surgical transplants become less needed.

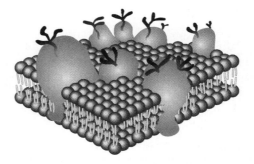

FIGURE 12.10 Antigens and the Immune System
A vast array of different HLA antigens are embedded in the outer membranes of cells, projecting beyond their surfaces. These antigens can be recognized by the body's immune cells and antibodies. Since every person's antigens are different, tissue transplanted from one person to another is usually rejected because the donor's HLA antigens are recognized as foreign and destroyed by the immune response of the recipient.

Blood Transfusions and Rh Factors

In the early part of the twentieth century, a blood transfusion often led to the patient's death. Because the patient's immune system recognized the donor's blood cells as being "foreign," it attacked them with both T-cells and antibodies. The antibodies caused clumps of blood cells to form in the veins and arteries, impeding the flow of blood and oxygen to, and waste products from, the body's tissues. If oxygen and nutrients are prevented from reaching essential tissues such as the heart or brain, death may occur from a heart attack or stroke.

Red blood cells have many different potential antigens on their cell surfaces, each of which can evoke an antibody response when recognized as "nonself." The two most important human red blood cell surface antigens are the ABO and Rh-positive/Rh-negative proteins. There are actually many other groups of antigens on red blood cells, but these two are by far the most important ones in evoking an immune response that can endanger health. Table 12.5 shows the pattern of donor-recipient ABO blood types that must be matched for a successful transfusion.

People with type O blood have neither A nor B antigens on their red blood cells. People with type O blood are **universal donors**; their blood cells will not stimulate an antibody response in the recipient, no matter what the blood type. People with type AB blood have both antigens present on their red blood cells and do not synthesize A or B antibodies, because these antigens are recognized as "self" and those antibody-producing cells are destroyed. People with type AB blood are **universal recipients**; they can accept blood from any of the four groups.

The Rh-positive antigen and the antibody that reacts against it cause problems primarily in pregnancy. A woman is termed Rh-negative if her red blood cells do not contain any of this antigen. If the red blood cells of a developing fetus have the Rh-positive antigen (inherited from the father), and if any of the fetus' red blood cells enter the mother's blood supply, production of anti-Rh antibodies can be stimulated by her immune system, which recognizes the fetal cells as foreign. This usually does not cause any difficulty during the first pregnancy and might even go unnoticed until the woman becomes pregnant again.

Now, if the second fetus is also Rh-positive, the Rh-positive antibodies (synthesized during the first pregnancy) in the mother's blood will attack the developing infant's red blood cells, resulting in anemia, brain damage, or even death. Fortunately, doctors can manage this problem safely and effectively. At the time the first child is delivered, the mother is given an injection of anti-Rh antibodies that destroys any Rh-positive antibodies in her blood. In this way any danger to the fetus during a subsequent pregnancy is avoided.

AIDS AND HIV

The infectious disease that has received the most public and research attention since it was first diagnosed in the early 1980s is **AIDS (acquired immune deficiency syndrome)**. It is important to understand that AIDS, like cancer or diabetes, is not a single disease. AIDS is defined by the U.S. Centers for Disease Control and Prevention (CDC) as consisting of more than two dozen specific diseases accompanied by a very low level of CD4 T-cells in the blood (see Chapter 11 for a discussion of AIDS). A normal CD4 T-cell level in the blood is 800–1200 cells per ml. An AIDS patient is defined as having less than 200 CD4 T-cells per ml plus one of the designated infectious diseases. In 1993, the CDC expanded the definition of AIDS to include twenty-seven different infectious diseases, which almost doubled the number of official AIDS cases in this country.

HIV (human immunodeficiency virus), the cause of AIDS, is an unusual virus because once it infects a cell it integrates its genetic information with a chromosome, thereby becoming a permanent resident of any cell it infects (Figure 12.11). Proteins on the surface of the virus recognize receptors on the surface of CD4 T-cells, allowing the virus to inject its genetic information (RNA). Once inside the cell the **RNA (ribonucleic acid)** is converted to DNA, which is integrated into a chromosome. Once integrated, the viral DNA cannot be eliminated from the cell any more than a normal human gene

TABLE 12.5   Blood Transfusions Are Determined According to ABO Blood Groups

Blood group	Genotype	Antigens on red blood cells	Transfusions cannot be accepted from	Transfusions are accepted from
O (universal donor)	OO	none	A, B, AB	O
A	AA, AO	A	B, AB	A, O
B	BB, BO	B	A, AB	B, O
AB (universal recipient)	AB	A, B	none	A, B, AB, O

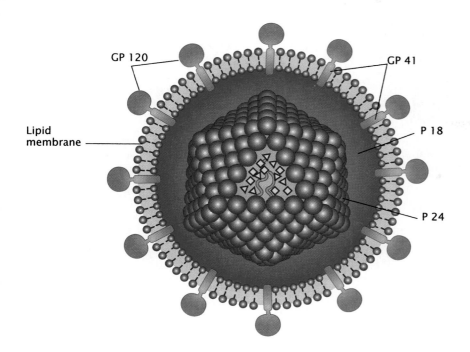

GP 120

GP 41

Lipid membrane

P 18

P 24

FIGURE 12.11 The Human Immunodeficiency Virus (HIV), the Cause of AIDS
Protein spikes extrude from the outer shell of the virus. The genetic information is carried in two RNA molecules in the core. Other proteins form protective layers. Reverse transcriptase is the enzyme that the virus uses to copy its genetic information and make new viruses.

in the chromosome can be eliminated. The integrated virus now is able to manufacture more viruses that can escape and infect other cells.

AIDS and the Immune System

The vital importance of the immune system in warding off infectious diseases became tragically apparent to the general public with the appearance of AIDS in the early 1980s. Long-term HIV infection eventually weakens the body's immune system by destroying particular helper T-cells called CD4 T-cells. Without a sufficient number of CD4 T-cells in the blood, other cells of the immune system also fail to function properly.

Infection by HIV gradually weakens the body's immune system exposing it to **opportunistic infections,** infection caused by any of a wide variety of microorganisms. AIDS patients become progressively weaker with each infection and eventually die. The course of HIV infection is unpredictable; some individuals progress to full blown AIDS and die within months. Others have no symptoms even after ten years or more of HIV infection (Figure 12.12). These long-lived, HIV-infected survivors are being studied to find out if they share a particular biological or behavioral characteristic that gives them the ability to fight off the infection for such a long time. It is hoped that these healthy, HIV-infected individuals will provide clues that can help in developing new drugs (Fackelmann, 1995).

T E R M S

universal donor: a person whose blood is accepted by everyone during transfusion

universal recipient: a person whose blood type is compatible with anyone else's blood

AIDS (acquired immune deficiency syndrome): a syndrome of more than two dozen diseases caused by HIV

HIV (human immunodeficiency virus): the virus defined as the cause of AIDS

RNA: (ribonucleic acid): a chemical substance found in some viruses such as HIV that also can carry genetic information; the RNA is converted to DNA when such viruses infect cells

opportunistic infections: any infectious disease in a patient with a weakened immune system; often occurs in AIDS patients

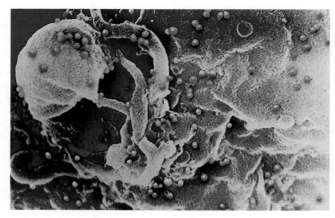

The AIDS virus as seen under the electron microscope. The red dots are presumed to be human immunodeficiency viruses being released from infected cells.

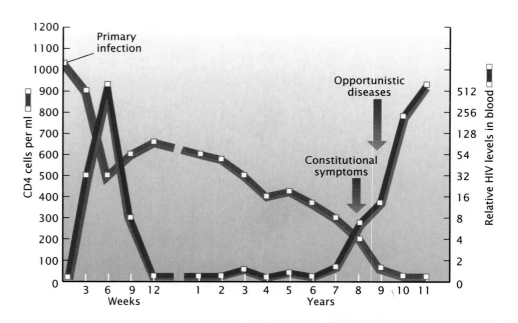

FIGURE 12.12 HIV and the Immune System After infection the virus level rises sharply in the blood, but within three months is undetectable. However, the virus is usually multiplying slowly in lymph nodes. The infected CD4 T-cells gradually decrease in number over many years. At some point the immune system is weakened so that the person becomes susceptible to any of dozens of infectious diseases. Although this figure shows a disease latency of eight years, many HIV-positive individuals have had no symptoms for more than ten years.

The AIDS Antibody Test

Upon infecting a person, HIV acts like all other viral infections by stimulating synthesis of antibodies capable of inactivating the virus. Detection of these antibodies is the basis of the **AIDS antibody test**. In reality, the test is only an indirect measure of HIV infection: it does not measure whether a person has AIDS or will get AIDS. During the first few weeks or months following HIV infection, antibodies are made by the immune system to combat the infection. However, this test is positive only after antibodies have reached a detectable level, which can take several weeks or even months following infection by HIV. In the interim, a person is highly infectious, but will show up negative on the AIDS antibody test. Thus even a recent negative AIDS antibody test may not mean that a person is uninfected if they have been sexually active or use injected drugs.

A major problem with the AIDS antibody test is frequent false positive results that create unnecessary anxiety in the recipient. A false positive means that the test shows that the person has antibodies in his or her blood that resemble ones produced in response to HIV. In reality, the person is not infected and the test is in error.

Infection by other viruses or bacteria whose antigens resemble those of HIV can give a positive result in the HIV antibody test. In some persons, a positive HIV test can result from a recent flu vaccination shot. Any positive AIDS test should always be rechecked by a more sensitive method. The most accurate test for HIV infection is the **Western blot test**, which tests for the presence of specific HIV proteins.

How Infectious Is HIV?

Compared to other viral infections, such as ones that cause colds, flu, or hepatitis, HIV is not very infectious. The virus is *never* transmitted by casual contact between an infected person and uninfected persons. Never, in this context, means that no well-documented cases of HIV infection have been reported except as a result of sexual intercourse or the receipt of HIV-contaminated blood (see Chapter 11 for a discussion of the sexual transmission of HIV). HIV is not transmitted in saliva, spit, sweat, air, water, or other objects that have been used by an HIV-infected person.

All testing for HIV infection is voluntary, primarily because the incidence of HIV infection in the general population (aside from the high risk groups) is very low. Many states have considered mandatory testing, but none except Illinois have actually done so. In 1988, Illinois required that all couples applying for a marriage license be tested for HIV. During the six months that the law was in effect, 70,848 persons applying for marriage licenses were tested for HIV; only 8 persons were positive giving a 0.011 percent rate of infection. Because of the high cost and the low rate of infection, Illinois repealed the law after six months.

Vaccination against HIV Infection

Because many viral diseases have been conquered by vaccination (smallpox, measles, polio), it was hoped that a vaccine would be developed to protect people at risk for HIV infection. However, the original hope is now quite dim. In 1994, clinical trials of two of the most promising HIV vaccines (more than a dozen are under development) were abandoned. Individuals at risk for HIV infection who received the vaccines not only were not protected, but the vaccines may have contributed to some AIDS deaths. While AIDS researchers still express optimism for finding a cure, no safe, effective treatment now exists for HIV infection nor can infection be prevented by vaccination.

Fortunately HIV is not an easily transmitted virus like the Epstein-Barr virus or the flu and cold viruses. You can protect yourself from HIV infection by understanding the facts about HIV and AIDS. HIV is transmitted only by sexual intercourse with an HIV-infected partner (the sexual transmission of HIV is discussed in Chapter 11), by sharing blood-contaminated needles during use of illegal drugs, or by receiving HIV-contaminated blood in transfusions. With care, these are all situations that can be avoided.

CHRONIC FATIGUE SYNDROME

A disease that has received much less publicity and public support than AIDS but which debilitates a comparable number of people is **chronic fatigue syndrome**

(CFS). Although the cause of CFS is unknown, it also involves abnormal functions of the immune system. In some respects, the changes that are observed in the immune system in CFS patients resemble those observed following infection by HIV. For this and other reasons, a viral infection is suspect as the underlying cause of CFS. However, no virus has consistently been shown to cause the symptoms of CFS.

In 1988 the Centers for Disease Control and Prevention published a set of criteria that can be used to establish a diagnosis of CFS. The primary criteria are 1) a debilitating fatigue that reduces a person's activities to less than half of their previous activities, and 2) elimination of other diseases that could account for the symptoms.

CFS can afflict anyone but is most common among children and women under age 45. There is no standard treatment for CFS and, as in the case of AIDS, there is no cure. The numerous symptoms of CFS wax and wane over a period of years and many victims of the disease improve with time, possibly as a result of improvement in immune system functions.

Despite extensive research into possible causes for these symptoms, no bacterium, virus, or other infectious organisms to account for the illness have been found in patients with CFS (Dawson and Sabin, 1993). At first Epstein-Barr virus, which causes mononucleosis, was thought to be implicated, but further scientific studies have ruled out EBV as the causative agent in CFS. The inability to identify an infectious organism causing the various symptoms of CFS frustrates both patients and the medical profession.

Health Update

Some Essential Facts about HIV Infection and AIDS

AIDS is a disease caused by HIV, a virus that infects immune system cells:
The greatest risk of getting AIDS is through unprotected sex or by sharing drug paraphernalia with an infected man or woman.

The AIDS virus can be passed from men to women, women to men, men to men or by a mother to a newborn.

The best protection against AIDS is:

- abstinence from sex
- participation in a sexually faithful relationship with an uninfected partner

- not shooting drugs
- using a latex condom during sexual intercourse to decrease the risk of giving or getting the HIV virus

You won't get AIDS from:

- a kiss or even a sneeze
- casual contact with an infected person
- a swimming pool or toilet seat
- a mosquito bite
- making a blood donation
- caring for someone with AIDS
- working with or going to school

with someone who is infected by the HIV virus

A test is available to tell if a person is infected by the HIV virus.

There is currently no cure for AIDS; medicines are available to help prolong the lives of people with AIDS.

Much of the fear about AIDS comes from lack of understanding and confusion about the risks.

AIDS INFORMATION HOTLINE:
24 hours: 1-800-344-7432
En Espanol 1-800-243-7889

What is clear from AIDS, CFS, and the many kinds of infectious diseases that occur in people, is the crucial role of the immune system in maintaining health. Thoughts and feelings affect the immune system in either positive or negative ways and make people more or less open to infections (Glaser and Kiecolt-Glaser, 1994). Depressed states of mind, chronic worry and stress, and poor social interactions all seem to depress immune system functions. On the other hand, positive emotional states seem to enhance the functions of the immune system. The key elements to a strong immune system are good nutrition, regular exercise, and positive mental attitudes.

HEALTH IN REVIEW

- Infectious diseases are caused by a myriad of pathogenic organisms: viruses, bacteria, fungi, protozoa, and worms. Growth of certain microorganisms in the body can cause a wide range of diseases and sickness; some produce only mild symptoms, but others produce serious disease and death.
- Some pathogenic microorganisms are easily passed from one person to another and cause communicable diseases.
- Some infectious diseases are caused by a vector, an insect or another animal that transmits the pathogenic microorganism to an uninfected person.
- Some major epidemics of the past include plague, smallpox, influenza, typhus, yellow fever, and polio.
- In the United States new epidemics are emerging: tuberculosis is on the rise; Lyme disease and chronic fatigue syndrome are growing problems; and AIDS is a major concern.
- Human immunodeficiency virus (HIV) is the infectious agent that causes AIDS (acquired immune deficiency syndrome). Infection by HIV can be prevented by not engaging in sexual intercourse with an HIV-infected person and by not being exposed to HIV-contaminated body fluid.
- Many pathogenic bacteria are becoming resistant to common antibiotics, making treatment of serious infectious diseases difficult to treat.
- Antibiotics kill microorganisms but do not kill viruses, which are not alive in the sense that cells are.
- Serious infectious diseases, nosocomial diseases, can be acquired in hospitals and are difficult to treat because the pathogenic bacteria are often antibiotic-resistant.
- Infectious disease is fought in four ways: sanitation, antibiotics, vaccination, and healthful living.
- The skin and mucous membranes keep harmful substances from entering the body.
- Specialized white blood cells circulate in the body attacking and destroying invading foreign organisms.
- The immune system produces cells that make antibodies, proteins that recognize any foreign substance or organism.
- Malfunctioning of the immune system causes autoimmune diseases and allergies.
- Each person carries a unique set of antigens on cells of the body that make tissues and organs unique to each individual.
- Transplantation of organs or blood requires that the donor and recipient be matched with respect to histocompatibility, the matching of HLA or ABO antigens.
- AIDS results from destruction of CD4 cells of the immune system, which opens the door to opportunistic infections.
- Currently there are no effective treatments or vaccines for AIDS, although researchers are working on both.
- Chronic fatigue syndrome also results from abnormalities in immune system functions and may be caused by an unknown virus.

REFERENCES

Barbour, A. G., and D. Fish (1993). "The Biological and Social Phenomenon of Lyme Disease." *Science,* June 11.

Beardsley, T. (1995). "Better Than a Cure." *Scientific American,* January.

Begley, S. (1994). "The End of Antibiotics." *Newsweek,* March 28.

Bender, G. A. (1966). *Great Moments in Medicine.* Detroit: Northwood Institute Press/Parke Davis Co.

Cohen, M. L. (1992). "Epidemiology of Drug Resistance: Implications for a Post-Antimicrobial Era." *Science,* 257: 1057.

Dawson, D. M., and T. D. Sabin (1993). *Chronic Fatigue Syndrome.* Boston: Little, Brown.

Diamond, J. (1992). "The Mysterious Origin of AIDS," *Natural History,* September.

Fackelmann, K. (1995). "Staying Alive: Scientists Study People Who Outwit the AIDS Virus." *Science News,* March 18.

Fendrick, A. M. (1994). "Toward a National Hepatitis B Vaccination Program (editorial)." *Hospital Practice,* 29(2).

Glaser, R., and J. Kiecolt-Glaser (1994). *Handbook of Human Stress and Immunity.* New York: Academic Press.

Gonzalez, E. (1992). "Latex Hypersensitivity: A New and Unexpected Problem." *Hospital Practice,* 27: 137–140.

Graham, D. Y. (1993). "Treatment of Peptic Ulcer Caused by Helicobacter Pylori." *New England Journal of Medicine,* February 4.

Jewett, D. L., G. Fein, and M. H. Greenberg (1990). "A Double Blind Study of the Symptom Provocation to Determine Food Sensitivity." *New England Journal of Medicine,* 323: 429–433.

McKeown, T. (1988). *The Origins of Human Disease.* New York: Basil Blackwell.

Norman, P. S. (1990). "Immunotherapy of IgE-Mediated Disease." *Hospital Practice,* 25(4).

Price, R. (1994). *A Whole New Life.* New York: Atheneum.

Sampson, H. A. (1987). "Late-Phase Response to Food in Atopic Dermatitis." *Hospital Practice,* 22: 121–122.

Selzer, R. (1993). *Raising the Dead: A Doctor's Encounter with His Own Mortality.* New York: Penguin Books.

Young, E., M. D. Stoneham, A. Petruckevitch, J. Barton, and R. Rona (1994). "A Population Study of Food Intolerance." *Lancet,* 343: 1127–1130.

SUGGESTED READINGS

Cowley, J. (1990). "Chronic Fatigue Syndrome: A Modern Medical Mystery." *Newsweek.* November 12. An in-depth article on chronic fatigue syndrome.

Kramer J. (1993). "Bad Blood." *The New Yorker,* October 8. Describes the infection of French hemophiliacs by blood contaminated with the AIDS virus.

"Life, Death, and the Immune System" (1993). *Scientific American,* September. An entire issue devoted to various aspects of the immune system, including allergies, AIDS, and autoimmune diseases.

McKeown, T. (1988). *The Origins of Human Disease.* New York: Basil Blackwell. The best account of the history and causes of all kinds of diseases.

Monmaney, T. (1993). "Marshall's Hunch." *The New Yorker,* September 20. The fascinating story of how the ulcer bacterium was discovered.

Preston, R. (1994). *The Hot Zone.* New York: Random House. The story of how the world's most dangerous virus, the Ebola virus, got loose in a laboratory in Maryland.

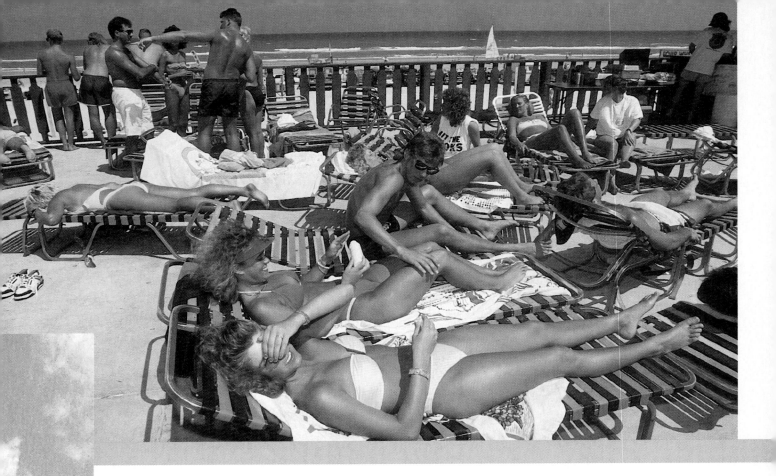

LEARNING OBJECTIVES

After reading this chapter you should be able to:

1. Identify and describe several ways in which you can prevent cancer.
2. Briefly discuss the incidence of cancer today.
3. Define the following terms: cancer, tumor, benign tumor, malignant tumor, and metastasis.
4. Compare and contrast inherited diseases and genetic diseases.
5. Discuss how environmental factors cause cancer.
6. Describe the three kinds of environmental agents that cause cancer.
7. Identify ways to prevent skin cancer.
8. Explain the factors associated with breast cancer.
9. Describe how to do a breast self-exam (BSE) and a testicular self-exam (TSE).
10. Describe how to reduce the risk of testicular and prostate cancer.
11. Discuss the association between diet and cancer.
12. Identify several ethical issues regarding determining cancer susceptibility genes.
13. Identify and briefly describe the three medical treatments for cancer.
14. Describe several coping mechanisms for someone with cancer.

13

Cancer
Understanding Risks and Measures of Prevention

Based on recent statistics, about two out of every five Americans will develop some type of cancer during their lifetime, and about one person in five will die from cancer. Despite this rather dismal outlook, the news about cancer is not all bad. Most cancers *are* preventable. Avoiding cigarettes and tobacco products in any form is the most important action anyone can take to prevent cancer, especially of the lung and pancreas. In addition to increasing the risk of lung cancer, cigarette smoke is estimated to cause approximately 30 percent of *all* forms of cancers.

A healthy diet that is low in animal fat and high in consumption of fresh fruits, vegetables, and whole grains also reduces the risk of cancer. Avoiding unnecessary exposure to ultraviolet radiation in sunshine helps to prevent cancer of the skin. Finally, knowing what chemicals in the environment are cancer causing can help you to avoid dangerous substances. Overall, if everything known about cancer prevention were practiced, up to two-thirds of cancers would not occur (American Cancer Society, 1995).

Although "prevention is the best medicine," about 50 percent of cancer patients can be cured if their cancer is detected at an early stage. Being "cured" means that a person's life expectancy is the same as a person who never had cancer. It is important to have cancer screening tests as indicated for your age and risk group, such as mammograms for breast cancer, exams for colon cancer, and

Pap tests for cervical cancer. The American Cancer Society recommends watching for certain warning signs that the body gives that may indicate a cancer is developing (Figure 13.1).

UNDERSTANDING CANCER

Incidence of Various Cancers

In the United States, the incidence of some types of cancer, such as cancer of the esophagus, bladder, and pancreas, have remained relatively unchanged over the past 50 years among both men and women. Stomach cancer, on the other hand, has declined in both sexes, although it seems to be on the rise again among white males. Liver, uterine, and colon cancers have been declining in women in recent years.

However, all of these modest declines in some cancers have been more than offset by the continuing rise in lung cancer in both men and women (Figure 13.2). Increases in lung cancer began to be noticed in men in the 1940s; in women, the rise did not become appreciable until the 1960s. As every reader of this book knows, the major reason for the increase in lung cancer is cigarette smoking. Unfortunately, gender equality has extended to cigarette smoking, and women now die from lung cancer about half as often as men and the rate is still increasing.

Statistics are like a bathing suit; what they reveal is interesting but what they conceal is significant.
Anonymous

In addition to lung cancer, increases are also being observed in breast, prostate, and skin cancers (Figure 13.2). Because most cancers that have developed beyond a certain stage still are not curable, more attention is now being paid to preventing cancer by discouraging the use of cigarettes and encouraging the use of more fresh fruits and vegetables in the diet. The "War on Cancer," declared in 1971 by President Richard Nixon, is still far from being won (Beardsley, 1994).

What Is Cancer?

The term *cancer* comes from the Latin word meaning crab. Cancer was characterized as a crablike disease by the Greek physician Hippocrates, who observed that cancers spread throughout the body eventually cutting off life. Now **cancer** generally is defined as the unregulated growth of specific cells in the body. The word cancer actually refers to over one hundred different diseases, but in all cases, certain body cells multiply in an abnormal, unregulated manner.

Normally the growth and reproduction of every cell in the body are regulated; this regulation in turn, determines the size and functions of tissues and organs. If a normal body cell begins to grow abnormally and reproduces too rapidly, a mass of abnormal cells eventually develops that is called a **tumor**. A tumor generally contains millions of genetically identical abnormal cells before it can be detected or felt.

Type of cancer	Warning sign
Skin	Change in a wart or mole
Throat	Hoarseness
Esophagus	Difficulty in swallowing
Lungs	Nagging cough
Breasts	Thickening or lump
Lymphoma	A sore that does not heal
Stomach	Persistent indigestion
Leukemia	Unusual bleeding or discharge
Colon or bladder	Change in bowel or bladder functions
Testicles	Thickening or lump

FIGURE 13.1 Some Warning Signs of Cancer If any of these symptoms occur, see a physician promptly.

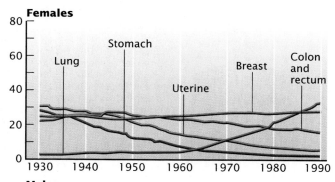

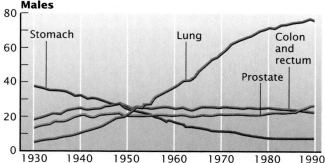

Rates are per 100,000 and are age-adjusted to the 1970 U.S. census population.

FIGURE 13.2 Cancer Death Rates by Site, Males and Females United States, 1930–1991 The rates of cancer deaths (per 100,000 people) for most sites have remained more or less unchanged. A few types, such as stomach, uterine, and colon cancer, have declined. However, lung cancer has increased almost ten-fold in both males and females, primarily due to cigarette smoking.

Source: Cancer Facts and Figures, 1995 (Atlanta: American Cancer Society, 1995).

If the cells of the tumor remain localized at the site of origin in the body and if the cells multiply relatively slowly, the tumor is said to be benign. **Benign tumors** such as cysts, warts, moles, and polyps do not spread to other parts of the body. Benign tumors usually can be removed surgically and generally are not a threat to life. In fact, benign tumors weighing several hundred pounds have been surgically removed from persons who then recovered fully. Benign tumors cannot regrow if all of the abnormal cells are removed by surgical excision of the tumor.

Malignant tumors are composed of cells that grow rapidly, have other abnormal properties that distinguish them from normal cells, and invade other normal cells. In particular, malignant cells may have altered shapes and cell-surface characteristics that contribute to their rapid proliferation. Many malignant cells also have abnormal chromosomes or altered genes, and they manufacture abnormal proteins. The numerous altered properties of malignant cells enable a **pathologist**, a physi-

cian who specializes in the causes of diseases, to determine whether the cells removed from a tumor are abnormal and to what degree.

The cells of most malignant tumors also undergo **metastasis**, a process in which cells detach from the original tumor, enter the lymphatic system and bloodstream, and are carried to other organs. Once the malignant cells spread to other organs, they develop into new tumors that often grow more rapidly than cells in the original tumor. Metastases and the growth of new tumors in many organs of the body eventually disrupt a vital body function that is the cause of death (Liotta, 1992).

Cancers are medically classified according to the organ or kind of tissue in which the tumor originates. The four major categories of cancers are *carcinomas, sarcomas, leukemias,* and *lymphomas* (Figure 13.3). Within these major categories are numerous subgroups that generally describe the organ in which the cancer originates, such as adenocarcinoma of the stomach or adenocarcinoma of the lung. About half of all human cancers originate in one of four organs: the lung, breast, prostate, or colon, which is why so much research is devoted to these particular forms.

Cancer does not develop suddenly but results from a series of genetic and cellular changes that occur in cells over many years (Figure 13.4). This slow development explains why even potent carcinogens such as cigarette smoke do not produce tumors for twenty years or more in most people. Some heavy smokers are lucky and never develop cancer. However, the risk of cancer is much, much greater among smokers than among nonsmokers.

Once a tumor has been detected, cells can be removed from it in a procedure called a **biopsy,** and examined under the microscope by a pathologist. In stage I, cancer cells can be distinguished from normal cells. The cancer cells are still localized and surgical

Lymphoma
About 5% of all cancers, most common being Hodgkin's disease
Cancer similar to leukemia; abnormal production of white blood cells by the spleen and lymph system.

Leukemia
About 4% of all cancers
Cancer of the organs and tissues (lymph glands, bone marrow, etc.) that form blood cells, causing an overproduction of immature white blood cells

Carcinoma
80–90% of all cancers
Cancer originating from epithelial tissues, such as skin, membranes around glands, nerves, breasts, linings of respiratory, urinary, and gastrointestinal tracts

Sarcoma
About 2% of all cancers
Cancer originating from connective tissues, bone, muscles, fat, and blood vessels

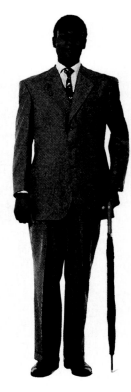

FIGURE 13.3   The Four Major Categories of Cancers and the Approximate Frequencies of Their Occurrence

removal of the tumor usually results in a cure. In stage II, the cancer cells have begun to metastasize and may have migrated to nearby lymph nodes. That is why lymph nodes near the tumor are removed and examined during surgery to determine if cancer cells have spread. By stage III the cancer cells have spread throughout the body and tumors may have begun to grow in other organs. In stage IV, often a terminal stage, tumors are found throughout the body and usually are resistant to treatment. (The leading causes of cancer deaths by organ and by sex are shown in Figure 13.5.)

Most Cancers Are Not Inherited

Many people live in fear of cancer, often because one or more closely related family members have died from some type of cancer. They believe that cancer is passed on in the genes or that, at least, the susceptibility to cancer is inherited. Neither of these beliefs is correct for the vast majority of people. However, a constant fear of developing cancer can generate stress that may weaken the immune system and contribute to the development of disease including cancer.

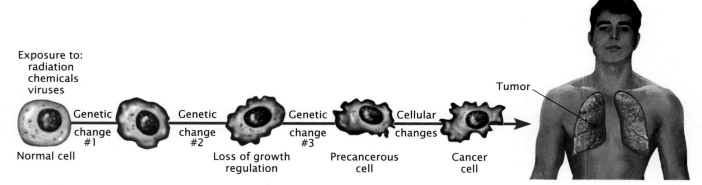

Exposure to: radiation chemicals viruses

Genetic change #1 — Genetic change #2 — Genetic change #3 — Cellular changes

Normal cell   Loss of growth regulation   Precancerous cell   Cancer cell   Tumor

FIGURE 13.4   A Cancer Cell Develops over Many Years from Accumulated Genetic and Cellular Changes

Female

Breast
182,000

Lung
73,900

Colon and rectum
67,500

Uterus
48,600

Ovary
26,600

Lymphoma
24,700

Melanoma of the skin
15,400

Bladder
13,200

Pancreas
13,000

Kidney
11,700

Leukemia
11,000

Oral
9,350

All sites
575,000

*Excluding basal and squamous cell skin cancer and carcinoma in situ.

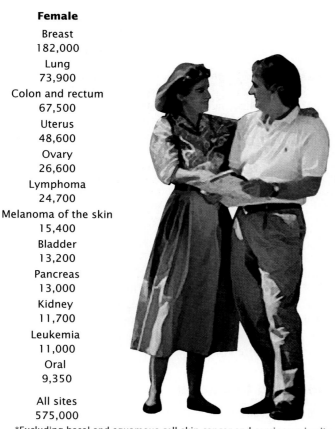

Male

Prostate
244,000

Lung
96,000

Colon and rectum
70,700

Bladder
37,300

Lymphoma
34,000

Oral
18,800

Melanoma of the skin
18,700

Kidney
17,100

Leukemia
14,700

Stomach
14,000

Pancreas
11,000

Larynx
9,000

All sites
677,000

FIGURE 13.5 Estimated Number of Cancer Cases by Site and Sex* in 1995
Source: Cancer Facts and Figures, 1995 (Atlanta: American Cancer Society, 1995)

Many scientific studies indicate that 90 to 95 percent of all cancers, including breast, lung, stomach, colon, skin, or prostate, are not inherited from parents except in a few families in which members do inherit one or more cancer-susceptibility genes (discussed in a later section).

Confusion often stems from misunderstanding the meanings of the words "genetic" and "inherited." The two are not synonymous. All body cells (except for red blood cells) contain chromosomes and genes: in fact, copies of the same chromosomes that were in the fertilized egg that develops in an individual. The genes in the chromosomes of any cell of the body, such as skin, lung, or stomach cells, can be chemically changed by environmental agents. These genetic changes in skin, lung, or stomach cells may transform them into cancer cells. Thus, cancer is a genetic disease in that genes are changed in a person's body cells, but is not an inherited disease because defective genes were not passed on from one's parents.

The fact that several close family members have died of cancer does not mean that cancer "runs in the family" and is an inherited disease. Currently, one out of every five deaths each year in the United States is due to cancer (American Cancer Society, 1995). If your parents and eight aunts or uncles died, probably two or three of them died of cancer simply by chance. If they all smoked

cigarettes, it would not be surprising if more than three close relatives out of ten died of cancer. For most people, life-style plays a far greater role in cancer than any genes that are passed on from parents.

ENVIRONMENTAL FACTORS

The causes of cancer or, more correctly, the risk factors associated with the development of cancer are numerous and complex (Shields and Harris, 1991). It often is difficult to point to a single cause of a cancer but certain environmental factors are strongly correlated with the occurrence of particular cancers. Two examples are the strong correlation between cigarette smoking and lung cancer and exposure to ultraviolet light (UV) and skin cancer. Even in these examples, not everyone who smokes heavily or stays in the sun day after day will get cancer.

Epidemiology is the branch of science that investigates the causes and frequencies of diseases in human

T E R M

epidemiology: a branch of science that studies the causes and frequencies of diseases in human populations

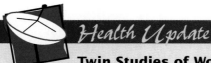
Twin Studies of World War II Veterans Show That Cancer Is Not Inherited

One of the impressive pieces of evidence showing that most cancers are not inherited comes from a study of World War II veterans conducted by the U.S. military. The health of approximately 15,000 pairs of identical or nonidentical (fraternal) twin brothers was followed for many years after the war. No difference was observed in the rates of cancer between the identical and fraternal twin pairs of brothers. That is, if one of an identical twin pair contracted cancer, the other twin brother was no more likely to get cancer than the average person.

Because identical twins have identical genes, they should both have inherited the same cancer-causing genes from their parents, if such genes existed. The fact that their rates of cancer were no different from fraternal twins who inherited a different set of genes means that most cancers are not caused by genes inherited from parents.

populations. Many epidemiological studies show that as many as 80 to 90 percent of cancers are caused by exposure to environmental factors that are known to increase the risk of cancer (Table 13.1). For example, smoking cigarettes while young puts a person at 10 to 20 times higher risk of developing cancer later in life than persons who do not smoke. Eating fat-laden hamburgers and pizza frequently may be convenient, but is ultimately unhealthy and may contribute to the development of certain cancers (Davis and Freeman, 1994). Because each of us can change our diets, stop smoking, and avoid other cancer-causing risks in the environment, preventing cancer is a realistic and attainable goal for most people.

Three classes of environmental agents—ionizing radiation, tumor viruses (viruses that cause cancer in animals), and chemical carcinogens (cancer-causing chemicals)—have been shown to increase the risk of cancer in both laboratory animals and people. Each of these agents increases the risk of cancer by producing chemical changes in genes, called **mutations,** that can occur in any cell in the body and cause it to grow abnormally. If a cell undergoes one or more mutations in genes that regulate its growth, it may begin to multiply rapidly and develop into a tumor. Environmental factors cause both mutations and also affect the rate of abnormal cell growth (Figure 13.6).

> *If what is to be found is really new, then it is by definition unknown in advance.*
>
> Francis Jacob,
> Nobel laureate, biology and medicine

Ionizing Radiation

Ionizing radiation consists of X-rays, UV light, and radioactivity whose energy can damage cells and chromosomes. The high rate of leukemia among survivors of the Hiroshima and Nagasaki atomic bomb blasts in 1945 leaves no doubt that radioactivity increases the risk of cancer. In the United States, among children born in southern Utah in the 1950s who were exposed to radioactive fallout from nearby atomic tests, leukemia deaths were two to three times greater than among children born in southern Utah before and after the atomic tests.

In a landmark legal decision in 1984, a federal court ruled that the U.S. government was negligent in conducting atomic bomb tests in southern Utah in the 1950s because they released radioactive material into the atmosphere. The court ruled that the families who were exposed to radioactivity as a result of these tests, and whose members died as a result of exposure to the

HEALTHY PEOPLE 2000

Reduce cigarette smoking to a prevalence of no more than 15 percent among people aged 20 and older.

In 1987, 29 percent of people over 20 smoked: 32 percent of men and 27 percent of women smoked. Among people aged 20 and older, cigarette smoking has been declining steadily at a rate of 0.5 points per year since 1965. The decline has been substantially slower among women. By the late 1990s, smoking rates for women will probably exceed the rates for men.

T E R M S

mutation: a permanent change in the genetic information in a cell; only mutations in sperm and eggs are inherited

ionizing radiation: radiation such as X-rays that can damage cells and cause cancer; also used to treat cancer

melanoma: a particularly dangerous form of skin cancer

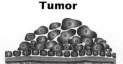

Factors that change genes in cells

Ionizing radiation

Tumor viruses

Carcinogenic chemicals

Tumor

Factors promoting growth of genetically abnormal cells

Hormones
Nutritional deficiencies
Reduced immune system
Aging
Immunosuppressive drugs

FIGURE 13.6 Environmental factors change both genes and the growth properties of cells that may lead to the development of cancer.

radioactivity, were entitled to compensation. The nuclear reactor accident at Chernobyl in the Ukraine in 1986 also resulted in a large amount of radioactive fallout over nearby cities.

In the 1940s and 1950s across the United States, several million children received large doses of X-rays to shrink tonsils and to treat neck and chest ailments. At that time X-ray treatments were considered harmless and part of standard medical practice. We now know that this group of X-ray-treated people has a much higher risk of developing thyroid and salivary gland tumors.

Because any amount of ionizing radiation, however small, has the potential for causing damage to chromosomes and genes, one should minimize exposure to X-rays. For example, if you are healthy, periodic chest X-rays are unnecessary. Dental X-rays with each six-month checkup also pose a cumulative risk. Many homes release radon, a radioactive gas present in some building materials. Long-term exposure to the invisible radon gas in some homes also contributes to the risk of cancer (see Chapter 24 for more on radon).

The most common source of radiation is the ultraviolet (UV) radiation in sunlight. Because children and

young people tend to play in the sun whenever possible, we are exposed to as much as 80 percent of our lifetime UV exposure by age 20. Also, many people are addicted to sun bathing and to acquiring a tan, which is associated with health and sexual attractiveness among white Americans.

As a result of overexposure to sunlight, the rate of skin cancers has increased appreciably in recent years. The rate of **melanoma,** a particularly dangerous form of skin cancer because abnormal skin cells grow rapidly and spread easily, has doubled over the past ten years. Regardless of skin color, exposure to UV in sunlight can increase the risk of various kinds of skin cancers as well as cause skin to wrinkle and age prematurely; however, there is lower risk in African Americans compared with Caucasians.

Any unusual looking sore on the skin or change in the appearance of a mole or freckle should be examined by a physician. Many skin cancers can be removed at an early stage and cause no further problem. However, melanoma cells grow rapidly, metastasize readily, and cause tumors to form in other organs that can lead to death. The most common skin cancer among people who are overexposed to sunlight is **squamous cell car-**

TABLE 13.1 Environmental and Life-style Risk Factors That Contribute to Cancer

Factor	Amount of risk	Types of cancer
Nutrition	About *half* of cancer deaths are due to nutritional problems: Excess calories Excess fat consumption Obesity Nutritional deficiencies, especially fiber and vitamin A	Cancers of the colon, rectum, stomach, breast, and ovaries
Cigarettes and alcohol	About *one-third* of cancer deaths are due to smoking cigarettes and excessive alcohol consumption	Cancers of the lung, mouth, larynx, liver, esophagus, and bladder
Occupation	About *5 percent* of cancer deaths are due to substances in the workplace such as asbestos, benzene, and vinyl chloride	Cancers of the bladder, lung, stomach, blood, liver, bones, and skin
Radiation	About *3 percent* of cancer deaths are due to ionizing radiation such as X-rays and ultraviolet light	Blood, skin
Other	Other cancer deaths are due to heredity, chronic disease, drugs, and chemotherapy	Various cancers

cinoma, which also is dangerous if not detected and treated surgically at an early stage.

Ultraviolet radiation in sunlight is characterized by two different wavelengths called UVA and UVB. Until recently it was thought that only UVB was dangerous, but now it appears that both forms of UV radiation are harmful. Reducing the time of exposure to intense sunlight and using sunscreen creams to protect exposed areas of the body can reduce the risk of skin cancer.

Tumor Viruses

In 1911 Peyton Rous, a scientist working at the Rockefeller Institute in New York, showed that cancer could be produced in chickens by injecting them with a virus isolated from tumors that occur in chickens. Since then, other viruses, called **tumor viruses**, have been found that cause cancer in animals such as mice, cats, and monkeys.

Finding tumor viruses that infect people has been generally unsuccessful despite a generation of research.

HEALTHY PEOPLE 2000

Increase to at least 60 percent the proportion of people of all ages who limit sun exposure, use sunscreens and protective clothing when exposed to sunlight, and avoid artificial sources of ultraviolet light (e.g., sun lamps, tanning booths).

Skin cancer is the most common form of cancer in the United States. The American Cancer Society (1995) estimates that 800,000 new cases will occur in 1995. Most skin cancers are basal cell and squamous cell carcinomas that are highly treatable and rarely metastasize. Of the two, basal cell cancer is most common. Squamous cell is more invasive and accounts for three-fourths of nonmelanoma skin cancer deaths. The most serious form of skin cancer is malignant melanoma.

Only four viruses have been associated with specific human cancers; in the vast majority of people infection by these viruses will not cause cancer, although it will increase their risk somewhat. Increased cancer risk is associated with hepatitis B virus (liver cancer), papilloma virus (genital cancer), human T-cell leukemia-lymphoma virus (leukemia and lymphoma), and Epstein-Barr virus (cancer of the nose or pharynx in Africans).

Early in the "war on cancer" there was great hope that if viruses were a main cause of human cancer, vaccines could be developed to prevent cancer. Currently, there is a vaccine for Hepatitis B. However, the causes of most cancer lie in environmental factors rather than tumor viruses.

Chemical Carcinogens

A **chemical carcinogen** is an environmental chemical that can interact with cells to initiate cancer, usually by chemically altering the chromosomes or genes in cells. Genes are responsible for manufacturing the enzymes and other proteins a cell needs to function properly. An altered gene usually makes an abnormal protein that may change the growth properties of a cell and cause it to become a cancer cell.

Many chemicals that are developed now are tested to determine their cancer-causing potential. Unfortunately, many thousands of chemical substances already in use

T E R M S

squamous cell carcinoma: a common form of skin cancer that is curable if detected early

tumor viruses: viruses that infect cells, change their growth properties, and cause cancer

chemical carcinogen: a chemical that damages cells and causes cancer

mesothelioma: a form of lung cancer caused by asbestos

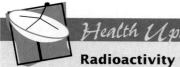
have not been adequately tested. Of the thousands of chemical substances that have been tested, many have been found to be carcinogenic and should be avoided if at all possible. These carcinogens include cigarette smoke, pesticides, asbestos, heavy metals (lead, mercury, cadmium), benzene, and nitrosamines (Table 13.2).

Despite the long list of carcinogenic substances, some scientists and public health officials argue that tobacco is the only substance of consequence with respect to the numbers of cancers caused. While the argument has some basis, it is of small consolation to those who acquire cancer from exposure, often without their knowledge, to other carcinogenic substances.

In some industries, workers suffer from cancers that

> *I don't want to achieve immortality through my work; I want to achieve immortality by not dying.*
> Woody Allen

almost never arise in the general population. For example, **mesothelioma** is a rare form of lung cancer that only occurs among persons exposed to asbestos fibers. Long-term exposure to the heavy metals beryllium and cadmium increases workers' risk of prostate cancer. Workers exposed to vinyl chloride, the starting material for polyvinyl chloride (PVC) pipes and other products, develop a rare form of liver cancer not found in the general public. Fortunately, with current regulations we do not see high numbers of these types of cancer.

Although the total number of cancers attributable to industrial chemicals is relatively small compared to the risks of tobacco smoke and dietary factors, the fact remains that cancers caused by industrial hazards are

Wellness Guide

Ways to Prevent Skin Cancer

Sunscreen products contain chemicals that provide sun protective factors (SPFs) to varying degrees. The SPF value indicates how much additional time you can expose yourself to the sun without burning. For example, if someone usually burns after 15 minutes exposure to intense sun, a sunscreen product with an SPF of 10 should give protection for ten times as long or 150 minutes of exposure; 30 SPF means thirty times more protection. Generally, SPF values above 30 are not considered useful because the cream or lotion wears off before its usefulness is exhausted. The effectiveness of a sunscreen product depends on the SPF number, how waterproof the product is, and how effectively it covers the skin.

The SPF number refers *only* to protection from UVB, so exposure to UVA still can harm the skin. The primary ingredients in sunscreen products are para-amino-benzoic acid (PABA) or Padimat-O, both of which absorb only UVB. Chemicals such as avobenzone or oxybenzone protect against UVA, so look for sunscreen products that contain these substances or that claim to protect against both forms of UV.

Fear of skin cancer is driving many people to use chemical tanning products marketed in the form of lotions, creams, gels, and mousses. This tan-in-a-bottle industry has grown from sales of about $5 million in 1988 to more than $86 million in 1993. Clearly, looking tan is still a desirable goal for many people. These products may be safe, but they have not been in use long enough to know.

TABLE 13.2 Possible Carcinogenic Substances

Substances in the environment that have been shown to cause cancer in experimental animals, and either directly or indirectly in people.

Substance	Site of cancer
Aromatic amines	Bladder
Arsenic	Skin and bronchus
Asbestos	Bronchus, pleura, and peritoneum
Benzene	Marrow
Beryllium	Prostate
Bis(chloromethyl) ether	Bronchus
Bis(chloroethyl) sulfide	Respiratory tract
Cadmium	Prostate
Chrome ores	Bronchus
Coke oven soot	Bronchus
Nickel ores	Bronchus and nasal sinuses
Soots, tars, and oils	Skin and lungs
Wood dust	Nasal sinuses
Vinyl chloride	Liver
Wood and leather dust	Respiratory tract
Alkylating agents	Bladder and hematopoietic tissue
Anabolic steroids	Liver
Chlornaphazine	Bladder
Diethylstilbestrol	Vagina
Immunosuppressive drugs	Lymphoid tissue
Phenacetin (acetophenetidin)	Kidney
Chloramphenicol, melphalan	Marrow
Aflatoxins	Liver
Tobacco smoke	Lung, esophagus, oral
Oral contraceptives	Liver
Betel nut and lime	Mouth
Nitrates, nitrites, and nitrosamines	Stomach, liver, bladder, kidney

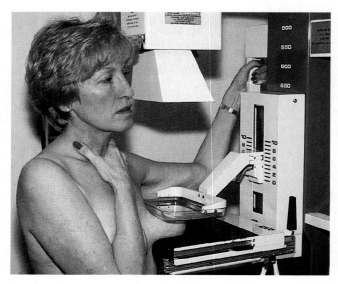

A woman having a mammogram to test for possible breast cancer.

association between a food and a higher rate of cancer among people who ingest it is not considered proof that the food causes cancer.

For example, there is a significant association between the rate of breast cancer and the amount of fat in the diet of people in various countries (Figure 13.7). This association has led to the hypothesis that dietary fat

preventable. Before you accept a job, it would be wise to determine what chemicals you may be exposed to for long periods.

REDUCING CANCER RISK

Reducing Risk of Breast Cancer

Even with the strong epidemiological evidence indicating that as many as half of all cancers are due to dietary excesses or deficiencies, it has been virtually impossible to identify specific foods that cause cancer. Finding an

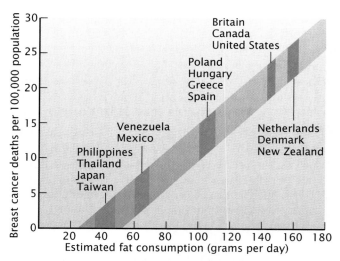

FIGURE 13.7 Dietary Fat and Breast Cancer A strong association is observed between consumption of fat in the diet and the number of breast cancer deaths in various countries. Asian and Central and South American countries have the lowest number of breast cancer deaths. European and North American countries have the highest. Epidemiological studies suggest diet is one of the important risk factors in breast cancer.

How to Examine Your Breasts

1. Lie down and put a pillow under your right shoulder. Place your right arm behind your head.

2. Use the finger pads of your three middle fingers on your left hand to feel for lumps or thickening. Your finger pads are the top third of each finger.

3. Press firmly enough to know how your breast feels. If you're not sure how hard to press, ask your health care provider. Or try to copy the way your health care provider uses the finger pads during a breast exam. Learn what your breast feels like most of the time. A firm ridge in the lower curve of each breast is normal.

4. Move around the breast in a set way. You can choose either the circle (a), the up and down line (b), or the wedge (c). Do it the same way every time. It will help you to make sure that you've gone over the entire breast area, and to remember how your breast feels.

5. Now examine your left breast using right hand finger pads.

6. If you find any changes, see your doctor right away.

Source: The American Cancer Society.

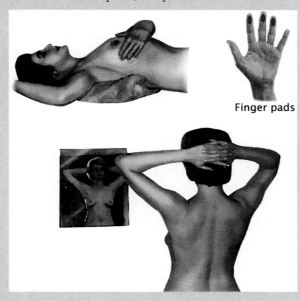

Finger pads

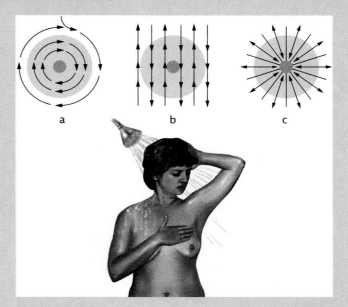

a   b   c

is a significant risk factor in breast cancer. While this may be so, studies have failed to show how fat causes breast cancer, so the association between the two does not prove that fatty foods cause breast cancer. Other factors associated with a higher-than-average risk of breast cancer include high radiation exposure, late childbearing, late menopause, and high lifetime exposure to estrogen.

To aid early detection, women should perform regular breast self-exams. In addition, the American Cancer Society (1995) recommends a screening **mammogram** by age 40. Women ages 40–49 should get a mammogram every 1–2 years, women ages 50 and older should get a mammogram yearly. Younger women who are concerned about breast cancer because they are in a high-risk group should also obtain yearly mammograms, which may detect small lumps in the breast that would go unnoticed in a breast self-exam.

HEALTHY PEOPLE 2000

Reduce breast cancer deaths to no more than 20.6 per 100,000 women.

Breast cancer is the second leading cause of cancer death among women. In 1995, an estimated 46,000 women will die of breast cancer, while an estimated 182,000 new cases will be diagnosed (American Cancer Society, 1995). Approximately one in every eight women will develop breast cancer in her lifetime. About 1,400 new cases of breast cancer will be diagnosed in men during 1995.

TERM

mammogram: an X-ray of the breast

TABLE 13.3 Detecting Cancer at an Early Stage

Age	Recommended frequency	Females	Males
18–20	Monthly	Skin self-exam	Skin self-exam
	Yearly	Pap test	Testis self-exam
20–40	Monthly	Skin self-exam, breast self-exam	Skin self-exam
	Yearly	Pelvic exam, Pap test	Testis self-exam
40–50	Monthly	Skin self-exam, breast self-exam	Skin self-exam, testis self-exam
	Yearly	Pelvic exam, Pap test, rectal exam, stool blood test	Rectal exam, stool blood test
	1 to 2 years	Mammogram	
50–65+	Monthly	Skin self-exam, breast self-exam	Skin self-exam, testis self-exam
	Yearly	Pelvic exam, Pap test, rectal exam, stool blood test	PSA blood test for prostate cancer rectal exam, stool blood test
	3–5 years	Proctosigmoidoscopy	Proctosigmoidoscopy

The amount of X-rays used in a mammogram are quite low, and generally the benefits outweigh the possible harm from the X-ray for women who are at risk for breast cancer. For young women who are not at high risk for breast cancer, mammograms are not recommended because of unnecessary X-ray exposure.

Men also can get breast cancer, but the incidence is extremely low. However, men also need to be alert to any unusual lumps or swellings around the nipples.

One possible reason for the increasing incidence of breast cancer is the exposure of women to environmental chemicals called **xenoestrogens** that mimic the effects of natural estrogen produced in the female body. These xenoestrogens include the pesticides DDT, heptachlor, and atrazine, as well as petroleum byproducts and polychlorinated biphenyls (PCBs).

Many of these chemicals produce mammary tumors in mice and other laboratory animals. Also, women with breast cancer often have higher levels of xenoestrogens in their blood than do women without breast cancer. Since 1976 in Israel, when chlorinated pesticides were banned and all residues eliminated from milk products, the rate of breast cancer has been falling. Israel is the only industrialized country without an increase in the rate of breast cancer in the past twenty years.

Reducing Risk of Testicular and Prostate Cancer

The rates of both testicular and prostate cancer have been increasing and, as with breast cancer, the causes are unknown. Testicular cancer is rare but can occur in young men, which is why a testicular self-exam should be performed regularly. Prostate cancer occurs primarily in men over 65, although some abnormal cells can be detected in younger men who die from other causes.

Generally, prostate cancers are very slow growing and may never become life-threatening.

Early diagnosis of prostate cancer is facilitated by two tests. One is the finger rectal exam in which a physician can feel the prostate and determine if it is enlarged or otherwise abnormal. A blood test also is useful in early detection of prostate cancer. The prostate-specific antigen (PSA) test can detect a protein in blood that is associated with abnormal growth of the prostate gland. A high PSA level may indicate prostate cancer, but also occurs with many other noncancerous disorders. Additional tests are necessary to confirm the presence of prostate cancer. Many prostate tumor cells are sensitive to male hormones, called androgens, that stimulate their rate of growth. Specific tests that facilitate the detection of several types of cancer are recommended for men and women at various ages (Table 13.3).

Regulating Diet

Many epidemiological studies show that the risk of certain cancers is influenced by diet (Shields and Harris, 1991). For example, stomach cancer is very high in Japan but low among white Americans in Hawaii. Japanese-Americans in Hawaii have stomach cancer rates that are almost as low as the white American population. Excessive consumption of smoked and pickled foods may contribute to the higher rates of stomach cancer in Japan. However, as with the association of dietary fat and breast cancer, it is not known what foods increase the risk of stomach cancer.

T E R M

xenoestrogens: environmental chemicals that mimic the effects of natural estrogen

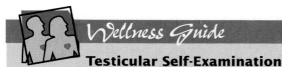

Wellness Guide

Testicular Self-Examination

How to Do TSE

A simple procedure called testicular self-exam (TSE) can increase the chances of finding a tumor early.

Men should perform TSE once a month—after a warm bath or shower. The heat causes the scrotal skin to relax, making it easier to find anything unusual. TSE is simple and only takes a few minutes:

- Examine each testicle gently with both hands. The index and middle fingers should be placed underneath the testicle while the thumbs are placed on the top. Roll the testicle gently between the thumbs and fingers. One testicle may be larger than the other. This is normal.
- The epididymis is a cord-like structure on the top and back of the testicle that stores and transports the sperm. Do not confuse the epididymis with an abnormal lump.
- Feel for any abnormal lumps—about the size of a pea—on the front or the side of the testicle. These lumps are usually painless.

If you do find a lump, you should contact your doctor right away. The lump may be due to an infection, and a doctor can decide the proper treatment. If the lump is not an infection, it is likely to be cancer. Remember that testicular cancer is highly curable, especially when detected and treated early. Testicular cancer almost always occurs in only one testicle, and the other testicle is all that is needed for full sexual function.

Routine testicular self-exams are important, but they cannot substitute for a doctor's examination. Your doctor should examine your testicles when you have a physical exam. You also can ask your doctor to check the way you do TSE.

Source: Testicular Self-Examination (Washington, D.C.: National Cancer Institute, 1994).

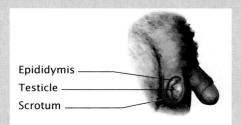

Epididymis
Testicle
Scrotum

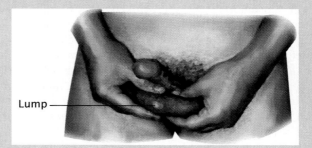

Lump

TABLE 13.4 Dietary Recommendations to Help Prevent Cancer About 50 percent of all cancers are thought to derive from nutritional deficiencies or excesses.

Substance or food	Effect on cancer risk	Advice
Fiber	Helps decrease colon and rectal cancer	Obtain fiber from vegetables, fruits, whole grains
Cruciferous vegetables (broccoli, cauliflower, brussels sprouts)	Phytochemicals in these vegetables may detoxify cancer-causing chemicals	Eat more; raw or undercooked is best
Allium vegetables (onion, garlic, chives)	Sulfur-containing chemicals in allium vegetables may help prevent cancer	Eat more
Beta-carotene (15 mg), vitamin E (30 mg), and selenium (50)	A daily supplement reduced cancer (mainly stomach and esophagus) in a large Chinese population	Use supplements in moderation; selenium in high dose is toxic
Folic acid	Deficiency in this vitamin increases genetic damage that may contribute to cancer	Supplement if diet is deficient
Green tea	Reduced esophageal cancer in Chinese population	Most tea drunk in U.S. is black tea; try green tea
Shitake mushrooms	Extracts of shitake mushrooms reduced tumors in laboratory animals; also reduces blood cholesterol	Add to diet
Vitamins C and E	Boost immune system and may help prevent cancer	Supplement diet if desired

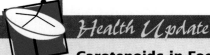

Carotenoids in Foods Help Protect against Cancer

Carotenoids refer to a class of chemical found in many fruits and vegetables. A number of studies have found that carotenoids in foods may reduce the risk of many forms of cancer, as well as heart disease and an eye disease called macular degeneration that can lead to blindness. So far scientists have identified six chemically different carotenoids, but it is not known which ones are important in preventing cancer. Carotenoids can be obtained from the foods shown in the table.

Pigmented vegetables	Green leafy vegetables	Fruits
pumpkin	spinach	orange
carrot	chard	pink grapefruit
sweet potato	romaine lettuce	tangerine
cantaloupe	kale	papaya
tomato	collard greens	watermelon
red pepper	okra	guava
winter squash	broccoli	apricot

Despite the scientific uncertainty over what specific foods increase the risk of cancer, certain dietary choices may help in preventing cancer (Table 13.4). Most of these dietary recommendations also help boost the immune system, which is the body's main defense against foreign cells (Chapter 12). B-vitamins, vitamin C, vitamin E, folic acid, and carotenoids have been shown to boost the immune system and, as a consequence, may also help destroy cancer cells. These vitamins and substances can be taken as supplements, but also are readily available in fresh fruits and vegetables.

Over the years vitamin C has received much attention both as a preventive agent and as a cure for cancer when taken in extremely high doses (Richards, 1991). Some cancer patients who received megadoses of vitamin C have survived much longer than expected, but other studies involving vitamin C and cancer have shown no positive therapeutic effect. However, keep in mind that the effects of any cancer treatment vary from person to person and vitamin C may help some people even if it acts only as a placebo.

Scientists continue to speculate over why certain kinds of cancer are so dependent on diet. One possibility is that we are asking the body to do things chemically for which it is unprepared by the course of human evolution. That is, cancer may be thought of as a disease of maladaptation.

Our ancestors foraged for their food. They collected and ate seeds, roots, fruits, vegetables, and occasionally meat. Refined sugar, salt, and animal fats were scarce or nonexistent. Meat, milk, and cheese were certainly a rarity in the ancestral diet. Thus, the diet we consume today, filled with excess sugar, salt, fat, and meat, may be incompatible with the body chemistry we have inherited from our ancestors. The modern diet, heavy with processed foods, may result in the accumulation of toxic chemicals or an insufficient amount of some essential nutrients found in fresh fruits and vegetables.

HEALTHY PEOPLE 2000

Reduce dietary fat intake to an average of 30 percent of calories or less and average saturated fat intake to less than 10 percent of calories among people aged two and older.

Evidence associates diets high in fat with increased risk of obesity, some types of cancer, and possibly gallbladder disease. Epidemiological and experimental animal studies suggest that dietary fat can influence the risk of some cancers, particularly cancers of the breast, colon, and prostate. The amount of fat consumed, rather than the specific type of fat, appears to be responsible for the risk of some types of cancer.

CONFRONTING CANCER

Cancer-Susceptibility Genes

To become a cancer cell, a normal cell must first undergo several genetic changes that alter its growth rate. These genetic changes usually accumulate over many years. For example, development of colon cancer requires changes

T E R M

cancer-susceptibility gene: gene responsible for familial breast cancer and genes which cause susceptibility to colon cancer; increases the risk of a person developing cancer in his or her lifetime

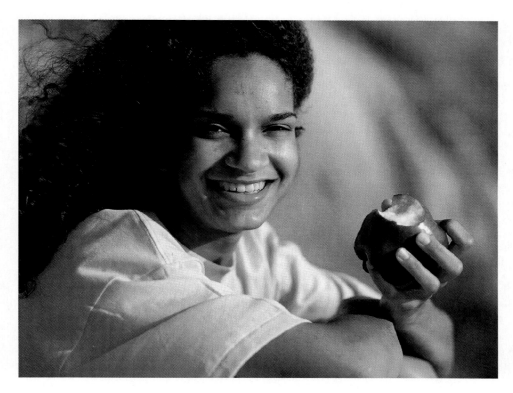

Fresh fruits and vegetables contain chemicals that help prevent cancer cells from developing.

in at least four different genes in a normal colon cell to convert it into a cancer cell.

Although only a fraction (estimates range between 5 to 10 percent) of all cancers are due to heredity, some people do inherit **cancer-susceptibility genes.** A cancer-susceptibility gene makes a person more vulnerable to the environmental factors that increase cancer risk. For example, in persons who have a gene called *adenomatous polyposis coli* (APC), colon cells grow slightly faster than usual. As a result, dietary factors or environmental agents are more likely to produce changes in colon cells that result in the conversion of a normal cell into a cancer cell. However, less than 1 percent of colon cancer patients carry the APC gene. For carriers of the APC gene frequent examination of the colon is recommended so that therapy can be initiated if abnormal changes are observed. Recently, two other inherited susceptibility genes for colon cancer have been identified that may account for some of the other cases.

Identification of colon cancer susceptibility genes in people raises very serious ethical questions, as well as offering potential benefits. People who want to know their colon cancer risk status may soon be able to request the genetic tests from their physicians, but what can they do if the test is positive? At present, nothing can be done to change any person's cancer-susceptibility genes; therefore, careful monitoring of such individuals for the earliest sign of colon cancer is the best approach to successful treatment.

Controversy in Health

Should the Presence of a Cancer-Susceptibility Gene Be Kept Secret from Other Family Members?

A young woman has been diagnosed with colon polyps (small growths in the colon) that, if left untreated, will develop into colon cancer. Genetic tests indicate that she has inherited one of the colon cancer-susceptibility genes. With aggressive treatment and frequent check-ups, she may be able to avoid dying from colon cancer. The woman refuses to inform her brothers, sisters, or other relatives of the cancer-susceptibility gene she has inherited, although they too may be at risk. She also refuses to have her two children tested.

STUDENT REFLECTIONS

- Does the woman's right to medical privacy outweigh the right of family members to know their status with respect to inheriting the colon cancer-susceptibility gene?

Controversy in Health

Should People Be Tested for Inherited Cancer-Susceptibility Genes?

Because all persons except identical twins are genetically different, it is not surprising that people differ in their susceptibility to inherited cancer factors. In 1994, cancer-susceptibility genes were identified that increase the risk of either colon or breast cancer. The presence of one of these susceptibility genes means a greater risk of developing cancer at a fairly young age.

What are the potential benefits and risks of knowing whether or not you carry a cancer-susceptibility gene? According to the experts, genetic testing for cancer-susceptibility genes is not yet warranted for the following reasons:

- If a person does carry a cancer-susceptibility gene, nothing can be done to correct it. All people should adopt the healthiest lifestyle possible and watch for any signs of cancer regardless of any susceptibility genes that they may carry.

- How accurate are the genetic tests for cancer susceptibility genes? How many false positive and false negative results do the tests produce? How are the standards of accuracy for these tests to be regulated? As yet, none of these concerns have been resolved.

- How can genetic discrimination in insurance and employment be avoided for people who are known to carry a cancer-susceptibility gene?

- A positive test will create emotional and psychological stress that in itself can harm health. Some people may not be able to cope with a positive result.

- Pregnant women might elect to have their fetuses tested for cancer-susceptibility genes and might elect to abort any fetus carrying such a gene.

STUDENT REFLECTIONS

- Considering all these issues, would you want to be tested for a cancer-susceptibility gene?
- Would you abort a fetus carrying such a gene?

Pharmaceutical companies plan to market a test for the breast cancer susceptibility gene (called BRCA1) in the near future. But based on current knowledge, if the test is positive there is nothing a woman can do to reduce her breast cancer risks other than not smoking and eating a healthy diet (which should be every person's goal regardless of cancer risk).

Certainly anxiety and stress will increase if a woman believes that she is likely to eventually get breast cancer. Also, the tests are highly unreliable since many different mutations have been discovered in the BRCA1 gene, not all of which are detected by the current genetic tests (Nowak, 1994). A few young women at high risk for breast cancer have opted to have their breasts surgically removed to avoid the possibility of breast cancer later.

Concerns about the reliability of the genetic tests for cancer-susceptibility genes, as well as concerns about the adverse psychological and social consequences, have prompted the National Advisory Council for Human Genome Research (1994) to recommend that the genetic tests not be used until many concerns are resolved. Widespread use of genetic tests for cancer-susceptibility genes entails both serious risks and possible benefits—both need to be widely discussed before such tests are marketed.

Seeking Cancer Treatments

The three medical treatments for cancer are surgery, **radiation therapy,** and **chemotherapy.** Surgical removal of all or as much of a tumor as possible is considered the best treatment for cancer, particularly if the tumor is small and cells have not spread throughout the body. If even a few cancer cells remain, however, they may grow into new tumors, which is the reason that surgery such as mastectomy often removes a great deal of tissue in addition to the tumor.

If there is evidence that tumor cells have spread, or if some of the tumor could not be removed surgically, then radiation and/or chemotherapy are used to kill the remaining cancer cells. X-rays or other forms of high-energy radiation can destroy cancer cells as can the pow-

T E R M S

radiation therapy: use of high-energy radiation such as X-rays to kill cancer cells and treat some forms of cancer

chemotherapy: use of toxic chemicals to kill cancer cells and treat some forms of cancer

immunotherapy: an experimental cancer therapy using immune system cells to kill cancer cells

erful chemotherapy drugs. Although both treatments kill both normal cells as well as cancer cells, the cancer cells sometimes are killed more readily than normal cells (which also recover better than cancer cells). Because radiation therapy and chemotherapy destroy normal cells, only limited amounts of each treatment can be tolerated by the body.

Despite improvements in surgical techniques and development of new chemotherapeutic drugs, cancer treatments today are not noticeably more successful than they were in the past, a fact that is reflected in the more or less unchanged death rates for most cancers. Because of the limited success of current cancer therapies, new approaches are being tested. There have been successes with childhood leukemia, testicular cancer, and Hodgkin's disease.

Cancer patients often become desperate and depressed about their condition, the pain of treatments, and the prospect of death. In this state, some patients turn to unconventional therapies and promises of "miracle" cures. Studies show that many cancer patients turn to alternative therapies in addition to conventional medical treatments (Downer et al., 1994). Although unconventional therapies may be helpful or at least produce more peace of mind, patients and their families need to be wary of practitioners who make unfounded claims for unlicensed drugs and unproven therapies. Things that are "too good to be true" usually are.

Coping with a Diagnosis of Cancer

A diagnosis of cancer raises serious problems for the patient and for family and friends. Often the patient enters a state of disbelief or shock. The family has to cope with new problems. The patient must face surgery or other treatment. Along with treatment, the patient usually must deal with fear of death, anger at the disease, loss of income, changes in living habits, and, above all,

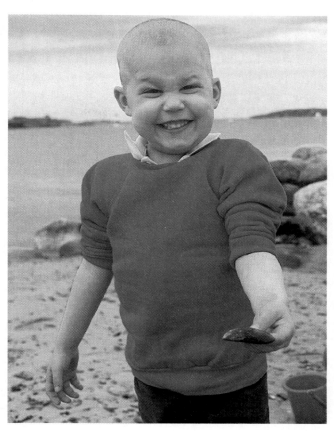

Some cancers can be cured with chemotherapy and other treatments. Temporary hair loss is one of the consequences of chemotherapy treatments.

the uncertainty of the outcome, which may last for months or years. These are some of the reasons why coping with cancer can be difficult. Stress and emotional upset can depress the normal functions of the immune system. There also is evidence that hostile feelings,

Health Update

New Cancer Therapies Involve the Immune System

In some seriously ill cancer patients, in rare instances tumors do disappear spontaneously. How these tumors suddenly disappear is not understood, but has been documented in hundreds of medical reports. It is thought that in these unusual cases, the person's immune system has been activated so that it recognizes and destroys tumor cells.

Because of these observations, **immunotherapy** is being investigated as an alternative approach in treating cancer (Rosenberg, 1990). In one experimental approach, the patient's immune system cells are removed and specific lymphocytes called "killer T-cells" are stimulated with a drug. After being grown in a test tube to increase the number of killer T-cells, the cells along

with the drug are injected back into the patient. A few cancer patients have responded favorably to these treatments, but many have experienced serious side effects and some have died. While immunotherapy remains a promising approach, it is not likely to offer significant help to cancer patients in the foreseeable future.

The Art of Visualization

The new field of psycho-neuroimmunology has provided some amazing insights into the mind-body-spirit connection. For example, several people diagnosed with terminal cancer so severe that no medical treatment was suggested, began to work with alternative methods of healing. To the surprise of many, their tumors went into remission. What was their secret? When these people were studied to find what they did to initiate their own healing process, one common theme emerged: a change in attitude. As director of Biofeedback Research at the Menninger Clinic in Topeka, Kansas, Dr. Patricia Norris has documented several cases where mental imagery and visualization were used successfully to complement traditional medical treatment. Dr. Norris cites eight specific characteristics which help to make mental imagery and visualization effective as a healing tool, specifically with regard to cancer. They include the following:

1. **Make the visualization personal.** The images must be self-generated. Images which are created by the practitioner and not the patient appear to be ineffective.

2. **Make the imagery "egosyntonic."** Egosyntonic means that the image must fit the values and ideals of that person. If, for example, the individual is pacifistic, then combative or warlike imagery will undermine the effectiveness of this type of treatment.

3. **Make the imagery positive.** Negative imagery reinforces negative thoughts, which are not conducive to healing. As an example, Norris notes that sharks, as a healing image, are not a good idea.

4. **Take an active role in the imagery.** Rather than imagining watching the imagery on a movie screen, you must feel the sensations of your images in the first person. You must have a sense that what you are seeing is happening inside your body, not "out there somewhere."

5. **Make the image anatomically correct and accurate.** Knowing exactly what body region and physiological system is in a disease state will dictate the type of imagery used. Consequently, you need to know whether to access the central nervous system or the immune system. Norris states that more than one image can be used in the healing process.

6. **Be constant, use dialogue.** Constancy means to be regular in generating your imagery. Norris suggests three 15-minute sessions per day, with intermittent shorter sessions throughout the day. When you feel pain, your body is communicating to you. She suggests making pain your friend. In the dialogue style of self-talk, she suggests thanking the pain for making you aware of the problem so that you may be able to fix it. Finally, she suggests "destroying" a tumor with its permission. Respond with love. Make peace with your body.

7. **Create a blueprint.** The concept of the blueprint is a strategy. A blueprint visualization is like time lapse photography where a flower (symbolizing a tumor) is shown to bloom within seconds, and then closes up again and fades away. An example would be to see the construction of a building, starting from the hole in the earth to opening day where you are cutting the ribbon at the front entrance.

8. **Include the treatment in the imagery.** Norris has found that patients who use mental imagery with chemotherapy treatment and radiation do better than those who "fight" these medical procedures. She notes that it helps to have benevolent feelings versus ambivalent feelings toward the treatment. She suggests one mentally "welcome the treatment into the body." Consider the treatment as a guest in your house. Based on her patient research, she offers these examples:

   a) *Chemotherapy*—a gold-colored fluid that healthy cells, acting as a bucket brigade, pass along to the cancer cells, who in turn drink up the chemotherapy.

   b) *Radiation treatment*—a stream of silver energy aimed at the cancerous tumor(s). Ask the white blood cells to move away or to shield themselves and act like mirrors to reflect the radiation toward the cancer cells, then watch the cancer cells die.

resentment, deeply felt personal loss, and feelings of hopelessness may be important factors in cancer development and lowering of disease resistance.

The coping strategies for dealing with the emotional distress resulting from cancer, AIDS, and other serious diseases are similar. They all depend on using the mind in positive ways. The effectiveness of any therapy and the ability to cope with a life-threatening illness depend on focusing the mind on ways to enhance the healing process. Meditation and relaxation techniques are important in reducing stress. Learning how to use visual imagery can help with the effectiveness of treatments. Along with mental relaxation techniques, the mind can focus on images and suggestions that may help the

Examples of Belief Causing Tumors to Disappear

A dramatic illustration of the power of belief in altering the course of cancer is the case of Mr. Wright, a patient in the 1950s. At that time, a drug called krebiozen was touted by some as a "miracle drug" that could cure cancer. Mr. Wright, who had terminal lymphosarcoma, was given a life expectancy of two weeks by his physician. However, Mr. Wright had enormous faith in the miracle drug and insisted that he be treated with it. After a single injection, his doctor noted that "the tumor masses had melted like snowballs on a hot stove, and in only these few days, they were half their original size" (Klopfer, 1957).

Mr. Wright was symptom free for two months until he read in the newspaper that krebiozen was worthless in treating cancer, whereupon he relapsed and was readmitted to the hospital. With nothing to lose, his doctor assured him that a fresh, double-strength injection of krebiozen would cure him. In actuality, Mr. Wright received an injection of water. Nevertheless, he again was symptom free for two months. Then headlines again proclaimed "nationwide tests show krebiozen to be a worthless drug in treatment of cancer." Mr. Wright relapsed and died in two days.

In 1994, a case was reported in which a 50-year-old man had been treated for three years for what he thought was a mild blood disorder. He actually had a very mild case of leukemia, but had never been told this. One day he saw the word "leukemia" in notes on his physician's desk. Three weeks later he was dead from having seen the diagnosis of leukemia (Hewlett, 1994).

STUDENT REFLECTIONS

- Provide an example of how faith was crucial in healing someone in your experience.
- Do you think Mr. Wright would have died if he had not heard that krebiozen was a worthless drug?

immune system fight and destroy cancer cells (Figure 13.8).

Studies have shown that psychosocial support and group therapy have a very positive effect on the survival rate of women with metastatic breast cancer (Spiegel et al., 1989). O. Carl Simonton, a physician, also pioneered the use of mental imagery in the healing process. He and his wife used meditation, biofeedback, hypnosis, and image visualization to help cancer patients fight their disease (Simonton and Shook, 1986). Hypnosis, medita-

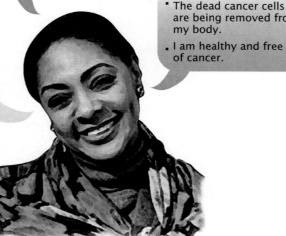

- The army of white blood cells is vast and destroys the cancer cells.
- The white blood cells are aggressive and destroy the cancer cells.
- The dead cancer cells are being removed from my body.
- I am healthy and free of cancer.
- The cancer cells are weak and confused.
- The treatment is strong and powerful.
- The healthy cells can repair any slight damage the treatment might do.

FIGURE 13.8 Positive Mental Images and Suggestions for Dealing with Cancer

tion, placebo effects, and faith can all affect the course of cancer, even cancer that is considered terminal.

Coping with cancer requires courage and conviction. A cancer patient must not give up hope despite what the statistics predict or what physicians say about the prognosis. The patient must believe that a cure is possible and work toward that end. For many people, coping with cancer is a transforming experience and gives renewed meaning to life.

The most important thing to remember to avoid getting cancer later in life is to abstain from using any tobacco and to follow a diet rich in fresh fruits and vegetables. Also avoid exposure to excess sunlight and to chemicals that are known to be carcinogenic.

HEALTH IN REVIEW

- Cancer refers to a number of different diseases, all of which share the common property of abnormal, unregulated cell growth in the body.
- Dietary factors and environmental agents, such as smoking and sunlight, act on the genetic material in cells to cause chemical changes that may initiate a tumor, which is a mass of abnormal cells.
- Both breast and testicular self-examinations are positive means of early cancer detection.
- The principal environmental agents that cause cancer are ionizing radiation, tumor viruses, and carcinogenic chemicals.
- If everything known about cancer prevention were practiced, up to two-thirds of cancers would not occur; thus cancer is largely a preventable disease.
- Only 5 to 10 percent of cancers are caused by genes that have been inherited. The genetic changes in body cells that result in cancer are not passed on to children, as these genetic changes have not occurred in sperm or eggs.

- The goal of all three cancer treatments is the removal or destruction of as many cancer cells as possible. The treatments for cancer include: surgery; radiation; and chemotherapy.
- Recovery from cancer depends on good nutrition, positive attitudes, healing mental images, and medical treatment appropriate for the particular cancer. A healthy, active immune system also is an essential component in cancer prevention and recovery.
- Cigarette smoking is responsible for about one-third of all cancers, especially lung cancer.
- Dietary deficiencies or excesses are responsible for about one-half of all cancers.
- Overexposure to sunlight causes skin cancer, which is increasing.
- Significantly reducing cancer requires major changes in peoples' life-styles, including more attention to a healthy diet, elimination of tobacco use, limiting alcohol consumption, and reducing exposure to intense sunlight and chemical carcinogens.

REFERENCES

American Cancer Society (1995). *Cancer Facts and Figures, 1995.*

Beardsley, T. (1994). "A War Not Won." *Scientific American,* January.

Davis, D. L., and H. P. Freeman (1994). "An Ounce of Prevention." *Scientific American,* September.

Downer, S. M., M. M. Cody, P. McCuskey, and P. D. Wilson (1994). "Pursuit and Practice of Complementary Therapies by Cancer Patients Receiving Conventional Treatment." *British Medical Journal,* 309: 6947.

Hewlett, C. (1994). "Killed By a Word." *The Lancet,* 344: 8923.

Klopfer, B. (1957). "Psychological Variables in Human Cancer." *Journal of Prospective Techniques,* 21: 331–340.

Liotta, L. A. (1992). "Cancer Cell Invasion and Metastasis." *Scientific American,* February.

Nowak, R. (1994). "Breast Cancer Gene Offers Surprises." *Science,* September 23.

Richards, E. (1991). *Vitamin C and Cancer: Medicine or Politics?* New York: St. Martin's Press, 1991.

Rosenberg, S. A. (1990). "Adoptive Immunotherapy for Cancer." *Scientific American,* May.

Shields, P. G., and C. C. Harris (1991). "Molecular Epidemiology and the Genetics of Environmental Cancer." *Journal of the American Medical Association,* 266(5): 681–687.

Simonton, S. M., and R. L. Shook (1986). *The Healing Family: The Simonton Approach for Families Facing Illness.* New York: Bantam.

Spiegel, D., J. R. Bloom, H. C. Kraemer, and E. Gottheil (1989). "Effect of Psychosocial Treatment on Survival of Patients with Metastatic Breast Cancer." *The Lancet,* 8668: 888–891.

SUGGESTED READINGS

American Cancer Society. *Cancer Facts and Figures.* Published yearly by the American Cancer Society and available at any branch of the society. Contains the latest statistics on all forms of cancer.

Beardsley, T. (1994). "A War Not Won." *Scientific American,* January. Explains why the "war on cancer" has been largely unsuccessful.

Cooper, G. M. (1993). *The Cancer Book.* Boston: Jones and Bartlett. Excellent explanations of all aspects of cancer and treatments.

Cowley, G. (1993). "Family Matters: The Hunt for a Breast Cancer Gene." *Newsweek,* December 6. Describes the search for cancer-susceptibility genes in high-risk families.

Lerner, M. (1994). *Choices in Healing: Integrating the Best of Conventional and Complementary Approaches to Cancer.* Cambridge, Mass.: MIT Press. Discusses both conventional and alternative treatments for cancer.

Price, R. (1994). *A Whole New Life.* New York: Atheneum. A famous author copes with a spinal tumor that leaves him paralyzed and in pain. An inspired story of overcoming cancer.

Richards, E. (1991). *Vitamin C and Cancer: Medicine or Politics?* New York: St. Martin's Press. The fascinating history of the health controversy over vitamin C.

Winawer, S. J., and M. Shike. (1995). *Cancer Free: A Comprehensive Prevention Program.* New York: Simon and Schuster. Everything you can do to reduce your risk of cancer.

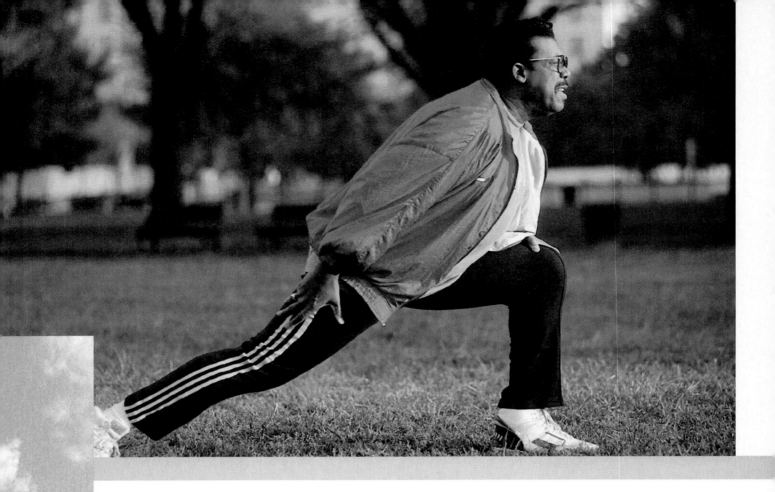

LEARNING OBJECTIVES

After reading this chapter you should be able to:

1. Describe how the heart functions.
2. Define cardiovascular disease, infarction, heart disease, stroke, and heart attack.
3. Explain the role atherosclerosis plays in heart disease.
4. Identify and explain several types of heart surgeries.
5. Identify the major risk factors of heart disease that cannot be changed, major risk factors that can be changed, and other contributing factors.
6. Identify three vitamins and explain their contribution to reducing heart disease.

Cardiovascular Diseases

Understanding Risks and Measures of Prevention

*T*he human heart has long been a symbol of human love expressed in poetry, stories, and everyday customs. Our language still reflects the idea that love and feelings reside in the heart. When love relationships collapse people refer to their "broken hearts" or the "heartlessness" of the former lover. People are described by the nature of their hearts—cruel, kind, warm, or cold; some are even referred to as having a heart of stone. When people refer to distressing experiences in life they talk of "heartache" and when they are happy, their heart may "leap with joy."

Today we know that emotions, thoughts, and feelings of every kind originate in the brain, not the heart. The heart's only function is to pump blood and circulate it throughout the body. The heart is an extraordinarily effective pump; it pumps slightly more than a gallon of blood per minute through approximately 60,000 miles of blood vessels in the body. In this gallon of blood are about 25 trillion red blood cells that carry oxygen from the lungs to all the body's cells and remove the carbon dioxide that is exhaled as waste. Each day about 200 billion new red blood cells are synthesized in bone marrow (the soft material at the center of large bones), and released into the circulation. Each day the heart expands and contracts (heart beat) 100,000 times and pumps about 2,000 gallons of blood (Heart and Stroke Facts, 1994). Maintaining healthy heart and blood vessels is essential for survival.

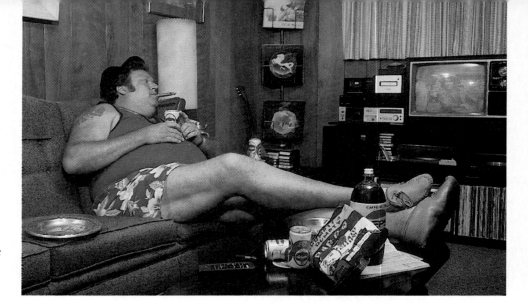

Risk factors for cardiovascular disease include being overweight, a sedentary life-style, smoking, and drinking alcohol.

UNDERSTANDING CARDIOVASCULAR DISEASES

Cardiovascular disease refers to any of a number of conditions that damage the heart or the arteries that carry blood to and from the heart. If the **coronary arteries** (the large blood vessels that carry blood to and from the heart) become diseased or blocked, a **heart attack** may result. If the cells of the heart do not receive a continual supply of blood and oxygen, the cells die, a condition known as an **infarction.** If the blood supply to the heart is only partially blocked, the process is known as **ischemia.**

According to current estimates more than 56 million Americans have some form of cardiovascular disease (Heart and Stroke Facts, 1994). More than 40 percent of all deaths each year in the United States are due to cardiovascular diseases that lead to heart attacks and **strokes.** A stroke occurs when there is damage to the brain due to an insufficient supply of blood to brain cells. While cardiovascular diseases tend to occur in the elderly, heart attacks can occur at any age, often without warning.

The rate of deaths due to cardiovascular diseases has been declining steadily in the United States for about 30 years (Figure 14.1). Certainly public awareness of the risk factors in cardiovascular disease has been a major contributor to the decline. Less fat and cholesterol in the diet, less cigarette smoking, and more exercising have all contributed to reducing deaths from cardiovascular disease. Like cancer, most heart disease is preventable and is caused primarily by unhealthy life-styles.

The Heart and Blood Vessels

The circulatory system consists of the heart (the pump) and the various blood vessels (Figure 14.2). **Arteries** carry oxygenated blood from the heart to all organs and tissues in the body. **Veins** return blood to the heart after oxygen and nutrients have been exchanged for carbon dioxide and waste products. **Capillaries** are tiny blood vessels that branch out from arteries and veins and circulate blood to all of the cells in the body. Blood vessels

FIGURE 14.1 Age-adjusted Death Rates from Heart Disease, Stroke, and Hypertension (high blood pressure) Note the steady decline in deaths from heart disease that began around 1965 and has continued to the present.
Source: Heart and Stroke Facts, 1994 (Dallas, Tex: American Heart Association, 1994).

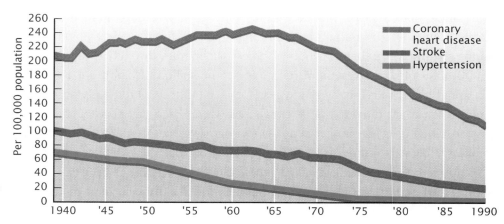

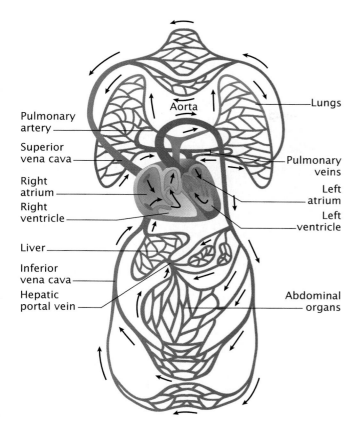

Pulmonary artery

Superior vena cava

Right atrium

Right ventricle

Liver

Inferior vena cava

Hepatic portal vein

Aorta

Lungs

Pulmonary veins

Left atrium

Left ventricle

Abdominal organs

FIGURE 14.2   The Circulatory System   Includes the heart, arteries, and veins. The heart receives oxygenated blood from the lungs and pumps it to all tissues in the body.

can be damaged by injury or by disease; this damage may obstruct the flow of blood carrying oxygen and nutrients.

The organ that keeps the blood circulating throughout the body is the heart, a highly specialized muscle about the size of an adult fist that pumps blood (Figure 14.3). The muscular wall of the heart is called the **myocardium.** If the blood supply to heart cells is blocked, cells begin to die and a heart attack results.

The heart consists of four separate chambers: the upper two chambers are called the left atrium and the right atrium; the lower two chambers are the right ven-

tricle and the left ventricle (Figure 14.4). Blood that is depleted of oxygen returns to the heart via the right atrium and then flows to the right ventricle. From there blood is pumped to the lungs where it is reoxygenated and returned via the pulmonary artery to the left atrium. Finally, the fresh blood is pumped throughout the body's tissues from the left ventricle through the large artery called the **aorta.**

The heart contracts from 65 to 70 times a minute depending on the body's activity. The entire volume of blood in the body is recirculated almost once every minute. During an average lifetime of 70 years, the heart will pump between 30 to 40 million gallons of blood, and it will beat 2.5 billion times!

A healthy heart beats rhythmically at a pace initiated by the heart itself. In the right atrium a region called the **sinoatrial node** (pacemaker) generates an electric signal that causes the heart to contract and pump blood. The pace of the heartbeat, however, is also influenced by electrical signals from the brain, which explains how emotions, excitement, or stress can suddenly change the rhythm of the heartbeat.

The heartbeat also can be affected by nerve impulses that originate in areas of the heart other than the sinoatrial node. If these signals interfere with the normal heartbeat, causing different areas of the heart to beat

TERMS

cardiovascular disease: any disease that causes damage to the heart or to arteries that carry blood to and from the heart

coronary arteries: two arteries arising from the aorta that supply blood to the heart muscle

heart attack: death of, or damage to, part of the heart muscle due to an insufficient blood supply

infarction: death of heart cells due to a blocked blood supply

ischemia: an insufficient supply of blood to the heart

stroke: an insufficient supply of blood to the brain resulting in loss of muscle function, loss of speech, or other symptoms

arteries: any one of a series of blood vessels that carry blood from the heart to all parts of the body

veins: blood vessels that return blood from tissues to the heart

capillaries: extremely small blood vessels that carry oxygenated blood to tissues

myocardium: muscular wall of the heart that contracts and relaxes

aorta: the large artery that transports blood from the heart to the body

sinoatrial node: the region of the heart that produces an electrical signal that causes the heart to contract

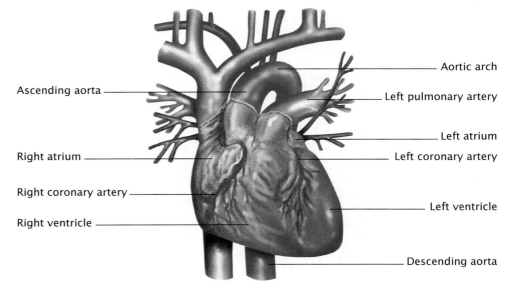

Aortic arch

Ascending aorta

Left pulmonary artery

Left atrium

Right atrium

Left coronary artery

Right coronary artery

Left ventricle

Right ventricle

Descending aorta

FIGURE 14.3   The Heart and the Major Arteries
Oxygenated blood is pumped through the arteries (red) and oxygen-depleted blood is returned to the heart via the veins (blue).

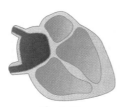
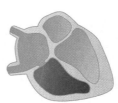
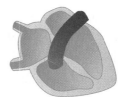

First stage
Entering right atrium from body

Second stage
Flowing to right ventricle

Third stage
Flowing to lungs through pulmonary artery

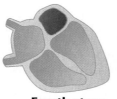
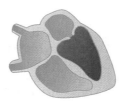
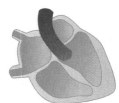

Fourth stage
Returning from lungs to left atrium

Fifth stage
Flowing to left ventricle

Sixth stage
Flowing out of aorta to body

FIGURE 14.4   Blood Circulates through the Four Separate Chambers of the Heart

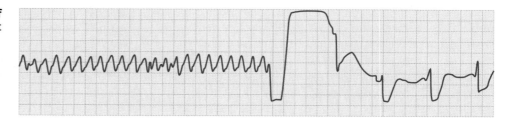

FIGURE 14.5   A Recording of a Heart Beating   The first part shows the heart in fibrillation, with weak, irregular beats. The second part shows the heart returned to a normal heartbeat.
Source: Heart and Stroke Facts, 1994 (Dallas, Tex.: American Heart Association, 1994).

independently of one another, the result is **fibrillation** (Figure 14.5). While fibrillation may precede a heart attack, many people have an irregular heartbeat without being at risk for a heart attack. Irregular heartbeat can be controlled by a **pacemaker,** a small electrical device that is implanted in a person's chest and provides a steadying electrical signal to the heart.

Regulating Blood Flow

To maintain uniform blood flow in the correct direction through arteries and veins, the cardiovascular system is equipped with one-way valves both in the chambers of the heart and in blood vessels (Figure 14.6). With every heartbeat, the valves in the heart open and close to allow

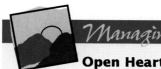

Managing Stress

Open Heart Meditation

Dr. Dean Ornish received much notice recently when he proved that the build-up of plaque along the inner linings of the coronary arteries could be reversed. Unlike others who created earlier rehabilitation programs combining exercise and nutrition, Ornish added support group interaction and meditation to the exercise and nutrition formula with great success. Ornish believed that meditation was a crucial factor in reversing heart disease, and was convinced there was a connection between the hardened arteries and one's level of anger or what he called a "hardened heart."

The following is a meditation exercise similar to that used by Ornish. Its aim is to increase our capacity to show compassion and understanding to all we encounter, and to forgive and let go of issues and feelings which hold us hostage.

- Sit in a comfortable position, keeping your back straight.

- Begin to concentrate on your breathing by sensing the flow of air into your mouth or nose, down into your lungs, and begin to feel your stomach extend as you inhale and return as you exhale. Repeat this five times.

- Focus on your upper chest, specifically the middle of your upper chest.

- Now for each breath, feel as though you are taking air in through this area of your chest, breathing slowly and easily, comfortably slow and deep. Follow this with five more breaths and feel a sense of relaxation each time you exhale.

- Now imagine that just outside your chest bone (sternum) there is a bud of flower (you can use any image you wish, such as an elevator door, a book, a window, etc.). Visualize this flower bud and allow yourself to see the bud begin to open into a wonderfully beautiful flower. What color petals do you see? Imagine the petals grow and expand.

- Think of this flower (or your chosen symbol) as a symbol of compassion. Imagine what compassion feels like. If this feeling does not come easily, imagine holding a newborn puppy, or recreate the feeling of the happiest moment of your life. Think of the feeling in your mind, but feel it in your heart.

- As you breathe, continue to breathe through your chest and with each exhalation, feel the sensation of compassion.

- Once you have this feeling, think of someone you would like to share this feeling with (e.g., a friend, a parent, a child, a pet) and imagine a rainbow from your heart to theirs. Take five slow breaths, and with each breath think and feel this expression of compassion to that person as you exhale.

- Sharing love with someone you care for is wonderful, but it's also easy compared to sending compassion to someone whom you feel violated against. Comb your mind for a moment and find someone with whom you are not at peace. Picture this person in front of you now. Realize that feelings of anger are toxic when left unresolved. Slowly take another deep breath through the heart area and as you exhale send a message of compassion to this person visualized in front of you. If it seems that a message of love is too difficult you can begin with a message of acknowledging his or her humanness.

- Remember to keep your symbolic image open as you send this thought and feeling to this person. And know that by opening up your heart you begin to release feelings associated with a hardened heart.

Try this meditation technique a couple of times per week. At first it may seem hard not to feel vulnerable, but with time you will find this exercise not only im-proves your emotional health, but your physical and spiritual health as well.

---

blood to circulate in one direction. In rare cases, one or more of the heart valves may be defective at birth because of developmental abnormalities. With modern techniques of open-heart surgery, defective heart valves can be repaired or replaced with artificial valves that allow the heart to function normally.

Heart valves can also be damaged by childhood throat infections caused by *streptococcus* bacteria. Repeated streptococcal infections can cause rheumatic heart disease (formerly called rheumatic fever), a serious inflammatory disease of the heart valves. In susceptible people, the immune system overreacts to the presence of the bacteria. Some proteins on the heart cells are similar in structure to proteins on the bacteria, so the immune

T E R M S

fibrillation: rapid, erratic contraction of the heart

pacemaker: an electrical device implanted in the chest to control the heartbeat

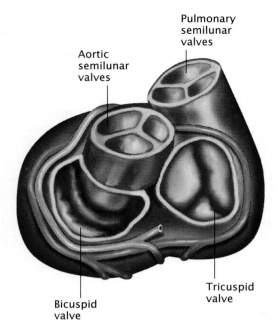

FIGURE 14.6 The heart's valves keep the blood flowing in one direction into and out of the chambers of the heart.

system attacks heart valve cells as well as the infectious bacteria.

The mitral and aortic valves are particularly susceptible to damage by infections. Scar tissue forms and prevents the valves from opening and closing correctly. By listening to the heartbeat, a **cardiologist,** a physician who specializes in heart diseases, can detect abnormalities in the heart's valves. Because of potential heart problems, it is important that all strep throats in children be treated with antibiotics to reduce the risk of developing rheumatic heart disease.

Another common, but less serious defect of the circulation, is in valves in the veins that cause **varicose veins.** These appear as unsightly, bluish bulges in veins and usually occur in the legs. Blood returning to the heart from the legs has to flow against the pull of gravity and one-way valves in the veins normally prevent the blood from draining downward. If the valves in the veins of the legs become weakened, blood tends to accumulate, distending the veins and producing visible varicose veins. The valve failures in the veins are not life threatening and often can be corrected by surgical removal of the damaged areas.

EFFECTS OF ATHEROSCLEROSIS

Arteriosclerosis, which literally means hardening of the arteries, includes all kinds of diseases that damage the arteries. However, the one form of arteriosclerosis that is of primary concern is **atherosclerosis** (Ross, 1993). This arterial disease begins with damage to cells of the heart's arteries and leads to the formation of a fibrous, fatty deposit called **plaque.** The arterial plaque slowly increases in size until eventually the amount of blood flowing through the artery is greatly reduced or completely blocked (Figure 14.7). The current model of how atherosclerosis blocks arteries indicates that the plaque ruptures and flips up like a "trap door" to effectively block the flow of blood through the artery.

Obstruction of blood flow in an artery is very serious because heart cells are deprived of oxygenated blood and die. Oxygen is supplied to the heart by the coronary arteries, which are the first to branch from the aorta. Despite its relatively small size, the heart uses about 20 percent of the total oxygenated blood circulated through the body.

If the coronary arteries become partially blocked and the heart cells do not get enough oxygen, chest pain called **angina pectoris** results. The drug nitroglycerin dilates blood vessels and is used to relieve the pain of angina. If a coronary artery becomes completely blocked, a person usually suffers a heart attack.

Health Update

New Blood Tests May Detect a Heart Attack Quickly

During a heart attack, the damaged tissues in the heart release certain proteins into the blood. Several tests are being developed that can detect changes in one or more of four different proteins: creatine kinase, tro- ponin, myoglobin, and myosin. Changes in the blood levels of these proteins can confirm or rule out a heart attack. With just a few drops of blood from the patient, the tests will give a result in minutes, so that appropriate life-saving procedures can be started. These tests are expected to be available in the near future (Hamm, 1994).

Diagnosing a Heart Attack

Each year in the United States more than a million people are admitted to hospitals because of possible heart attacks. Tests eventually rule out a heart attack in about 50 percent of those admitted. Chest pains that mimic those of a heart attack can be brought on by severe indigestion (heartburn), panic, and stress.

Distinguishing between a heart attack and less serious causes of chest pains is crucial if appropriate treatment is to be started. At present diagnosing a heart attack involves time-consuming and costly procedures. By the time a heart attack has been confirmed, it may be too late to save the patient. Generally, about 15 percent of patients admitted with a heart attack die in the hospital (Manson et al., 1992). Tests that could quickly distinguish heart attack from other causes of chest pain would save many lives.

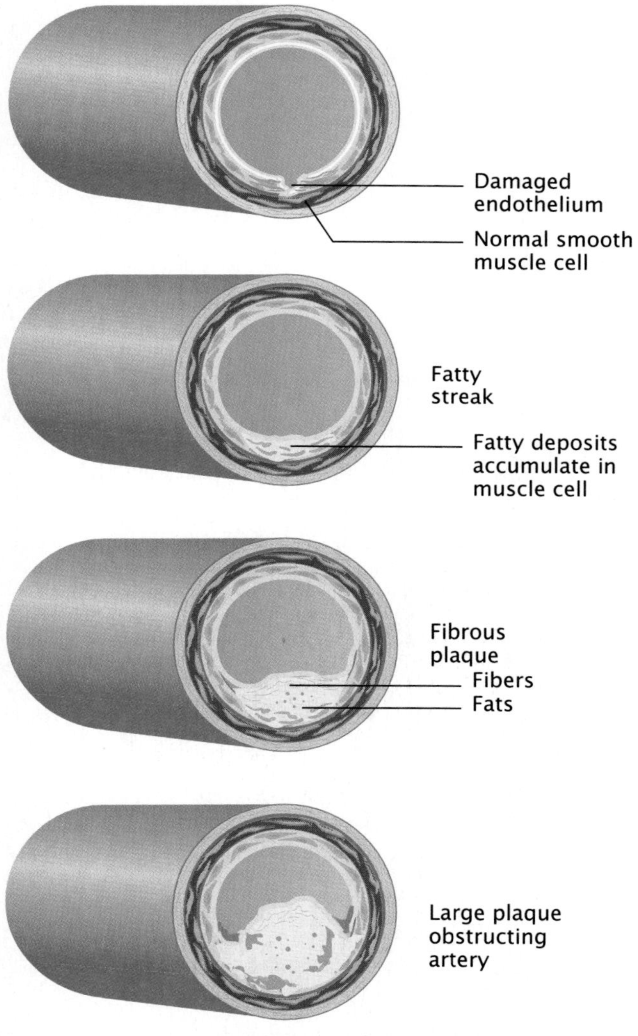

Repairing Blocked Arteries

When medical tests such as an **angiocardiography**, a procedure for visualizing the flow of blood through the coronary arteries and chambers of the heart, confirm that one or several coronary arteries are blocked and that blood flow to the heart is restricted, various kinds of surgery are usually recommended. In **coronary bypass surgery**, the diseased segment of an artery is cut out and a segment of a healthy vein or artery is grafted onto the damaged artery to restore normal flow of blood to the heart. If one graft is made into a blocked artery, the surgery is called a single coronary bypass; if four grafts are made it is called a quadruple bypass.

Coronary bypass surgery is a form of **open-heart surgery** and usually requires several months of recuperation. In open-heart surgery, while the heart is exposed and being repaired, the bloodstream is diverted through a heart-lung machine. More than 350,000 bypass surgeries are performed every year in the United States at an average cost of approximately $50,000. Although bypass surgeries are successful and save many lives, as many as half of bypass patients experience another arterial blockage within five years, especially if they do not modify their life-style to reduce the risk factors contributing to heart disease.

FIGURE 14.7 Development of an Atherosclerotic Lesion (Plaque) inside an Artery These plaques can eventually block blood flow, causing a heart attack or stroke. Many factors are suspected in the formation of a plaque, but none has been proven.

Labels on figure:
- Damaged endothelium
- Normal smooth muscle cell
- Fatty streak
- Fatty deposits accumulate in muscle cell
- Fibrous plaque
- Fibers
- Fats
- Large plaque obstructing artery

T E R M S

cardiologist: a physician who specializes in diseases of the heart

varicose veins: swelling of veins (usually in the legs) due to defective valves

arteriosclerosis: hardening of the arteries

atherosclerosis: a disease process in which fatty deposits build up in the arteries and block the flow of blood

plaque: deposit of fatty substances in the inner lining of arteries

angina pectoris: medical term for chest pain due to coronary heart disease; a condition in which the heart muscle doesn't receive enough blood, resulting in chest pain

angiocardiography: an X-ray examination of the coronary arteries and heart

coronary bypass surgery: surgery to improve blood supply to the heart muscle. Most often performed when narrowed coronary arteries reduce the flow of oxygenated blood to the heart

open-heart surgery: surgery performed on the opened heart while the blood supply is diverted through a heart-lung machine

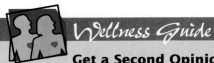
Get a Second Opinion before Undergoing Heart Surgery

High-tech surgical procedures, such as coronary bypass, angioplasty, and pacemaker implantation, have revolutionized the treatment of coronary heart disease (CHD). Each year in the U.S. approximately 300,000 coronary bypass operations are performed to unplug arteries that supply blood to the heart as shown in the figure below. While these surgeries prevent some heart attacks and save lives, in many instances they are performed for heart conditions that do not warrant surgery. Many CHD problems such as angina (chest pain) can be controlled with medications.

In the 1950s, angina pain from partially blocked coronary arteries was relieved by an operation in which a chest artery was tied off in the hope that more blood would be supplied to the patient's heart. About 40 percent of the patients felt better following this operation. To determine whether the relief of angina pain was a placebo effect or actually resulted form the surgery, a number of mock operations were performed. (In the 1950s, informed consent was not mandatory in most hospitals.) Patients were given anesthesia, the chest was cut open, but nothing else was done to correct blood flow to the heart. Patients who underwent mock surgeries had just as much relief from angina as patients who had the chest artery tied-off (Frank, 1975). As a result, this operation was abandoned.

In a similar fashion, coronary bypass operations may relieve angina due to the long period of rest and recuperation that patients undergo; life-style changes that people make also may contribute to their relief. A large part of the success of bypass surgery may be due to a placebo effect (Chapter 2).

Studies of the medical records of patients who were referred for a second opinion on their heart condition indicate that many coronary angiography tests are performed without sufficient medical justification. These tests are used to determine if bypass or angioplasty operations are necessary. The study found that at least 50 percent of all the angiograms performed to measure the extent of blockage in arteries were unnecessary. In addition to excessive use of diagnostic angiograms, overuse of balloon angioplasty operations, especially in the relief of angina, is very common and patients are advised to obtain another opinion before undergoing either procedure.

Another overused procedure is the implantation of pacemakers.

About one in 500 Americans has a permanent heart pacemaker in their chest to maintain a regular heartbeat. A large study of pacemaker implantation, paid for by Medicare, showed that at least 20 percent of the 1983 implants were "definitely medically unjustified." An additional 36 percent were "judged to be probably unnecessary" (Greenspan, 1988).

The overuse of high-tech medical diagnostic and surgical procedures has greatly inflated the costs of American health care. Unnecessary medical procedures also cause suffering and risk to life.

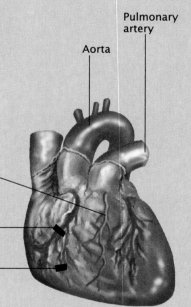

Block in coronary artery

Saphenous vein graft to left artery distal to block

Saphenous vein graft to diseased right coronary artery

Aorta

Pulmonary artery

Diagram of the coronary arteries showing where grafts are made to correct blockages.

An alternative surgical approach to opening a blocked artery is **balloon angioplasty.** In this procedure a thin wire is threaded from the femoral artery in the thigh up to the point of blockage in a coronary artery. Another thin tube containing a deflated balloon is then slipped over the wire and threaded up to the area of the arterial plaque. The balloon is inflated and pushes the plaque back into the wall of the artery thereby opening

T E R M S

balloon angioplasty: a procedure to open blocked arteries

aneurysm: a ballooning out of a vein or artery

carotid endarterectomy: removal of fatty deposits in arteries in the neck to prevent a stroke

angiogram: the X-ray image that is obtained from angiocardiography

it up. Angioplasty costs much less than a bypass operation, but the frequency with which the blockage recurs is quite high, making a repeat procedure necessary. About 300,000 angioplasty operations are performed each year in the United States.

Other high-technology devices for opening clogged arteries are being developed and clinically tested. These include high-speed rotary scrapers that grind away plaque and lasers that are threaded into the artery to melt or burn away plaque. Although these techniques for opening blocked arteries are valuable, in many instances heart and artery surgery may not be necessary.

Until recently, it was universally believed that atherosclerosis was a progressive and irreversible disease. However, an experiment with a small group of volunteers who had partial blockage of their arteries showed that this longstanding conviction is not necessarily correct. This study showed that over a period of a year, life-style changes could significantly reduce arterial blockage in over 80 percent of the experimental group (Ornish, 1990). While this study has been criticized for its methodology by some cardiologists, it does show that healthy life-style changes can halt or reverse the effects of heart disease.

Stroke

Stroke is a form of cardiovascular disease that affects arteries supplying blood to the brain. If a brain artery becomes blocked or ruptures, brain cells die within minutes due to lack of oxygen. Parts of the body that depend on these damaged or dead cells in the brain for functioning also are affected. Thus, a person suffering a stroke can lose the ability to speak, become paralyzed in an arm or leg, or lose the use of one whole side of the body. Strokes can result from injuries to the head or from weak spots in the arteries called **aneurysms** that balloon out and rupture. Strokes also can result when the heart beat is weak and the heart does not pump enough blood through the arteries to the brain. The effects of strokes vary greatly ranging from mild or unnoticed symptoms to sudden death.

Four kinds of strokes are defined medically; two are caused by the rupture and hemorrhage of an artery supplying blood to the brain, and two are caused by clots that block the flow of blood. Cerebral thrombosis and cerebral embolism are the most common types of stroke, accounting for about 70–80 percent of all strokes. These strokes are caused by clots that plug an artery. Cerebral and subarachnoid hemorrhages are caused by ruptured blood vessels. Although these types of strokes occur less frequently, they have a much higher fatality rate than strokes caused by clots (Heart and Stroke Facts, 1994).

The warning signs of a stroke are any of the following conditions that occur suddenly. Immediate medical attention is needed if any of the symptoms of stroke occur:

- Sudden weakness or numbness of the face, arm, or leg on one side of the body
- Sudden dimness or loss of vision, especially in one eye
- Loss of speech, difficulty understanding speech, or trouble talking
- Sudden, severe headaches with no known cause
- Unexplained unsteadiness, dizziness, or sudden falls, especially with one of the other symptoms

A surgical procedure called **carotid endarterectomy** removes fatty deposits from the main arteries in the neck that supply blood to the brain and is effective in reducing the risk of stroke (Fackelmann, 1994). Blocked neck arteries that pose a risk of stroke can be detected with a stethoscope or with an ultrasound scan. People over age 50 or with a family history of cardiovascular disease should have their physician examine their neck arteries for any sign of blockage.

The best way to prevent a stroke is to reduce the risk factors. There are five controllable risk factors for a stroke: 1) high blood pressure; 2) heart disease; 3) cigarette smoking; 4) transient ischemic attacks, and 5) high

Health Update

Life-style Changes Can Reverse the Effects of Heart Disease

It has long been known that habits such as smoking and overeating contribute to the risk of heart disease. What was not known until recently is that life-style changes can reverse the disease of atherosclerosis and reduce the risk of heart attack. The life-style changes that the patients agreed to make were: 1) adopt a low-fat vegetarian diet, 2) stop smoking, 3) attend a stress management training group, and 4) adhere to a moderate exercise program.

Angiograms are X-ray images of the arteries that show the extent of blockage. Angiograms were done before and after the life-style changes and showed that the amount of blockage in the arteries had been reduced after the changes had been maintained for a year. The important lesson from this study is that a healthy life-style can reverse cardiovascular disease to some degree in highly motivated patients. Other studies show that a healthy life-style helps to prevent the development of cardiovascular disease.

red blood cell count. These risk factors can, for the most part, be controlled by one's life-style. Factors resulting from heredity or natural processes can't be changed. Risk factors for a stroke that cannot be changed include: 1) increasing age; 2) being male; 3) race; 4) diabetes mellitus; 5) prior stroke; 6) heredity, and 7) **asymptomatic carotid bruit.**

Elevated blood cholesterol and lipids, physical inactivity, and obesity are considered controllable factors that indirectly increase the risk of stroke. These factors are referred to as secondary risk factors, because they affect the risk of stroke indirectly by increasing the risk of heart disease.

RISK FACTORS FOR CARDIOVASCULAR DISEASE

What starts the development of plaques in arteries that lead to cardiovascular disease, heart attacks, and strokes? No one knows for certain. Arterial plaques are found in the hearts of healthy young people who die accidentally, suggesting that the disease process begins early in life in some individuals. We also know that atherosclerosis is primarily a disease of modern, industrialized societies. Tribal people in New Guinea, !Kung tribes in Africa, and Eskimos in Greenland have a low incidence of cardiovascular disease. Tarahumara Indians in Mexico have virtually no heart disease or high blood pressure as long as they consume their native diet. However, when researchers switched a group of Tarahumara Indian volunteers to a typical American diet, they gained weight and had dramatic increases in lipid and cholesterol levels in their blood (McMurry et al., 1991).

Some studies indicate that environmental chemicals and pollutants may damage cells in the lining of the blood vessels and initiate the formation of plaques. Thus, the same factors that trigger changes in cells that lead to cancer may also be risk factors in cardiovascular disease. In particular, cigarette smoking, high blood cholesterol levels, and high blood pressure are well documented **risk factors** that contribute to the development of both atherosclerosis and heart disease (Figure 14.8).

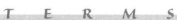

T E R M S

asyptomatic carotid bruit: an abnormal sound when a stethoscope is placed over the carotid artery

risk factor: an element or condition involving certain hazard or danger

high-density lipoprotein (HDL): the carrier of cholesterol from tissues to the liver for removal from the circulation; carrier of "good" cholesterol

low-density lipoprotein (LDL): the carrier of "bad" cholesterol in blood

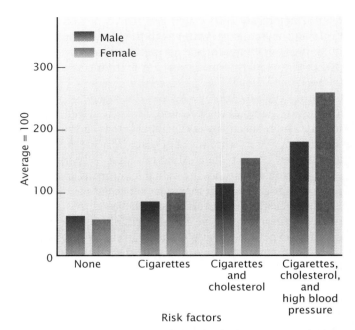

FIGURE 14.8 The increased risk of a heart attack from a cholesterol level above 260, a blood pressure of 150 systolic, and a pack-a-day smoker. The calculation is for a 55-year-old male or female.

TABLE 14.1 Amount of Cholesterol in Various Foods

Food	Cholesterol
Cream, 1 oz.	20 mg
Cottage cheese, 1/2 cup	24 mg
Ice cream, 1/2 cup	27 mg
Cheddar cheese, 1 oz.	28 mg
Whole milk, 1 cup	34 mg
Lard, 1 tablespoon	12 mg
Butter, 1 tablespoon	35 mg
Oysters, salmon, 3 oz.	40 mg
Clams, tuna, 3 oz.	55 mg
Beef, pork, lobster, chicken, turkey, 3 oz.	75 mg
Lamb, veal, crab, 3 oz.	85 mg
Shrimp, 3 oz.	130 mg
Beef heart, 3 oz.	230 mg
Egg, one yolk	250 mg
Liver, 3 oz.	370 mg
Kidney, 3 oz.	680 mg
Brains, 3 oz.	1,700 mg

The most common source of cholesterol in the diet is from egg yolk. The American Heart Association recommends a maximum daily cholesterol consumption of 300 mg. Only about half of the consumed cholesterol is absorbed. Additionally, the human liver itself synthesizes 1,000 to 1,500 mg a day.

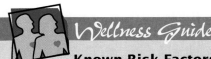
Known Risk Factors for Heart Disease

Major Risk Factors That Cannot Be Changed

- **Heredity:** Both heart disease and atherosclerosis appear to be linked to heredity. If your parents have had heart disease, or if you are an African-American, your risk of heart disease is greater than that of the population at large.

- **Being male:** Men have a greater risk of heart disease than women early in life. However, after women reach menopause their death rate due to heart disease increases. Research indicates the potential reason for this is the decrease in estrogen after menopause.

- **Increasing age:** The majority of people who die from heart attacks are age 65 or older.

Major Risk Factors That Can Be Changed

- **Cigarette/tobacco smoke:** People who smoke are two times at risk of a heart attack than those who do not smoke. Cigarette smoking is the greatest risk factor for sudden cardiac death. Studies also indicate that chronic exposure to environmental tobacco smoke exposure increases the risk of heart disease.

- **High blood cholesterol:** As your blood cholesterol level increases, so does your risk of coronary heart disease. A person's cholesterol level is affected by age, gender, heredity, and diet. With other risk factors such as high blood pressure and cigarette/tobacco smoke, your risk of coronary heart disease increases even more.

- **High blood pressure (HBP):** High blood pressure is sometimes referred to as the "silent killer," because there are no specific symptoms or early warning signs. Eating properly, losing weight, exercising, and restricting sodium all will help reduce HBP. People with high blood pressure should work with their doctor to control it.

- **Physical inactivity:** Physical inactivity is a risk factor for heart disease. Regular aerobic exercise plays a significant role in preventing heart disease; even modest levels of low intensity physical activity are beneficial if done regularly and long term.

Other Contributing Factors

- **Diabetes:** More than 80 percent of people with diabetes die of some form of heart disease or blood vessel disease.

- **Obesity:** If you are overweight, overfat, or obese you are more likely than a person of normal weight to have heart disease, despite the fact you may not have any other risk factors.

- **Individual response to stress:** There is some evidence of a relationship between coronary heart disease and stress, behavior habits, and socioeconomic status.

Source: Adapted from *Heart and Stroke Facts* (1994) (Dallas, Tex.: American Heart Association).

Physical inactivity, stress, and high levels of glucose in the blood are additional factors that contribute to the occurrence of heart attacks once the blood supply to the heart has been restricted.

Cholesterol

Cholesterol is an essential component of body cells and is synthesized in the body as well as being obtained from food (Table 14.1). Cholesterol circulates in the blood mostly in the form of particles consisting of proteins, triglycerides (fats), and cholesterol. These particles are divided into two kinds. Called **high-density lipoproteins (HDL)** and **low-density lipoproteins (LDL)**, their functions are different and, in some sense, are opposite to one another. Other kinds of cholesterol-carrying particles also are found in the blood, but these are ultimately converted into LDL particles.

The cholesterol that gets deposited in plaques and blocks the arteries comes mainly from LDL particles. As LDL particles circulate in the blood, cholesterol is used by tissues to build new cells. Any excess cholesterol is processed in the liver and the cholesterol level in the blood is maintained by regulatory mechanisms in the liver. Receptor proteins on the surface of liver cells bind

HEALTHY PEOPLE 2000

Increase to at least 75 percent the proportion of adults who have had their blood cholesterol checked within the preceding five years.

Data from 1988 indicates that only 59 percent of people ages 18 and older had "ever" had their cholesterol checked. Identifying those with high blood cholesterol not only allows the health profession to help control the cholesterol but also allows them an opportunity to educate about the risk factors of coronary heart disease.

Cardiac Risk Assessment

Changing Your Habits

Take the cardiac risk assessment test. Make a list of any habits you have that might contribute to heart disease. Resolve to change at least one of these habits for a given period of time. Then try to make the healthy new habit a permanent part of your life-style.

Cardiac Risk Assessment Test

Listed below are eight categories that pertain to the health of your heart. Select the number in each category that applies to you. If you don't know your blood cholesterol level, assume that it is less than 200 mg, which is the case for most college students of normal weight. You can estimate your risk by comparing your score with the risk table shown at the end of the test.

1. *Age*	10 to 20	21 to 30	31 to 40	41 to 50	51 to 60	61 to 70 and over
	1	2	3	4	6	8
2. *Heredity*	No known history of heart disease	1 relative with cardio-vascular dis-ease over 60	2 relatives with cardio-vascular dis-ease	1 relative with cardio-vascular dis-ease under 60	2 relatives with cardio-vascular dis-ease under 60	3 relatives with cardio-vascular dis-ease under 60
	1	2	3	4	6	8
3. *Weight*	More than 5 lbs below standard weight	Standard weight	5–20 lbs overweight	21–35 lbs overweight	36–50 lbs overweight	51–65 lbs overweight
	0	1	2	3	5	7
4. *Tobacco smoking*	Nonuser	Cigar and/or pipe	10 cigarettes or less a day	20 cigarettes a day	30 cigarettes a day	40 cigarettes a day or more
	0	1	2	3	5	8

LDL particles and remove excess cholesterol. If the liver is overwhelmed with LDL particles, it may not be able to process all of them. When that occurs, too much cholesterol circulates in the blood and may be deposited in the walls of the arteries. Because LDL particles carry the cholesterol that is deposited in plaques, they are often referred to as carrying "bad" cholesterol.

HDL particles are produced in the liver and intestines and are released into the bloodstream. As HDL particles circulate through the body, they pick up cholesterol and return it to the liver for removal. Thus, HDL particles scavenge excess cholesterol from the blood and arteries, thereby reducing the buildup of plaques. For these reasons, HDL particles are often referred to as carriers of "good" cholesterol (Figure 14.9).

People differ markedly in their ability to process excess cholesterol, just as they differ in other traits governed by genes. The most dramatic example of cholesterol metabolism is that of an 88-year-old man who had eaten twenty-five eggs a day for over fifteen years and yet

had completely normal blood cholesterol levels (Kern, 1991).

At the other extreme of the body's ability to process cholesterol are persons with a rare inherited disease called **familial hyperlipidemia (FH)** that results in markedly elevated levels of cholesterol in the blood. People with this disease have two defective genes, one inherited from each unaffected parent. The normal forms of these genes are responsible for synthesizing LDL receptor proteins on liver cells that bind LDL particles and remove cholesterol from the blood. As a result of their defective genes, people with FH cannot synthesize these essential LDL receptor proteins. Cholesterol cannot be removed and processed in the liver, and it accumulates to exceptionally high levels in the blood. People with

T E R M

familial hyperlipidemia (FH): an inherited disease causing extremely high levels of cholesterol in the blood

5. *Exercise*	Intensive occupational and recreational exertion **1**	Moderate occupational and recreational exertion **2**	Sedentary work and intense recreational exertion **3**	Sedentary occupational and moderate recreational exertion **5**	Sedentary work and light recreational exertion **6**	Complete lack of all exercise **8**
6. *Cholesterol or percent fat in diet*	Cholesterol below 180 mg. Diet contains no animal or solid fats **1**	Cholesterol 181–205 mg. Diet contains 10% animal or solid fats **2**	Cholesterol 206–230 mg. Diet contains 20% animal or solid fats **3**	Cholesterol 231–255 mg. Diet contains 30% animal or solid fats **4**	Cholesterol 256–280 mg. Diet contains 40% animal or solid fats **5**	Cholesterol 281–330 mg. Diet contains 50% animal or solid fats **7**
7. *Blood pressure*	100 upper reading **1**	120 upper reading **2**	140 upper reading **3**	160 upper reading **4**	180 upper reading **5**	200 or over upper reading **7**
8. *Sex*	Female under 45 **1**	Female over 45 **2**	Male **3**	Bald male **4**	Bald, short male **6**	Bald, short stocky male **7**

Your total score _____

Degree of risk

6 to 11 = Very low risk   26 to 32 = High risk
12 to 17 = Low risk   33 to 42 = Dangerous risk
18 to 25 = Average risk   42 to 60 = Extremely dangerous risk

Source: Adapted from a test designed by John L. Boyer.

this disease usually suffer heart attacks at an early age. In a few cases, transplant of a normal liver has successfully reversed the effects of FH to a significant degree.

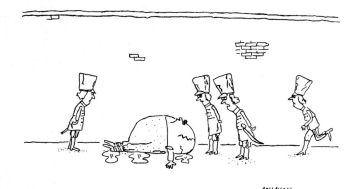

FIGURE 14.9 "Someone Said He Was Depressed about His Cholesterol Level"
Copyright John Callahan, courtesy Levin Represents.

Cholesterol and lipid levels in the blood are measured in various ways. Total cholesterol levels are measured in milligrams per deciliter (mg/dl) of blood. Generally, a cholesterol level below 200 mg/dl indicates relatively low risk of coronary heart disease (CHD); 240 mg/dl or higher doubles the risk of CHD. Blood cholesterol values between 200–239 mg/dl indicate moderate and increasing risk of CHD. However, the total cholesterol level may not be a reliable indicator of cardiovascular disease risk because the level of HDL in the blood is also important and can modify the risk due to high cholesterol levels.

For example, a cholesterol level of 240 might not be considered dangerous if your HDL level also was high. Generally, if the ratio of the total cholesterol divided by the HDL level is about 4.5, the risk is said to be average. A ratio above 4.5 increases the risk of heart disease; a ratio below 4.5 reduces it. The various numbers used to establish the risk of heart disease are quite confusing but the general rules are explained in the Wellness Guide,

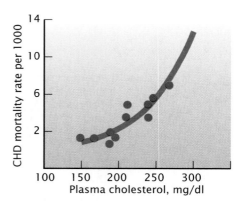

FIGURE 14.10 Death from heart disease in males increases as the level of cholesterol in blood increases. The relative risk is three times greater in a man with a cholesterol level of 250 compared to a man with a level of 200. These data were obtained by studying thousands of men over many years in the Multiple Risk Factor Intervention Trial.

"How to Interpret Blood Cholesterol and Lipid Measurements."

Research on human populations that consume different diets has shown a strong association between blood cholesterol levels and cardiovascular disease deaths (Figure 14.10). However, many epidemiological studies also show either no connection or little connection between the kind of diet and blood cholesterol levels. For example, the French enjoy a diet laden with eggs, meats, and fats. They have cholesterol levels that, on average, are much higher than those of Americans. Yet the French die of heart disease at less than half the rate observed in the United States (sometimes called the "French paradox"). Nobody can give a satisfactory explanation for the discrepancy; some heart experts attribute it to drinking wine with meals (which may reduce stress) and eating more vegetables (which may be protective in some way). Cholesterol level is a risk factor for cardiovascular disease, but the level at which it becomes a risk is still extremely controversial.

High Blood Pressure

Medical surveys indicate that one in every four Americans suffers from **hypertension**, blood pressure that is above the range that is considered normal. About one-third of these individuals is unaware of their hypertension, which contributes to development of heart disease.

 Wellness Guide

How to Interpret Blood Cholesterol and Lipid Measurements

In evaluating your risk of heart and artery disease, the level of four different "fat" molecules are measured: cholesterol, high-density lipoprotein (HDL), triglycerides, and low-density lipoprotein (LDL). The range of values for each is indicated below.

Cholesterol

• Below 200 mg/dl: safe. Unless the HDL level is below 35 mg/dl.

• 200 to 239: borderline high. If you have other risk factors for heart disease such as high blood pressure or an HDL level below 35 mg/dl, then you are at risk and some corrective action is needed.

• Above 240: high. Further tests are needed; dietary changes, as well as drugs to lower the level, may be recommended.

High-density Lipoprotein

• 35 mg/dl: low. Exercise and other steps may be needed to raise the level. Women generally have higher levels of HDL than men.

• 35 to 60: considered protective, especially if cholesterol levels are below 240.

Triglycerides

• Below 200 mg/dl: considered normal range.

• 200 to 400 mg/dl: borderline high.

• Above 400 mg/dl: high. Dietary changes recommended.

Low-density Lipoprotein

LDL is not measured directly, but levels are calculated according to the following formula:

$$LDL = \text{Total cholesterol} - HDL - (\text{Triglycerides}/5)$$

Using this formula, a LDL value below 130 is considered safe; a value above 160 is considered high and lipid-lowering drugs may be prescribed. However, even this formula does not satisfy all the experts, some of whom believe that the ratio of LDL to HDL is the really significant measure of risk for heart disease.

Controversy in Health

What Do High Cholesterol Levels in Blood Really Mean?

Attributing the risk of heart disease to particular lipid levels is rather arbitrary and has attracted vigorous criticism. At stake is the credibility of the medical establishment and the federal government that establishes guidelines, as well as the health of millions of people. If the guidelines of the National Heart, Lung, and Blood Institute are accepted (see the Wellness Guide on p. 302). then about 25 percent of all Americans between the ages of 20 and 74, more than 60 million people, will need to reduce their cholesterol levels by diet, drugs, or both.

The "cholesterol controversy" has been going on for years and is far from being settled. When Gulliver's travels took him from Lilliput he encountered the big enders and the little enders, who argued furiously, to the point of war, over the best end of the egg for extracting the contents. This comes to mind when one contemplates arguments over cholesterol, not because eggs contain it but because in much of the debate facts seem to be used as missiles to defend entrenched positions rather than elements in a solution to a scientific problem of profound importance clinically and for public health.

—Marmot, 1994

STUDENT REFLECTIONS

- If you knew there was a tendency toward high cholesterol in your family, would you alter your eating habits?
- Do you believe the federal government should determine cholesterol level guidelines to be used by health-care professionals?

The cause of high blood pressure in 90–95 percent of the cases is unknown; the medical term for this is **essential hypertension.** Some factors have been identified that contribute to the elevation of the blood pressure. They include atherosclerosis, hypertrophy of the artery wall, and excess contraction of arterioles.

The remaining cases of high blood pressure are symptoms of a recognizable problem such as a kidney abnormality, congenital defect of the aorta, or adrenal gland tumor. This type of high blood pressure is called **secondary hypertension.** Generally, when the cause of secondary hypertension is determined and corrected, blood pressure returns to normal.

In addition, high blood pressure may be caused by psychosocial factors, although the mechanisms by which these factors could cause high blood pressure are not understood. For example, people with low income and poor education are at higher risk for high blood pressure. The stress of being poor or jobless may generate stress and raise blood pressure. Black and Hispanic Americans have a higher rate of high blood pressure than white Americans (Heart and Stroke Facts, 1994). The stress of being a member of a minority group may also increase the risk of high blood pressure and heart disease, although there is no definitive scientific evidence that proves that being socially or economically disadvantaged causes hypertension. According to the Harvard Health Letter, "Hypertension is a disease of civilized life. Growing up in New Guinea or the northern forests of Brazil is a fine way to avoid the disease."

High blood pressure is a major risk factor for heart attacks and stroke because blood vessels in the heart or brain are more likely to rupture under increased pressure. Hypertension is often called the "silent killer" because it is a disease without symptoms until something serious occurs. As many as 50 million Americans have high blood pressure, which can occur even in young children.

Each time the heart contracts, blood is pumped through the arteries and exerts pressure on the arterial walls (Figure 14.11). In fact, there are two pressures that are measured. The maximum pressure in the arteries occurs when the heart contracts **(systole)**, pumping blood from the heart to the lungs and body. Between contractions, the pressure falls **(diastole)** as blood flows from one chamber of the heart to another. Normal blood pressure is defined as a value less than 140/90 (systole/diastole). Generally, the diastolic pressure is considered the more significant of the two with respect to health risk. A person with a diastolic pressure of 120 has double the risk of a heart attack or stroke compared to a person with a diastolic pressure of 90.

T E R M S

hypertension: high blood pressure

essential hypertension: high blood pressure that is not caused by any observable disease

secondary hypertension: high blood pressure due to a recognizable disease or problem

systole: the pressure in the arteries when the heart contracts

diastole: the pressure in the arteries when the heart relaxes

Factors such as obesity, heredity, cigarette smoking, caffeine, excessive alcohol use, stress, and excessive consumption of salt have all been associated to some degree with hypertension. Salt consumption was considered a major hypertension risk factor for years, but recent evidence indicates that only a tiny fraction of people with hypertension are sensitive to salt intake.

Since race is also a risk factor for hypertension, considerable effort has been devoted to finding genetic or biological differences between black and white Americans that could account for the higher prevalence of hypertension among black Americans. However, others believe that black and Hispanic Americans suffer from high blood pressure more frequently than white Americans because of social and economic factors.

Blood pressure is the result of two forces. The first is created by the heart as it pumps blood into the arteries, the second created by the arterial blood vessels as they resist blood flow from the heart. Tiny receptors in the walls of the arteries respond to changes in blood pressure. If blood pressure rises, these receptors send signals to the nerves to relax the arteries and to slow down the heartbeat, thus returning blood pressure to normal levels. However, these regulatory mechanisms can be overcome by signals from the brain. Arteries can be constricted and blood pressure raised by thoughts and emotions. Fear, tension, anger, and anxiety activate the sympathetic nervous system, which sends signals to the arteries causing them to constrict. If one's life is overly stressful or full of anger and frustration, arteries may stay constricted and blood pressure remain elevated.

While drugs are the most expedient (and profitable) means of controlling hypertension, mental relaxation techniques are also effective. Elmer and Alyce Green (1980) worked with a group people who suffered from severe hypertension. By using biofeedback equipment that displayed blood pressure values, this group learned how to develop mental relaxation states that lowered their blood pressure. In fact, many studies demonstrate that a variety of different relaxation techniques is effective in lowering blood pressure in hypertensive patients (Steptoe, 1988).

However, working with people to lower blood pressure through relaxation techniques is time-consuming and costly in a modern medical setting, so physicians

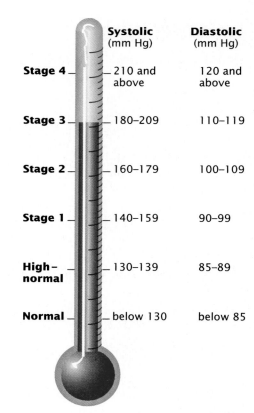

FIGURE 14.11   The Stages of High Blood Pressure
According to current guidelines, normal blood pressure is 130/90 (systolic/diastolic) or below. High blood pressure (hypertension) is defined in four stages, the risk of heart disease being greater the higher the blood pressure. Weight loss, exercise, not smoking, and stress reduction are recommended ways to control hypertension at earlier stages; drugs may also be necessary at later stages.

prescribe antihypertensive drugs even though most of them have undesirable side effects (Table 14.2). Rather than take a drug for a lifetime, people with hypertension can make other choices of how to cope with their high blood pressure. Everyone can start by taking control of one's diet, by exercising regularly, by finding ways to reduce stress, and by taking an aspirin daily if recommended by a physician.

Smoking Cigarettes

Smoking cigarettes is another major risk factor contributing to the development of cardiovascular disease, heart attacks, and strokes. Smokers are at two to four times greater risk of dying from a heart attack than nonsmokers. The risk of heart disease from tobacco smoke extends to those who breathe second-hand smoke at work or at home (He et al., 1994). The more tobacco smoke a person is exposed to, the greater the risk of cardiovascular disease and a heart attack. Tobacco smoke is the most dangerous environmental pollutant known and is a major contributor to both heart disease and cancer.

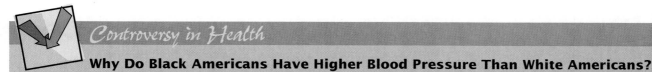

Controversy in Health

Why Do Black Americans Have Higher Blood Pressure Than White Americans?

It is well documented that black Americans have a higher incidence of hypertension and stroke than white Americans. In 1990 the death rate per 100,000 population from hypertension was 6.1 for white males and 29.6 for black males; 4.7 for white females and 22.5 for black females. In the same year, the death rates from stroke among black Americans were double that for white Americans (American Heart Association, 1994).

For years, medical researchers have tried to account for these differences between black and white Americans in terms of biological factors, but have been unsuccessful in finding significant differences until recently. Some research points to genetically determined sensitivity to salt that is specific to Americans of

African descent. Supporting this claim is the idea that people with this gene need less salt and would have survived better under the horrible conditions of heat and water deprivation that existed on the slave ships that transported Africans to America. As a result, the gene for salt retention (if one exists) should be more prevalent among black Americans than among white Americans. So far, this proposed biological difference is purely speculative.

Recent studies of blood vessels removed from African-Americans during bypass surgery suggests that their blood vessels are less flexible than those removed from white Americans. The reduced flexibility of blood vessels may make them more susceptible to hypertension and to damage from the high blood

pressure. Whether these differences in flexibility are due to genetic or environmental factors has not been determined. Nor is it clear that less flexible blood vessels is a common characteristic of black Americans.

In the midst of all the arguments and explanations, it often is forgotten that in their original environments, before the intrusion of Western culture and habits, Africans did not have hypertension. A physician working on a tribal reservation in Kenya in the 1930s measured blood pressure in all patients admitted to his hospital. Among 1800 African patients of all ages there was not a single case of high blood pressure (Donnison, 1938). He concluded then that hypertension is a problem of culture and life-styles. That conclusion still seems valid today.

STUDENT REFLECTIONS

- Do you believe that socioeconomic factors affect the prevalence of high blood pressure?
- Knowing this information, how might you counsel an African-American friend concerning his or her high blood pressure?

TABLE 14.2 Side Effects of Antihypertensive Drugs

Drug category	Side effect
Diuretics	Low blood potassium levels (except for potassium-sparing diuretics) Excess uric acid and sugar in blood (thiazide diuretics) Breast enlargement
Sympatholytics (beta-adrenergic blockers)	Edema (water retention) Depression Diarrhea Fever (methyldopa) Impotence Lethargy
Vasodilators (hydralazine) (calcium channel blockers)	Palpitation Edema Rapid heartbeat Drug-induced lupus erythematosus
Angiotensing converting enzyme (ACE) inhibitors	May affect kidney function

Cigarette smoke also damages the blood vessels that carry blood to the arms and legs, causing them to narrow and to lose elasticity. Heavy cigarette smokers are at risk for **gangrene**, the decay of tissue when the blood supply is obstructed. Gangrene is particularly common in smokers' legs, which may have to be amputated. Cigarette smoke also decreases the level of HDL, which acts to protect blood vessels from damage, and reduces the survival and functioning of **platelets**, blood cells that are essential in the clotting process.

Stopping smoking at any time can reverse many of the harmful physiological effects of tobacco on the cardiovascular system. After several years of not smoking, ex-smokers have about the same risk of cardiovascular

TERMS

gangrene: decay of tissue when the blood supply is restricted
platelets: cells in the blood that are essential for clotting

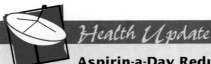
Aspirin-a-Day Reduces the Risk of a Heart Attack

One commonly used drug reduces the risk of heart attacks significantly. It has been known for years that aspirin helps to "thin" blood and prevent blood clots that can cause of heart attacks and stroke. To confirm this relationship between aspirin and heart attacks, hundreds of studies have been carried out involving both healthy people and people who have already had a heart attack or stroke. In all instances, small amounts of aspirin taken daily (one-half tablet or one baby aspirin) reduce the risk of a heart attack.

An analysis of all the aspirin studies determined that if everyone in the world took half an aspirin a day, 100,000 deaths and 200,000 nonfatal heart attacks would be prevented annually (Aldhous, 1994). However, whether healthy individuals who are at low risk of heart attack should take aspirin daily is still an open question. As with taking vitamin supplements or indulging in an occasional drink of alcohol, this is a personal decision that each person must make.

---

disease as nonsmokers. One key to protecting your heart is not smoking and not living or working in a smoke-filled environment.

Stress

In the 1960s two physicians, Meyer Friedman and Ray Rosenman, created a furor by suggesting that almost all heart disease is of behavioral origin. They claimed that in the absence of a pattern they called **type A behavior,** all the other risk factors would not cause cardiovascular disease. They argued that these other factors—smoking, lack of exercise, high cholesterol, hypertension—contribute to the development of heart disease, but that the main risk factor was stress caused by how people live and act.

In 1981, type A behavior was officially recognized by medical experts as a heart disease risk factor. Type A behavior is characterized by the following traits:

- becoming irritated and impatient while waiting in lines
- constantly feeling pressed for time
- insisting that everything always be done on time
- not letting other people finish what they are saying
- always trying to show others how to do things correctly
- playing games to win every time
- not allowing time for relaxation

The association between type A behavior and heart attacks has been difficult to prove because of the difficulty in measuring the subjective behaviors associated with type A people. At least five large studies failed to find any connection between type A behavior and cardiovascular disease; however, other studies did find an association. Recent studies, using more sophisticated interviewing procedures, indicate that anger and hostility are key psychological factors associated with an increased risk of cardiovascular disease. Whatever the scientific evidence for a connection between type A behavior and cardiovascular disease, all health research indicates that persistent stress is unhealthy. If the stress is accompanied by anger and hostility, high blood pressure and other unhealthy changes in the cardiovascular system may also occur.

> *A man's worst enemies can't wish on him what he can think up himself.*
> Yiddish proverb

VITAMINS HELP PREVENT HEART DISEASE

As already mentioned, diet plays a major role in heart disease, especially as it contributes to being overweight and overfat, and to elevated levels of cholesterol. However, certain vitamins in the diet seem to provide some protection from cardiovascular disease. Studies show that oxidized LDL particles are more likely to cause damage to blood vessels than the unoxidized form of LDL. Oxidized LDLs seem to initiate plaque formation and hasten the process that results in blocked arteries.

Vitamin E

Vitamin E acts as an antioxidant in blood and reduces the amount of oxidized LDL that is formed. When volunteers took vitamin E supplements (800 IU), their LDL particles were more resistant to oxidation. Also, a study of about 40,000 men in which other risk factors were taken into account found that those who took 100 to 250 IU of vitamin E every day for two years had a 37

T E R M S

type A behavior: behaviors characterized by traits such as anger or hostility that contribute to the risk of heart disease

free radicals: oxidizing substances in the body that can damage blood vessels and tissues

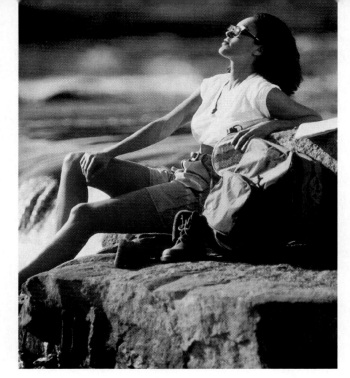

Taking a break from activities is good for the mind, good for the body, and good for the heart.

Vitamin C

For years, Nobel laureate Linus Pauling advocated using vitamin C (ascorbic acid) in megadoses to prevent or help minimize the effects of colds and cancer. Although the ability of vitamin C in warding off these illnesses has never been proved, vitamin C's value in protecting against cardiovascular disease is much greater. Like vitamin E, vitamin C is an antioxidant and can neutralize destructive oxygen atoms and other oxidizing substances called **free radicals.**

Free radical compounds in the blood may damage the elastic tissues in arteries that allow blood vessels to expand and contract. If a blood vessel is damaged and cannot relax, blood pressure rises. Vitamin C prevents such damage from occurring by eliminating the free radical compounds in blood. Taking up to a gram of vitamin C supplement a day is safe; any that is not used is excreted in urine. However, taking megadoses of vitamin C (10 grams a day) can cause serious side effects such as stomach irritation and kidney stones.

Other studies that support the role of vitamin C in preventing heart disease were done with a group of hypertensive patients. These studies showed that people with the highest levels of vitamin C in their blood had the lowest blood pressure. The evidence that vitamin C helps to prevent heart disease is now strong enough that the president of the American Heart Association has recommended large clinical trials to test the efficacy of vitamin C supplements in reducing heart disease. However, other dietary recommendations, especially with respect to alcohol, are still controversial.

With the increased attention given to risk factors that cause cardiovascular disease, people are now armed with knowledge about reducing their chances of heart attacks and stroke. People should reduce consumption of foods containing large amounts of saturated fats and cholesterol. Understanding the dire consequences of cigarette smoking should encourage smokers to quit. Also, taking supplements of vitamins C, E, B_6, B_{12}, and folic acid in the amounts present in a multivitamin tablet seems prudent. Finally, for those who like garlic, the more garlic you eat the better it is for your heart and arteries. Many studies have shown that garlic reduces both blood pressure and cholesterol levels. Preventing cardiovascular disease can be accomplished by adopting good health habits now!

percent lower risk of heart disease compared to a group of men who did not take the vitamin supplement (Rimm et al., 1993). A similar benefit from vitamin E was also reported for women.

While the oxygen gas that we breathe is essential to life, uncombined oxygen atoms in cells can react with many substances and cause damage. For example, consider what happens to iron that is exposed to the oxygen in air under moist conditions; it quickly rusts and disintegrates. Body tissues also can be destroyed by oxygen atoms. The body has many mechanisms for protecting cellular constituents from oxidation, among them the antioxident action of vitamin E (Liebman, 1994).

Vitamin B

Other vitamins that protect against heart disease are three B-vitamins, B_6, B_{12}, and folic acid (folate). Years ago it was observed that high levels of the amino acid homocysteine were associated with atherosclerosis and heart disease (Stampfer and Willett, 1993). People with high levels of homocysteine in their blood also had low levels of the three B-vitamins. On the other hand, people with low homocysteine levels had high levels of the B-vitamins and were less likely to develop heart disease.

The key B-vitamins can be obtained from food; however, many people do not obtain enough in their diets (Table 14.3). The evidence that B-vitamins do, in fact, protect against heart disease is now strong enough that some health authorities recommend taking them in a daily multivitamin supplement.

TABLE 14.3 Food Sources for B-Vitamins

Vitamin	Foods
B_6	Meat, poultry, nuts, whole grain cereals, fish, green leafy vegetables
B_{12}	Meat, organ meats, eggs, dairy products, fish
Folic acid	Green leafy vegetables, fruits, liver, brewer's yeast, dried beans and peas, wheat germ

One Drink of Alcohol a Day Reduces the Risk of Heart Attacks

Alcohol is a drug to which more than 18 million Americans are addicted. Many alcoholics suffer from malnutrition, diseased pancreas or liver, high blood pressure, and other problems (Chapter 18). Although the dangers of alcohol overuse are well documented, there may be benefits in limited amounts. A study of 44,000 male health professionals showed that those who reported having one-half to two drinks a day had a 26 percent *lower* risk of developing cardiovascular disease compared to people who rarely or never drank (Hurley and Schmidt, 1992).

An even larger study of 275,000 middle-aged men showed that one to two drinks a day over twelve years reduced their risk of dying from a heart attack by 20 percent compared to men who never drank. However, more than two drinks a day *increases* the risk of a heart attack considerably, as shown in the accompanying graph.

Women also benefit from an occasional drink with respect to reducing the risk of a heart attack; but the slight benefit is offset by a slightly increased risk of cancer (Friedman and Klatsky, 1993). A 30-year-old woman who drinks moderately (three to nine drinks a week) has a slightly higher risk of breast

and large bowel cancer than a non-drinking woman. The slight reduction in heart disease risk is offset by the slight increase in cancer risk. These are generalizations for large populations and individuals who may have disease risk factors that far outweigh the slight benefits or risks of moderate drinking.

Moderate alcohol consumption seems to exert its beneficial effects by raising HDL levels in the blood. (High HDL levels counteract the

effects of high cholesterol in the blood.) Although moderate drinking has some health benefits, the issue is very controversial considering the many harmful effects of alcohol use. We can't recommend that anyone take up drinking alcohol as a means of reducing the risk of a heart attack, as there are other more effective steps. On the other hand, people who take an occasional drink need not feel guilty and may even accrue some health benefits.

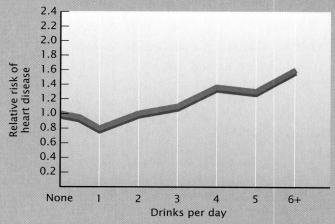

The relative risk of cardiovascular disease in white males aged 40–59 with varying amounts of alcohol consumption. Up to two drinks a day has a protective effect. More than two drinks a day, however, increases the risk, which rises appreciably with each added drink. (A drink is 1¼ oz. of 80 proof alcohol, a 12 oz. beer, or a 5 oz. glass of wine.)

STUDENT REFLECTIONS
- Do the harmful effects of alcohol outweigh the potential benefits of drinking alcohol moderately?
- What message best describes how much alcohol one should drink based on the information provided?

HEALTH IN REVIEW

- The heart is a pump that maintains blood circulation in the arteries and veins. The arteries carry oxygen and nutrients to cells and the veins carry carbon dioxide back to the lungs.
- Damage to the heart or arteries is called cardiovascular disease, which is the leading cause of death in the United States.

- Major risk factors of heart disease that cannot be changed are: heredity, gender, and age.
- Major risk factors of heart disease that can be changed are: cigarette/tobacco smoke, high blood cholesterol, high blood pressure, and physical inactivity.
- Other factors that contribute to heart disease are: diabetes, obesity, and stress.

- Various surgeries are performed to repair clogged arteries. These include coronary bypass surgery and balloon angioplasty.
- Vitamins E, C, B_6 and B_{12}, and folic acid all help protect against heart disease.

- Heart disease is caused by modern life-styles and can be prevented. Making changes in your diet, smoking behaviors, and exercise behaviors while you are young can help keep the heart and arteries healthy throughout life.

REFERENCES

Aldhous, P. (1994). "A Hearty Endorsement for Aspirin." *Science,* January 7.

Donnison, C. P. (1938). *Civilization and Disease.* New York: Wood.

Facklemann, K. A. (1994). "Artery Surgery Slashes Risk of Stroke." *Science News,* October 8.

Frank, J. D. (1973). *Persuasion and Healing.* Baltimore: Johns Hopkins University Press.

Friedman, G. D., and A. I. Klatsky (1993). "Is Alcohol Good for Your Health?" *New England Journal of Medicine,* December 16.

Green, E., et al. (1980). "Self-Regulation Training for Control of Hypertension." *Primary Cardiology.*

Greenspan, A. M., K. R. Harold, and B. C. Berger (1988). "Incidence of Unwarranted Implantation of Permanent Cardiac Pacemakers in a Large Medical Population." *New England Journal of Medicine,* 318: 158–163.

Hamm, C. W. (1994). "New Serum Markers for Acute Myocardial Infarction." *New England Journal of Medicine,* 331(9).

He, Y., T. H. Lam, and L. S. Li (1994). "Passive Smoking at Work a Risk Factor for Coronary Heart Disease in Chinese Women Who Never Have Smoked." *British Medical Journal,* 308(6925).

Heart and Stroke Facts, 1994. Dallas, Tex.: The American Heart Association Publications.

Heart and Stroke Facts, Statistical Supplement (1994). Dallas, Tex.: The American Heart Association Publications.

Hurley, J., and S. Schmidt (1992). "A Drink a Day?" *Nutrition Action Health Letter,* November.

Kern, F. (1991). "Normal Plasma Cholesterol in an 88-Year-Old Man Who Eats 25 Eggs per Day." *New England Journal of Medicine,* 324(13).

Liebman, B. (1994). "The Heart Health-E Vitamin." *Nutrition Action Health Letter,* January/February.

Manson, J. E., et al. (1992). "Medical Progress: The Primary Prevention of Myocardial Infarction." *New England Journal of Medicine,* 326(21): 1406–1416.

Marmot, M. (1994). "The Cholesterol Papers." *British Medical Journal,* 308(6925).

McMurry, M. P., M. T. Cerqueira, S. L. Connor, and W. E. Connor (1991). "Changes in Lipid and Lipoprotein Levels and Body Weight in Tarahumara Indians after Consumption of an Affluent Diet." *New England Journal of Medicine,* 325(24).

Ornish, D. (1990). "Can Lifestyle Changes Reverse Coronary Heart Disease?" *World Review of Nutrition and Dietetics,* 72: 38–48.

Rimm, E. B., M. J. Stampfer, A. Ascherio, E. Giovannucci, G. A. Colditz, and W. C. Willett (1993). "Vitamin E Consumption and the Risk of Coronary Heart Disease in Men." *New England Journal of Medicine,* 328(20): 1450–1456.

Ross, R. (1993). "The Pathogenesis of Atherosclerosis: A Perspective for the 1990s." *Nature,* 362: 801–810.

Stampfer, M. J., and W. C. Willett (1993). "Homocysteine and Marginal Vitamin Deficiency: The Importance of Adequate Vitamin Intake." *Journal of the American Medical Association,* 270(22).

Steptoe, A. (1988). "The Processes Underlying Long-Term Blood Pressure Reduction in Essential Hypertension Following Behavioral Therapy," in T. Elbert, W. Langosch, A. Steptoe, and D. Vaitl (eds.), *Behavioral Medicine and Cardiovascular Disease.* New York: John Wiley.

SUGGESTED READINGS

American Heart Association (AHA). *Heart and Stroke Facts, Statistical Supplement, 1994.* Published yearly and obtainable from any AHA office. Contain the latest information on cardiovascular diseases, treatments, and statistical data.

Hurley, J., and S. Schmidt (1992). "A Drink a Day?" *Nutrition Action Health Letter,* November. Discusses the evidence for the protective value of small amounts of alcohol in heart disease.

Liebman, B. (1994). "The Heart Health-E Vitamin." *Nutrition Action Health Letter,* January/February. Discusses the evidence that vitamin E and antioxidants prevent cardiovascular disease.

Moore, Thomas J. (1990). *Heart Failure.* New York: Random House. A critical appraisal of the heart treatment industry and especially of the cholesterol controversy.

Ornish, D., et al. (1990). "Can Lifestyle Changes Reverse Coronary Heart Disease?" *The Lancet,* July 21. Concludes that it can.

Simon, H. B. (1994). *Conquering Heart Disease: New Ways to Live Well Without Drugs or Surgery.* New York: Little, Brown Publishers. A physician with heart disease presents a life-style approach to conquering heart disease.

Winston, M. (ed.) (1993). *American Heart Association Cookbook.* New York: Times Books. Information on meal planning and recipes for maintaining a healthy heart.

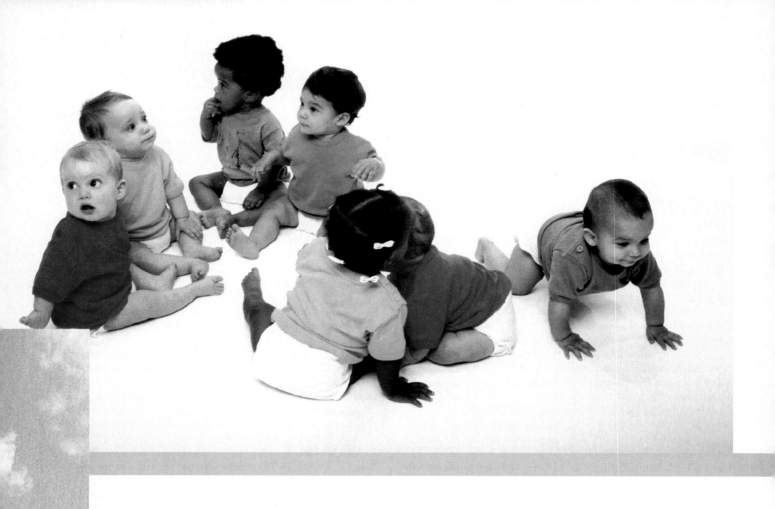

LEARNING OBJECTIVES

After reading this chapter you should be able to:

1. Identify and describe several congenital birth defects.
2. Identify and describe several chemical substances that cause birth defects.
3. Explain what a hereditary disease is.
4. Discuss the importance of chromosomes in one's genetic makeup.
5. Discuss prenatal testing for genetic disease.
6. Discuss the importance of genetic counseling.
7. Describe how some hereditary diseases can be treated.

Understanding Birth Defects and Genetic Diseases

*M*ost babies are born healthy. However, in about one of every fifty births in the United States, a physical defect or biological abnormality is observable immediately or shortly after birth. Birth defects can be caused by both hereditary factors (genes) and environmental agents, such as certain chemicals, that affect the normal development of the fetus. In many cases of birth defects it is difficult to sort out the relative contribution of genetic and environmental factors. With further medical tests, about half of birth defects can be traced to specific defective genes that were passed from one or both parents.

The past two decades have witnessed an explosion of new information pertaining to human genetic (inherited) disorders and the mechanisms by which defective genes produce physical abnormalities and diseases in people who inherit them. The extraordinary advances in diagnosing and detecting inherited disorders in adults and in fetuses have generated complex economic, personal, social, and ethical problems.

Ethical and social problems arise mainly around genetic information that may be used as a basis for aborting a fetus. As more human genes become identified, prospective parents will be able to find out if they or their fetus carry defective versions of these genes. For example, in the foreseeable future, genes that increase the risk of cancer, heart disease, or mental disorders may become diagnosable. Other genes may be discovered that contribute to the risk of alcoholism, obesity, or violent behavior. People will be able to find out if they carry such genes. They also will be able to find out if those genes are present in a fetus. Individuals and society will have to determine whether to allow testing for such genes and whether such information can be used to justify an abortion.

From an economic perspective, for example, individuals identified as carrying a defective gene could have problems obtaining life or health insurance, as well as finding employment. Given a choice, few companies want to insure or hire a person at high risk of becoming sick because of a known genetic defect that might lead to a disease. Because of the inherent economic hazard in having one's genetic profile generally available to insurance companies or employers, genetic privacy laws are being considered in several states and by the U.S. Congress.

On a personal level, knowing about defective genes that one carries may cause severe stress and emotional problems. For example, Huntington's disease is a severe neurological disease that begins at mid-life or later in persons who carry the defective gene. The disease progresses inexorably, is untreatable, and leads to death within a few years after symptoms appear. It is now possible to test fetuses, children, or adults to determine if they carry the Huntington's disease gene. If those tested have the gene, they must live with the knowledge that later in life, at an unknown age, they will experience symptoms and die prematurely. Such information is not always welcome and, in fact, some persons at risk for Huntington's disease and other hereditary disorders prefer not to know their genetic risk or genetic status (Nowak, 1994).

> *Knowledge about one's genetic makeup is one of the most personal and private pieces of information one can possess about oneself. It vies with private thoughts, fantasies, and dreams as being the essence of self-identity.*
>
> Margery W. Shaw,
> professor of law and genetics

In the near future, scientists expect to identify defective genes that increase a person's risk of cancer, heart disease, diabetes, or Alzheimer's disease (a form of brain degeneration). Some scientists even predict that they will be able to find genes that make people susceptible to obesity, alcoholism, or criminality. The possible results of identifying these genes are highly controversial, but do emphasize why people need to understand enough about genetics to be knowledgeable users of the new genetic tests and gene therapies that are being developed (Nelkin and Tancredi, 1989).

CONGENITAL DEFECTS AND TERATOGENS

Each newborn is examined immediately after birth for any observable physical or biological abnormalities, which are called **congenital defects**. Such defects are not necessarily inherited, although defective genes passed from parents may play some role. Most congenital defects are due to a complex interaction of genes and environmental factors (Figure 15.1). Examples of congenital defects are cleft lip, cleft palate, and spina bifida (cleft spine), which result from developmental abnormalities in the formation of the oral cavity and the spine, respectively. Cleft lip has been known to occur in only one of a pair of identical twins, so environmental factors other than genes must contribute to this abnormality. The importance of environmental factors during fetal development is borne out by the observation that even though identical twins are genetically identical, they usu-

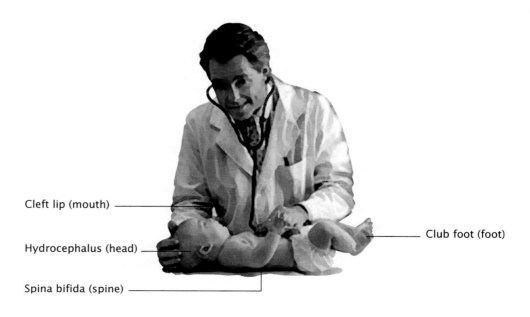

FIGURE 15.1 Congenital defects arise in different areas of the body during fetal development.

Cleft lip (mouth)

Hydrocephalus (head)

Spina bifida (spine)

Club foot (foot)

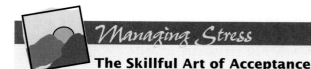
The Skillful Art of Acceptance

Sometimes we encounter stressors in our lives. One such case would occur if we faced a hereditary disease. How do we learn to cope with such a situation? Those who consider themselves most successful in coping are those who have learned how to accept their situation and get on with their lives. Perhaps it was said best by Reinhold Niebuhr in the now famous Serenity Prayer: *"Lord, grant me the serenity to change the things I can, accept the things I cannot change, and the wisdom to know the difference."*

When people hear the word "acceptance," there is often a sense of resignation. There is also a sense of anger and victimization. "Why me? Why did this have to happen to me? What did I do to deserve this?" True, or unconditional, acceptance is an understanding of the existing conditions; a receptivity to the things that cannot be changed and a discarding of the feelings of pity. True acceptance is not giving up; rather it is a recognition of the

particular situation. In the stage of acceptance, there is no trace of anger or pity, no feelings of victimization. Unconditional acceptance allows you to move on with your life. With acceptance may come hope and a sense of faith that it will all work out.

As we are now learning, not all hereditary diseases are evident at birth. Many surface in the second, third, or fourth decades of life. For some people unprepared for what lies ahead, a diagnosis translates into a major obstacles. In terms of spiritual wellness, roadblocks on the human path may actually be the path itself, meaning that sudden stressors, like hereditary diseases or a significant loss of some kind, are not a punishment. Rather, they may be an opportunity to learn about life from a different perspective. Unfortunately, many people facing major changes in their life feel a sense of personal violation. Rather than overcoming the obstacle, they choose to sit and become immobilized by it.

Some of our greatest role models are people born with great odds against them. They not only overcome adversity, but do it with great distinction. Consider the physicist Steven Hawking, author of *A Brief History of Time.* Recognized as a genius at an early age, he was struck with a crippling disease in his twenties. Although he was unable to use his body, he never stopped exercising his mind. Now recognized as one of the world's leaders in quantum physics, Hawking showed that roadblocks in life can be a test of true character.

The art of acceptance is not a skill acquired overnight. It takes practice over a lifetime. Nor do all problems go away once we accept them. But when we learn the skill of unconditional acceptance, we learn to direct energy where it will serve the highest good. In the words of Richard Bach, author of *Illusions,* "There is no such thing as a problem without a gift for you in its hands. You seek problems, because you need their gifts."

---

ally are born with quite different birth weights. This shows that identical twins are affected differently by environmental factors in the same uterus.

Spina bifida is a congenital defect that affects one of every 1,000 newborns. It occurs when one or more spinal vertebrae fail to close and the spinal cord and nerves bulge through the cleft, forming an easily damaged, fluid-filled sac. The protruding spinal nerves are vulnerable to paralysis-causing damage and also to life-threatening infections. The most serious congenital defect of the nervous system is *anencephaly,* which refers to very abnormal brain development; affected babies are either stillborn or die soon after birth. Surgery can repair some of the damage resulting from spina bifida; however, nothing can be done for anencephaly. More important, the risk of spina bifida and other birth defects can be significantly reduced by a simple vitamin supplement taken before and during pregnancy.

Any chemical substance that causes a defect in a developing fetus is called a **teratogen** (Table 15.1). Many environmental agents such as prescription and illegal drugs, viral and bacterial infections, alcohol consump-

tion during pregnancy, and smoking cigarettes act as teratogens during pregnancy and may cause abnormal development in a fetus (Robinson, 1990). With a little care, many teratogens can be avoided, thereby increasing the likelihood of a healthy baby. In particular, smoking cigarettes and drinking alcohol should be avoided by any woman who is pregnant or attempting to become pregnant. Alcohol is concentrated in crossing the placenta so that even one or two drinks can lead to high alcohol levels in the fetus and affect its development.

Thalidomide

Thalidomide is a sedative used as a sleeping pill and to quell morning sickness early in pregnancy. It was con-

T E R M S

congenital defect: any physical or biological abnormality observed in a newborn

teratogen: any environmental agent that causes abnormal development of a fetus

TABLE 15.1 Teratogens Environmental agents (infectious viruses and other microorganisms, chemicals, medicines, and other substances) can act as teratogens and cause birth defects. Many agents in addition to those listed below are suspected of causing abnormal development of the fetus.

Environmental agent	Effects
Accutane (acne drug)	Spontaneous abortion, stillbirth, malformation of the brain and heart
Alcohol	Growth deficiencies, mental retardation
Cocaine	Fetal death, nervous system and genital abnormalities
Diethylstilbestrol (DES)	Masculination of female, abnormalities of vagina and cervix, risk of vaginal cancer
Cytomegalovirus, Herpes simplex virus, Varicella Zoster virus	Growth deficiencies, mental retardation
Lithium carbonate	Heart and blood vessel defects
Polychlorinated biphenyls	Growth deficiencies, pigment abnormalities
Poor nutrition during fetal development	Growth deficiency, mental retardation
Ionizing radiation	Growth deficiencies, mental retardation, organ malformation depending on dose
Rubella virus (German measles)	Heart and eye abnormalities, mental retardation
Tetracycline (antibiotic)	Teeth and bone abnormalities
Thalidomide	Limb malformation
Tobacco smoke	Growth deficiencies, increased risk of sickness and death soon after birth

sidered safe and was widely prescribed in Europe in the early 1960s. It had been tested in animals and no teratogenic effects were discovered; however, the drug was not approved for distribution in the United States. By 1961, it was clear that thalidomide was causing serious birth defects. Thalidomide interferes with the normal development of the bones of the arms and legs of the fetus as well as other developmental abnormalities. Between

Health Update

Prevent Birth Defects with Vitamins

Supplementing the diet of pregnant women with the vitamins folic acid and B_{12} can reduce the risk of spina bifida and other birth defects by as much as half (Rosenberg, 1992). Folic acid supplement seems to be the most important and most beneficial if taken during the first few weeks of pregnancy, so women who plan to become pregnant should begin taking the vitamin on a regular basis. Folic acid also is found in green leafy vegetables, meats, and fruits, but many people still obtain a suboptimal amount from their diets.

Worldwide, folic acid deficiency is the most common vitamin deficiency and the greatest cause of birth defects.

The current recommended daily amount of folic acid is 200 micrograms, but experts suggest that women who plan to become pregnant should take multivitamin tablets with twice that amount. While this amount of folic acid is safe, women should not overdose with vitamins during pregnancy. Although the benefits of folic acid and vitamin B_{12} supplementation for

pregnant women are now well documented, supplementing foods with folic acid to raise everyone's intake is still controversial. Too much folic acid can have adverse consequences for some women; for example, it complicates the diagnosis of pernicious anemia.

Since the benefits of folic acid are now well established and the risks of overdose quite small, it is likely that some foods, particularly flour, will be supplemented with folic acid in the future.

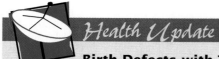

Health Update

Birth Defects with Two Drugs

Methotrexate and Tegison (etretinate), both of which are approved by FDA to treat severe psoriasis, can cause severe birth defects in children born to women who are or who become pregnant while taking either drug.

Warnings in the labeling of both drugs state that they should not be prescribed to women who are pregnant or who are likely to become pregnant. Couples are advised to avoid pregnancy for at least three months after the man takes methotrexate and for at least one menstrual cycle after the woman takes it.

The period during which a woman should avoid pregnancy after treatment with Tegison is not known. It is known that, in some women, etretinate may still be detected in blood three years after they stopped taking the drug.

Birth defects associated with Tegison include high palate, fused bones, webbed hands and feet, and malformed skull, spinal cord, face, fingers, and toes. Tegison is a retinoid, chemically similar to vitamin A.

Both drugs also should not be used by nursing women. Despite the risks, doctors can prescribe these drugs to women of childbearing age in cases where other treatments have been unsuccessful and both the doctor and patient consider that the medical benefits of treatment outweigh the risks.

Source: *FDA Consumer* (April 1995): 29(3): 15.

1960 and 1962, in many countries several thousand babies were born with deformed arms and legs before the teratogenic effects of the drug were established. Aside from its teratogenic effects in pregnant women, thalidomide is a very safe drug and is still being used to treat certain diseases today.

DES

In the 1950s and 1960s, the synthetic hormone *DES* (diethylstilbestrol) was prescribed to help prevent miscarriage. DES was not identified as a teratogen until the 1970s. Many daughters of women who took DES before or during pregnancy discovered that they had abnormalities in their reproductive organs when they tried to become pregnant. These daughters also have a higher risk of developing vaginal cancer. Although the drug did not cause abnormalities in all children of DES mothers, the risk is sufficiently great that most DES women carry the psychological burden of their potential for reproductive problems and cancer.

Accutane

Isotretinoin is an analog of vitamin A and is sold as a drug called Accutane that is used to treat severe acne and other skin disorders. Accutane was tested in laboratory animals and labeled a teratogen because it caused birth defects when administered to pregnant mice and rats. The drug was finally released with the warning that it should not be used during pregnancy. However, during the 1980s, hundreds of babies with congenital defects were born to women who became pregnant while taking Accutane for skin problems. In some cases, the women may have become pregnant by accident while taking the drug; in others the desire to improve their skin condition may have caused them to disregard the warning. This points out a dilemma that is faced by Food and Drug Administration (FDA), the government agency that regulates drugs. Should an effective drug that is known to be a teratogen be released with a warning or should it be banned entirely?

Alcohol and Other Drugs

Chronic use of alcohol during pregnancy may cause the newborn to be affected with fetal alcohol syndrome (FAS) (see Chapter 18 for more information). This birth defect is characterized by abnormal facial features and mental retardation (Figure 15.2). Although most babies with fetal alcohol syndrome are born to women who consume large amounts of alcohol during preg-

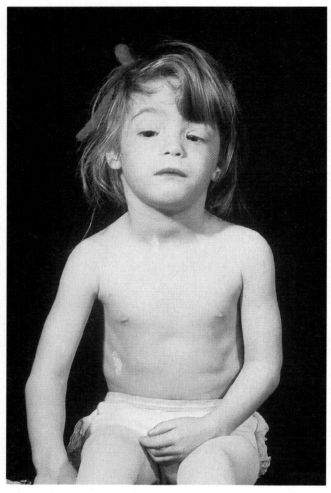

FIGURE 15.2 A Child with Fetal Alcohol Syndrome
Such children, born to women who consumed significant amounts of alcohol while pregnant, are undersize and have eyes and facial features that are abnormally proportioned or positioned. Many have heart defects, and most are mentally retarded.

nancy, studies show that even moderate drinking during pregnancy increases risk.

The drinking of alcohol by pregnant women who give birth to a handicapped child raises questions about individual rights. Does a mother have a right to do with her body as she sees fit even if it means harming the baby? Does society have the right to regulate the consumption of alcohol and other harmful substances by a pregnant woman? Some people argue that a pregnant woman who irresponsibly takes drugs during pregnancy should be imprisoned while pregnant so that her use of dangerous substances can be controlled. The ethical and legal questions surrounding pregnancy and drugs, including alcohol, are very complex.

Many congenital defects could be prevented if women took more care with their diets and drug use during pregnancy. Smoking cigarettes and drinking alcohol should be eliminated since they greatly increase the risks of spontaneous abortion, a low birth-weight, or congenital defects. The most critical period of development for the fetus is the first months of pregnancy, so if a pregnancy is anticipated, the consumption of alcohol, and cigarettes should be discontinued. Over-the-counter and prescription drugs should be monitored carefully by a physician during this time.

Hereditary Diseases

A **hereditary (genetic) disease** results from the following sequence of events. A defective gene (one whose chemistry has been altered in some way in the chromosomes of one or both parents) is passed on to a child in sperm, egg, or both. As a result of inheriting the defective gene or genes, a protein is produced that is abnor-

 Wellness Guide

Do Not Mix Alcohol and Pregnancy

Babies born to mothers who are chronic alcoholics have significant risk of being born with congenital defects, mental retardation, and other health problems known as fetal alcohol syndrome (FAS). Alcohol in the pregnant woman's blood acts as a teratogen during development of the fetus. The potential for alcohol to cause problems was observed by physicians in ancient

Greece, but generally has been ignored until recent scientific studies established alcohol as a cause of congenital defects.

Although most babies with FAS are born to women who are chronic alcoholics, some studies indicate that even moderate drinking (two drinks a day) during pregnancy can increase the risk of FAS. Also, babies born to women who drink moder-

ately tend to have lower than average birth weights, which puts them at risk for a number of health and developmental problems. While there is no evidence that an occasional drink during pregnancy puts the fetus at risk, most pregnant women avoid all alcohol during pregnancy to give their babies the best environment for healthy development.

mal or a necessary protein is entirely absent in certain tissues or organs. For example, if an essential muscle protein is defective or missing in a fetus, muscle tissues develop abnormally. Several forms of *muscular dystrophy* are inherited in this way. If a protein necessary for bone formation is defective, short stature or *dwarfism* results.

If the defective protein is an enzyme, an essential chemical reaction in the body will be affected and some aspect of metabolism will be abnormal. For example, in *hemophilia,* an enzyme called Factor VIII, required for normal blood clotting, is defective due to an altered gene on an X chromosome. *Phenylketonuria* (PKU) is an inherited disease caused by a defect in an enzyme that is needed to digest the amino acid phenylalanine present in food. If excess phenylalanine in the blood is not broken down, it accumulates in tissues and causes abnormal brain development and mental retardation.

Sickle cell disease is caused by a defect in hemoglobin proteins present in all red blood cells. Hemoglobin molecules pick up oxygen as blood circulates through the lungs. In sickle cell disease, the defective hemoglobin proteins change the shape of red blood cells so that they tend to clog small blood vessels. As a result, essential oxygen cannot reach tissues and organs.

> *Genetic explanations for intelligence, sex role differences, or aggression lead to absolving of society of any responsibility for its inequities, thus providing support for those who have interest in maintaining these inequities.*
>
> Jon Beckwith,
> geneticist

Hereditary diseases are *always* due to defective chromosomes or genes that change body structure or chemistry in some way. However, determining if a disease or physical abnormality is inherited is not a simple matter. As indicated, many birth defects are due to infections, teratogens, or other environmental factors, as well as to defective genes.

Sometimes a disease is said to "run in the family," which means that several members of a family have the same disease. Allergies, obesity, or alcoholism may run in the family, but this does not mean that these diseases are inherited or are caused by defective genes. Families share many environmental factors as well as genes. For example, families share the same water, food, and air, any one of which may contain harmful or toxic substances. When parents have a poor diet, children usually do also. To appreciate the difference between an inherited disease and one that "runs in the family" consider these examples. Being a Protestant or a Catholic runs in families as does being a Republican or a Democrat, but these traits clearly are not determined by any genes that have been inherited.

To unambiguously classify a disease as resulting from an inherited defect, at least one of the following criteria must be satisfied: 1) the disease must show a pattern of inheritance over several generations conforming to the laws of inheritance; 2) the chromosomes in cells of affected individuals must be visibly abnormal; 3) a biochemical defect such as the loss of an enzyme or protein must be demonstrated in cells from the affected individual; or 4) a defective gene can be shown to exist in chromosomes in cells from the affected individual. Only a physician trained in medical genetics can determine if a disease or defect is due to inherited genes, to environmental factors, or to a combination of both.

Chromosomes

Each person carries 23 pairs of chromosomes (46 total) in every cell of his or her body. Men and women differ only in a pair of chromosomes called the sex chromosomes; men have an XY pair and women have an XX pair. In both men and women the chromosomes that were present in the fertilized egg are also present in skin, brain, heart, lung, or liver cells. Half of each parent's chromosomes is passed on to progeny in the sperm and egg that join during fertilization. Occasionally, errors are made when the chromosomes are distributed to sperm or egg, resulting in too few or too many chromosomes; different chromosomal abnormalities cause different hereditary diseases (Table 15.2).

Human chromosomes have a characteristic size, shape, and banding pattern that shows up when they are stained with dyes. In this way, each of the 23 different chromosomes can be distinguished and identified. Human chromosomes are visualized under the microscope and then are photographed and arranged in pairs in a standardized display called a **karyotype.** Visualization of chromosomes in cells removed from a fetus, child, or adult can identify chromosomal abnormalities, such as the extra chromosome 21 that causes *Down syndrome* (Figure 15.3).

This serious inherited birth defect occurs in about one in every 700 babies born in the United States. However, the rate increases dramatically in women over age 35 who bear a child. Because of the increase in Down syndrome with maternal age, all pregnant women over age 35 are advised to undergo genetic tests of fetal cells (see section below on Prenatal Testing) to determine if they are carrying a fetus with Down syndrome. If the tests are positive, women can elect to have an abortion or continue the pregnancy.

T E R M S

hereditary (genetic) disease: any disease due to the inheritance of defective genes or chromosomes from one or both parents

karyotype: visual display of all of a person's chromosomes that can detect chromosomal abnormalities characteristic of inherited diseases

TABLE 15.2 Chromosomal Abnormalities Genetic diseases associated with an extra or missing chromosome. Most abnormalities in chromosome number (more or less than 46) are incompatible with long-term survival; in most cases, affected babies die before birth. However, abnormalities in chromosome 21, X, or Y are compatible with survival but usually produce serious physical and mental abnormalities.

Genetic disease/disorder	Chromosomal defect	Incidence per live births	Symptoms
Turner syndrome (female)	Missing X	1/1000	Absence of ovaries, short stature, underdeveloped breasts
Klinefelter syndrome (male)	Extra X	1/1000	Small, undeveloped testes, sterility, mental retardation
Down syndrome (male or female)	Extra chromosome 21	1/700	Physical abnormalities, mental retardation, heart defects
XXX syndrome (female)	Extra X	uncertain (1/1000)	No clinical abnormalities, height above average, possible mental retardation
XYY (male)	Extra Y	uncertain (1/1000)	No clinical abnormalities, height above average, controversy over "criminal" tendency

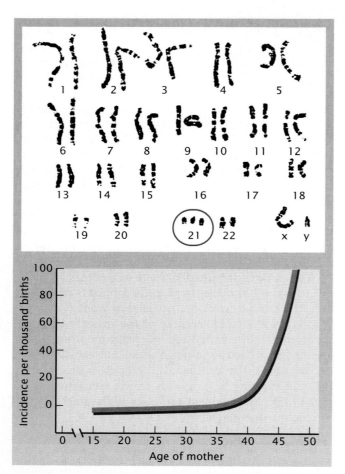

FIGURE 15.3 Karyotype of Individual with Down Syndrome Note three copies of chromosome 21. Frequencies of children born with Down syndrome are shown in relation to the age of the mother. At age 35 the risk of this particular chromosomal defect begins to rise sharply.
Source: Data from E. B. Hook, 1977.

The extra chromosome 21 carried in all cells of individuals with Down syndrome causes heart defects, altered facial features, and mental retardation. With modern medical care, the life expectancy of a person with Down syndrome is 40 to 50 years. However, caring for a Down syndrome person beyond childhood is taxing on families both emotionally and financially. Eventually, most individuals with Down syndrome are placed in special living situations with trained caregivers.

Genes

Genes are present in chromosomes in a chemical substance called **DNA (deoxyribonucleic acid)**. Each chromosome, depending on its size, contains hundreds or thousands of different genes. Together the 46 human chromosomes contain about 200,000 genes that uniquely determine a human being. Since chromosomes occur in pairs, each person carries two copies of each gene; these may be identical or slightly different from one another. When the chemistry of a gene is significantly different from that in healthy people, the defective

T E R M S

DNA (deoxyribonucleic acid): the chemical substance in chromosomes that carries genetic information

enzymes: proteins in cells that carry out and speed up chemical reactions

genetic counseling: information to help prospective parents evaluate the risks of having or delivering a genetically handicapped child

amniocentesis: a procedure in which amniotic fluid is removed from the uterus and tested to determine if genetic or anatomical defects exist in the fetus

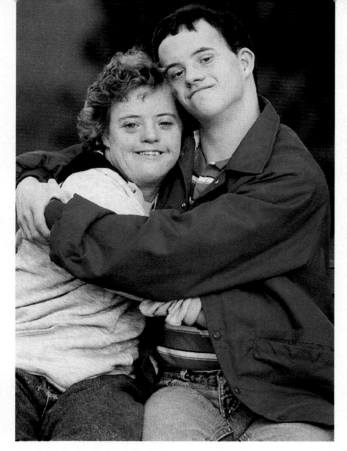

Down syndrome is caused by inheriting an extra chromosome 21 from the mother. Individuals with Down syndrome are capable of living fulfilling and productive lives.

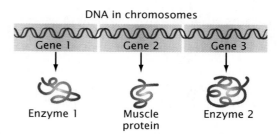

FIGURE 15.4 DNA in Chromosomes Genes direct the synthesis of proteins in cells. Each gene in a chromosome codes for a different protein. Most proteins are enzymes that speed up chemical reactions in cells. Other proteins are used to construct bone, muscle, hair, and nails. Genes consist of sequences of chemical substances called bases in DNA. Proteins consist of sequences of amino acids that fold and twist to form specific shapes according to their function.

gene usually alters or eliminates a chemical reaction in the body and may produce an inherited disease.

Almost all of the different human genes direct the synthesis of uniquely different proteins. Some of these proteins are used to construct the bones and muscles of the body. However, most genes direct the synthesis of special proteins called **enzymes** (Figure 15.4). Enzymes catalyze (speed up) the thousands of different chemical reactions in cells that keep them (and us) alive.

PREVENTING GENETIC DISEASES

Prenatal Testing

An important goal of modern medicine is preventing inherited diseases caused by defective genes or chromosomes. **Genetic counseling** of couples who are at risk for having a child with a hereditary disorder can help prevent them from having a handicapped child by counseling them before and during pregnancy. Genetic counseling can provide useful information for parents, but in the end the parents make the decisions. Prenatal testing is not advised or necessary for all pregnant women or couples planning to have a child. Only those who are at higher-than-average risk for bearing a child with a hereditary defect are advised to undergo prenatal testing and genetic counseling.

Hundreds of single gene defects that cause hereditary diseases now can be diagnosed *in utero* with a prenatal surgical procedure called **amniocentesis** (Figure 15.5). In this procedure fetal cells are obtained by removing a sample of amniotic fluid from the womb around the fifteenth week of pregnancy. Although amniocentesis is very safe, there is still a small risk of harming the fetus or inducing a miscarriage. The physician should discuss the risks and benefits of the procedure as part of the genetic counseling.

The fetal cells obtained by amniocentesis are grown in the laboratory and tested for biochemical and genetic abnormalities (Rennie, 1994). Examination of the chromosomes in the karyotype analysis also identifies the sex of the fetus, but this information is only provided if the pregnant woman specifically requests it. (While most people in American society are joyful at the birth of

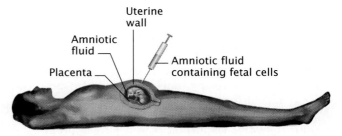

FIGURE 15.5 Amniocentesis In the diagnostic procedure called amniocentesis, a sample of the fluid that surrounds the developing fetus is collected. Both the fluid and the fetal cells it contains are then analyzed for biochemical or chromosomal defects. Amniocentesis is performed so that prospective parents can decide whether to continue the pregnancy or abort the fetus. The decision is generally made after discussion with their physician and a counselor.

Determining If You Are at Risk for Bearing a Genetically Disabled Child

Prenatal testing and genetic counseling are advised if a person falls into any one of the risk categories listed below:

- Maternal age over 35 years (risk of Down syndrome).

- High or low levels of alpha-fetoprotein during pregnancy (risk of neural tube defect).

- Woman had a previous child with a chromosomal abnormality or neural tube defect.

- Woman had a previous stillbirth or neonatal death.

- Woman or mate carries a previously diagnosed chromosomal or genetic abnormality.

- Woman carries a previously diagnosed defective gene.

- Woman and mate carry the same previously diagnosed defective gene.

- Close relatives have a child with an inherited disorder.

- Woman has been exposed to a teratogenic agent during pregnancy.

- Woman has recently been infected by rubella (measles) virus or cytomegalovirus.

---

either a boy or a girl, in many other countries, male children are still considered more desirable. In fact, determination of a female fetus by amniocentesis and karyotype analysis is the most common cause of elective abortion in many countries of the world, particularly in India. Another prenatal procedure called **chorionic villus analysis** can be performed as early as eight weeks after conception. This earlier test provides information regarding the health of the fetus, allowing the parent(s) to make decisions such as taking pregnancy to term or terminating the pregnancy.

An advance in safe prenatal testing is **ultrasound scanning**, used to visualize the fetus developing in the womb (Figure 15.6). Ultrasound scans use high frequency sound waves that bounce back from the various tissues in the fetus with different intensities. The sound waves reflected from the fetus are displayed on a screen and the image is interpreted by a physician trained in the use of this technique.

Ultrasound scans are used to detect multiple fetuses and to determine the location of the placenta, which is important if amniocentesis is to be performed. The scans can gauge the fetus' head size, thereby providing determination of the age of the fetus. Abnormal brain development and neural tube defects also can be diagnosed with an ultrasound scan. Despite their safety, pregnant women are advised not to have an ultrasound scan unless their health or that of the fetus requires one. Even though ultrasound does not use radiation as in X-rays, the effects of the sound waves on the fetus and its development are unknown (Berkowitz, 1993).

Genetic Counseling

Genetic counseling is necessary both before a pregnancy occurs and after a pregnancy develops to help high-risk prospective parents determine the genetic risks to the fetus. Although genetic counseling begins with objective calculations of risk to a fetus (which in some cases approach certainty that an abnormal fetus is present), from that point on subjective values inevitably influence the decisions (Wertz and Fletcher, 1989). For example, religious convictions lead some women to deliver babies determined by testing to have Down syndrome.

Although genetic counselors strive to be objective, the counseling process is subtle and counselors may inadvertently convey personal opinions. For example, prospective parents who carry certain genes can be told that any child that they bear will have one chance in four of being abnormal, or they can be told that the odds are three to one that the child will be normal. Both statements express the same truth about the probabilities, but the prospective parents may well interpret the two statements differently.

Giving advice or making recommendations that affect the life of another person inevitably necessitates moral decisions—decisions that are influenced by many factors. Ideally, the personal views of the genetic counselor

---

HEALTHY PEOPLE 2000

Increase to at least 95 percent the proportion of newborns screened by state-sponsored programs for genetic disorders and other disabling conditions and 90 percent the proportion of newborns testing positive for disease who receive appropriate treatment.

Almost all states screen infants for genetic and metabolic disorders and refer for treatment those with a confirmed diagnosis. Some disorders are more uniformly screened for than others, and follow-up testing and early initiation of preventive treatment is uneven.

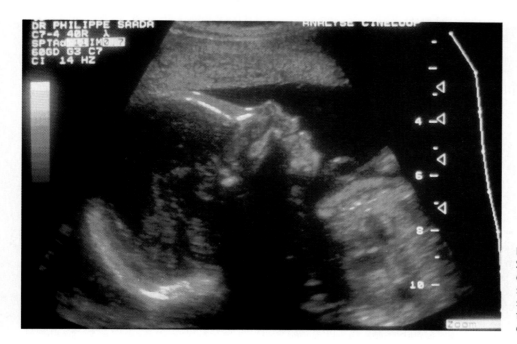

FIGURE 15.6 Ultrasound Scanning Image of a fetus obtained by ultrasound scanning. Such ultrasound scans reveal the position of the fetus and may also indicate certain physical abnormalities.

should not influence the families' decisions. Clients should arrive at their own decision after careful consideration of all medical options that have been explained to them.

Treating Hereditary Diseases

Very few of the thousands of known hereditary diseases can be treated effectively. Phenylketonuria (PKU) is an exception, and can be managed if the affected newborn is diagnosed at birth. Because PKU is treatable and because the test is accurate and inexpensive, all newborns in the United States are tested for PKU. The amino acid phenylalanine is present in any normal diet and if it is eaten by a PKU child, phenylalanine accumulates in the blood, brain development is affected, and mental retardation follows. A person with PKU carries two defective genes and lacks an enzyme that is essential for the chemical breakdown of the phenylalanine present in most proteins, including proteins in milk. Thus, any baby with PKU is immediately put on a phenylalanine-free diet, which must be maintained at least until and often beyond puberty.

T E R M S

chorionic villus analysis: a prenatal procedure used to determine if genetic or anatomical defects exist in a fetus; an alternative to amniocentesis

ultrasound scanning: use of sound waves to visualize the fetus in the womb

gene therapy: a technique for replacing defective genes with normal ones in certain tissues of a person affected with a hereditary disease

Another genetic disease that can be treated successfully is hemophilia, which is caused by a defective blood-clotting protein called Factor VIII. The normal Factor VIII protein is now manufactured and hemophiliacs take the drug to prevent bleeding. Another important drug produced by biotechnology is human growth hormone (HGH). Individuals who inherit a defective gene that causes dwarfism can now be treated with HGH during childhood. Children treated with HGH will grow to near normal height.

While the treatments noted above do not cure genetic diseases, they do alleviate symptoms in the same way that a tranquilizer relieves, but does not cure, symptoms of anxiety or depression. To cure a genetic disease requires replacement of the defective genes by normal ones in many cells of the affected person: this is the goal of **gene therapy**, which is in the early stages of development.

It is an extremely difficult process to insert genes into the human body and get them to function correctly in the proper organs. Gene therapy is being used experimentally to treat persons with cystic fibrosis, muscular dystrophy, some forms of immune system diseases, and for certain cancers (Thompson, 1993). For gene therapy to be successful, a number of steps must be carried out with great care and precision:

1. The normal gene is isolated in a chemically pure form (as a piece of DNA) and the gene is inserted into a harmless virus.
2. Cells from the patient are removed and are exposed to the viruses carrying the normal gene. The viruses transport the genes into millions of cells, some of which pick up the gene and insert it into a chromo-

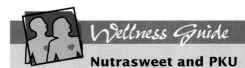
some. In a few of those cells, the gene may manufacture the normal protein.

3. The genetically modified cells are injected back into the patient, where it is hoped that some of them will function and produce the missing protein and correct the symptoms of the disease.

Most of the thousands of known hereditary diseases are not suitable candidates for gene therapy because permanent damage has occurred by the time the baby is born. In other cases too many different cells of the body would have to be genetically altered to correct the disease. In addition to the many technical problems, aspects of gene therapy and new genetic technologies raise fears in some people regarding potential abuses.

COMPLEX DISEASES AND TRAITS

Although hundreds of human diseases and physical defects are known to be caused by abnormalities in just a single gene, many others are caused by several, even hundreds, of different genes that act in unknown ways. Diseases such as hypertension, diabetes, schizophrenia, allergies, and depression are often described as having a hereditary basis although no genes have been found that cause these **complex diseases.** Many normal traits, such as height, skin and eye color, and intelligence, are also determined by many genes; these are called **complex**

traits. These terms mean that the disease or trait in question is determined by an unknown number of genes interacting with an unknown number of environmental factors.

For example, intelligence is determined by an unknown number of genes (it could be hundreds or even thousands), as well as by environmental factors such as nutrition, stimulation, love, and education. Hypertension may be partly due to genes but also is caused by environmental factors such as stress, obesity, and excess salt in the diet. Among identical twins if one twin has schizophrenia (a severe form of mental illness), the other twin does not get the disease in at least half of the twin pairs, proving that genes alone are not the cause of the disease.

Research to quantify the relative contribution of genes and environmental factors to complex traits and diseases, is very difficult to do and the results are invariably controversial. For example, some studies indicate that intelligence is as much as 80 percent determined by genes and some scientists have argued that people of

African ancestry have fewer of the so-called intelligence genes than Caucasians based on their different scores on IQ tests. However, the data used to support claims of differences in intelligence between races have been challenged in considerable detail and have been consistently debunked (Gould, 1995; Kamin, 1995). Arguments over the genetic basis of intelligence have raged for at least a century, and some studies supporting such a basis have been shown to be fraudulent (Gould, 1981).

In recent years, some psychologists and biologists have increasingly characterized abnormal or undesirable human behaviors as being genetically determined. For example, health problems such as alcoholism, obesity, phobias, even suicide, have been ascribed to defective genes. Although no genes have been isolated that cause these problems, scientists continue to search for them. While some peoples' genes may make them more susceptible to obesity or alcoholism than others, the fact remains that these problems

> *All disease is a clash between the environment and our endowment for withstanding the environment. Thus all disease is environmental, and all disease is genetic.*
> Edmond A. Murphy, M.D.

are behavioral and *are* cured by changes in mental attitude and life-styles (Peele, 1990).

Alcoholism is cured by not drinking alcohol, obesity is cured by reducing caloric intake and by exercise, and drug abuse is cured by not using drugs. No genes need to be changed to cure these problems. Because of advances in genetic technologies, scientists continue to look for biological solutions to these serious human problems. Even if some genes are discovered that predispose some people to these problems, the solutions still will require changes in life-styles (Alper and Beckwith, 1994).

Advances in diagnosing hereditary diseases and in identifying human genes that help determine specific complex diseases are going to have a profound effect on the lives of people in the future (Spaulding, 1995). Understanding how genetic tests can affect your life and reproductive decisions is essential if people want to make the best health choices.

Controversy in Health

Will New Genetic Discoveries Cause a Return to Eugenic Ideas?

Francis Galton, a cousin of Charles Darwin, concluded over a century ago that what we are is almost entirely a product of our genes. Rich people are rich because of their genes and poor people are poor because of their genes. He considered the environment a rather insignificant element in most human traits and abilities. Since then, scientists have argued over the relative contribution of genes (nature) and the environment (nurture) to the talents, intelligence, and disease susceptibilities of people.

Galton was a member of English aristocracy; all of his relatives were well-educated, wealthy, and talented. The average Englishman, Galton believed, was poor, stupid, and boorish. Galton developed statistical methods for measuring differences in physical, behavioral, and mental abilities among people, particularly between the upper class and the rest of society. His studies led him and others to conclude that the rich and famous had superior genes to those inherited by poor or unsuccessful people.

Galton's work led to the development of **eugenics**, which is based on the idea that nature (genes) was of overwhelming importance in determining human characteristics. Eugenics advocated the bearing of children by couples with desirable genes, generally white, upper-class, wealthy English men and women. Eugenics also discouraged the bearing of children by poor, undesirable classes of people. Galton and other eugenicists argued that in this way the human species would be improved and those with undesirable traits would eventually be eliminated.

The tragic outcome of eugenic ideas was their use by the Nazis before and during World War II to justify exterminating groups deemed undesirable, such as Jews, Gypsies, the mentally retarded, and homosexuals. Eugenics led to the idea of racial hygiene and genocide. The ideas of eugenics have largely fallen into disfavor, but some people worry that the new genetic and reproductive technologies may again encourage such ideas (Hubbard and Wald, 1993).

STUDENT REFLECTIONS

- A new genetic industry is poised to inform us of the harmful genes we carry that may lead to an early death or to aberrant behavior. Do we want this information? Do we need this information? Can we use it wisely?
- Are we ready as a society to use information about our genes in positive ways to improve the health and lives of everyone, and not just that of an elite class?

HEALTH IN REVIEW

- Congenital defects are observed at birth in about one out of fifty newborn babies in the United States. Abnormal development of the fetus during pregnancy can be caused by environmental factors, chemically defective genes that were passed on from one or both parents, or a combination of both.
- Ultrasound, amniocentesis, and chorionic villus analysis are prenatal diagnostic procedures that can determine if fetal development is normal or if there is a physical or biological defect.
- About 1 to 2 percent of all newborns have a genetic disease resulting from inheriting an abnormal chromosome or defective gene.
- Taking prescriptions or illegal drugs, drinking alcohol, or becoming infected by viruses during pregnancy also can harm the fetus. If these substances are used by a pregnant woman, especially in early pregnancy,

the fetus may abort spontaneously or the newborn may suffer growth deficiencies, mental retardation, or other problems.
- To establish that a disease is inherited requires testing affected individuals and identifying abnormal chromosomes, genes, or proteins.
- Couples who are at higher-than-average risk for having a disabled child should undergo genetic counseling before and after pregnancy is established.
- Modern genetic diagnostic tests can detect hundreds of different hereditary diseases; only a few can be treated successfully.
- Gene therapy is a new method of treatment that may find application in the future.
- Health problems such as alcoholism and obesity may be partly due to genes but behavioral changes are still the best medicine.

REFERENCES

Alper, J. S., and J. Beckwith (1994). "Genetic Fatalism and Social Policy: The Implications of Behavior Genetic Research." *Yale Journal of Biology and Medicine,* 66: 511.

Berkowitz, R. L. (1993). "Should Every Pregnant Woman Undergo Ultrasonography?" *New England Journal of Medicine,* September 16, 329(12): 874–875.

Gould, S. J. (1995). "Curveball." *The New Yorker,* November 28.

Gould, S. J. (1981). *The Mismeasure of Man.* New York: W. W. Norton.

Hook, E. B. (1977). "Differences between Rates of Trisomy 21 (Down's Syndrome) and Other Chromosomal Abnormalities Diagnosed in Live Births and in Cells Cultured after Second Trimester Amniocentesis—Suggested Explanations and Implication for Genetic Counseling and Program Planning," in D. Bergsma and R. L. Summitt (eds.), *Proceedings of the 1977 Birth Defects Conference.* New York: Alan R. Liss.

Hubbard, R., and E. Wald (1993). *Exploding the Gene Myth.* Boston: Beacon Press.

Kamin, L. J. (1995). "Behind the Curve." *Scientific American,* January.

Nelkin, D., and L. Tancredi (1989). *Dangerous Diagnostics: The Social Power of Biological Information.* New York: Basic Books.

Nowak, R. (1994). "Genetic Testing Set for Takeoff." *Science,* July 22.

Peele, S. (1990). "Second Thoughts About a Gene for Alcoholism." *The Atlantic Monthly,* August.

Rennie, J. (1994). "Grading the Gene Tests." *Scientific American,* June.

Robinson, A. D. (1990). "Teaching about Teratology," *The American Biology Teacher,* November/December.

Rosenberg, I. H. (1992). "Folic Acid and Neural Tube Defects—Time for Action." *New England Journal of Medicine,* December 24: 327(26).

Spaulding, K. (1995). "Knowing Isn't Everything." *Newsweek,* April 3.

Thompson, L. (1993). "The First Kids with New Genes." *Time,* June 7.

Wertz, D. C., and J. C. Fletcher (1989). "Disclosing Genetic Information: Who Should Know." *Technology Review,* 92: 12–13.

SUGGESTED READINGS

Beckwith, J. (1993). "A Historical View of Social Responsibility in Genetics." *Bioscience,* May. A discussion of genetic abuses in the past.

Henry III, W. A. (1993). "Born Gay?" *Time,* July 26. An article on the possibility of a "homosexual" gene.

Hubbard, R., and E. Wald (1993). *Exploding the Gene Myth.* Boston: Beacon Press. Explains why genes are not the ultimate cause of human sickness and disease.

Milunsky, A. (1992). *Heredity and Your Family's Life.* New York: Bantam: 1992. An excellent guide to understanding the risks of hereditary diseases.

Robison, A. D. (1990). "Teaching about Teratology." *The American Biology Teacher,* November/December. Discusses the most serious teratogenic agents.

Thompson, L. (1993). "The First Kids with New Genes." *Time,* June 7. Explains how an immune system gene was inserted into several children to treat a rare genetic disease.

Explaining Drug Use and Abuse

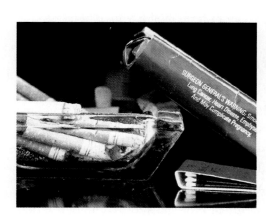

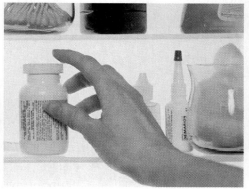

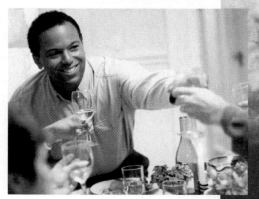

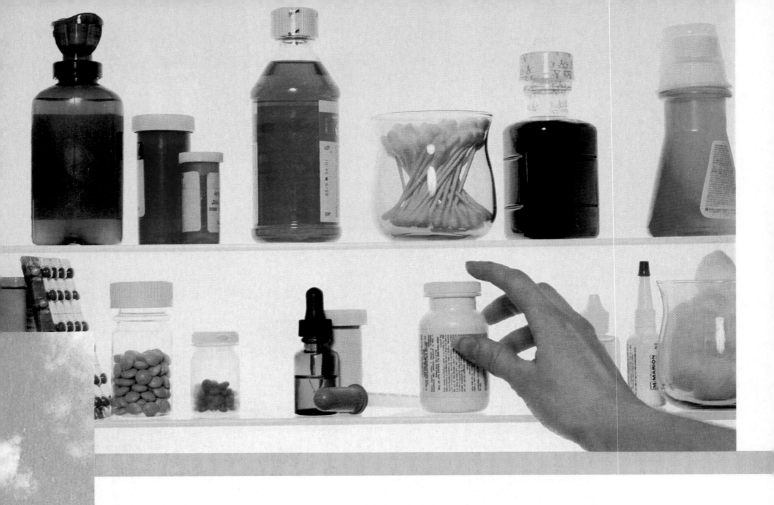

LEARNING OBJECTIVES

After reading this chapter you should be able to:

1. Define the following terms: over-the-counter drug, medicine, dose, drug abuse, drug misuse, drug addiction, and tolerance.
2. Explain how drugs work and their potential side effects.
3. Discuss the effectiveness of drugs.
4. Discuss why Americans take so much medication.
5. Compare and contrast physical and psychological dependence.
6. Identify the effects of cocaine, amphetamines, caffeine, opiates, marijuana, hallucinogens, inhalants, and PCP.

16

Using Drugs Responsibly

*T*hroughout the centuries, potions, herbs, elixirs, and extracts have been used to heal the sick and wounded, change consciousness, produce sleep, drive out evil spirits, and promote tribal and family harmony. Today, drugs and medicines in industrialized societies are no longer folk remedies, but instead result from advances in modern chemical and biological technologies. In the United States, about two billion drug prescriptions are filled each year, or an average of seven for every person in the country. The annual cost of prescription drugs is about $30 billion, and another $10 billion is spent on nonprescription **over-the-counter (OTC) drugs.** About 100 million Americans use alcohol regularly, and another 53 million smoke cigarettes, which contain chemicals that act as drugs. Many adult Americans ingest caffeine daily for its stimulatory effects.

The use of drugs in our society has become so commonplace and accepted that many people automatically turn to drugs to solve their physical, mental, and emotional problems, failing to understand their dangers and health hazards. When people have symptoms such as headache, backache, fatigue, stomach upset, colds, and allergies, many believe that taking drugs is the *only* source of relief. Although many medicines are extremely valuable, and occasional and responsible use of caffeine and alcohol is acceptable, reliance on drugs to solve problems opens the way for chemical dependency. Many people do not consider the possible consequences of drug use, which may have a negative impact on their well-being.

WHAT IS A DRUG?

A **drug** is a single chemical substance in a medicine that alters the structure or function of some of the body's biological processes. The alteration can be to start, stop, speed up, or slow down a process, depending on the specific drug and its effect on biological processes. A **medicine** is a drug (or combination of drugs) that is intended to: 1) prevent illness, as vaccines do; 2) cure disease, as antibiotics do; 3) aid healing, as ulcer medications do; or 4) suppress symptoms, as pain relievers do. Not all drugs—for example, alcohol and nicotine—are medicines.

Drugs are usually classified according to the particular biological process they affect rather than by their chemical properties. For example, all substances that increase urine production, regardless of their chemical structure, are called **diuretics**; those that reduce pain are **analgesics**; and those that produce nervous system excitation are **stimulants**.

How Drugs Work

Many drugs act by interacting with specific cells in the body that carry **receptors**, usually proteins with which the drugs interact; a drug-receptor interaction is akin to the way a key fits into a lock (Figure 16.1). When a drug binds to a receptor, it affects the biological process or processes of cells and organs. Frequently a drug may

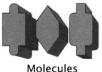
Molecules

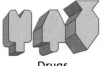
Drugs

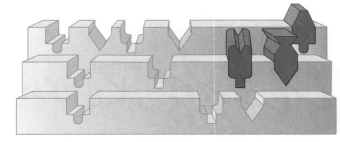

FIGURE 16.1 Bindings of Drugs to Cellular Receptor Sites The molecular structures of many drugs are similar to molecules normally produced in the body. The drugs compete for binding sites on cells and alter the physiological functioning of organs and tissues.

chemically resemble a natural body component, such as a hormone or a neurotransmitter, which interacts with the receptor as part of normal functioning. The drug, acting like a counterfeit key, binds to the receptor in place of the natural substance, and thereby alters physiology.

For example, many antibiotics cure bacterial infections by binding to receptors in bacteria and blocking their reproduction. Many chemotherapeutic drugs used in cancer treatment also work by blocking cell reproduction. In this instance the reproduction of the body's cancer cells are the target (Chapter 13). The aim of chemotherapy is to destroy the cancer cells, which tend to reproduce rapidly, while affecting normal, healthy cells to a lesser degree, allowing them to recover.

Side Effects of Medication

Even though a drug may be intended to have a single effect, it often does not because it binds to different kinds of receptors on different cells. Unintended drug actions are called **side effects** (Figure 16.2), which may be minor or severe. Some side effects include allergic reactions (**drug hypersensitivity**); harm to developing embryos and fetuses (**teratogen**); or physical dependence (addiction).

In addition to side effects, a drug also may be harmful if the drug-taker has a condition that will be aggravated by that drug. A medical reason for not taking a drug is called a **contraindication.** For example, a history of blood vessel disease is a contraindication for taking birth control pills. The need to screen for contraindications is one reason why many medicines are available only by prescription.

Medical practitioners should be knowledgeable about the side effects and contraindications of drugs, but sometimes these are overlooked. About one-third of hos-

---

T E R M S

over-the-counter (OTC) drugs: drugs that do not require a prescription

drug: a single chemical substance in a medicine that alters one or more of the body's biological functions

medicine: drugs used to prevent, treat, or cure illness; medicines are drugs that are prescribed by a physician

diuretics: drugs that increase the urine production

analgesics: drugs that relieve pain without affecting consciousness

stimulants: drugs that produce nervous system excitement; including cocaine, caffeine, amphetamines

receptor: protein on the surface or inside a cell to which a drug or natural substance can bind and affect cell function

side effects: unintended and often harmful actions of a drug

drug hypersensitivity: an allergic reaction to a drug

teratogen: a drug that affects the development of a fetus causing birth defects

contraindication: any medical reason for not taking a particular drug

dose: amount of drug that is administered

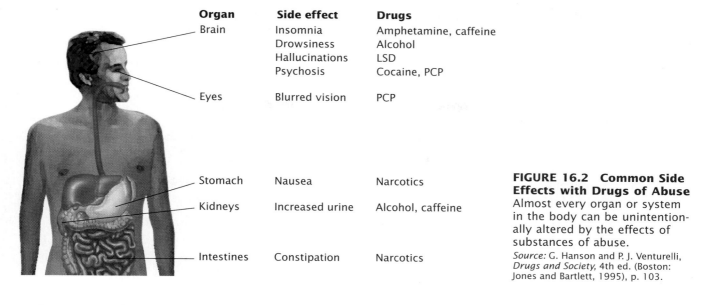

Organ	Side effect	Drugs
Brain	Insomnia	Amphetamine, caffeine
	Drowsiness	Alcohol
	Hallucinations	LSD
	Psychosis	Cocaine, PCP
Eyes	Blurred vision	PCP
Stomach	Nausea	Narcotics
Kidneys	Increased urine	Alcohol, caffeine
Intestines	Constipation	Narcotics

FIGURE 16.2 Common Side Effects with Drugs of Abuse Almost every organ or system in the body can be unintentionally altered by the effects of substances of abuse.
Source: G. Hanson and P. J. Venturelli, *Drugs and Society,* 4th ed. (Boston: Jones and Bartlett, 1995), p. 103.

pital stays are needlessly extended because inappropriate medications are administered or managed improperly by medical staff. Consumers of medications should learn as much as they can about the intended and side effects of their drugs, and they should ask their medical providers to explain the rationale for the medications that they are taking.

Routes of Administration

Drugs can be taken by mouth, inhalation, or injection into the muscles, under the skin (from which they diffuse into surrounding tissues and blood), or injected directly into the bloodstream. Drugs also can be absorbed through the skin and the mucous membranes of the nose, eyes, vagina, and anus. Regardless of the route of entry, most drugs remain active in the body for a relatively short time, often only a few hours.

Once in the body, drugs are broken down by the liver, (metabolized). Drugs are also filtered by the kidneys and passed out of the body in urine. Drugs such as inhalatory anesthetics or nitrous oxide can be eliminated in expired air.

Effectiveness of Drugs

The **dose** of a drug is the amount that is administered or taken. The effectiveness of a particular dose of a drug is influenced by a person's body size, how rapidly the drug breaks down and is eliminated, and sometimes by the presence of other drugs and foods recently consumed (Table 16.1). A drug's effectiveness also depends on the person's expectations of the drug's efficacy (placebo effect) (Chapter 3) and the person's mental state. For example, when stressed or anxious, many people require higher doses of analgesics to relieve pain than when they

More over-the-counter drugs are available in the United States than anywhere else in the world.

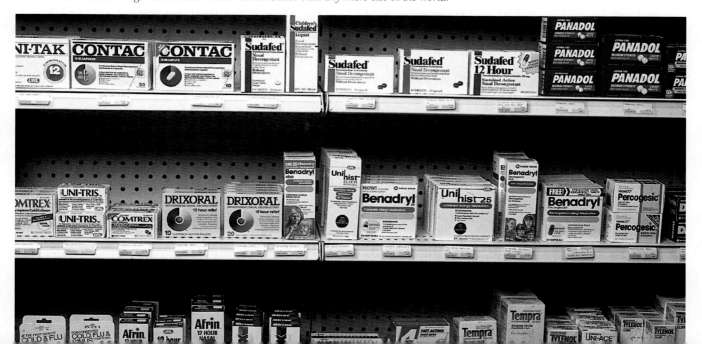

TABLE 16.1 Drug and Food Interactions That Should Be Avoided

If you take	Avoid	Because
Erythromycin- or penicillin-type antibiotics	Acidic foods; pickles, tomatoes, vinegar, colas	These antibiotics are destroyed by stomach acids
Tetracycline-type antibiotics	Calcium-rich foods: milk, cheese, yogurt, pizza, almonds	Calcium blocks the action of tetracycline
Antihypertensives (to lower blood pressure)	Natural licorice (artificial is OK)	A chemical in natural licorice causes salt and water retention
Anticoagulants (to thin blood)	Vitamin K: green leafy vegetables, beef liver, vegetable oils	Vitamin K promotes blood clotting
Antidepressants (monoamine oxidase inhibitors)	Tyramine-rich foods: colas, chocolate, cheese, coffee, wine, avocados	Tyramine elevates blood pressure
Diuretics	Monosodium glutamate (MSG)	MSG and diuretics both increase water elimination
Thyroid drugs	Cabbage, brussels sprouts, soybeans, cauliflower	Chemicals in these vegetables depress thyroid hormone production

are relaxed. Most drugs have a narrow range of effectiveness, that is, doses that produce intended results. In excess many drugs are toxic and some are lethal (Figure 16.3). If the dose is too low, insufficient therapeutic effect may result.

The effects of a drug or medicine are often determined scientifically by performing double-blind clinical trials, which involve administering the drug and a look-and-taste-alike placebo to matched groups of patients. Neither the people administering the drug nor the patients know who is receiving the drug and who is receiving the placebo (thus the expression **double-blind**). Only after the trial is the code revealed that tells which patients received the drug. What is most remarkable about many of these drug trials is not that drugs show a therapeutic effect, but that placebos often come very close to giving the same relief or results as do the drugs (Chapter 2).

In 1984, ibuprofen was introduced into the OTC market. Because aspirin and acetaminophen compounds commanded over 90 percent of the pain-reliever market, manufacturers of ibuprofen advertised heavily in medical journals to get physicians to recommend or prescribe the new drug. One advertisement showed that after four hours Nuprin, the trade name for an ibuprofen drug, relieved headaches about 8 percent more effectively than acetaminophen (Figure 16.4). From a holistic health perspective, however, the more significant result is that 40 percent of headache sufferers got the same relief with a placebo. Thus, four out of ten headache sufferers found relief simply by believing that they had taken a pain relief medicine.

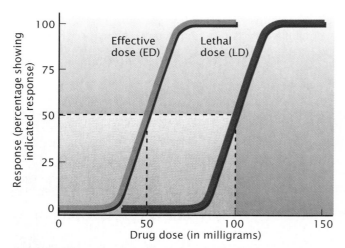

FIGURE 16.3 Method for Calculating a Drug's Therapeutic Index (LD-50/ED-50) The LD-50 is the drug dose that causes lethality in 50 percent of the users (100 mg in figure). In this example, the therapeutic index is 2 (100/50 + 2). The greater the therapeutic index, the safer the drug.
Source: G. Hanson and P. J. Venturelli, *Drugs and Society*, 4th ed. (Boston: Jones and Bartlett, 1995), p. 106.

T E R M

double-blind: when neither the person receiving the drug nor the person administering the drug know whether it is a placebo or the real drug

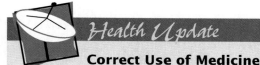

Health Update

Correct Use of Medicine

Americans have made significant progress over the past 10 years in using medicines correctly, according to a report by the National Council on Patient Information and Education (NCPIE). People have learned to ask more questions about their medicines, senior citizens are getting their medicines reviewed, and health-care professionals are counseling patients better, the report says.

The report, "Making Proper Medicine Use a National Priority," credits this progress to education efforts of consumer groups, physicians, pharmacists, nurses, drug manufacturers, voluntary health organizations, and FDA. Through the efforts of these groups:

- Eighty-eight percent of patients were told by their doctors how much medicine to take and how often to take it.
- Eighty-one percent of patients received instructions on how long to continue use.
- Eighty-one percent of persons 45 and older were "very likely or somewhat likely" to ask the doctor questions about a new prescription.
- Eighty-four percent of persons 45 or older were told by or asked their doctor about how and when to take their prescription medicine.
- Fifty-nine percent were told or asked about precautions.
- Fifty-five percent were told or asked about side effects.

Source: FDA Consumer, January–February, 1994.

An even more remarkable placebo effect is shown by the ability of balding men to stimulate hair growth simply by believing that they are using a hair-stimulating drug called Rogaine. The Upjohn Company, manufacturer of Rogaine, advertises extensively in the most prestigious medical journals and on TV. In these ads, the company emphasizes the effectiveness of Rogaine compared to a placebo solution applied to the scalp. Rogaine produces minimal to moderate growth of new hair in 33 percent of patients receiving the drug. However, a placebo containing no active ingredient produces minimal to moderate hair growth in 20 percent of patients. While this fact is ignored by the advertising, it means that one out of five men who have pattern baldness (an inherited trait) can stimulate new hair growth simply because they believe they are using a drug. How

the mind changes physiology to accomplish this is unknown. The point, however, is never to underestimate the power of your mind to act like a drug and help you to heal an injury or illness.

THE OVERMEDICATING OF AMERICANS

Americans consume an enormous quantity of drugs, often to their detriment. A few years ago, the American Medical Association concluded that "the abuse of prescription drugs results in more injuries and death to Americans than all illegal drugs combined. Prescription drugs are involved in almost 60 percent of all drug-related deaths."

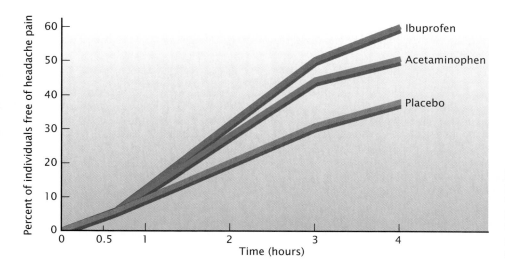

FIGURE 16.4 A Study of the Effectiveness of Ibuprofen versus Acetaminophen in Relieving Headaches Note that 40 percent of headache sufferers get relief with no drug at all.

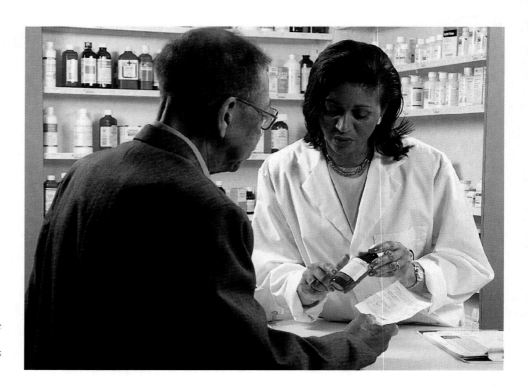

It is important to understand possible side effects a drug may cause and its interactions with other drugs or foods that are ingested.

People over 65 are the largest consumers of both prescription and OTC drugs, which explains why TV drug ads usually show older persons. Older persons often take numerous drugs for a variety of complaints, and these drugs may interact in unforeseen ways to cause additional problems. It is not uncommon for older people to take ten or more different medications daily, which may have been prescribed by different physicians at different times. Older people are physiologically less able to tolerate drugs than younger people and often suffer more serious side effects. Quite often elimination of all drug use for a brief period will cause many symptoms to disappear, a clear indication that the combination of drugs is causing problems. Patients need to ask for and use fewer drugs; physicians need to become less willing to prescribe drugs for any and all complaints.

Pharmaceutical companies now spend $2 billion dollars each year promoting their products to physicians and to the general public (Cornacchia and Barrett, 1993). During winter, the TV screen and the pages of popular maga-

---

Health Update

Older Americans Take Inappropriate Drugs

At least 1 in 4 older Americans not living in nursing homes may take a prescription drug considered inappropriate, a national study concludes.

The study's authors defined an inappropriate drug as any of 20 identified by an expert panel as drugs that older Americans should avoid because of adverse effects, such as daytime sedation or cognitive impairment, resulting in an increased risk of falls.

The study's authors said their findings probably underestimate the incidence of inappropriate prescribing because the study did not consider other prescribing practices, such as excessive drug dosage or duration, and medication interactions.

The study report appeared in the July 27, 1994, issue of the *Journal of the American Medical Association,* with information from 6,171 people in the 1987 National Medical Expenditure Survey by the Agency for Health Care Policy and Research, a part of the U.S. Department of Health and Human Services.

According to the study, 24 percent of people 65 and older who do not live in nursing homes received at least one of the 20 inappropriate drugs in 1987. Of those receiving the inappropriate drugs, nearly 80 percent received only one drug, while 20 percent received two or more.

The [study's] authors recommend "more vigorous" doctor education and increased drug regulation to improve the safety of prescribing medicines.

Source: FDA Consumer, October, 1994.

zines are loaded with inducements to buy products for coughs and colds. In the summer TV ads for sunburn and tanning creams and lotions. Ads for pain relievers are incessant. The Food and Drug Administration (FDA) regulates advertising and requires that print media ads carry information about effectiveness, side effects, precautions, contraindications, and potential reactions. The FDA also requires that these ads include "adequate directions for use." The regulations for print media ads surpass the regulations for TV advertisements, which say little about effectiveness, side effects, precautions, contraindications, and potential reactions.

Because most clinical drug sales come from prescription medications, the heaviest drug company advertising is directed toward physicians. Drug companies spend thousands of dollars per year per physician trying to persuade doctors to prescribe the drugs that they manufacture. Drug companies send sales representatives to doctors' offices, hospitals, and health maintenance organizations to inform them of the company's products and to leave free samples. Drug companies sponsor seminars and courses often accompanied by free lunches or vacations to update health care providers on the diagnosis and treatment of particular diseases (for which the company manufactures a drug). And drug companies deluge physicians with pharmaceutical "junk" mail: one doctor received over 500 pounds of drug company junk mail in one year.

When confronted with a person in distress but not physically sick, many physicians feel obligated to offer some remedy, even if a medically legitimate one does not exist. People expect doctors to prescribe something. The answer to this dilemma has been neatly provided by pharmaceutical companies that manufacture and advertise mood-altering drugs just for this situation. If a person is anxious, drug ads tell the physician to prescribe a tranquilizer. If depression is a problem, an antidepressant should be prescribed. If the person cannot sleep, a barbiturate or hypnotic may help. As people become more informed and aware of the undesirable consequences of taking drugs and how infrequently drugs are really necessary, they will elect to cope with stress and anxiety in ways that do not involve drugs.

Indeed, in some cases, the tranquilizer or sleeping pill may help temporarily. Sometimes people become so depressed or upset over a life situation that they cannot muster the clear thinking and action necessary to deal

> One out of six TV commercials tells you and me and our youngsters that if you're not feeling well there is a substance that will make you feel better, be it something for a headache, something to give you energy, or something to lose weight.
>
> John C. Lawn,
> Drug Enforcement Administration

with the problem. In such instances, a sleeping medication, tranquilizer, or antidepressant may help achieve a calmer psychological state in which appropriate action can be taken. Unfortunately, too many people and their doctors mistakenly assume that the drug itself will solve the problem, whereas it may, instead, substitute for proper help and treatment.

Drugs and medications are highly useful substances. We have vaccines to prevent viral infections, antibiotics to help cure bacterial infections, and a variety of medications that treat serious illnesses. However, the availability of so many medications has fostered the belief that drugs can help solve just about any problem. Most people expect some form of medication to be assured that their illness is being treated. And doctors may prescribe unnecessary medications to assure patients and themselves that they are providing treatment and care.

Many physicians recognize this problem. They would prefer to deal only with physically ill people—the patients whose problems they were educated to treat. But many patients resist the suggestion that they do not have a diagnosable disease, and insist that they receive some form of treatment even if only the prescribing of a tranquilizer. This is a serious form of current drug abuse.

Being healthy means, among other things, being responsible for the drugs you use. You do not have to resort to "chemical coping" for emotional problems. You can resist being pushed into "pill popping" by drug company advertising. You should question a drug from your doctor for a condition that stems from anxiety, stress, or emotional problems. Seeking alternatives to prescription or over-the-counter drug use may be the most healthful action you can take (Chapter 20).

PREVENTING DRUG ABUSE

The human body is capable of tolerating and eliminating small quantities of virtually any substance or drug with no permanent harmful effects. However, it may be harmful to ingest large doses or to use a drug frequently even in small quantities. Generally, using any drug to the point where health is adversely affected or the ability to function in society is impaired can be defined as **drug abuse.**

H E A L T H Y   P E O P L E   2 0 0 0

Reduce drug-related deaths to no more than 3 per 100,000 people.

Drug-related deaths are an important indicator of the adverse consequences of drug use.

T E R M

drug abuse: persistent or excessive use of a drug without medical or health reasons

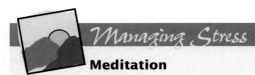

Meditation

It's fair to say that most people experiment with drugs out of curiosity, peer pressure, or a combination of the two. What may begin as an innocent experiment, however, often ends up a struggle for self-sovereignty.

People who have given up drugs will give a number of reasons, the most common being that although the trips may have been exciting, the side effects were horrendous, if not tragic. This was the case with the Beatles, who found that drug use stifled rather than promoted their creative efforts. Seeking a way to gain passage through the door to objective reality they met Maharishi Mahesh Yogi, the founder of transcendental meditation (TM). And so began a journey of exploration of human consciousness, natural highs, and profound revelations without the unwanted baggage of side effects and addiction.

Today we know that there are many ways to meditate. What is important is to find a style that's right for you. The standard definition of meditation is "increased con-centration leading to increased awareness," and indeed with repeated practice some experiences may occur that will surpass any drug-induced high.

Meditation isn't so much thinking about something as it is *not* thinking about anything. Meditation is a way to clear the thoughts from your mind and deactivate the censoring process of the ego to open the way for new insights, wisdom, intuition, or enlightenment that otherwise go unnoticed in the course of a hectic day.

The steps to meditation are easy. They require nothing more than 1) a quiet environment, 2) a comfortable sitting position, 3) a passive attitude, and 4) a meditative object (like monitoring your breathing, or listening to the sound of ocean waves.

After accomplishing the first three steps, try this exercise:

Imagine yourself standing in a cylinder, about four feet in diameter, made of concrete blocks. As you look up, you see the walls are high, too high to climb. The walls repre-sent the walls of your ego. Each block has etched in it a description of an issue you are dealing with or an unresolved conflict with another person. The way out is not through physical means, but rather through your mental, emotional, and spiritual energies. First, you take a few slow deep breaths to relax your mind and body. By trying to address each issue in your mind (e.g., patience, detachment, forgiveness, acceptance, etc.), you slowly see the walls begin to descend, eventually to a point where you are no longer held captive by your thoughts and feelings of anger and anxiety. You are free of the limitations of your own mind. As these walls disappear, what do you see in front of you, and all around you? What do you experience? Take a moment to sense all that you can.

This is just one of many types of meditation exercises to help you shift your way of thinking and explore the realms of consciousness without the aid or complications of drugs.

Drug abuse refers not just to the type or amount of a drug taken. Rather it occurs when the drug is used to mask personal problems. If a drug is used to mask anxiety or facilitate undesirable behaviors, it is being abused. If a drug is used continually to combat the effects of stress, it is being abused. If pleasure is experienced only when a drug is taken, the drug is being abused. If a person cannot control the use of a drug, it is being abused.

There are many dangers of continual drug use; it can cause **physical dependence**, commonly called addiction. Physical dependence means that frequent use of a drug causes physical changes in the tissues with which the drug interacts and generates further need for the drug. Many tranquilizers and sedatives cause addiction.

Both legal and illegal drugs can cause physical dependence. The legality of a drug is more a function of social, political, and economic considerations than the drug's toxicity or pharmacology (Kleber, 1994). From a personal and community health standpoint, alcohol causes far more harm than all other drugs combined (Angell and Kassirer, 1994), yet it is legal.

The legal status of drugs changes with social customs and people's beliefs. In the 1920s and 1930s alcohol was illegal in the United States, but marijuana was legal. During the early twentieth century, opium, morphine, and cocaine were openly advertised and sold in the form of tonics and cough syrups. Coca-Cola, concocted by a Georgia pharmacist in 1886, was sold as both a remedy and an enjoyable drink. "Coke" contained cocaine until 1906, when the cocaine was replaced by caffeine.

Withdrawal Symptoms

One consequence of physical dependence is the experience of **withdrawal symptoms** (or abstinence syndrome) after the drug is no longer used. Withdrawal symptoms are often uncomfortable and may be fatal. For example, someone physically dependent on heroin may experience anxiety, pain, sweating, muscle cramps, and several other unpleasant reactions when deprived of the drug. Indeed, for those who have experienced withdrawal, the fear of experiencing it again may become a greater motivator to continue drug use than the effects of the drug itself. Another example is caffeine withdrawal, where headaches and shakiness may be experienced.

With many drugs, withdrawal symptoms are the opposite of the drug's primary effects. In general, withdrawal from nervous system depressants such as alcohol, opiates, tranquilizers, and sedatives leads to symptoms such as hyperexcitivity, anxiousness, irritability, and susceptibility to seizures. Withdrawal from stimulants such as cocaine, amphetamines, and caffeine, on the other hand, can produce sleepiness, depression, and loss of consciousness.

Psychological Dependence

Besides physical dependence, drugs can create **psychological dependence**, called **habituation**, which does not involve changes in cells and organs, but is manifested as an intense craving for the drug. Habituation becomes injurious when the person becomes so consumed by the need for the desired drugged state that all of one's energy is siphoned into compulsive drug-seeking behavior. Physically addicting drugs like heroin, alcohol, nicotine, and caffeine invariably also produce habituation. As a consequence of this compulsive drug-seeking behavior, relationships, jobs, and families can be destroyed.

Tolerance is an adaptation of the body to a drug such that larger doses are needed to produce the same effect. Because not all parts of the body become tolerant to the same degree, these higher doses may cause harmful side effects to less tolerant parts. For example, a heroin or barbiturate user can become tolerant to the psychological effects of the drug but the brain's respiratory center, which controls breathing, does not. If the dose of heroin, barbiturate, or other depressant becomes high enough, the brain's respiratory center ceases to function and the person stops breathing.

PSYCHOACTIVE DRUGS

Most of the commonly abused drugs are **psychoactive** substances, meaning they affect thoughts, perceptions, feelings, and moods; in other words, they change consciousness (Table 16.2). Consciousness is the state of being aware of one's mental processes. Each of us has a "normal" state of consciousness, although many people would have difficulty describing what they mean by "normal." However, everyone knows when his or her state of consciousness deviates from normal—for example, when drunk, extremely angry, sad, or depressed. High fever can alter consciousness even to the point of hallucinations.

There are numerous activities not generally regarded as consciousness-altering that produce changes comparable in many respects to those produced by psychoactive drugs. Long-distance runners may experience a change of consciousness that is described as "runners' high"; dancing can produce psychic "highs" and even ecstatic states of consciousness, which is the goal of whirling dervishes who practice particular forms of Sufi dancing. Fasting can produce profound changes in consciousness, which is why prolonged fasts are often part of religious training. Many "thrill" activities, such as riding on roller coasters or shooting the rapids on river rafts, change consciousness and presumably are enjoyed for that reason. Put into this perspective, ingesting psychoactive drugs is only one of many ways people use to change consciousness.

THE EFFECTS OF STIMULANTS

Stimulants are substances that act on the central nervous system (CNS). Pleasant effects are experienced initially after taking some stimulants, such as increased energy and a state of euphoria or a "high." But a user can also feel restless, talkative, and have difficulty sleeping. Long-term use can produce personality changes or even dangerous behaviors if high doses are taken. Because the initial effects are pleasant, stimulants are frequently abused leading to dependence.

Cocaine

Cocaine is a stimulant obtained from the leaves of the coca shrub, *Erythroxylum coca,* a plant indigenous to the Andes. For thousands of years, inhabitants of Peru,

T E R M S

physical dependence: a physiological state that depends on the continuous presence of a drug; absence of the drug may cause discomfort, nervousness, headaches, sweating (withdrawal symptoms) and sometimes death

withdrawal symptoms: uncomfortable and sometimes dangerous reactions that occur after a person stops taking a physically addicting drug

psychological dependence: dependence that results because a drug produces pleasant mental effects

habituation: repeating certain patterns of behavior until they become established or habitual

tolerance: a condition in which increased amounts of a drug or increased exposure to an addictive behavior are required to produce desired effects

psychoactive: a substance that primarily alters mood, perception, and other brain functions

cocaine: a stimulant drug obtained from the leaves of the coca shrub that causes feelings of exhilaration, euphoria, and physical vigor

TABLE 16.2 Classifications of Drugs That Affect the Central Nervous System

Drug classification	Common and trade names	Medical uses	Effects of average dose	Physical dependence	Tolerance develops
Narcotics	Codeine Demerol Heroin Methadone Morphine Opium Percodan	Analgesic (pain relief)	Blocks or eases pain; may cause drowsiness and euphoria; some users experience nausea or itching sensations	Marked	Yes
Analgesics	Darvon Talwin	Pain relief	May produce anxiety and hallucinations	Marked	Yes
Sedatives	Amytal Nembutal Phenobarbital Seconal Doriden Quaalude Halcion Xanax	Sedation, tension relief	Relaxation, sleep; decreases alertness and muscle coordination	Marked	Yes
Minor tranquilizers	Dalmane Equanil/Miltown Librium Valium	Anxiety relief, muscle tension	Mild sedation; increased sense of well-being; may cause drowsiness and dizziness	Marked	No
Major tranquilizers (phenothiazines)	Mellaril Thorazine Prolixin	Control psychosis	Heavy sedation, anxiety relief; may cause confusion, muscle rigidity, convulsions	None	No
Alcohol	Beer Wine Liquor	None	Relaxation; loss of inhibition; mood swings; decreased alertness and coordination	Marked	Yes
Inhalants	Amyl nitrite Butyl nitrite Nitrous oxide	Muscle relaxant, anesthetic	Relaxation, euphoria; causes dizziness, headache, drowsiness	None	?
Stimulants	Benzedrine Biphetamine Desoxyn Dexedrine Methedrine Preludin Ritalin	Weight control, narcolepsy; fatigue and hyperactivity in children	Increased alertness and mood elevation; less fatigue and increased concentration; may cause insomnia, anxiety, headache, chills, and rise in blood pressure; organic brain damage after prolonged use	Mild to none	Yes
Cocaine	Cocaine hydrochloride	Local anesthetic, pain relief	Effects similar to stimulants	Marked	No
Cannabis	Marijuana Hashish	Relief of glaucoma, asthma, nausea accompanying chemotherapy	Relaxation, euphoria, altered perception; may cause confusion, panic, hallucinations	None	No
Hallucinogens	LSD PCP Mescaline Peyote Psilocybin	None	Altered perceptions, visual and sensory distortion; mood swings	None	Yes
Nicotine	(In tobacco)	None	Altered heart rate; tremors; excitation	Yes	Yes

Bolivia, and Colombia have chewed coca leaves to obtain stimulant and other beneficial effects. After the Spanish conquest of the Inca empire in the sixteenth century, use of coca leaves was introduced to Europe and later to North America. In the late nineteenth century, Angelo Mariani, a Corsican, received a medal from the pope for manufacturing an extract of coca leaves that "freed the body of fatigue, lifted the spirits, and induced a sense of well-being." In the United States in the 1880s, Atlanta pharmacist J. C. Pemberton mixed extracts of coca leaves and kola nuts to produce Coca-Cola, claimed at the time to be not only refreshing but also "exhilarating, invigo-

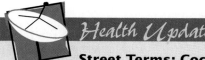

rating, and a cure for all nervous afflictions." Today, of course, Coke no longer contains cocaine, although cocaine-free extracts of coca leaves are still used for flavoring. Sigmund Freud extolled the use of cocaine as a mood elevator, a possible antidote to depression, and a treatment for morphine addiction. However, witnessing a friend's severe and terrifying psychotic reaction to cocaine tempered Freud's enthusiasm for the drug.

In the doses common to **illegal recreational use** today, cocaine induces euphoria, a sense of power and clarity of thought, and increased physical vigor. The effects vary depending on the route of administration (snorting or "sniffing" a cocaine-containing powder, injection, or smoking). The duration of effects is also dependent on the administration route, after which the user usually experiences a letdown and a craving for another dose of the drug.

Cocaine increases heart rate and blood pressure. Continued use of the drug can result in appetite and weight loss, malnutrition, sleep disturbance, and altered thought and mood patterns. Frequent cocaine sniffing can inflame the nasal passages and cause permanent damage to the nasal septum. An overdose can cause seizures or death.

Cocaine does produce tolerance, physical dependence, and withdrawal. The potential for psychological dependence is great, probably the greatest among all psychoactive drugs. Some people develop such a strong craving for the drug that their lives are consumed by their cocaine habit.

Amphetamines

Amphetamines are manufactured chemicals that stimulate the central nervous system. The most common

T E R M S

illegal recreational use: taking illegal drugs for fun, pleasure, or to experience an altered state of consciousness

amphetamines: synthetic drugs that stimulate the central nervous system and sometimes produce hallucinogenic states

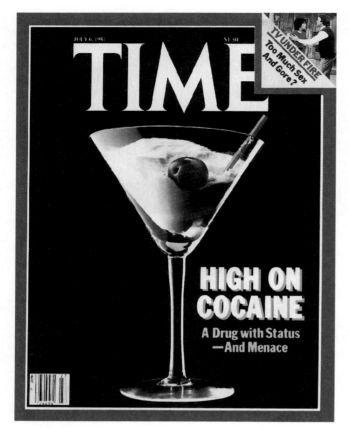

Although accepted as a part of popular culture since the early 1980s, cocaine use has long been known to destroy health and lives.

HEALTHY PEOPLE 2000

Reduce the percent of young people who have used alcohol, marijuana, and cocaine in the past month.

Mind-altering substances and addictive substances have been shown to jeopardize physical, mental, and social development during the formative years and to endanger the successful transition from school to workplace. Moreover, use of these substances, including alcohol, is illegal for young people and thus may have long-term implications for employment and schooling.

amphetamine substances are dextroamphetamine, methamphetamine, dextromethamphetamine, and amphetamine itself. MDA (*methylenedioxyamphetamine*), another psychoactive amphetamine, is manufactured and sold illegally; it produces a hallucinogenic state lasting several hours. Amphetamines are usually taken orally but they can also be injected ("mainlined") and smoked. The effects of an oral dose usually last several hours. Slang terms for amphetamines include dexies, footballs, orange, bennies, peaches, meth, speed, and ice.

Although amphetamines may be prescribed by a physician, their medical use is limited. The legal use of amphetamines is restricted to three medical conditions: 1) narcolepsy, 2) hyperkinetic behavior (attention-deficit hyperactivity disorder), and 3) short-term weight reduction programs (Hanson and Venturelli, 1995).

The principal uses of amphetamines are recreational. These drugs produce feelings of euphoria, increased energy, greater self-confidence, an increased ability to concentrate, increased motor and speech activity, and perceived improved physical performance. Besides being used by those wishing to experience an amphetamine high, these drugs are frequently abused by people who fight sleep, such as truck drivers, students who cram for exams all night, and nightclub entertainers. Athletes believe amphetamines improve their physical performance and increase their self-confidence; however, these are the user's perceptions not the reality.

Excessive amphetamine use can cause headaches, irritability, dizziness, insomnia, panic, confusion, delirium, and crash. The user often experiences a "crash," which occurs when the stimulants wear off, during which he or she usually is very depressed, tired, and sleeps for long periods.

Prolonged use of amphetamines can lead to tolerance, especially for the euphoric effects and for appetite suppression. Amphetamines can cause mild physical dependence, and create a psychological dependence and a particular pattern of use called the "yo-yo," which is a cycle of amphetamine use for the stimulatory effect followed by a depressant in order to sleep, followed by more amphetamines the next day to get going. Chronic use can cause an amphetamine psychosis, consisting of auditory and visual hallucinations, delusions, and mood swings.

A particularly dangerous form of amphetamine is "ice"—a smoked form of pure methamphetamine hydrochloride. The inhaled drug reaches the brain almost immediately, producing a high that can last for several hours. Because the drug can be so easily inhaled, the potential for compulsive use, tolerance, and abuse is also very great. This amphetamine is manufactured at clandestine laboratories; the purity of the drug varies considerably from one laboratory to another, which adds to its risks.

Caffeine

Caffeine is a natural stimulant found in a variety of plants used in coffee, tea, chocolate, and soft drinks (Table 16.3). These beverages and foods are an integral part of American eating habits and may be enjoyed partly for their psychoactive properties.

The effects of caffeine are familiar to most people. They include decreased drowsiness and fatigue (especially when performing tedious or boring tasks), faster and clearer flow of thought, and increased capacity for

TABLE 16.3 Caffeine Content of Beverages and Chocolate

Beverage	Caffeine content (mg)/cup	Amount
Brewed coffee	90–125	5 oz.
Instant coffee	14–93	5 oz.
Decaffeinated coffee	1–6	5 oz.
Tea	30–70	5 oz.
Cocoa	5	5 oz.
Coca-Cola	45	12 oz.
Pepsi-Cola	30	12 oz.
Chocolate bar	22	1 oz.

Source: G. Hanson and P. J. Venturelli, *Drugs and Society,* 4th ed. (Boston: Jones and Bartlett, 1995), p. 285.

sustained performance (for example, typists work faster with fewer errors). In higher doses, caffeine produces nervousness, restlessness, tremors, insomnia, and potentially have a negative effect when performing complex tasks. In very high doses (10 grams, or 60 cups of coffee) it can produce convulsions, which can be fatal.

In the past, caffeine was prescribed for a variety of complaints, but it is rarely used medically any more. However, it is still a key ingredient in over a thousand over-the-counter drugs. For example, many "energizers" and "stay-awake" products are pure caffeine. Pain relievers, cough medicines, and cold remedies contain caffeine to counteract the drowsiness produced by other ingredients in these medications. Caffeine is also put into weight control and menstrual pain products because it increases urine output and water loss.

Psychological dependence can result from chronic use of caffeine, and tolerance to the stimulant effect can gradually develop. Mild withdrawal symptoms such as

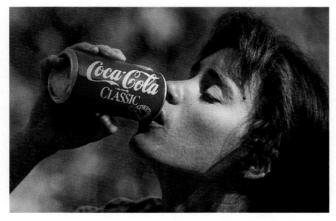

Most Americans consume more soft drinks than glasses of water. This can mean a significant daily intake of caffeine.

headache, irritability, restlessness, and lethargy may occur when caffeine use is stopped.

DEPRESSANTS

Depressants comprise a vast number of drugs whose common effects include reducing level of arousal, motor activity, and awareness of the environment, while increasing drowsiness and sedation. The depressants include alcohol (Chapter 18), and drugs that affect sleep, **sedatives, tranquilizers,** and **hypnotics.** A number of other drugs, such as opiates, antihistamines, and some medications used in the treatment of high blood pressure or heart disease may also act as depressants. In low doses, depressants produce a mild state of euphoria, reduce inhibitions, or induce a feeling of relaxation. In high doses they may impair mood, speech, and motor coordination.

Depressants are dangerous. All carry the potential for physical and psychological dependency, tolerance, unpleasant withdrawal symptoms, and toxicity from continual use or overuse. Acute overdoses may produce coma, respiratory or cardiovascular collapse, and even death. Aggravating the potential for lethal overdose is the synergistic actions of depressants. That is, when taken together, two or more different depressants can produce a much stronger effect than either drug produces if taken alone. The most common synergistic effect occurs when people drink alcohol while taking depressant medications, such as barbiturates or tranquilizers.

Opiates

The **opiates** are a group of chemically related drugs that depress the central nervous system. These substances cause physical dependence, habituation, and tolerance and produce serious withdrawal symptoms. Opiates are derived from the opium poppy, *Papaver somniferum,* extracts of which have been used for thousands of years in a variety of cultures to produce euphoria, to relieve pain, and to treat various diseases.

T E R M S

caffeine: a natural stimulant found in a variety of plants; commonly found in tea, coffee, chocolate, and soft drinks

sedatives: CNS depressants used to relieve anxiety, fear, and apprehension

tranquilizers: central nervous system depressants that relax the body and calm anxiety

hypnotics: CNS depressants used to induce drowsiness and encourage sleep

opiates: derived from the opium poppy, they are drugs that depress the central nervous system

Opium is a complex mixture of plant alkaloids; its principal psychoactive substances are morphine and, to a much lesser degree, codeine. Heroin is derived from morphine. Morphine and other opiates block nerve transmission in the central nervous system, thereby suppressing mental and physiological functions. Opiates bind to the nerve cell receptors and mimic the actions of the body's natural pain-relieving substances, endorphins, and enkephalins. Morphine and codeine are used medically for pain relief and as a cough suppressant, while heroin is used primarily as an illegal recreational drug.

The sensations produced by injecting heroin into the circulatory system are markedly different from those of morphine and codeine, even though the opiate drugs are similar in chemistry. As one heroin user described the sensation: "It's so good, don't even try it once." Regular use of opiates can produce many unwanted effects in addition to the psychological high. Among the adverse reactions are constipation, loss of appetite, depression, loss of interest in sex, constriction of the pupil of the eye, disruption of the menstrual cycle, and drowsiness. Very large doses or prolonged use can be lethal because of respiratory failure.

Street heroin may contain as little as 1 to 3 percent heroin; the rest is sugar, cornstarch, cleansing agents, strychnine, or almost any white powder. Heroin is converted to morphine in the body, and the morphine is eventually excreted in urine, saliva, sweat, and the breast milk of lactating women. Because morphine crosses the placenta, a developing fetus can become addicted even before birth and will experience withdrawal symptoms after it is born.

Marijuana

Marijuana, or *Cannabis sativa*, grows in temperate climates all over the world. Species of cannabis have been cultivated for thousands of years, principally as a source of hemp fiber used in rope. Other species have been cultivated for the psychoactive drug marijuana found in leaves and flowers, and a derivative called **hashish.**

The principal psychoactive ingredient in marijuana and hashish is a chemical called delta-9-tetrahydrocannabinol, or THC. Ingestion of THC occurs by inhaling smoke from marijuana cigarettes or hashish pipes, taking pills, or eating food (such as cookies or brownies). Once ingested, THC is absorbed rapidly in the tissues. In most individuals, low doses of THC produce euphoria, a sense of relaxation, and occasionally altered perception of space and time. Speech may be impaired and short-term memory is affected. Because perception, motor coordination, and reaction time are also impaired, driving a car or operating other machines while intoxicated with THC is unsafe.

Sometimes marijuana use may evoke confusion, anxiety, panic, hallucinations, and paranoia. Sometimes there is no effect at all. Marijuana may also aggravate an existing mental health problem or negative mood. Long-term use does not cause permanent changes in brain function or impaired cognitive abilities. Some of the possible health dangers of long-term marijuana use include the risk of bronchitis caused by marijuana smoke, increased heart rate and blood pressure, and possibly a slight depression of immune system functions. Research concludes that there are carcinogens in

 Wellness Guide

Specific Signs of Marijuana Use

1. An odor similar to burnt rope in room, on clothes, etc.
2. Roach—small butt end of a marijuana cigarette.
3. Joint—looks like a hand-rolled cigarette, usually the ends are twisted or crimped.
4. Roach clips—holders for the roach. These could be any number of common items such as paper clips, bobby pins or hemostats. They could also be of a store-bought variety in a number of shapes and disguises.
5. Seeds or leaves in pockets or possession.
6. Rolling papers or pipes, usually hidden somewhere.
7. Eye drops—for covering up red eyes.
8. Excessive use of incense, room deodorizers, or breath fresheners.
9. Devices for keeping the substance such as boxes, cans, or even concealed containers like a soft drink can with a screw-off lid.
10. Eating binges—an after effect in some marijuana users.
11. Appearance of intoxication yet no smell of alcohol.
12. Excessive laughter.
13. Yellowish stains on finger tips from holding the cigarette.

Source: L.A.W. Publications, "Let's All Work to Fight Drug Abuse," rev. ed. (Addison, Tex.: C&L Printing, 1985): 39.

marijuana. Contrary to what was once-popular belief, marijuana does not turn users into crazed murderers and rapists, nor does it cause genetic damage.

In an exhaustive study, *Marijuana and Health,* conducted by the National Academy of Sciences, a panel of experts concluded that "the verdict of the experts is—that there is no verdict. . . . Marijuana cannot be exonerated as harmless, but neither can it be convicted of being as dangerous as some have claimed." The study stated that there was no evidence supporting the belief that marijuana use inevitably leads to the use of any other drug.

Marijuana has been shown to be effective in treating glaucoma (by reducing ocular fluid pressure), and in relieving the nausea and vomiting that frequently accompany cancer chemotherapy and AIDS treatments. However, federal laws prohibit the medical use of marijuana, a situation that many patient-advocate groups are working to change.

Hallucinogens

The **hallucinogens** comprise a variety of chemical substances derived from as many as 100 kinds of plants as well as by chemical synthesis in the laboratory (Table 16.4). Despite their chemical differences, hallucinogens share the ability to alter perception, thought, mood, sensation, and experience. The similarity of their effects to psychotic hallucinatory experience is one reason they are called hallucinogens, but in many respects the psychedelic drug experience is not the same as a psychotic hallucination. Psychotic hallucinations are generally auditory and frightening, and the hallucinator believes them to be real. Drug-induced hallucinations tend to be visual, usually are enjoyable, and the individual is aware that the experience is unusual and is not part of his or her normal state of consciousness.

Hallucinogens are most often ingested orally, either by eating the plant itself or by ingesting powder containing the active chemical. Normally, a hallucinogenic

TABLE 16.4 Substances Considered to Be Hallucinogenic or Psychedelic

Substance/Active ingredient	Common name
D-lysergic acid diethylamide	LSD
Trimethoxyphenylethylamine	Mescaline (peyote)
2,5-Dimethoxy-4-methyl-amphetamine	STP
Dimethyltryptamine	DMT
Diethyltryptamine	DET
Tetrahydrocannabinol	Marijuana (Cannabis)
Phencyclidine	PCP
Psilocybin	Mushrooms

drug begins to take effect in 45 to 60 minutes. The first effects are physical: sweating, nausea, increased body temperature, and pupil dilation. These symptoms eventually subside, and the psychological effects become manifest within an hour or two of ingestion. Depending on the particular substance and the amount ingested, the "trip" will last anywhere from 1 to 24 hours. Perhaps the most commonly used hallucinogen is **LSD** (D-lysergic acid diethylamide), commonly called "acid."

A common feature of the hallucinogenic experience is the suspension of the normal psychic mechanisms that integrate the self with the environment. The distortion of self-environment interactions makes the user extremely open to conditions in the surroundings. For this reason, experience in any particular drug episode is highly influenced, for better or worse, by the environmental setting in which the trip takes place and by the "psychic set"—the expectations and attitudes—of the user. This is why someone may think they can fly and jump out of a fifth-floor window of a building.

A designer amphetamine drug called "Ecstasy" (also called Adam, MDMA, and MDM) has become popular in recent years. This drug is a chemical hybrid of mescaline and an amphetamine and has some of the properties of both. Users of Ecstasy experience hallucinogenic effects, as well as feelings of euphoria, become more verbal, and find it easier to express feelings. A few psychiatrists have used the drug as part of therapy to relieve patients' anxieties and help them gain emotional insights. However, the drug is illegal and potentially dangerous. It affects the release of neurotransmitters, particularly serotonin, in the brain. It also may cause neurological damage. Like other hallucinogenic drugs, MDMA can be abused and has the potential to be toxic to nerve cells.

Hallucinogenic drugs produce tolerance to the psychedelic effect but do not create physical dependence or produce symptoms of withdrawal, even after long-term

---

T E R M S

marijuana: a psychoactive substance present in the dried leaves, stems, flowers, and seeds of plants of the genus *Cannabis*

hashish: the sticky resin of the *Cannabis* plant

hallucinogens: psychoactive substances that alter sensory processing in the brain; produce visual or auditory sensations that are not real (are hallucinatory)

LSD: a powerful hallucinogenic chemical; ingestion alters brain chemistry and produces a variety of hallucinogenic and behavioral effects

The following description was shared with Dr. Glen Hanson by one of his students in 1992. The student describes a psychedelic "trip" caused by consuming a slurry of grain grown with a hallucinogen-producing fungus.

> The effect started about 45 minutes after drinking the slurry and was extraordinary. While it lasted (about three hours), the trip caused by consuming the fungus was the most sublime, ineffable experience I've ever had. Unlike cocaine, this experience could easily have been considered religious. Indeed, it was the closest thing to the Beatific Vision I can imagine. The intoxication I experienced was truly singular. I tasted colors, I saw beautiful lights with my eyes closed, my hands could pass through solid objects, I felt extraordinary compassion for other living things. I laughed and cried over a tomato I ate, for giving its life so that I might sustain mine. I looked at my little

> daughter crawling on the floor and could remember being a toddler, surrounded by a vast floor and large objects towering above me. The antics of my 2-year-old son made me laugh till I had to leave the room for fear of going into hysterics. . . .

> Then it wore off. I didn't have any particular hangover or headache afterward—I just slid back into reality. Easy come, easy go, I guess.

STUDENT REFLECTIONS

- Do experiences like this—when no real problems or harm result—encourage continued drug use?
- What potential dangers could have occurred with a child present?

Source: G. Hanson and P. J. Venturelli, *Drugs and Society,* 4th ed. (Boston: Jones and Bartlett, 1995), p. 337.

---

use. However, as with most psychoactive drugs, there is a danger of psychological dependence. There is no evidence that hallucinogens have permanent harmful effects on health, and they do not cause genetic damage or birth defects in humans.

> *Addictive drugs owe their market not to the pleasure of using them, but to the pain of giving them up.*
> David Jones,
> columnist

Phencyclidine (PCP)

Phencyclidine, also known as **PCP,** angel dust, hog, crystal, and killer weed, was developed originally for medical use as an animal anesthetic. But because of the drug's many adverse effects, it was removed from legal sale and became an illegal recreational drug. In the 1960s, phencyclidine was called the PeaCePill—a serious misnomer in view of the drug's effects.

The effects of PCP are variable: depending on the

dose and the route of administration, it can be a stimulant, a depressant, or a hallucinogen. Some of the intended effects are heightened sensitivity to external stimuli, mood elevation, relaxation, and a sense of omnipotence. Some of the frequent unintended effects are paranoia, confusion, restlessness, disorientation, feelings of depersonalization, and violent or bizarre behavior. In high doses the drug can cause coma, interruption of breathing, and psychosis.

Many admissions to psychiatric emergency rooms are for PCP intoxication. The drug impairs perception and muscular control, and users are prone to accidents such as falling from heights, drowning, walking in front of moving vehicles, and collisions while driving under the influence of the drug. PCP does not induce tolerance or physical dependence, but because it is eliminated slowly from the body, chronic users may experience the drug's effects for an extended period.

The effects of PCP are unpredictable and frequently unpleasant, if not terrifying and life-threatening. PCP produces more unwanted and dangerous symptoms of drug intoxication than any other psychoactive substance. Drug dealers often surreptitiously mix PCP with marijuana or cocaine or sell PCP while claiming it to be LSD, DMT, or some other drug. Because PCP is relatively easy to manufacture, it is one of the more readily available and dangerous of the illegal recreational drugs.

T E R M S

phencyclidine (PCP): drug that, depending on the route of administration and dose, can be a stimulant, depressant, or hallucinogen; originally developed as an anesthetic

inhalants: vaporous substances that, when inhaled, produce alcohol-like intoxication

Inhalants

Inhalants are a wide variety of chemical substances that vaporize readily and when inhaled, produce various kinds of depressant effects similar to those of alcohol. Like alcohol, inhalants are depressants of the central nervous system. Generally, their intended effect is loss of inhibition and a sense of euphoria and excitement. Unintended effects include dizziness, amnesia, inability to concentrate, confusion, impaired judgment, hallucinations, and acute psychosis.

Inhalants commonly used for recreational purposes include:

1. Commercial chemicals such as model airplane glue, nail polish remover, paint thinner, and gasoline, and substances such as acetone, toluene, naphtha, hexane, and cyclohexane.
2. Aerosols—found in aerosol spray products.
3. Anesthetics such as amyl nitrite, nitrous oxide ("laughing gas"), diethyl ether, and chloroform.

Because they are vaporous, these substances enter the body rapidly. The fumes are usually inhaled from plastic bags. The intoxicant effects are often felt within minutes, and the high lasts less than an hour. Regular users tend to be preteens and others without the money to buy other drugs. Some adults use amyl nitrite ("poppers") during sexual relations, believing that the drug enhances the sexual experience. Some medical personnel are frequent users of nitrous oxide or "laughing gas" because it is available.

The inhalant chemicals do not produce tolerance or withdrawal, nor do they induce physical dependence. However, they are dangerous. In addition to any harm resulting from uncontrolled behavior (such as driving while intoxicated), these chemicals damage the kidneys, liver, and lungs and can upset normal rhythmic heartbeat. Some users have suffocated while inhaling the fumes from plastic bags, and the potential for explosion is always present.

Health Update

Ecstasy Update

Ecstasy—A derivative of nutmeg or sassafras, causing euphoria and sometimes hallucinations; also known as XTC, Adam, MDMA, decadence, essence, or the hug-drug.

Background

- 1914: Ecstasy was shelved as an appetite suppressant.
- 1967: Ecstasy became popular because of its mild euphoria and lightbulb-like flashes of self discovery it produced.
- 1970: Ecstasy broke out into the streets, and by the mid 1980s, up to 30,000 doses were sold on the street per month.
- 1985: The U.S. Drug Enforcement Administration banned Ecstasy due to possible brain changes related to the drug; Ecstasy was classified as an illegal drug not having any legitimate uses.

Chemical Make-Up

- Ecstasy is closely related chemically to mescaline and the amphetamines.

- It is synthesized as a white to light brown powder or as an amber liquid.
- Ecstasy is sold in powder, tablet, or capsule form. It is inhaled, swallowed, or injected.
- A typical dose of Ecstasy is 50-150 mg; effects begin within 30 minutes, lasting 4–6 hours.

Effects of Ecstasy

- Lightens up the body's arousal system
- Causes calming and relaxation
- Affects a variety of physical and emotional states
- Feelings of empathy and togetherness
- Up-all-nite amphetamine rush
- Boosts insight and enhances communication
- Possible illusions, hallucinations, and poor perception of time and distance

Side Effects

- Dilated pupils

- Dry mouth and throat
- Nervousness
- Physical tension
- Due to the quick tolerance Ecstasy is capable of producing, overdose and death are possible

Possible Long-Term Effects

- Liver and brain damage
- Exhaustion and/or anxiety
- Delusions
- Paranoia; psychosis

Federal Penalties

- *First offense:* up to one year imprisonment and/or a fine of up to $5,000
- *Second offense:* up to two years imprisonment and/or a fine of up to $10,000

Manufacture, distribution, or possession with the intent to distribute is punishable by imprisonment of 10 years to life, and/or a fine of up to $4 million.

Source: Illinois State University, Student Health Services, 1995.

ANABOLIC STEROIDS

Characteristics and Use

Anabolic steroids are synthetic derivatives of the male hormone testosterone. The full name is androgenic (promoting masculine characteristics) anabolic (building) steroids (the class of drugs). These derivatives of testosterone promote the growth of skeletal muscle and increase lean body muscle. Anabolic steroids were first abused nonmedically by elite athletes seeking to improve performance. Today, athletes and nonathletes use steroids to enhance performance, and also to improve physical appearance. A recent national survey revealed:

- 2.1 percent of high school seniors had used anabolic steroids at least once in their lifetimes.
- 1.7 percent of both 8th and 10th graders had used anabolic steroids at least once and 1.1 percent had used them within the past year.
- Males accounted for more users of anabolic steroids than females.
- Over 90 percent of those surveyed disapprove of people who use steroids.
- 15.1 percent of 8th graders, 25 percent of 10th graders, and 51.7 percent of twelfth graders believed it would be fairly or very easy for them to get steroids (National Institute on Drug Abuse, 1993).

Steroids are taken orally or injected. Athletes and other abusers use them typically in cycles of weeks or months, rather than continuously, in patterns called cycling. Cycling involves taking multiple doses of steroids over a specified period, stopping for a while, and starting again. In addition, users frequently combine several different types of steroids to maximize their effectiveness while minimizing negative side effects, a process known as stacking.

Health Hazards

Anabolic steroids produce increased lean muscle mass, strength, and ability to train longer and harder; but the long-term effects of high-dose steroid use are largely unknown. Many, but not all, of the hazards of short-term use are reversible. Side effects of anabolic steroid use include liver tumors, jaundice, fluid retention, and high blood pressure, severe acne, and trembling. Shrinking of the testicles, reduced sperm count, infertility, baldness, and development of breasts have been observed in males. In females, growth of facial hair, changes or cessation of menstrual cycle, enlargement of the clitoris, and deepened voice are among the side effects.

REDUCING DRUG USE

Almost everyone takes drugs of one kind or another at one time or another. People take drugs to relieve headaches, heartburn, tension, cramps, fatigue, and anxiety. Drugs are used to get to sleep and to stay awake. They are used for body problems and emotional problems. When used appropriately, drugs can play a vital role in the treatment and prevention of disease.

However, as a society we are overmedicated and overly dependent on drugs. The healthiest approach is to be as free of drugs as possible. Wellness is not achieved by taking drugs. No drug should ever be taken casually, whether prescribed, over-the-counter, or offered in a social setting. Each person should learn when drugs are necessary to maintain or restore health and when the benefits of the drug outweigh the risks.

All drugs are dangerous, and illegal recreational drugs are especially so, since you cannot be sure of either the quality or the strength. The use of most recreational drugs is illegal, and if caught, users and sellers are prosecuted as criminals. Still many people in American society, especially young people, experiment with one or more illegal drugs. Experimenting with drugs is just that: you are taking a chance of getting caught, or getting high and causing an accident, or getting the wrong dose and dying.

HEALTH IN REVIEW

- People have been ingesting drugs throughout recorded history for a variety of reasons, including curing illness and facilitating social purposes.
- A drug is a chemical substance capable of producing a change in physiology. Most drugs react by binding to receptor sites in or on cells, which alters biological activity.

- Legal and illegal, medical and nonmedical drug use in the United States is widespread. Drug use is encouraged by extensive advertising by pharmaceutical, alcohol, and tobacco industries.
- Drug abuse is the overuse of a drug, often to the point of loss of control. Many drugs-of-abuse are psychoactive, meaning that they alter thoughts, feelings, and

perceptions. Many psychoactive drugs cause physical dependence; some cause psychological dependence.

- Tolerance is the adaptation of the body to repeated drug use so that ever increasing doses of the drug are required to produce an effect.

- The most commonly used psychoactive drugs in the United States include stimulants (cocaine, amphetamine, caffeine); depressants (sedatives, tranquilizers, hypnotics); opiates; marijuana; hallucinogens; PCP; and inhalants.

REFERENCES

Anabolic Steroid Abuse (NIDA Capsule 43) (1993). Washington, D.C.: National Institute on Drug Abuse.

Angell, M., and J. P. Kassirer (1994). "Alcohol and Other Drugs: Toward a More Rational and Consistent Policy." *New England Journal of Medicine,* 331: 537–538.

Bureau of Justice Statistics (1992). *A National Report: Drugs, Crime and the Justice System,* U.S. Department of Justice, Office of Justice Programs. Washington, D.C.: U.S. Government Printing Office.

Cornacchia, H. J., and S. Barrett (1993). *Consumer Health: A Guide to Intelligent Decisions.* St. Louis: Mosby.

"Correct Use of Medicine" (1994). *FDA Consumer,* January–February.

Hanson, G., and P. J. Venturelli (1995). *Drugs and Society,* 4th ed. Boston: Jones and Bartlett.

Illinois State University (1995). Student Health Services. *Let's All Work to Fight Drug Abuse* (rev. ed.) (1985). Addison, Tex.: C & L Printing.

Kleber, H. D. (1994). "Our Current Approach to Drug Abuse: Progress, Problems, Proposals." *New England Journal of Medicine,* 330: 361–364.

"Older Americans Take Inappropriate Drugs" (1994). *FDA Consumer,* October.

SUGGESTED READINGS

Begley, S. (1994). "One Pill Makes You Larger, and One Pill Makes You Small." *Newsweek,* February 7. A discussion of Prozac, one of the most controversial drugs now being taken by prescription for psychiatric problems.

Hanson, G., and P. J. Venturelli (1995). *Drugs and Society,* 4th ed. Boston: Jones and Bartlett. Provides an excellent overview of drug use in our society, including both legal and illegal drugs.

Murray, M. T. (1994). *Natural Alternatives to Over-the-Counter and Prescription Drugs.* New York: Morrow.

Explains how naturopathic remedies and life-style changes can replace drug use.

Volker, R. (1994). "Medical Marijuana: A Trail of Science and Politics." *Journal of the American Medical Association,* June 1. Discusses the politics that prevent the medical use of marijuana.

Yesalis, C. E., et al. (1993). "Anabolic-Androgenic Steroid Use in the United States." *Journal of the American Medical Association.* Discusses the dangers of using drugs to enhance athletic performance.

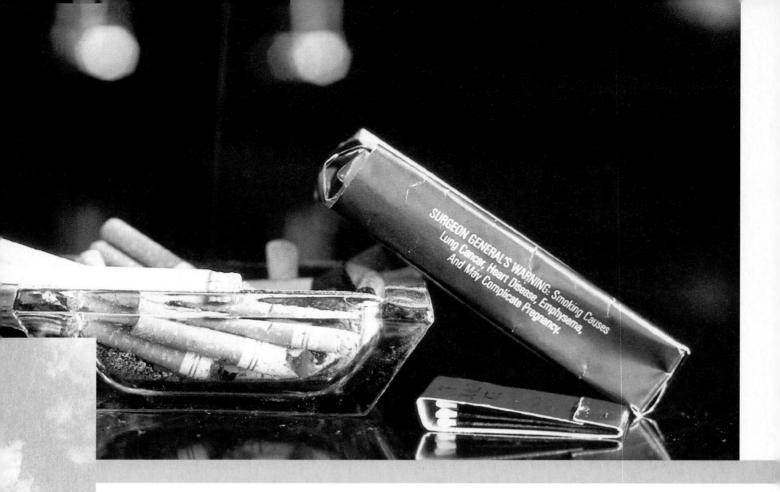

LEARNING OBJECTIVES

At the end of the chapter you should be able to:

1. Describe the hazards of cigarette smoking.
2. Describe the hazards of smokeless tobacco use.
3. Identify and explain the physiological effects of tobacco.
4. Differentiate the different types of smokeless tobacco.
5. Discuss the health and social consequences of tobacco use.
6. Discuss the effects of smoke on nonsmokers, and the implications for both groups.
7. Identify why some people smoke.
8. Identify ways to quit smoking.
9. Discuss the role of the U.S. government in tobacco production and laws regulating tobacco use.

Eliminating Cigarette and Tobacco Use

"Warning: The Surgeon General Has Determined That Cigarette Smoking Is Dangerous to Your Health." This message and other warnings from government officials and medical experts have reached just about everyone. Yet 53 million Americans smoke cigarettes regularly, thereby damaging not only their own health and well-being, but also the health and well-being of their family members, friends, and everyone else within breathing range of their smoke. The incidence of smoking among American adults has declined by almost half over the past 30 years (Figure 17.1), but the United States still has a long way to go to become a smokeless society by the year 2000.

PROFILE OF TOBACCO USE

The health costs of smoking are staggering. Each year about 420,000 Americans die as a result of smoking; this is 50 times as many as die from all illegal drugs combined. Another 10 million suffer from diseases caused by smoking. Cigarette smoking causes 30 percent of all human cancers, including about 85 percent of lung cancers. Government officials estimate that cigarette smoking costs the nation about $68 billion annually in health-care expenses and time lost from work. Economists estimate that around $30 billion of those costs are covered by smokers

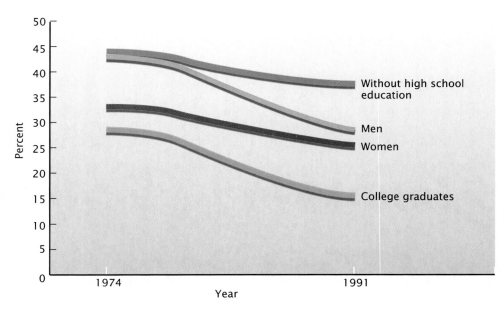

FIGURE 17.1 Cigarette Smoking among Adults Aged 18 and Over, 1974 and 1991 Data from the National Health Interview Survey (NHIS) indicates cigarette smoking among adults ages 18 and over has declined.

Source: Cancer Facts and Figures, 1995 (Atlanta: American Cancer Society, 1995).

themselves in the form of cigarette taxes, direct costs, and health insurance. The remaining $38 billion in smoking-related costs is borne by nonsmokers. The cost of treating smoking-related diseases and lost productivity is approximately $2.59 per package of cigarettes sold in the United States.

Tobacco companies steadfastly maintain that cigarettes have not been proven harmful, and the tobacco industry spends approximately $2.5 billion a year in advertising. To combat declining sales, U.S. tobacco companies target women, teenagers, and non-Caucasian males in the U.S. Tobacco companies also contribute to smoking-related diseases in other countries by promoting cigarette use around the world. U.S. export of cigarettes has increased almost threefold

since 1985. China, in particular, is expected to experience a major epidemic of lung cancers in the near future.

The 1994 Executive Summary of the U.S. Surgeon General's report, *Preventing Tobacco Use Among Young People,* presented the following conclusions:

- Nearly all first use of tobacco occurs before high school graduation; this finding suggests that if adolescents can be kept tobacco-free, most will not start using tobacco.
- Most adolescent smokers are addicted to nicotine and report that they want to quit but cannot; they experience relapse rates and withdrawal symptoms similar to those reported by adults.

Controversy in Health

How Much Are You Willing to Pay?

According to economist Jeffrey Harris of the Massachusetts Institute of Technology, cigarettes are responsible for 20 percent of deaths in the United States and approximately 8 percent of all health-care spending.

Harris estimates that smoking-related costs to society total $88 billion, of which $33 billion is borne by smokers and their insurance companies; nonsmokers pick up the largest portion of the tab. Harris further estimates that for every package of cigarettes sold, nonsmokers pay $2.59 to cover the medical costs incurred by smokers.

STUDENT REFLECTIONS
- Are you willing to pay for the health-care expenses of people who smoke?
- Are you willing to tax cigarettes to cover their full cost to society, which could lessen tobacco consumption, put tobacco growers out of business, and drastically reduce tobacco companies' profits?

- Tobacco is often the first drug used by young people who later use alcohol, marijuana, and other drugs.
- Adolescents with low school achievement levels often turn to cigarettes to improve their self-image; adolescents with low self-image are more likely to use tobacco.
- Community-wide efforts that include tobacco tax increases, enforcement of minors' access laws, youth-oriented mass media campaigns, and school-based tobacco-prevention programs are successful in reducing adolescent use of tobacco (U.S. Department of Health and Human Services, 1994).

Smoking is the most preventable cause of death in our society and tobacco use is responsible for almost one in five deaths in the United States. The World Health Organization estimates that 3 million people die worldwide each year as a result of smoking.

> *Cigarettes are the only legal product that when used as intended cause death.*
> Louis W. Sullivan,
> former Secretary of Health and Human Services

Tobacco Use Yesterday and Today

Tobacco was introduced to European societies in the sixteenth century by the Spanish returning from voyages to the Americas. The Spanish had learned about smoking from Native Americans, who used tobacco much as it is used today. In fact, the word "tobacco" is an Indian word referring to the pipe used to smoke the minced or rolled leaf of the tobacco plant.

The smoking habit spread quickly in Europe, fueled by tobacco imports from Spain's colonies. By the nineteenth century, changing social customs had caused tobacco smoking to be replaced largely by tobacco chewing; even more popular was the habit of sniffing tobacco in the form of snuff. Not until the 1880s, when the cigarette-making machine was invented in the United States, did cigarette smoking became the predominant form of tobacco use worldwide. Camel cigarettes, introduced in 1913, ushered in the modern era of smoking in the United States. By coincidence, the American Cancer Society was established in the same year.

Tobacco used for smoking, chewing, or snuff is the processed product of the leaves of the plant *Nicotinia tabacum*. This plant is indigenous to the Western Hemisphere, where it grows best in semitropical climates. Since its distribution by European explorers, it has been cultivated in many regions of the world. In the United States today, tobacco is grown primarily in thirteen southern states where the tobacco industry is vital to their economies.

Tobacco Characteristics

Processing tobacco for consumption involves harvesting the tobacco leaves and curing them by any one of several drying methods. The cured tobacco leaves are shredded, and various types of leaves are blended into commercially desirable mixtures. Often flavorings and colorings are added, as well as chemicals that facilitate even burning. Finally, the mixture is used to manufacture cigarettes, pipe tobacco, and chewing tobacco, or is wrapped in specially cured tobacco leaves to make cigars.

The most familiar chemical constituent of tobacco is **nicotine,** but when tobacco is burned, approximately 4,000 other chemical substances are released and carried in the smoke. These chemicals include acetone, acrolein, carbon monoxide, methanol, ammonia, nitrous dioxide, hydrogen sulfide, traces of various mineral elements, traces of radioactive elements, acids, insecticides, and other substances. Besides these chemical compounds, tobacco smoke also contains countless microscopic particles that contribute to the yellowish brown residue of tobacco smoke known as **tar,** a documented cause of lung cancer.

PHYSIOLOGICAL EFFECTS OF TOBACCO

Most of the physiological effects of tobacco smoking are attributable to the pharmacological effects of nicotine. The most prominent effects include increased heart rate, increased release of adrenaline, and a direct stimulatory effect on the brain, which combine to produce the mild "rush" cigarette smokers may experience when they light up. Nicotine is also responsible for the nausea and vomiting experienced by most beginning smokers. Addiction to nicotine is probably responsible for perpetuating a smoker's habit. Nicotine addiction has been determined to be as powerful as addiction to heroin.

Some harmful cardiovascular effects of cigarette smoking probably result from nicotine and carbon monoxide, which are believed to contribute to the development of heart and blood vessel disease. A host of other harmful chemicals contribute to the development of cancer and diseases of the respiratory tract. Among these chemicals are benzoapyrene, aza-arenes, N-nitrosamines, and radioactive polonium. Polonium is a product of the breakdown of radioactive lead, a natural constituent of soil. Radioactive particles in the soil become deposited on sticky tobacco leaf hairs and eventually become part of tobacco smoke. Radon, a radioactive gas, is also present in tobacco smoke inhaled both by the smoker and nonsmoker via second-hand smoke. These radioactive substances can become trapped in tiny air sacs in the lungs, where they induce cancerous changes in lung tissue.

SMOKELESS TOBACCO

Smokeless tobacco is available in two main forms: **chewing tobacco** and **snuff.** Chewing tobacco is processed into three different forms: loose leaf, firm/moist plug, and twist/rope chewing tobacco. A portion of chewing tobacco is either chewed or placed in the mouth and held in place between the lower lip and gum. Snuff is made from powdered or finely cut tobacco leaves and is available in two forms, dry and moist. In many European countries dry snuff is inhaled through the nose. However, in the United States a pinch of snuff is placed in the

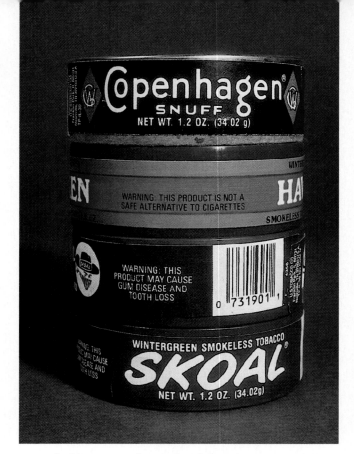

Despite health warnings, the use of smokeless tobacco is increasing, especially among young adults.

mouth and held in place between the cheek and gum, referred to as "snuff dipping." **Moist snuff** is made from air- and fire-cured tobacco leaves that are processed into fine particles, flavored, and packaged in moist form in round, flat containers. Moist snuff is considered the most hazardous form of smokeless tobacco because of the methods used in processing it.

History of Smokeless Tobacco

Tobacco for chewing and sniffing has been used for many centuries. Smokeless tobacco use by both men and women flourished until the end of the nineteenth century. At this time scientists discovered that tuberculosis bacillus and other harmful organisms could survive in saliva and be spread by air. Spitting into spittoons and onto barroom floors became unacceptable and even unlawful in many public places. Cigarettes replaced chew and snuff. Chewing became a habit retained mainly by older men.

Chewing tobacco became fashionable again in the 1970s when the dangers of cigarette smoking became clear. Smokeless tobacco again became popular, but this time with a much younger group of users (Connolly, Orleans, and Blum, 1992; National Cancer Institute, 1993). Smoking tobacco, not smokeless tobacco, was

T E R M S

chewing tobacco: a form of shredded smokeless tobacco; chewed or placed in mouth between lower lip and gum

snuff: a form of smokeless tobacco; made from powdered or finely cut leaves

moist snuff: a form of snuff made from air- and fire-cured tobacco leaves; most hazardous form of smokeless tobacco

publicized as a carcinogenic agent and people began to believe smokeless tobacco was a safer alternative to smoking. But as former U.S. Surgeon General C. Everett Koop made clear, "the public must be made aware that there is no safe form of tobacco use."

Prevalence of Smokeless Tobacco Use

Chewing tobacco has been replaced by moist snuff, the most hazardous form of tobacco. From 1980 to 1989, U.S. consumption of snuff increased by 57 percent, especially among young people ages 17 to 19 (Connolly, Orleans, and Blum, 1992). About 5 million adults use smokeless tobacco. According to the Centers for Disease Control and Prevention's 1993 Youth Risk Behavior Survey, 20 percent of male high school students use smokeless tobacco (American Cancer Society, 1995). The U.S. government's 1992 National Household Survey on Drug Abuse showed that 5 percent of American male teens and 12 percent of American young adult males use smokeless tobacco regularly (Figure 17.2).

Targeting young people, advertisers have promoted smokeless tobacco at sporting events to athletes as being healthy. Between $100 to $500 million has been spent on this type of advertisement since 1971 (Wichman and Martin, 1991). Forty-five percent of professional baseball players use smokeless tobacco, mainly chewing tobacco (Connolly, Orleans, and Blum, 1992). Football players, wrestlers, and runners tend to dip snuff (Strauss, 1991). These men serve as role models

for young people; children and adolescents believe if athletes chew, it must be healthy, safe, and enhance performance. Not only has tobacco been promoted to youth, but shredded chewing gum called Big League Chew encourages young children to get into the act of chewing.

Smokeless tobacco ads have been all too successful in getting the young to use these dangerous products. However, in 1986, Congress passed a law banning TV advertising of smokeless tobaccos (cigarette advertising on TV had been banned since the 1970s). Congress also required companies to put warning labels on packages as well as stating that consumers must be at least 18 years old.

Health and Social Consequences

Smokeless tobacco, or spit tobacco as it is now called, is not a safe alternative to smoking. Smokeless tobacco mixes with saliva, and the nicotine and other chemicals are absorbed into the bloodstream. Tobacco in this form leads to nicotine addiction just as cigarette smoking does. Smokeless tobacco causes various kinds of oral cancer. It also causes other less serious diseases of the mouth, such as hard white patches on the gums (leukoplakia) and inflammatory lesions of the gum (gingivitis). The majority of these lesions are benign, but about 2 to 6 percent of the cases develop into cancer (Greer, 1994). Some users show a marked increase in blood pressure, which is a major factor in heart disease.

Health Update

Trends in Tobacco Use among Youth

- Each day, more than 3,000 young people begin to smoke—or more than 21 million each year. Most of the new smokers are children or teens.

- The prevalence of cigarette smoking among high school seniors remained virtually unchanged from 1981 through 1990. In 1992, 17 percent of both male and female high school seniors were daily cigarette smokers.

- Almost 75 percent of daily smokers in high school still smoke 7 to 9 years later, even though only 5 percent had thought they would definitely be smoking 5 years later.

- Use of smokeless tobacco among youth is a growing problem. Between 1970 and 1986, the use of snuff increased 15 times and the use of chewing tobacco 4 times among males ages, 17-19 years.

- Many factors interact to encourage cigarette smoking among youth, including smoking by peers and family members, advertising and promotion, and easy availability of cigarettes.

- About half of adolescent smokers have parents who smoke. Teenagers are three times more likely to smoke if their parents and at least one older sibling smoke.

- About 85 percent of adolescent smokers who buy their own cigarettes usually buy Marlboro, Newport, or Camel cigarettes, the most heavily advertised brands.

- White high school seniors are on average five times more likely to smoke than black high school seniors. Smoking prevalence among Hispanics falls in between.

- Among male high school seniors, the prevalence of smoking half a pack of cigarettes or more a day is 18 percent among Native Americans, compared with 12 percent among whites, 5 percent among Mexican-Americans, 4 percent among Asian-Americans, and 2 percent among African-Americans.

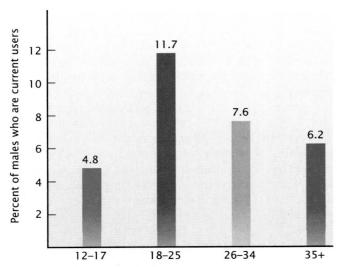

FIGURE 17.2 Smokeless Tobacco Use among American Men The prevalence among American women is about 0.5% for all age groups 12 and above.
Source: Cancer Facts and Figures, 1995 (Atlanta: American Cancer Society, 1995).

The risk of developing oral cancers—cancers of the throat, larynx, mouth, and esophagus—is much greater among smokeless tobacco users than nonusers (National Cancer Institute, 1992). In 1995 the American Cancer Society predicted 28,150 new cases of oral cancer and nearly 8,400 deaths due to oral cancer. An estimated 75 percent of all oral cancers can be correlated to tobacco use, whether it be cigarettes, cigars, pipes, chewing tobacco, or snuff (Greer, 1994). The greatest cancer risk is for people who use both alcohol and tobacco (National Cancer Institute, 1993).

Oral cancers account for about 3 percent of all cancers. Because of the increased use of smokeless tobacco by young people since 1970, physicians and health professionals believe oral cancer will account for an even larger percentage of cancers in the near future (National Cancer Institute, 1992).

Smokeless tobacco has also been linked to other health problems. Taste-enhancing sugars and sweeteners found in loose chewing tobacco may lead to tooth decay. Abrasive ingredients found in tobacco cause receding gums in areas where the tobacco is held for long periods between the teeth and lower lip or the teeth and the cheek. Tobacco users often experience halitosis and/or a loss of taste and smell (Haywood and Benson, 1993).

Social consequences for using smokeless tobacco include yellow and brown stains on the teeth, clothing, and automobile; the tobacco may cling to teeth, lips, tongue, and clothing. Spitting tobacco juice poses problems for users, thus some have learned to swallow the juice, which can contribute to stomach disorders (Haywood and Benson, 1993).

Health Update

Youth and Tobacco Advertising

- The Surgeon General concluded in 1989 that tobacco advertising and promotion do appear to stimulate cigarette consumption.

- Tobacco companies spent nearly $4 billion in 1990—or about $11 million a day—to advertise and promote cigarettes. Increasingly, these marketing dollars are going toward promotional activities that may have special appeal to young people, such as sponsorship of public entertainment, distribution of specialty items bearing product names, and the issuing of coupons and premiums.

- Cigarette advertisements tend to emphasize youthful vigor, sexual attraction, and independence—themes that are likely to appeal to teenagers and young adults struggling with these issues.

- About 85 percent of adolescent smokers prefer either Marlboro, Newport, or Camel, the three most heavily advertised cigarette brands.

- Cigarette promotions of televised sporting and entertainment events heavily expose large numbers of youth to explicit prosmoking messages. During the 1989 Marlboro Grand Prix Telecast, for example, the Marlboro logo was seen or mentioned nearly 6,000 times and was visible for 46 of the 94 minutes the race was broadcast.

- Tobacco company spending for specialty gift items (such as T-shirts, caps, sunglasses, key chains, calendars, and sporting goods) bearing a cigarette brand logo increased 17 percent, from $262 million to $307 million, between 1989 and 1990.

- "Old Joe," the cartoon camel used to advertise Camel cigarettes, is as familiar to children aged 6 years as Mickey Mouse's silhouette. A study found that 91 percent of 6-year-olds recognized Old Joe and linked him with his product. This was the same recognition level measured for the Disney icon.

- Cigarette advertisements appear in publications with large teenage readerships. In *Glamour*, 25 percent of whose readers are females 18 years old and under, cigarette advertising expenditures were $6.3 million in 1985. In *Sports Illustrated*, 33 percent of whose readers are males under 18, cigarette advertising expenditures were $29.9 million in 1985.

Smokeless tobacco is psychoactive and addictive (Chapter 16) because it contains numerous chemicals including nicotine. Users build up a tolerance to nicotine and require greater amounts to produce the same effect. Most youth do not realize how addictive smokeless tobacco is and when they attempt to quit they suffer anxiety, irritability, and decreased ability to concentrate (symptoms of withdrawal) (Riddle, 1994; Haywood and Benson, 1993).

> At present just under 20 percent of all deaths in developed countries are attributed to tobacco, but the percentage is still rising.
>
> *The Lancet*

Reducing Smokeless Tobacco Use

The health risks of smokeless tobacco have become increasingly apparent and various steps have been taken to alert the public of this problem. Federal legislation has been enacted to help combat smokeless tobacco use.

In 1986 the Comprehensive Smokeless Tobacco Health Education Act was passed. This bill banned all smokeless tobacco ads on television and radio, and mandated that health hazard warnings be placed on all tobacco packages. However, advertisements in print media and at car races and rodeos have increased the use of smokeless tobacco among young people.

SMOKING AND DISEASE

Almost from the beginning of tobacco use in Europe and America, people have been concerned about the possible harmful effects of smoking. Several articles in the medical literature of the eighteenth and nineteenth centuries claimed tobacco smoking as a cause of cancer of the lip, tongue, and lung. Modern research on the health consequences of cigarette smoking has provided overwhelming evidence that among smokers as a group, the incidence of certain diseases is greater, sometimes much greater, than among nonsmokers. Smoking has been established as a factor in the development of coronary artery disease, lung cancer, bronchitis, emphysema, cancer of the larynx, lip, and oral cavity, cancer of the bladder and stomach, duodenal ulcer, and allergies (Kessler, 1995).

An enormous amount of data demonstrate that the death rate from cancer, heart disease, and respiratory diseases is higher among cigarette smokers than among nonsmokers. The data also show that death rates for smokers are greater than for nonsmokers whatever the listed cause of death.

Babies born to mothers who smoke weigh less than babies born to nonsmoking mothers; smokers' babies also show a higher risk of dying early in infancy. There is evidence that pregnant women who smoke are more likely to have spontaneous abortions than those who do not. A father who smokes a pack a day risks having his baby's weight reduced by over four ounces at birth due to second-hand smoking effects.

All these findings confirm that the risk of developing smoking-related disease and other complications depends in part on the nature, as well as the extent, of exposure to tobacco smoke. For example, pipe and cigar smokers' incidence of death and disease for the smoking-related illnesses is somewhere between that for cigarette smokers and nonsmokers, presumably because pipe and cigar smokers inhale less smoke than cigarette smokers. Light smokers (4-10 cigarettes per day) are at less risk than heavy smokers (more than 25 cigarettes per day). Mortality rates for heart disease and cancer for those who stop smoking for 15 years are about the same as for nonsmokers. Cessation of smoking also improves breathing and reduces the chance of premature death from noncancerous respiratory disease.

Smokers' apparent concern for their health has produced a demand for low tar and nicotine cigarettes. Approximately 60 percent of all cigarettes now sold in North America are of the "low-yield" variety. While the use of low tar and nicotine cigarettes does reduce the risk of developing lung cancer, it apparently does not lessen the risk of developing heart disease (Figure 17.3).

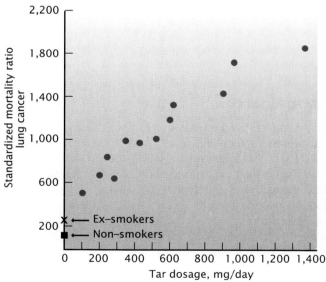

FIGURE 17.3 Deaths from Lung Cancer as a Function of Tar in Cigarettes Smoked The amount of tar in cigarettes has been shown to be one cause of lung cancer. Smokers who inhale the most tar have a 20 fold higher risk of lung cancer.

Source: S. D. Stellman and L. Garfinkel, "Lung Cancer Risk Is Proportionate to Cigarette Tar Yield," *Preventive Medicine,* 18 (1989): 518-525.

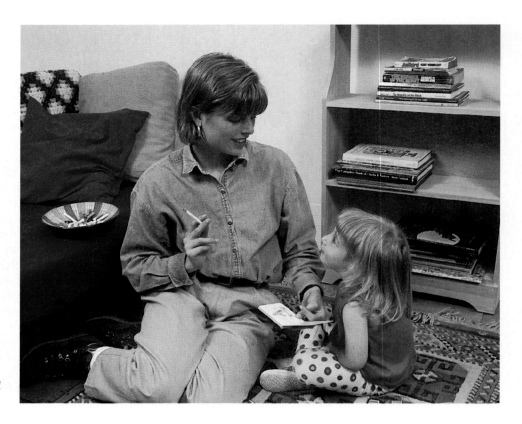

Children who live in homes where adults smoke have more respiratory problems than children who are raised in smoke-free environments.

The health risks of cigarette smoking can be eliminated only by quitting. For those who continue to smoke, some reduction in cancer risk may occur from a switch to lower tar and nicotine cigarettes, if the smoker does not increase the number of cigarettes smoked or inhale more deeply to compensate for the lower tar and nicotine. The National Cancer Institute indicates that research has shown that there is no such thing as a "safe" cigarette.

Lung Cancer

Lung cancer has long been the most common form of cancer among men and recently among women (Chapter 13). Each year approximately 170,000 persons are diagnosed with lung cancer and about 158,000 people die of this disease. The number of men dying of lung cancer has increased steadily since 1940. While the rate of increase among men is beginning to decline because fewer men are smoking cigarettes, the increase among women is rising because more women have been smoking during the last three decades. Thirty-year trends in cancer death rates show an increase for both men and women (Figure 17.4). In 1984, for the first time in U.S. history, lung cancer passed breast cancer as the leading cancer-related cause of death in women.

The increase in lung cancer deaths is the principal reason that the overall cancer death rate continues to rise. If lung cancer death rates are excluded from the sta-

tistics, the death rate from cancer has been falling steadily for many years, principally because of preventive efforts and improved diagnosis and treatment of cancers. This situation is ironic as well as tragic, for lung cancer

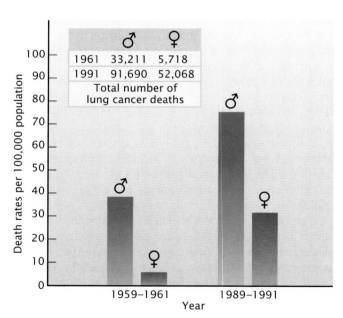

	♂	♀
1961	33,211	5,718
1991	91,690	52,068
Total number of lung cancer deaths		

FIGURE 17.4 30-Year Trend in Lung Cancer Death Rates per 100,000 People, 1959–1961 to 1989–1991

Source: Cancer Facts and Figures, 1995 (Atlanta: American Cancer Society, 1995).

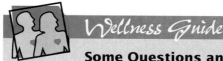
Some Questions and Answers about Oral Cancer

Q. What is the most common oral cancer?

A. Oral cancer of the tongue accounts for 30 percent of oral cancers.

Q. How is oral cancer diagnosed?

A. Oral cancer, like other cancers, is diagnosed by biopsy. A piece of tissue is removed from the area in question and sent to a pathologist for examination. This may be done after a dental or medical professional has continued to check a lesion to see if it warrants such a procedure.

Q. How widespread is oral cancer?

A. In 1995, an estimated 28,150 individuals will be diagnosed with cancers of the oral cavity and pharynx. Approximately 8,370 deaths are expected to result from oral cancers.

Q. Are any areas of the country more at risk than others?

A. In the southeastern rural United States, the incidence of oral cancer is four times as high among snuff users, most of whom neither smoke nor drink. For this group, risks can be 50 times as high for cheek and gum cancer.

Q. Who is most at risk for developing oral cancer?

A. Persons over 40 years of age and those who use tobacco—smoked or smokeless—in combination with drinking alcohol.

Q. Are there mouth lesions that are not cancerous?

A. Yes, many are not cancerous. However, certain noncancerous mouth conditions, such as leukoplakia, can become malignant. Leukoplakia is a painless white patch that can form on the lip, tongue or lining of the mouth. It usually occurs among tobacco users from cigarette and pipe smoking or from chewing tobacco.

Q. Can oral cancer be prevented?

A. Yes, most oral cancers can be prevented by not using tobacco in any form, and limiting or stopping the intake of alcohol.

Q. Can oral cancer be detected early?

A. Yes, regular mouth and throat examinations can detect oral cancer in its earliest, most curable stage. Five-year survival rates are around 75 percent if detected at this stage. Without periodic examinations, risks increase and survival rates decrease.

Source: Centers for Disease Control and Prevention, National Center for Prevention Services.

---

is one of the most preventable of all diseases. People simply need to stop (or never start) smoking cigarettes.

A full biological explanation of how smoking causes lung cancer (and contributes to cancer in other sites) is not yet available. A number of known **carcinogens** are found in tobacco smoke that are thought to cause the cellular changes leading to cancer.

Not all lung cancer deaths are attributable to cigarette smoking. The data suggest that about 80 percent of lung cancer deaths are related to smoking; the other 20 percent are likely due to a variety of environmental factors, including air pollution (some studies indicate that twice as many city dwellers die of lung cancer as do people who live in rural areas), airborne substances encountered in work environments such as particles of chromate, iron, radon, or asbestos, and breathing **sidestream smoke (passive smoking)** at home or at the worksite.

Bronchitis and Emphysema

Bronchitis and **emphysema** are respiratory diseases sometimes classified with asthma as **chronic obstructive pulmonary diseases (COPD)**. Each of these diseases is associated with breathing difficulty caused by obstruction of or destruction of some part of the respiratory system. Often persons suffer from more than one of these conditions at the same time.

Bronchitis is an inflammatory condition of the upper part of the respiratory tract, principally the **trachea** which is part of the larger bronchial airways. Bronchitis is characterized by excessive production of mucus by

T E R M S

carcinogens: any substances that can cause cancer in people and other animals

sidestream smoke (passive smoking): smoke released into the environment directly from lighted tip of cigarettes

bronchitis: inflammation of the bronchi of the lungs as a result of irritation; often accompanied by a chronic cough

emphysema: a progressive degeneration of the lung alveoli, causing breathing and oxygen assimilation to become more and more difficult

chronic obstructive pulmonary diseases (COPD): diseases that restrict the ability of the body to obtain oxygen through the respiratory structures (bronchi and lungs); these diseases include asthma, bronchitis, and emphysema

trachea: upper part of respiratory tract

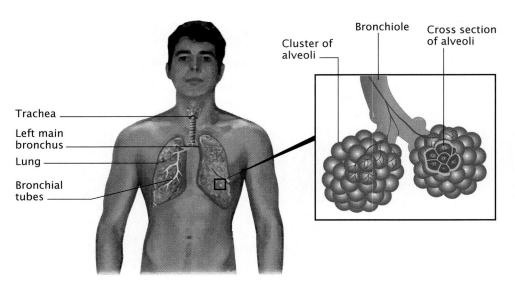

FIGURE 17.5 The Respiratory System
Provides the body with oxygen and removes carbon dioxide. Oxygen enters and carbon dioxide leaves the body via tiny air sacs in the lungs called alveoli. The rest of the respiratory system functions to facilitate gas exchange in the alveoli.

cells that line the airways, which causes the major symptoms of bronchitis—such as a continual cough (smoker's cough) and the production of large amounts of sputum. Some affected people also experience shortness of breath, particularly during exertion.

Unquestionably, smoking is a factor in the development of chronic bronchitis; however air pollution, passive smoke, and breathing hazardous chemicals and asbestos particles also contribute to developing the disease. Apparently, excessive production of mucus by the glands of the bronchi is a reaction to irritation caused by cigarette smoke and other air pollutants.

Fortunately, the pathology that produces the symptoms of bronchitis can be almost completely reversed by quitting smoking, reducing exposure to polluted air, or both. However, many people "live with" their persistent cough for many years and are not concerned with the message their body is giving them. If the disease is left to run its course, sufferers increase their vulnerability to other respiratory illnesses, and the airways may become irreversibly damaged.

Emphysema results from the destruction of the tiny air sacs deep in the lungs called **alveoli** (Figure 17.5).

Each lung contains millions of alveoli: across their thin membranes the function of breathing is accomplished—the exchange of the respiratory gases, oxygen, and carbon dioxide.

When the alveoli are destroyed due to emphysema, they lose their shape and become distended with trapped air, which ultimately impairs gas exchange. Emphysema involves a slow, irreversible process of alveoli destruction; as the disease progresses, affected people have greater and greater trouble breathing.

As with lung cancer, the exact mechanism by which tobacco smoking or air pollution contribute to emphysema is unknown. One hypothesis suggests that cells in the lung (macrophages and leukocytes produced by the immune system) (Chapter 12) normally engaged in the destruction of material foreign to the body release enzymes which inadvertently destroy lung tissue, thereby causing emphysema. Normally, a protein in the blood called **alpha-one-protease inhibitor** inhibits the activities of destructive enzymes in the lungs. The inhibitory protein blocks the action of the enzyme elastase which, if not properly regulated, destroys alveoli and results in emphysema. Some people have low levels

Health Update

Effects of Environmental Tobacco Smoke on Children

- Tobacco smoke contributes each year to 150,00 to 300,000 respiratory infections in babies, resulting in 7,500 to 15,000 hospitalizations

- Tobacco smoke causes 8,000 to 26,000 new cases annually of asthma in previously unaffected children

- Tobacco smoke worsens asthma symptoms in 400,000 to 1 million asthmatic children each year

Source: Environmental Protection Agency.

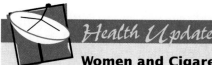
Women and Cigarette Advertising

For over 50 years tobacco company ads have tried to entice women to smoke cigarettes by emphasizing sexiness, slimness, elegance, and fun. The success of such ads over the years in getting women to smoke is borne out by the current number of lung cancer deaths among women smokers. Currently about 26 million American women smoke cigarettes. Between 1935 and 1993 the percentage of women who smoked increased from 18 percent of all women to 25 percent. (During the same interval the percentage of men who smoked actually decreased from 52 to 28 percent.)

About 40,000 women die from cigarette-caused lung cancer. Lung cancer has surpassed breast cancer as the leading cause of cancer deaths among women. Smoking also increases women's chances of heart disease and cervical cancer. And if that's not enough, the beauty editor of *Harper's* magazine points out that

"smokers' skin wrinkles up to 10 years sooner than that of nonsmokers." As long as tobacco is legal, companies have a right to advertise.

You also have the right to not smoke, which is one of the single most important health decisions you can make.

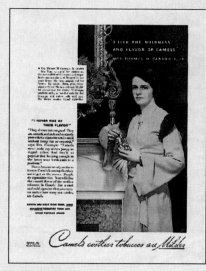

1934 advertisement

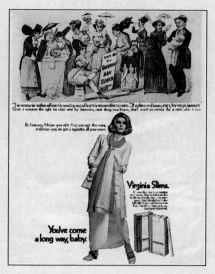

1969 advertisement

of the inhibitor due to a defective gene, and they are particularly at risk for emphysema. Approximately 100,000 emphysemics have this hereditary defect and smoking dramatically increases their chances of developing emphysema.

Tobacco Smoke's Effects on Nonsmokers

Nonsmokers, especially children, who are exposed to tobacco smoke run a health risk. People who work or live in environments heavily laden with tobacco smoke inhale the same smoke-borne substances as do smokers. In fact, about two-thirds of the smoke from a burning cigarette enters the environment. Anyone who has been in a roomful of smokers can attest that the room is con-

siderably more polluted than the worst smoggy day in a big city.

A nonsmoker in a smoke-filled room can inhale in one hour the equivalent of a cigarette's worth of nicotine, carbon monoxide, and carcinogenic substances. Also, many people are allergic to tobacco smoke, which can produce eye irritation, headache, cough, nasal congestion, and asthma. Nonsmokers forced to inhale tobacco smoke for long periods, such as workers in enclosed

T E R M S

alveoli: tiny air sacs in the lungs that exchange oxygen and carbon dioxide

alpha-one-protease inhibitor: a blood protein that inhibits destructive enzymes implicated in causing emphysema

H E A L T H Y   P E O P L E   2 0 0 0

Reduce to no more than 20 percent the proportion of children aged 6 and younger who are regularly exposed to tobacco smoke at home.

Environmental tobacco smoke is a cause of disease, including lung cancer, in healthy nonsmokers; it is also a significant health risk for children. The children of smokers are more likely to develop lower respiratory tract infections, to be hospitalized, or see a doctor for these conditions during their first year of life.

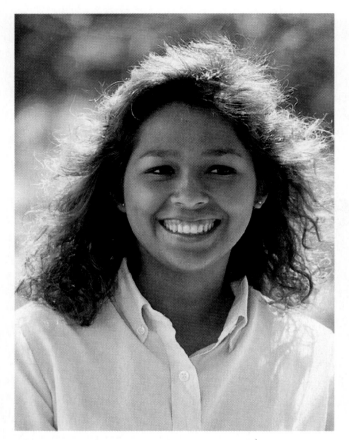

Passive cigarette smoking can also affect children. According to reports from the Environmental Protection Agency, children of smokers have increased rates of bronchitis, pneumonia, chronic cough, missed school days, and hospital admissions. Maternal cigarette smoking has been shown to hinder the development of the lungs of the fetus and to impair respiratory function, which may predispose these children to respiratory illnesses later in life. Smoking during pregnancy also impairs a child's body stature, cognitive development, learning ability, and predisposes them to later cigarette use.

WHY PEOPLE SMOKE

Most people begin to smoke in their teen years, emulating parents, others who smoke, or cigarette ad models. Teenagers also smoke to attain acceptance in their peer group. About half of those who experiment with smoking continue the habit into adulthood. There must be some very compelling reasons that people continue to smoke despite the unpleasant taste, the initial adverse physiological reactions to smoke and nicotine, and the knowledge—now widespread—that tobacco smoke causes cancer and other life-threatening diseases.

According to the American Cancer Society, the motivations of smokers fall into six general categories:

- **Stimulation.** Some people experience a psychological lift from smoking. They say that smoking helps them to wake up in the morning and organize their energies. They often report that smoking increases their intellectual capacities.

- **Handling.** Some people enjoy the mere handling of cigarettes and smoking paraphernalia, such as lighters.

- **Pleasurable relaxation.** Some smokers say they smoke simply because they like it. Smoking brings them true pleasure and relaxation, and is often prac-

Nonsmokers who live or work in close proximity with smokers are subject to the same health threats as those who inhale cigarettes directly.

smoke-filled workplaces, can suffer impaired lung function equivalent to that of smokers who inhale ten cigarettes a day. A study of the risks of passive smoking found that spouses of smokers had a 30 percent higher cancer mortality rate compared with spouses of nonsmokers.

Health Update

Waiting to Exhale

By the time most students enter high school, they have seen hundreds of antismoking ads and have listened to many lectures on not smoking. For the past several decades equal percentages of white and black students smoked. However, a recent report indicates that 22.9 percent of white teens smoked—about the same since 1977; only 4.4 percent of black youth smoked, which is 6 times fewer than in 1977. Why? The study reports it's all in the way kids define "cool." Apparently, smoking is seen as a white thing; black kids don't smoke to be accepted. How did this happen? A few years ago, Harold Freeman, director of surgery at Harlem Hospital in New York, began putting up posters to counter the tobacco advertisements targeting black youth. The poster showed a skeleton of the Marlboro man lighting a cigarette for a black youth and the slogan "They used to make us pick it. Now they want us to smoke it."

Source: Adapted from M. Ingrassia and K. Springen, "Waiting to Exhale," *Newsweek* (May 1, 1995).

ticed to enhance other pleasurable sensations, such as the taste of food and alcoholic beverages. However, smoking actually dulls the tastebuds.

- **Reducing negative feelings (crutch).** Approximately one-third of smokers say they smoke because it temporarily helps them deal with stress, anger, fear, anxiety, or pressure.
- **Craving.** Some people crave cigarettes and have no other explanation for their habit other than that they have a frequent need to smoke, regardless of the tension-relieving effects that smoking might bring.
- **Habit.** Some smokers light up only because of habit. They no longer receive much physical or psychological gratification from smoking; often they smoke without being aware of whether or not they really want the cigarette.

The question that still eludes a definitive answer is: What distinguishes people who smoke from those who do not? The list of suggested answers includes a biological susceptibility to dependence on nicotine, a variety of personality, sociological, and environmental traits, and a need to deal with stress via smoking. There may be as many reasons as there are smokers. Whatever the case, people smoke by choice. In the final analysis, smoking, like any other habitual, health-threatening behavior, is a personal matter. In the case of smoking, the choice can ultimately be—and often is—fatal.

LEARNING TO QUIT SMOKING

There's an old joke among smokers: "It's easy to quit. I've done it over fifty times!"

Each year millions of smokers try to kick their habit. The major problem they face, as the little joke recognizes, is that stopping for a while is not nearly as difficult as permanently eliminating the habit. However, by 1991 almost 44 million Americans, nearly half of all living adults who ever smoked, had quit smoking (American Cancer Society, 1995). People stop smoking for a variety

 Wellness Guide

Quitting Tips

Getting Ready to Quit

- Set a date for quitting. If possible, have a friend quit smoking with you.
- Notice when and why you smoke. Try to find the things in your daily life that you often do while smoking (such as drinking your morning cup of coffee or soda, or driving a car).
- Change your smoking routines. Keep your cigarettes in a different place. Smoke with your other hand. Don't do anything else when smoking. Think about how you feel when you smoke.
- Smoke only in certain places, such as outdoors.
- When you want a cigarette, wait a few minutes. Try to think of something to do instead of smoking, you might chew gum or drink a glass of water.
- Buy one pack of cigarettes at a time. Switch to a brand of cigarettes with a lower tar content.

On the Day You Quit

- Get rid of all your cigarettes. Put away your ashtrays.

- Change your morning routine. When you eat breakfast, don't sit in the same place at the kitchen table. Stay busy.
- When you get the urge to smoke, do something else instead.
- Carry other things to put in your mouth, such as gum, hard candy, or a toothpick.
- Reward yourself at the end of the day for not smoking. See a movie or go out and enjoy your favorite meal.

Staying Quit

- Don't worry if you are sleepier or more short-tempered than usual; these feelings will pass.
- Try to exercise—take walks or ride a bike.
- Consider the positive things about quitting, such as how much you like yourself as a non-smoker, health benefits for you and your family, and the example you set for others around you. A positive attitude will help you through the tough times.

- When you feel tense, try to keep busy, think about ways to solve the problem, tell yourself that smoking won't make it any better, and go do something else.
- Eat regular meals. Feeling hungry is sometimes mistaken for the desire to smoke.
- Start a money jar with the money you save by not buying cigarettes.
- Let others know that you have quit smoking—most people will support you. Many of your smoking friends may want to know how you quit. It's good to talk to others about your quitting.
- If you slip and smoke, don't be discouraged. Many former smokers tried to stop several times before they finally succeeded. Quit again.
- For more information about quitting, call: 1-800-4-CANCER or 1-800-ACS-2345.

Source: "Smoking Facts and Tips for Quitting," National Cancer Institute and the American Cancer Society, 1993.

Why Do You Smoke?

Here are some statements made by people to describe what they get out of smoking cigarettes.

How often do you feel this way when smoking? Circle one number for each statement.

Important: Answer every question.

	Always	Frequently	Occasionally	Seldom	Never
A. I smoke cigarettes in order to keep myself from slowing down.	5	4	3	2	1
B. Handling a cigarette is part of the enjoyment of smoking it.	5	4	3	2	1
C. Smoking cigarettes is pleasant and relaxing.	5	4	3	2	1
D. I light up a cigarette when I feel angry about something.	5	4	3	2	1
E. When I have run out of cigarettes I find it almost unbearable until I can get them.	5	4	3	2	1
F. I smoke cigarettes automatically without even being aware of it.	5	4	3	2	1
G. I smoke cigarettes to stimulate me, to perk myself up.	5	4	3	2	1
H. Part of the enjoyment of smoking a cigarette comes from the steps I take to light up.	5	4	3	2	1
I. I find cigarettes pleasurable.	5	4	3	2	1
J. When I feel uncomfortable or upset about something, I light up a cigarette.	5	4	3	2	1
K. I am very much aware of the fact when I am not smoking a cigarette.	5	4	3	2	1
L. I light up a cigarette without realizing I still have one burning in the ashtray.	5	4	3	2	1
M. I smoke cigarettes to give me a "lift."	5	4	3	2	1

of reasons: to reduce the risk of early death from heart or lung disease; to enjoy, once again, the unpolluted taste of food; to please nonsmoking loved ones; to eliminate ever-present ashes and smell of cigarette smoke from their homes; and to fulfill a simple commitment to personal health. Frequently, a positive change in other aspects of life leads to cessation of smoking. For example, many people who take up meditation, t'ai chi ch'uan, jogging, or other physical activity automatically stop smoking. They simply lose the desire to smoke.

Finding a "quitter's magic bullet"—a single therapeutic approach that will help smokers stop, not only during the several weeks of treatment, or the six months to a year after the treatment has stopped, but for the rest of their lives—has proved elusive. Many different therapies can help people stop smoking. Often these strategies are applied in special stop-smoking clinics, where smokers are exposed to health information, counseling, encouragement, support, social pressure, and suggestions about how to resist the temptation to light up.

Chemically based therapies use the idea that many people smoke because they are addicted to nicotine. The therapy provides smokers with nicotine or a nicotine-like drug that dulls their craving for nicotine. Chemical approaches provide nicotine in the form of chewing gum or a skin patch from which nicotine is slowly and

	Always	Frequently	Occasionally	Seldom	Never
N. When I smoke a cigarette, part of the enjoyment is watching the smoke as I exhale it.	5	4	3	2	1
O. I want a cigarette most when I am comfortable and relaxed.	5	4	3	2	1
P. When I feel "blue" or want to take my mind off cares and worries, I smoke cigarettes.	5	4	3	2	1
Q. I get a real gnawing hunger for a cigarette when I haven't smoked for a while.	5	4	3	2	1
R. I've found a cigarette in my mouth and didn't remember putting it there.	5	4	3	2	1

How to Score

1. Enter the numbers you have circled in the spaces below, putting the number you have circled to Question A over line A, to Question B over line B, etc.

2. Add the three scores on each line to get your totals. For example, the sum of your scores over lines A, G, and M gives you your score on *Stimulation,* lines B, H, and N give the score on *Handling,* and so on.

	+		+		=	**Totals**
A		G		M		Stimulation
B	+	H	+	N	=	Handling
C	+	I	+	O	=	Pleasurable relaxation
D	+	J	+	P	=	Crutch: tension reduction
E	+	K	+	Q	=	Craving: psychological addiction
F	+	L	+	R	=	Habit

Scores of 11 or above indicate that this factor is an important source of satisfaction for the smoker. Scores of 7 or less are low and probably indicate that this factor does not apply to you. Scores in between are marginal.

Source: Smoker's Self-Testing Kit developed by Daniel Horn, Ph.D. Originally published by National Clearinghouse for Smoking and Health, Department of Health, Education, and Welfare.

continually absorbed into the skin. Chemical alternatives are usually unsuccessful unless they are combined with counseling to discover and combat the underlying reasons for the smoking habit.

Other therapies are based on the idea that smoking is a response to stress. Stress reduction techniques such as meditation and biofeedback are employed to give the smoker an alternative way to deal with stress.

Whatever the specific technique, most people involved in helping smokers quit agree that the major factor in stopping smoking is the personal resolve of the smoker. No single therapeutic technique in itself breaks the smoking habit. This does not mean that smokers have to employ unusual behaviors like putting money in a piggy bank each time they resist the urge to smoke. Such artificial practices rarely stop smoking permanently. Successful quitting can be accomplished by becoming aware of personal motives for smoking. It is possible to reprogram the mind to eliminate the thoughts and behaviors that lead to smoking. A person can then integrate positive and rewarding activities, thoughts, and feelings in place of those that lead to smoking. People stop smoking because they want to feel good. Once smokers stop smoking, they feel good. After all, smokers really do not want to kill themselves, yet smoking cigarettes is potentially lethal.

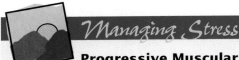

Progressive Muscular Relaxation

Of all the relaxation techniques known to help people quit smoking, progressive muscular relaxation (PMR) seems to be the most effective. PMR is a technique for learning how to relax muscles made tense by stressors confronted in a normal day. Muscle tension is the number one symptom of stress. Learning to relax your muscles helps promote the relaxation response. In turn, feeling relaxed helps negate some of the most obvious symptoms of stress, and may, in fact, also help you quit smoking.

People who do smoke may tell you that they do so to relieve stress and tension. Perhaps you are one of these people. Although smoking may seem to calm your nerves, the chemicals in cigarette smoke actually keep the body's nervous system in a heightened state of stress. In an effort to kick the habit, smokers often adopt another, healthier behavior in place of smoking to deal with stress, in this case PMR. Here is how they do it:

When feelings of stress and tension begin to surface, give yourself some positive feedback, by saying to yourself *"I have the ability to control my stress levels without any outside help."* Next, do a quick body scan to determine if any one area is more tense than others, like your facial muscles, your neck and shoulders, or your stomach area. Then, before you light up try the following:

1. Squeeze the muscles of your eyes and forehead really tight, as if you were squinting as hard as you can. Hold this position for about 5-10 seconds and then let go by relaxing those same muscles around your face. Feel the difference between the levels of tension and relaxation. Think to yourself: the muscles of my face and eyes feel calm and relaxed.

2. Tense the muscles of your jaws as hard as you can, like you are biting on something really hard. Hold this position for about 5-10 seconds and then let go by relaxing the muscles of the jaws. Feel the difference between the levels of tension and relaxation. Think to yourself: the muscles of my jaws feel calm and relaxed.

3. Contract the muscles of your neck and shoulders really hard. Hold this position for about 5-10 seconds, and then let go by completely relaxing the neck and shoulder muscles. Feel the difference between the levels of ten-sion and relaxation. Think to yourself: the muscles of my neck and shoulders feel calm and relaxed.

4. Make a fist with both hands and tighten them both really hard. Hold this tension level for about 5-10 seconds, and then let go by relaxing your hands completely, opening and spreading the fingers wide. Feel the difference between the levels of tension and relaxation. Think to yourself: the muscles of my hands and fore-arms feel calm and relaxed.

5. Tense the muscles of your stom-ach area as hard as you can. Hold this position for about 5-10 seconds and then let go by relax-ing the muscles and organs in your abdominal area as much as you can. Feel the difference between the levels of tension and relaxation. Think to yourself, my stomach area feels calm and relaxed.

It may take a few tries with this technique to both reduce levels of stress and tension and rid your desire for a smoke, but with time you may find this to be just the technique to stop the smoking habit.

HEALTHY PEOPLE 2000

Eliminate or severely restrict all forms of tobacco product advertising and promotion to which youth younger than age 18 are likely to be exposed.

Public health concern about tobacco advertising is based on the premise that such advertising perpetu-ates and increases cigarette consumption. Cigarette advertising may increase cigarette consumption by recruiting new smokers, inducing former smokers to relapse, making it more difficult for smokers to quit, and increasing the level of smokers' consumption by acting as an external cue to smoke.

THE WAR OF WORDS

A longstanding war of words exists between antismoking groups (most notably, the American Cancer Society and the American Heart Association) and the tobacco indus-try (tobacco growers and other businesses involved in the production and sale of smoking products). At stake is influencing the behavior of millions of smokers and prospective smokers. The health groups try to persuade these people not to smoke; the tobacco industry encour-ages them to smoke more and more (Califano, 1994).

The health war of words takes place in relative obscurity compared with tobacco advertising. Each year

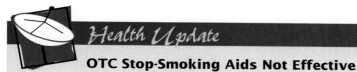

Health Update

OTC Stop-Smoking Aids Not Effective

No over-the-counter smoking deterrent products now on the market are effective, the FDA has concluded. Pills, tablets, lozenges, and chewing gum claiming to eliminate nicotine addiction can be sold until supplies are exhausted, but new shipments of these products will be prohibited after Dec. 1, 1993.

Some manufacturers of these nonprescription products have suggested conducting clinical trials on lobeline sulfate and silver acetate—two ingredients in current products. Past studies of these and other ingredients have not shown that they are effective in helping people stop or reduce smoking.

Several prescription products are approved as smoking cessation aids. One drug company has expressed interest in switching its prescription chewing gum product, Nicorette, to nonprescription status. Before allowing a switch, the agency would need to consider carefully Nicorette's own potential for addiction, since it contains nicotine.

Source: FDA Consumer, September, 1993.

the tobacco industry spends hundreds of millions of dollars to promote its products and to recruit new smokers. Perusal of many major magazines and newspapers reveals that cigarette advertising relies heavily on imagery portraying smoking as enjoyable and smokers as attractive, sexy, slim, and of high social status. Many magazines depend heavily on the income from cigarette advertising. When cigarette advertising was banned from radio and television in 1970, tobacco companies increased their advertising budgets and directed them to newspaper and magazine ads. They also developed costly promotional campaigns (such as the Virginia Slims Tennis Tournament) in an attempt to associate smoking cigarettes with health, fun, and fitness. Tobacco companies began to support health research, exotic travel excursions, rock concerts, and major athletic events to promote the virtues of smoking. To combat this promotional blitz by the tobacco industry, antismoking groups put forth hundreds of messages each year about the health consequences of smoking, using print media, radio, and television (Todd et al., 1995).

> *Why can't our government get tough with tobacco? Too many people are making too much money growing tobacco, peddling cigarettes, advertising them, and representing tobacco's corporate interests in Washington.*
>
> Arthur Caplan,
> medical ethicist

In other parts of the world, particularly Eastern Europe, Africa, and Asia, cigarette advertising has an enormous impact and smoking is increasing. Many governments do not warn their citizens of the health risks of smoking, and some are in economic partnership with tobacco companies. If this trend continues, the World Health Organization expects that by 2015, deaths from cigarette smoking worldwide will triple to one every 20 minutes (Sesser, 1993).

The U.S. government plays a paradoxical role in the smoking war. It supports both sides. Through the Department of Agriculture, the government provides price supports and other financial aids to tobacco growers and the tobacco industry. Through the Public Health Service, the government supports antismoking educational programs and finances research into the health effects of smoking. The pluralistic nature of our governmental system explains this dichotomy, which also illustrates why it would be foolish to depend entirely on the federal government—or on any other organization—to be the guardian of your personal health. If you value your health, don't smoke or use smokeless tobacco!

HEALTH IN REVIEW

- No public health message is disseminated as widely as that appearing on every package of cigarettes and in every cigarette advertisement: "Warning: The Surgeon General Has Determined That Cigarette Smoking Is Dangerous to Your Health."

- Despite the overwhelming evidence that cigarette smoking is associated with higher death rates from cancer, heart disease, and respiratory diseases, approximately 53 million Americans smoke. Smoking also is associated with a higher risk of emphysema and bronchitis.

- Users of smokeless tobacco also have increased health risks, particularly for lip and oral cancer.

- Besides smokers, nonsmokers who breathe smoke-laden air also have greater risk for lung cancer and other respiratory diseases. Children are harmed by breathing parents' cigarette smoke. Children of women who smoke during pregnancy tend to weigh less at birth (which is a health risk) and have developmental problems during childhood.

- Despite nicotine's capacity to cause physical dependence, ultimately the main reason people smoke is the desire to do so. For some, that desire results from the stimulation they receive from smoking; for others, smoking is a means to increase pleasure or to decrease stress.

- The fact that smoking is a matter of personal choice means that people can stop smoking if they choose. An abundance of stop-smoking programs are available to assist the motivated quitter. The success of any attempt relies on the smoker's resolve to quit and on replacing the unhealthy smoking habit with personally rewarding behaviors.

- One reason people continue to smoke is multi-million dollar advertising and promotional programs of the tobacco industry. The federal government shares blame. While the Public Health Service campaigns against smoking, the Department of Agriculture provides tobacco growers with price supports for their crop.

- The war of words will probably continue for a long time. But you need not be confused by the real issue: smoking is a serious risk to your health. Anyone who smokes, and anyone who is thinking of trying it, should keep in mind the dangers and understand these facts: there is no cure for heart disease, emphysema, or lung cancer.

REFERENCES

American Cancer Society (1995). *Cancer Facts and Figures.* Atlanta: American Cancer Society.

Califano, J. A. (1994). "Revealing the Link Between Campaign Financing and Deaths Caused by Tobacco." *Journal of the American Medical Association*, 272(15): 1217–1218.

Centers for Disease Control and Prevention (1995). "Some Questions and Answers about Oral Cancer." Atlanta: National Center for Prevention Services.

Connolly, G. N., C. T. Orleans, and A. Blum (1992). "Snuffing Tobacco Out of Sport." *American Journal of Public Health*, 82: 351–353.

Greer, R. O. (1994). "Oral Cancer and Molecular Biological Trends." *Dental Hygiene News*, 7(1): 3–8.

Haywood, C. C., and R. A. Benson (1993). "Lessons Reinforce Dangers of Smokeless Tobacco." *RDH*, 13(4): 20–24.

Ingrassia, M., and K. Springen (1995). "Waiting to Exhale." *Newsweek*, May 1.

Kessler, D. A. (1995). "Nicotine Addiction in Young People." *New England Journal of Medicine*, 333(3): 186–189.

National Cancer Institute (1993). *Chew or Snuff Is Real Bad Stuff: A Guide to Make Young People Aware of the Dangers of Using Smokeless Tobacco* (U.S. Department of Health and Human Services). Washington, D.C.: U.S. Government Printing Office.

National Cancer Institute (1992). *Tobacco Effects in the Mouth.* (NIH Publication 93–330) (U.S. Department of Health and Human Services). Washington, D.C.: U.S. Government Printing Office.

"OTC Stop-Smoking Aids Not Effective" (1993). *FDA Consumer,* September.

Riddle, S. G. (1994). "A Cancerous Epidemic." *RDH,* 14(7): 14–18.

Sesser, S. (1993). "Opium War Redux." *The New Yorker,* September 13: 78–89.

Strauss, R. H. (1991). "Spittin' Image." *The Physician and Sportsmedicine,* 19(11): 46–48.

Todd, J. S. et al. (1995). "The Brown and Williamson Documents: Where Do We Go From Here?" *Journal of the American Medical Association,* 274(3): 256–258.

U.S. Department of Health and Human Services (1994). *Preventing Tobacco Use among Young People: A Report of the Surgeon General* (U.S. Department of Health and Human Services). Washington, D.C.: U.S. Government Printing Office.

Wichman, S. A., and D. R. Martin (1991). "Sports and Tobacco." *The Physician and Sportsmedicine,* 19(11): 125–131.

SUGGESTED READINGS

Bartecchi, C. E., et al. (1994). "The Human Cost of Tobacco Use." *New England Journal of Medicine,* March 31. Documents the diseases and deaths that result from tobacco.

Bartecchi, C. E., T. D. MacKenzie, and R. W. Schrier (1995). "The Global Tobacco Epidemic." *Scientific American,* May, 44–51. Discusses the marketing strategies of tobacco companies around the world.

Farquhar, J. W., and G. A. Spillar (1990). *The Last Puff.* New York: W. W. Norton. Accounts of people who successfully quit smoking after years of addiction.

Hilts, P. J. (1994). "Is Nicotine Addictive? It Depends on Whose Criteria You Use." *New York Times,* August 2. Reviews how a drug is defined as being addictive.

Mansnerus, L. (1992). "Smoking: Is It a Habit or Is It Genetic?" *Good Health Magazine,* October 4. Examines research seeking to determine if smoking is behavioral or biological.

Raloff, J. (1994). "The Great Nicotine Debate." *Science News,* May 14. Examines the evidence that nicotine is the cause of smoking addiction.

Schwartz, J. (1994). "Smoking under Siege: Once Chic, Tobacco Now Is Defending Itself against a Revolution." *Washington Post National Weekly Edition,* June 27–July 3. The antitobacco revolution has been successful in passing laws to curtail smoking in public places; what's next?

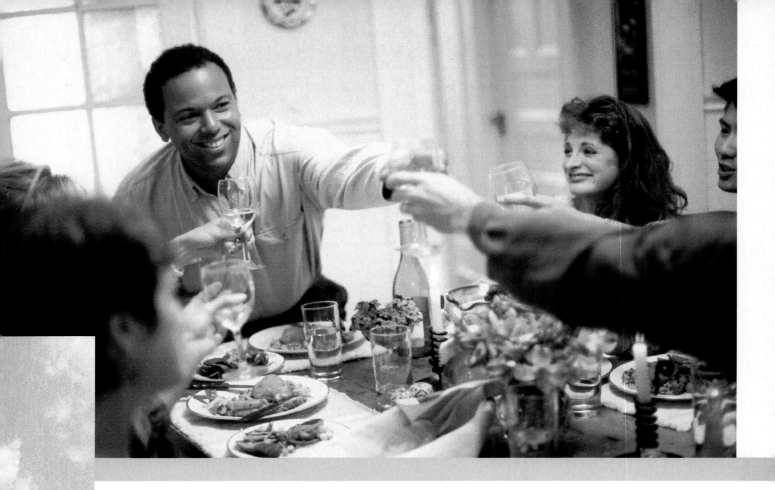

LEARNING OBJECTIVES

After reading this chapter you should be able to:

1. Discuss the prevalence of drinking, types of drinking, reasons for drinking, and attitudes toward drinking among youth.
2. Explain the effects of alcohol on the body.
3. Describe how alcohol is absorbed into the body and how this absorption relates to blood alcohol concentration.
4. Discuss the effects of alcohol on behavior including sexual behavior.
5. Describe the long-term effects of alcohol consumption.
6. Define alcohol abuse, alcohol addiction, and alcoholism.
7. Explain the phases of alcoholism.
8. Describe how alcohol affects one's significant others and the help that is available for both the family and alcoholic.

CHAPTER

Using Alcohol Responsibly

$\mathcal{A}$ lcohol abuse is one of the most significant health-related drug problems in the United States and in many other countries. Although cocaine and other illegal drugs receive much more attention from governments and the news media, these drugs affect far fewer people and cause far fewer health problems than alcohol (Chapter 16). Each year, over 100,000 deaths are alcohol related, many due to auto fatalities, and alcohol abuse is responsible for billions of dollars in health and social costs. Excessive alcohol use is also associated with thousands of divorces, perhaps as many as 50 percent of the incidents of family violence, and millions of hours of school and job absenteeism. In addition, alcohol abuse is linked to a long list of diseases and disorders (Figure 18.1).

Alcohol use has long been a part of social events such as parties, dinners, weddings, ball games, and picnics. The liquor industry encourages alcohol use by advertising in newspapers and magazines, and on radio and television. No direct link between advertising alcoholic products and alcohol abuse has been established. However, public health authorities and organizations such as the American Medical Association are concerned that advertising associating drinking with athletic prowess, material wealth, social prestige, and sex encourages irresponsible drinking behavior. Beer breweries and liquor distributors are especially active on college campuses, spending millions of dollars each year on advertising in campus newspapers and promoting their products by sponsoring "pub nights,"

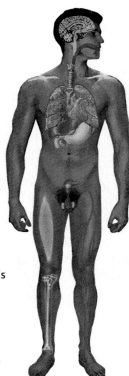

Brain *Wernicke's syndrome,* an acute condition characterized by ataxia, mental confusion, and ocular abnormalities. *Korsakoff's syndrome,* a psychotic condition characterized by impairment of memory and learning, apathy, and degeneration of the white brain matter.

Esophagus Esophageal varices, an irreversible condition in which the person can die by drowning in his own blood when the varices open.

Liver An acute enlargement of the liver, which is reversible, as well as the irreversible alcoholic's liver (cirrhosis).

Muscles Alcoholic myopathy, a condition resulting in painful muscle contractions.

Blood and bone marrow Coagulation defects and anemia.

Eyes Tobacco-alcohol blindness. Wernicke's ophthalmoplegia, a reversible paralysis of the muscles of the eye.

Pharynx Cancer of the pharynx is increased tenfold for drinkers who smoke.

Heart Alcoholic cardiomyopathy, a heart condition.

Lungs Lowered resistance is thought to lead to greater incidences of tuberculosis, pneumonia, and emphysema.

Spleen Hypersplenism.

Stomach Gastritis and ulcers.

Pancreas Acute and chronic pancreatitis.

Rectum Hemorrhoids.

Testes Atrophy of the testes.

Nerves Polyneuritis, a condition characterized by loss of sensation.

FIGURE 18.1 Diseases and Disorders Associated with Alcohol Abuse

giving away items with product logos, and underwriting some of the costs of college athletic events.

Alcohol's positive public image makes many people doubt that they need to learn about alcohol use and abuse. Most people who drink believe that they can "hold their liquor" and that alcoholic beverages, especially beer, are no more harmful to health than soft drinks. As with so many other aspects of health, for most people responsible and moderate alcohol consumption is more desirable than over zealous adherence to a single course of action. Everyone can benefit from knowing more about the effects of alcohol.

HISTORY OF ALCOHOL USE

It is likely that humans have been drinking alcohol since someone accidentally noticed the psychological effects of drinking fermented liquids. Archaeological evidence indicates that Stone Age people drank the fermented juice of berries. Perhaps this first fruit wine was produced when some berry juice was left too long in a covered earthen jar and yeasts began fermentation, converting the sugar in the juice to alcohol. The first recorded use of alcohol dates from the Mesopotamian agrarian cultures of around 2000 B.C.

Through the ages, drinking fermented grains (beer); fermented berries, grapes, and fruits (wine); and the distilled products of natural fermentation ("hard" liquors) has become commonplace in almost every human society

(with the important exception of Islamic societies). Alcohol is used in some religious ceremonies, is taken as medicine, is used to seal contracts, agreements, and treaties, and is offered to display hospitality. Alcohol consumption has been an integral part of American life since the landing of the *Mayflower* at Plymouth Rock. Yet over the years, many people have come to regard drinking as a social evil and drunkenness as a sin. The United States government tried to legislate alcohol use out of American lives in 1919 by the Volstead Act, a constitutional amendment that prohibited the sale and consumption of alcoholic beverages. This attempt to control alcohol consumption failed, however, and in 1933, Prohibition was repealed by another amendment to the Constitution.

Today, alcoholic beverages are available in many varieties. Not only are there the old standbys of beer, wine, and traditional hard liquors, but beverage manufacturers also market a variety of premixed cocktails, often sweetened with sugar and containing various flavors, wine coolers, and malt liquors.

PREVALENCE AND TRENDS REGARDING DRINKING

There is much drinking on most college campuses. According to a 1990 national survey, college students generally have a slightly higher drinking prevalence than their noncollege counterparts (Johnston, O'Malley, and Bachman, 1991). On a typical campus, 74.5 percent of

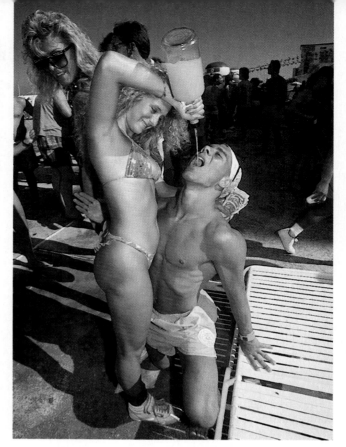

For most young people, drinking is part of socializing. Annual "spring break" vacations are viewed by some college students as an opportunity to do both to excess.

students consume alcohol, while 71 percent of their noncollege counterparts do.

Evidence shows that the percentage of students drinking increases between the freshman and senior year of college (Flynn and Brown, 1991). The social environment of college campuses often encourages and supports drinking. Studies show that 80 to 95 percent of all college students consume alcohol as a social activity in a new environment and as a rite of passage into adulthood.

One positive development shows a small, but significant, downward trend in the prevalence of alcohol use among college students. In 1980, 82 percent of college students had used alcohol in the last 30 days. By 1985, this figure was down to 80 percent, and in 1990, had declined to 74.5 percent. This trend mirrors a similar pattern of a small reduction in the national consumption of alcoholic beverages by all age groups (Johnston, O'Malley, and Bachman, 1991).

Types of Drinking

Forty-one percent of the nation's college students engaged in a bout of heavy drinking (five or more in a row) in the previous two weeks, while only 34 percent of their noncollege counterparts did so. Four percent of all college students drank every single day for a month. Many college students tend to drink in a binge style, particularly on weekend evenings (Baer, Stacy, and Larimer, 1991).

College students report a higher quantity and frequency of alcohol consumption than the general population. According to the National Institute on Drug Abuse, 22 percent of the drinkers ages 18 to 25 reported gulping down drinks quickly in order to get the desired effect.

> If alcoholism were a communicable disease, a national emergency would be declared.
> William C. Menninger, M.D., founder of Menninger Clinic

Reasons for Drinking

Approximately 20 percent of young people who drink first drink when they reach college. It is rare for a student to enter college as a nondrinker and remain an abstainer throughout the college years (Lo and Globetti, 1993). The culture of the campus, the opportunity to be independent of daily parental control, the need to conform, and insecurity of being on one's own all make a young adult particularly vulnerable (USDHHS, 1991).

According to government studies, there are a number of factors making the college alcohol environment risky for students. These reasons include:

- The high concentration of young men and women at a point in their lives where risk taking is common and peer acceptance is particularly important.
- The cultural traditions of the college campus.
- The heavy marketing of alcoholic beverages on college campuses.
- The limited alternative activities to drinking (according to students).

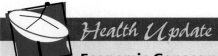

Attitudes toward Drinking

Social and normative influences on drinking behavior are evident in specific drinking patterns and practices observed among college students. College students who drink heavily tend to view campus attitudes toward drinking as liberal (Baer, Stacy, and Larimer, 1991). Students with the most positive attitudes toward drinking are typically the heaviest drinkers.

People's perceptions of the appropriateness of consuming alcoholic beverages in different social contexts is a strong predictor of the amount of alcohol they consume. Recent research indicates that many young people consider it acceptable to drink to "get by" in their social world. Students drink to belong to certain organizations (i.e., fraternities, sororities), to be accepted by peers, and to be a part of the college campus scene. Students perceive alcohol as an effective mechanism for enhancing sociability and for helping young adults feel like they are in control (Klein, 1992).

Media's Influence on Alcohol Consumption

A person's choice to drink may be influenced by the media. A college campus is not an island isolated from the rest of society. College TV stations and newspapers advertise alcoholic beverages. A study by the National Institute of Mental Health has estimated that approximately ten episodes per hour of typical television involve drinking (USDHHS, 1991).

A typical campus newspaper usually contains advertisements for alcoholic beverages and bar events. Slogans such as "Think when you drink," "Know when to say when," and "Friends don't let friends drive drunk" are frequently seen and heard in print and radio campaigns. These messages assume that after drinking alcohol you "think," you know "when" to say "when," and that you don't need to be responsible, just "let a friend drive." The alcohol industry states it is advocating responsible use of alcohol with these campaigns; others such as former Surgeon General Antonia Novello disagree (Scheel, 1994).

Pro-alcohol messages are everywhere: newspapers, radio, magazines, billboards, and television. Next to peer pressure, research has demonstrated that exposure to beer advertising is second only to peer influence in predicting alcoholic beverage consumption (USDHHS, 1991).

HOW ALCOHOL AFFECTS THE BODY

Alcoholic Beverages' Composition

The alcohol in beverages is a chemical called **ethyl alcohol (ethanol)**. There are many other kinds of alcohol, such as **methyl alcohol** and **isopropyl alcohol.** Most alcohols are poisonous if ingested in small amounts. In large amounts, even ethanol is toxic, but the body has ways to detoxify and eliminate it given enough time.

The amount of ethanol in a commercial alcoholic product usually is listed on the product label (beer is the exception). The amount of alcohol in beer and wine is usually given as the percentage of the total volume. Beer, for example, is generally about 4 percent alcohol, although some contain more or less (so-called light beers have nearly the same alcohol content as regular beers). Wine is about 12 percent alcohol. The amount of alcohol in distilled liquors (scotch, vodka, bourbon, tequila, rum, etc.) is given in terms of **proof,** a number that represents twice the percentage of alcohol in the product.

T E R M S

ethyl alcohol (ethanol): the consumable type of alcohol that is the psychoactive ingredient in alcoholic beverages; often called grain alcohol

methyl alcohol: wood alcohol or methanol

isopropyl alcohol: rubbing alcohol, sometimes used as an anesthetic

proof: a number assigned to an alcoholic product that is twice the percentage of alcohol in that product

blood alcohol content (BAC): the percent of alcohol in the blood

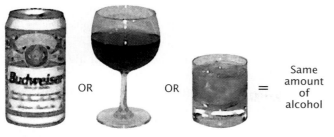

FIGURE 18.2 A can of beer, glass of wine, and a mixed drink have about the same amount of alcohol. So don't be fooled by the type of drink.

Thus, an 80 proof whiskey is 40 percent alcohol; 100 proof vodka is 50 percent alcohol.

Most standard portions of alcoholic drinks contain about ½ ounce of ethanol. For example, a 12-ounce can of beer that is 4 percent alcohol contains 0.48 ounce of alcohol. The same amount of alcohol is contained in a 4-ounce glass of wine. The alcohol content of a cocktail mixed with one shot (1 ounce) of a 100 proof bourbon is 0.5 ounce. So, a can of beer, a glass of wine, and a highball contain approximately the same amount of alcohol (Figure 18.2).

How Alcohol Is Absorbed, Excreted, and Metabolized

After alcohol is ingested, it is readily absorbed into the body through the gastrointestinal tract. About 20 percent of ingested alcohol is absorbed by the stomach and the rest by the small intestine. The alcohol is then carried through the bloodstream to all the body's tissues and organs. Although not strictly a food (it contains no protein, vitamins, or minerals), alcohol does contain calories—in fact, almost twice as many calories per gram as sugar.

Several factors affect the rate at which alcohol is absorbed into the body tissues. For example, food in the stomach—especially fatty foods or proteins—slows the absorption of alcohol. Nonalcoholic substances in beer, wine, and cocktails can also slow absorption of alcohol. The presence of carbon dioxide in beverages such as champagne, sparkling wines, beer, and carbonated mixed drinks increases the rate of alcohol absorption. That is why people feel intoxicated more quickly when drinking champagne or beer, especially on an empty stomach. The higher the alcohol content in a drink, the faster it is absorbed.

The concentration of alcohol in the blood is called the **blood alcohol content (BAC)**. A simple way to estimate BAC is to assume that ingesting one standard drink per hour (one beer, one glass of wine, one mixed drink), which contains approximately ½ ounce of ethyl alcohol, produces a BAC of 0.02 in a 150-pound male. Thus, the BAC of an average-sized man who drinks five beers during the first hour at a party will be 0.10; this level of alcohol in the blood violates the drinking-and-driving laws of most states. This shorthand method of approximating BAC changes depends on the body size, body composition (e.g., muscle, fat), and gender. All other things being equal, the BAC of a large person is less than that of a smaller person because the alcohol is diluted more in the large person's tissues. Women tend to have a higher BAC from the same number of drinks as men because they generally weigh less than men, have proportionately more body fat (which does not absorb alcohol as readily as muscle and other tissues), have sex hormones that tend to increase alcohol absorption and decrease its elimination, and tend to absorb more alcohol from the stomach.

Alcohol is eliminated from the body in two ways. About 10 percent is excreted unchanged through sweat, urine, or breath (hence the use of breath analyzers to test

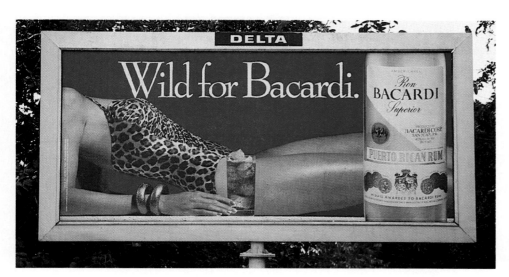

Alcohol advertisements, like cigarette ads, emphasize the connections among drinking, sex, and fun.

for drinking). The portion of alcohol that is not excreted (about 90 percent) is broken down primarily by the liver (metabolized), ultimately winding up as carbon dioxide and water. The liver detoxifies alcohol at a rate of about ½ ounce per hour; there is no way to speed up the process. Sobering-up remedies, such as drinking a lot of coffee, taking a cold shower, or engaging in vigorous exercise, do not accelerate the rate at which the liver removes alcohol from the body.

The Hangover

An occasional consequence of drinking alcohol is a **hangover,** which may involve stomach upset, headache, fatigue, weakness, shakiness, irritability, and sometimes vomiting after drinking too much. The frequency and severity of hangovers vary. The particular factors in alcohol that cause a hangover are unknown, but several causes have been suggested:

- When alcohol is present in the body, normal liver functions may slow in order to break down the alcohol. This slowdown may reduce the amount of sugar the liver releases into the blood, resulting in temporary hypoglycemia and its resultant fatigue, irritability, and headache.
- Alcohol may inhibit REM sleep, resulting in fatigue, irritability, and trouble concentrating.
- **Congeners,** which are other chemical substances in an alcoholic beverage, or the breakdown products produced in the liver may cause a hangover.
- **Acetaldehyde,** a toxic intermediate produced when the liver breaks down alcohol, may be responsible for hangover symptoms.

The best way to deal with a hangover is to sleep, to drink juice to replace lost body fluid and blood sugar (alcohol increases urine output), and perhaps to take an analgesic for a headache. Ingesting more alcohol will only prolong the hangover symptoms.

THE EFFECTS OF ALCOHOL ON BEHAVIOR

Pharmacologically, alcohol acts as a central nervous system depressant, which means that it slows certain functions in some parts of the brain. In moderate amounts, alcohol may affect the parts of the brain that control judgment and inhibitions, which is why many people have a drink or two at a party to help "loosen up," to become less shy and more able to interact freely with others. While some people may talk or laugh more than usual, others may become boisterous, argumentative, irritable, or depressed.

The behavioral effects of alcohol depend on the BAC (Table 18.1). At a BAC of 0.05, the "loosening-up" effects of alcohol become manifest. At a BAC of 0.10, the depressant effects of the drug become pronounced, the

TABLE 18.1   Behavioral Effects of Alcohol

Number of drinks	Ounces of alcohol	BAC (g/100 ml)	Approximate time for removal	Effects
1 beer, glass of wine, or mixed drink	½	0.02	1 hour	Feeling relaxed or "loosened up"
2½ beers, glasses of wine, or mixed drinks	1¼	0.05	2½ hours	Feeling "high"; decrease in inhibitions; increase in confidence; judgment impaired
5 beers, glasses of wine, or mixed drinks	2½	0.10	5 hours	Memory impaired; muscular coordination reduced; slurred speech; euphoric or sad feelings
10 beers, glasses of wine, or mixed drinks	5	0.20	10 hours	Slowed reflexes; erratic changes in feelings
15 beers, glasses of wine, or mixed drinks	7½	0.30	15–16 hours	Stuporous, complete loss of coordination; little sensation
20 beers, glasses of wine, or mixed drinks	10	0.40	20 hours	May become comatose; breathing may cease
25–30 beers, glasses of wine, or mixed drinks	15–20	0.50	26 hours	Fatal amount for most people

person may become sleepy, and motor coordination is affected. Speech may become slurred and postural instability may become noticeable. Alcohol's effects on motor skills, judgment, and reaction times make driving after drinking extremely dangerous. Approximately *half* of the more than 50,000 highway fatalities each year involve people who are intoxicated. Highway accidents are among the ten leading causes of death in the United States.

Two out of every three undergraduates admitted to driving while intoxicated. Driving while intoxicated is by no means the only dangerous driving practice related to alcohol. After just one or two drinks, an individual may not be legally drunk, but will likely have impaired driving capabilities such as slower reaction time, impaired perception, and poorer judgment (USDHHS, 1991).

Physical and psychological tolerance of the effects of alcohol can be acquired through regular use. The nervous system can adapt to the effects of alcohol so that greater amounts are required to produce the same physiological and psychological effects. Some people learn to modify their behaviors so that they appear sober even though their BAC is high. This phenomenon is called **learned behavioral tolerance.** In general, the more experience a person has with certain behaviors, the less likely it is that alcohol will impair those behaviors, although not all behaviors are affected by alcohol to the same degree.

Other socially undesirable consequences of drinking alcohol include arguments and fights, jeopardized relationships, failed exams and/or courses, college dropouts, and lost jobs. According to the National Institute on Drug Abuse (1988), 30 percent of 18- to 25-year-old drinkers reported that they had become "aggressive" while drinking; 19 percent had been in "heated arguments"; and 11 percent had been absent from school or work as a result of drinking.

Drunkenness and the consequent rowdiness and violence on college campuses is not a new phenomenon. Hundreds of years ago, the president of the University of Paris rode around with a squad of mounted archers to discipline unruly students. In 1858, the president of the University of Alabama appealed to the state legislature

> To put alcohol in the human brain is like putting sand in the bearings of an engine.
> *Thomas A. Edison*

for authority to deal with dissipation and rowdiness. The history of academic institutions here and in Europe is replete with attempts to deal with alcohol abuse on campus. In a sense, these earlier attempts viewed campus drinking as a discipline or moral problem rather than today's view of it as a health, educational, informational, or cultural problem as is the trend today.

Sexual Behavior

The relationship between alcohol consumption and sexual behavior is a topic of concern for college health educators. This relationship is most significant with respect to unintended pregnancies, the spread of HIV and other sexually transmitted diseases, interpersonal relationship issues, and unintended sexual experiences (Meilman, 1993).

For example, one study revealed that 23 percent of men and 14 percent of women had engaged in unintended sexual activity related to their alcohol use (Meilman, 1993). Also, twice as many women as men abandoned safer sex techniques due to their use of alcohol. Alcohol use has been a factor in failure to use condoms, with significant implications for the spread of sexually transmitted diseases, including HIV (Chapter 11).

The effects of alcohol on sexual desire and performance vary from person to person, and depend on the BAC. In some individuals, small amounts of alcohol may dispel uncomfortable feelings about sex and may facilitate sexual arousal. Higher amounts of alcohol (0.10 BAC or greater) may cause problems for males, such as getting and maintaining an erection or ejaculating, and for females, such as a reduction in vaginal lubrication and difficulty reaching orgasm. Even at moderate BACs, some individuals are too intoxicated to effectively give and receive sexual pleasure.

Sexual Assaults

"In both animal and human studies, alcohol, more than any other drug, has been linked with a high incidence of

Early in the morning last summer, I was arrested for driving under the influence of alcohol.

It's not easy to recall what actually happened—I see it through a fog, as if I was watching someone else.

The actual arrest is the blurriest. I was running for those few moments on pure adrenalin and fear. For awhile I don't even think I was breathing.

It's hard to explain the exact emotions.

It's hard to explain what it feels like to want more than anything to be sober.

It's hard to explain losing complete control of your life for even a short time.

It is hard to explain the feeling of handcuffs.

It's hard to explain what it feels like to sit in a holding cell and bite your lip in the hopes of not going to sleep.

One thing for sure is that when those flashing lights appeared in my rearview mirror, all the rationalizations that got me into that car vanished. "It's just around the corner," "I need to get a friend home," or "No one is on the road at this hour"—none of them mean a thing—zero.

At the jail, it took what seemed like days to be fingerprinted and photographed and to fill out the required forms. Each step was just a little more humiliating than the last.

I am still overwhelmed at how a single, incredibly poor judgment could affect so many parts of my life.

The ramifications will be with me in various ways for the next three years—which is as far ahead as I have ever cared to plan.

These shock waves include probation for three years, an exorbitant increase in the cost of my car insurance, restricted driver's license for 90 days (which was agreed upon in lieu of two days in jail) and a $600 fine, to name a few.

Many of the ramifications cannot be quantified. There was the call home, a couple of days of generally feeling lousy and the unshakable sense that I had proven myself a fool.

Through all of it, however, I have some things to be thankful for.

On the top of that very short list is the fact that I didn't kill anyone.

Having struggled to come to terms with the arrest, it is impossible to imagine . . . for that there is no atonement.

Also on that list is the discovery of some very supportive people in my life, all of whom said not that what happened was OK, but that I was going to be OK. I turned to my parents and friends for help, and no one turned away—I am thankful.

Whether this column will keep anyone from driving drunk is doubtful. If I had read this column before my arrest, I would have thought of a hundred reasons why it would never have applied to me—but I would have been wrong.

Source: The Aggie, University of California, Davis.

Weight	Drinks (two-hour period) 1½ oz. liquor or 12 oz. beer											
100	1	2	3	4	5	6	7	8	9	10	11	12
120	1	2	3	4	5	6	7	8	9	10	11	12
140	1	2	3	4	5	6	7	8	9	10	11	12
160	1	2	3	4	5	6	7	8	9	10	11	12
180	1	2	3	4	5	6	7	8	9	10	11	12
200	1	2	3	4	5	6	7	8	9	10	11	12
220	1	2	3	4	5	6	7	8	9	10	11	12
240	1	2	3	4	5	6	7	8	9	10	11	12

Be careful driving BAC to 0.05%

Driving will be impaired 0.05% – 0.09%

Do not drive 0.10% & up

Effects of drinking on driving

violence and aggressive behavior" (National Institute on Alcohol Abuse and Alcoholism, 1990). Every year college students are involved in thousands of acts of violence, either as perpetrators, as victims, or both. According to a 1987 study, 285,000 serious crimes were committed on America's college campuses, including 31 murders, 600 reported rapes, 13,000 assaults, and over 23,000 robberies and burglaries. In addition, there were tens of thousands of incidents of brawling, fighting, unreported rape, vandalism, and other acts of violence that were never reported or treated as crimes (*New York Times,* 1990).

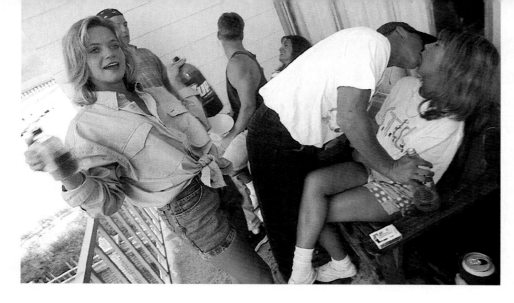

Drunken parties often lead to actions and feelings that one regrets the next day—and sometimes for much longer.

Acquaintance rape has been linked to alcohol consumption on college campuses (Chapter 23). A sexual assault study revealed that 26 percent of men who acknowledged committing sexual assault on a date reported being intoxicated; 29 percent reported being slightly intoxicated. In this same study, 21 percent of the women who were victims of sexual aggression on a date reported being intoxicated; 32 percent were slightly intoxicated. A woman's alcohol consumption may prevent her from realizing that her friendly behavior may be perceived as seduction; men may be inclined to perceive friendly cues from a woman as a sign of sexual interest (Abbey, 1991).

OTHER EFFECTS OF ALCOHOL

Alcohol can impair the functioning of other body organs other than the brain. Alcohol can irritate the organs of the gastrointestinal (GI) tract—the esophagus, stomach, intestine, pancreas, and liver—causing upset or irritability, nausea, vomiting, or diarrhea. Alcohol can also dilate arteries and cause bloodshot eyes. Dilation of arteries in the arms, legs, and skin can cause a drop in blood pressure and decrease body heat, explaining why people occasionally feel flushed and their faces redden when they drink. Giving people alcohol to "warm them up" actually produces the opposite physiological effect.

Alcohol should not be ingested simultaneously with other central nervous system depressants such as tranquilizers, sedatives, and antihistamines found in cold medicines. In many instances, the depressant effects of alcohol and the other drug interact so that the combined effects of the two drugs is greater than the simple additive effects of either drug taken separately. Seemingly reasonable amounts of alcohol taken with another depressant drug can dangerously suppress brain function and respiration (Table 18.2).

Long-Term Effects

Long-term heavy drinking can affect the immune, endocrine, and reproductive functions, and can cause neurological problems, including dementia, blackouts, seizures, hallucinations, and peripheral neuropathy (NIAAA, 1990). Various cancers associated with heavy drinking include cancers of the lip, oral cavity, pharynx, larynx, esophagus, stomach, colon, rectum, tongue, lung, pancreas, and liver. Long-term heavy drinking can also increase the risk of chronic gastritis, **hepatitis**,

T E R M

hepatitis: inflammation of the liver

TABLE 18.2   Alcohol and Drugs That Don't Mix*

Drug	Dangerous interaction
Acetaminophen (Tylenol, Anacin-3)	Moderate use plus alcohol can cause liver damage.
Aspirin (Anacin, Excedrin)	Heavy use plus alcohol can cause bleeding of stomach wall and GI tract.
Antihistamines (Chlor-Trimeton, Benadryl)	Drowsiness and loss of coordination increased by alcohol.
Tranquilizers, sedatives (Valium, Dalmane, Miltown)	Alcohol increases their effects.
Painkillers (codeine, Percodan, morphine)	Alcohol increases sedation and reduces ability to concentrate.
Barbiturates (Amytal, Seconal, phenobarbital)	Potentially FATAL. NEVER use with alcohol.

*Alcohol should NOT be consumed when taking drugs such as those listed.

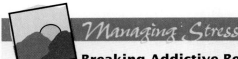
Breaking Addictive Behaviors

It's a little known fact but it was psychologist Carl Jung who inspired the Alcoholics Anonymous program. Frustrated with a client unable to change his alcoholism, Jung suggested that his only hope for recovery was to purposefully have a spiritual experience to rid himself of this addictive habit. So, Roland H. did just that. After conquering his addiction, he went on to share this experience with Edwin T., then Bill W., who then went on to co-found Alcoholics Anonymous.

In response to a letter from Bill W., Jung wrote, "His craving for alcohol was the equivalent, on a low level, of the spiritual thirst of our being for wholeness, expressed in medieval language: the union with God. You see alcohol in Latin is *spiritus,* and we use the same words for the highest religious experience as well as for the most depraving poison. The helpful formula therefore is: *Spiritus contra spiritum.*" (Spiritual crises require spiritual cures).

hypertension, cirrhosis of the liver, and coronary heart disease (NIAAA, 1987).

Chronic alcoholic men may become "feminized," with breast enlargement and female hair patterns. Chronic alcoholic women may experience menstrual disturbances, loss of secondary sex characteristics, and infertility. Women who drink heavily experience more gynecological problems and have surgery more often than women who do not (NIAAA, 1987).

Fetal Alcohol Syndrome

Alcohol can harm the health of anyone, man or woman, young or old. Even the fetus can be damaged by alcohol. Over the last ten years evidence has accumulated showing that numerous kinds of birth defects and mental retardation may result from ingestion of alcohol by pregnant women—a condition known as **fetal alcohol syndrome** (Chapter 15). Fetal alcohol syndrome is estimated to be the third leading cause of birth defects and mental retardation among newborns. Since the harmful effects on fetal development are believed to occur during the first few weeks or months of prenatal development, a time during which much of the nervous system is being formed, women should refrain from drinking if they are trying to become pregnant or if they suspect they are pregnant. Studies have also shown that the level of alcohol in the fetus' blood may be ten times greater than the BAC of the mother. This explains why even a couple of drinks early in pregnancy can endanger normal fetal development.

ALCOHOL ABUSE AND ALCOHOLISM

Alcohol abuse is the principal drug problem in the United States. Approximately 12 million Americans of different ages, religions, races, educational backgrounds, and socioeconomic status have problems with alcohol. Over 3 million American teenagers between 14 and 17 have a drinking problem. More than a third of all sui-

cides involve alcohol. Approximately 6 million adults have personal and health problems associated with alcohol that are severe enough to warrant the label **alcoholic** and to suffer from **alcoholism.** These people are unable to control their drinking; some are physically dependent on alcohol and may experience withdrawal symptoms, including **delirium tremens (DTs),** when deprived of alcohol. Delirium tremens is characterized by hallucinations and uncontrollable shaking.

Problem drinking can cause numerous negative consequences. Job and school performance can be impaired, family relationships and friendships can be destroyed, and drunk driving may cause financial problems, injuries, legal problems and fatalities. Because alcohol supplies calories, alcoholics are rarely hungry. They may suffer from vitamin deficiency syndromes, which result in loss of muscular coordination and mental confusion.

The cause or causes of problem drinking and alcoholism are unknown, although hypotheses abound. Before the advent of modern psychology and medicine, alcohol abuse was thought to be a manifestation of immorality and irreligiousness. Some people still hold that view, but many professionals (and problem drinkers) interpret alcohol abuse as a behavioral disorder or a medical disease. For example, some people with low self-esteem or seemingly unmanageable life conflicts may

T E R M S

fetal alcohol syndrome: birth defects caused by ingestion of alcohol during pregnancy

alcohol abuse: frequent, continued use of alcohol; binge drinking

alcoholic: a person dependent on alcohol

alcoholism: loss of control over drinking alcohol

delirium tremens (DTs): hallucinations and uncontrollable shaking sometimes caused by withdrawal of alcohol in alcohol-dependent individuals

blackout: failure to recall normal or abnormal behavior or events that occurred while drinking

drink in order to feel better about themselves or to try to cope with adversities. Instead, they may add a drinking problem to their other problems.

Some evidence indicates that, at least for some people, alcoholism may have a biological basis, either because people metabolize alcohol differently or because their brains respond differently to alcohol. Some experts resist considering alcohol abuse a disease because doing so may remove the sense of personal and social responsibility for problem drinking (Peele, 1990). Others argue that calling alcohol abuse a "disease" fosters successful treatment because it removes the stigma, lessens guilt, and offers a supervised and presumably scientifically based plan for treatment.

> *Is the disease model of alcoholism scientific? No. Simply calling behavior a disease process does not make it one.*
>
> *Jeffrey A. Schaller,*
> *psychotherapist*

The Phases of Alcoholism

Alcoholism usually develops from a prealcoholic stage of needing to drink to relieve tensions and anxieties. The prealcoholic phase may last for years, during which tolerance to alcohol gradually develops. Progression to a state of alcoholism is characterized by three phases:

- **The warning phase.** In this first stage of alcoholism, problem drinkers increase tolerance for alcohol and become more preoccupied with drinking. For example, when they are invited to a party they may ask what alcoholic beverages will be served rather than who is going to be there. In this stage problem drinkers may sneak drinks often and may deny that they are drinking too much. **Blackouts** may also occur. Blackouts are periods in which others observe the drinker as behaving normally, or abnormally, but the drinker has no recall of events that happened while drinking.

- **The crucial phase.** This phase of alcoholism is characterized by loss of control over how much alcohol is consumed. The person may not drink every day, but cannot control the amount of alcohol consumed once

Health Update

Women and Alcohol

Did You Know . . .

- Women achieve a higher blood alcohol level (and therefore become more intoxicated) than men do when drinking the same amount of alcohol proportionate to body weight.

- Women who drink are more likely than men to develop liver cirrhosis and die from it.

- Even three drinks a week increases the risk of breast cancer.

- Drinking during pregnancy leads to a range of disabilities in the baby; this is known as fetal alcohol syndrome and is the third leading cause of birth defects and mental retardation.

- Alcohol can lead to accidents, arrests, health and emotional problems, problems on the job and with friends and family.

- Among the most persistent myths about alcohol is that it is an aphrodisiac. Because it relaxes inhibitions, people believe it intensifies sexual pleasure. In fact,

drinking alcohol makes orgasm more difficult to achieve and lessens its intensity because it depresses the central nervous system.

- Alcohol inhibits the body's ability to use vitamins and calcium. Thus, its habitual use can result in dull hair and skin, aggravated acne, and dandruff.

- In some areas of the U.S., women make up to 50 percent of those seeking treatment for alcoholism.

- Sex under the influence of alcohol can include sexual acts which may betray a woman's commitment to herself and to the people she loves. Today, sex can also be fatal. Alcohol use makes safer sex difficult. People may ignore protecting themselves from sexually transmitted diseases such as HIV, the virus that causes AIDS.

- Women may be the recipients of increased aggression due to drinking. The growing incidents of rape documented on campuses

across the country frequently involve the use of alcohol and other drugs by both the men and the women.

- Although the rapist is usually not drunk, he has almost always been drinking; and since the victim, too, has often had something to drink, she may feel responsible for the attack. Therefore, most attacks are never reported.

- Studies of alcoholism and suicide show that women outnumber men in both completed and attempted suicides.

- Women who suffer from PMS often try to relieve their symptoms by drinking. However, alcohol, a depressant, only worsens the symptoms instead of alleviating them.

- Alcohol is potentially more damaging to women than it is to men!

Source: "Women and Alcohol," Illinois State University, Student Health Service (1995).

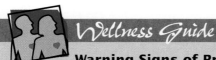

Wellness Guide

Warning Signs of Problem Drinking or Alcoholism

1. Gulping drinks.
2. Drinking to modify uncomfortable feelings.
3. Personality or behavioral changes after drinking.
4. Getting drunk frequently.
5. Experiencing "blackouts"—not being able to remember what happened while drinking.
6. Frequent accidents or illness as a result of drinking.
7. Priming—preparing yourself with alcohol before a social gathering at which alcohol is going to be served.
8. Not wanting to talk about the negative consequences of drinking (avoidance).
9. Focusing social situations around alcohol.
10. Sneaking drinks or clandestine drinking.
11. Preoccupation with alcohol.

drinking has begun. In this stage, the problem drinker may rationalize drinking behavior and actually believe that there are good reasons for heavy drinking. Alcoholics may still carry out responsibilities (housework, job, schoolwork) for some time, and they may employ a series of strategies to keep the family from rejecting them, including promises to stop drinking. Often alcoholics' extravagant measures to prove they do not have a drinking problem appear successful, but eventually they begin drinking heavily again. At this point the problem with alcohol is sometimes blamed on the kind of drinks preferred or on the usual place of drinking; as a result, problem drinkers may change to a different form of alcoholic beverage or to a different place in which to drink.

- **The chronic phase.** In this phase, the alcoholic is dependent on the drug, and drinking behavior consumes all aspects of life. Friends and family have resigned themselves to the problem and may be angry or ignore the alcoholic. At this stage of alcoholism the person may miss work or school occasionally. The health consequences of alcohol abuse may intensify and the person may need medical attention and even hospitalization. When physical addiction to alcohol occurs, continual drinking is needed to prevent withdrawal symptoms. Drinking for days at a time (a **bender**) may take place. The great majority of alcoholics do not wind up on "skid row," but instead struggle with their problem within their families and communities.

The Effects of Alcoholism on the Family

Alcoholism can severely disrupt marital and family relationships. One family member's drinking problem can put stress on all the other members, causing them mental and emotional suffering and sometimes financial hardship. Alcoholism is costly to many people, not just the alcoholic.

> *Our children are being taught that they should avoid all drugs, yet come home to see beer, wine, and spirits being consumed by their parents.*
>
> R. Curtis Ellison,
> epidemiologist

Close relatives of a problem drinker can experience a variety of emotions, ranging from joy and relief when the problem drinker stops drinking for a time to feelings of failure and depression when the problem drinker begins drinking again. In between the highs and lows, family members can feel anger, shame, guilt, pity, and constant anxiety. They may try to cope with the situation in different ways. Some may try to assume responsibility for the problem; others may be designated as scapegoats and blamed for it, while some family members blame others (i.e., other family members, other people) for the drinker's problem. Some may withdraw in silence while others try to maintain their sense of humor. These behaviors are all defense mechanisms against the family's psychological pain.

Like the problem drinker, family members may deny the problem, try to rationalize it, isolate themselves from friends and relatives, and in some cases actually feel responsible for the other's drinking problem. This **enabling** or protection process keeps the alcoholic from feeling responsible for his or her drinking—which is part of the paradox experienced by families of alcoholics. In their attempts to protect the alcoholic, family members may unwittingly contribute to the drinking problem; they may try to protect the alcoholic from serious social consequences of excessive drinking, for instance, making excuses for absenteeism from work or school.

Family members of alcoholics may attend Alanon, an organization that helps spouses, families, and friends of

TERMS

bender: several days of binge drinking

enabling: denial of, or excuses for, the excessive drinking by an alcoholic to whom one is close

denial: refusal to admit you (or someone else) have a drinking problem

codependency: a relationship pattern in which the nonaddicted family members identify with the alcoholic

alcoholics. Alateen is a similar organization that helps children of alcoholics. Alanon and Alateen help family members understand how alcoholism has affected their lives and help them to explore the family relationships that contribute to the alcohol problem. Family therapy (with or without the problem drinker's participation) may help a family find ways to cope with the problem and regain harmony in their family life.

Children of Alcoholics

The National Clearinghouse for Drug and Alcohol Information (1992) estimates that there are 28 million children of alcoholics (COAs) in the United States, 6.6 million of whom are under the age of 18. Adult children of alcoholics (ACOAs) and COAs grew up in families in which one or both parents had a drinking problem. As children many of these individuals experienced neglect, emotional deprivation, an unstable family environment, and sometimes violence and abuse. As a result they may have developed ways of thinking and behaving that impair personal and relationship harmony in adulthood. Children of alcoholics are at a high risk of becoming alcoholics themselves.

To numb the emotional pain stemming from parental alcoholism, many ACOAs learn as children to block from their awareness the truth of their situation—both the fact of a parent's alcoholism and also the emotional pain resulting from it. This tendency is referred to as **denial.** The consequences of denial by the ACOA go beyond issues of parental alcoholism to become a generalized way of approaching life. As adults, many ACOAs are constricted in their capacities to see the world as it really is and also to experience emotional fulfillment.

Denial gives many ACOAs a negative self-image and a tendency to be hypercritical of themselves. Rather than face the painful truth, many ACOAs when children believed themselves to be the cause of their parent's erratic, violent behavior. Indeed, sometimes the troubled parents reinforced this assumption by blaming their children for their problems. The children not only come to believe themselves to be "bad," but they also tend to believe they are responsible for everyone else's emotions. Thus, they become very other-focused, a behavior called **codependency.**

Another consequence of growing up in an alcoholic family is the tendency to try to control situations and other people. Because family life was unstable and painful, many ACOAs come to believe that their interpersonal environment is likely at any moment to become emotionally painful, violent, or disruptive. Thus, ACOAs tend to be constantly anxious and hypervigilant for signs of danger. To minimize the threat (experienced as criticism, abandonment, or abuse), ACOAs tend to be compliant and agreeable and actively try to please. Believing that others cannot be trusted and that the world must be made safe, ACOAs also try to be totally self-reliant and in control of their lives.

Denial, a negative self-image, the tendency to take responsibility for others, the need to control oneself and the environment, and other characteristics help an ACOA survive childhood in an alcoholic family. Unfortunately, in adulthood these same "survival" mechanisms limit the opportunity to grow and develop unique individual qualities and to experience healthy interpersonal relationships. Fortunately, these self-limiting beliefs and behaviors can be changed through counseling, twelve-step programs such as Codependents Anonymous, and various spiritual practices.

Seeking Help: Treatment Options

The situation of problem drinkers and alcoholics is serious but not hopeless. Recovery is possible if the person

---

Wellness Guide

Some Characteristics of Adult Children of Alcoholics

Guessing at what normal behavior is and having a higher tolerance for abusive behavior

Tendency to perceive things as all good or bad ("all-or-none" thinking)

Feeling different and cut-off from other people

Mercilessly self-critical

Fearful of losing control of one's feelings and behaviors

Trying to control others

Resisting and overreacting to change

Constantly seeking approval and affirmation

Lack of awareness of emotions

Fearful of expressing one's true thoughts and feelings

Being overly responsible for others' feelings

A tendency toward compulsive behavior: overeating, drug or alcohol abuse, workaholism

A tendency to be a "rescuer" or "victim" in interpersonal relationships

Difficulty relaxing, letting go, and having fun

Do You Have a Drinking Problem?

This questionnaire is designed to help you determine whether you have a problem with alcohol. Answer each question yes or no and record your choice in the right-hand column.

	Yes	No
1. Do you feel you are a normal drinker?	___	___
2. Have you ever awakened the morning after drinking the night before and found that you could not remember a part of the evening before?	___	___
3. Does your wife, husband, a parent, or other near relative ever worry or complain about your drinking?	___	___
4. Can you stop drinking without a struggle after one or two drinks?	___	___
5. Do you ever feel bad about your drinking?	___	___
6. Do friends or relatives think you are a normal drinker?	___	___
7. Do you ever try to limit your drinking to certain times of the day or to certain places?	___	___
8. Are you always able to stop drinking when you want to?	___	___
9. Have you ever attended a meeting of Alcoholics Anonymous?	___	___
10. Have you gotten into fights when drinking?	___	___
11. Has drinking ever created problems between you and your wife, husband, boyfriend, girlfriend, a parent, or other near relative?	___	___
12. Has your wife, husband, boyfriend, girlfriend, a parent, or other near relative ever gone to anyone for help about your drinking?	___	___
13. Have you ever lost friends because of drinking?	___	___
14. Have you ever gotten into trouble at work because of drinking?	___	___
15. Have you ever lost a job because of drinking?	___	___
16. Have you ever neglected your obligations, your family, or your work for two or more days in a row because you were drinking?	___	___
17. Do you drink before noon fairly often?	___	___
18. Have you ever been told you have liver trouble? Cirrhosis?	___	___
19. After heavy drinking have you ever had delirium tremens (DT's) or severe shaking?	___	___
20. After heavy drinking have you ever heard voices or seen things that weren't really there?	___	___
21. Have you ever gone to anyone for help about your drinking?	___	___
22. Have you ever been in a hospital because of drinking?	___	___
23. Have you ever been a patient in a psychiatric hospital or in a psychiatric ward of a general hospital?	___	___
24. Have you ever been in a hospital to be "dried out" (detoxified) because of drinking?	___	___
25. Have you ever been in jail, even for a few hours, because of drunk behavior?	___	___

Scoring: Item keying for alcoholic responses are 1. N; 2. Y; 3. Y; 4. N; 5. Y; 6. N; 7. Y; 8. N; 9–25, Y.

To score, add one point for each alcoholic response. The total score is the number of alcoholic responses.

No. of Alcoholic Responses	Interpretation
0–2	No problem with alcohol
3–5	Early warning signs that drinking is becoming problematic
6 or more	Problem drinker/alcoholic

is strongly motivated to stop drinking. Moreover, as in other aspects of health, "an ounce of prevention is worth a pound of cure."

Sometimes the motivation to stop drinking comes in the form of a threat—a drinking-related legal problem or illness, severe disruption of family life, the loss of a job.

The motivation to stop drinking can also come from the person's own resolve to stop his or her self-destructive behavior and to stop feeling helpless, hopeless, and confused.

Alcoholics Anonymous (AA), the worldwide non-profit self-help organization, has assisted many people to get on the road back to wellness and enjoyment of life. AA bases its program on total sobriety, anonymity, and a step-by-step program of recovery. The environment at AA meetings is relaxing, caring, and open. Members share their experiences, strengths, and hopes with each other, with the goal of helping new and old members identify and learn more about their own problems with alcohol. Practical tips on how to remain sober are shared, and telephone numbers are exchanged so that a member can contact another member if stressful situations arise that previously led to drinking.

Alcoholics Anonymous emphasizes that sobriety is a state of mind, which means that recovering from a drinking problem involves changing values, attitudes, and life-styles. The AA program helps problem drinkers honestly examine their feelings, recognize their limitations, and accept responsibility for past wrongs. For problem drinkers, remaining sober is an ongoing process, which involves finding new ways to satisfy emotional, spiritual, and social needs. Of course, AA may not be the answer for everyone who has a drinking problem. Individual and group psychotherapy with a therapist skilled in helping problem drinkers can also be successful.

> *Alcoholism is the most common social disease picked up in a bar.*
> *Anonymous*

RESPONSIBLE DRINKING

Each person has the option of drinking or abstaining from alcohol. Each of you has the responsibility for determining the occasions for drinking and the amounts of alcohol that you consume. If you are one of the millions of people who already enjoy drinking, here are some guidelines to remember:

- Make sure that alcohol use improves your social interactions and does not harm or destroy them.
- Drink slowly and avoid mixing alcohol with other drugs.
- Be sure that using alcohol enhances your general sense of well-being and does not make either you or other persons feel disgusted with your actions.
- If you plan to drink, decide beforehand that you will not drive and designate someone who will not drink to be the driver.

In addition to being responsible for your own drinking habits, you can also help others to drink responsibly. Respect the wishes of the person who chooses to abstain from drinking and don't push drinks on people at parties. If you are giving a party, be sure to provide alternatives to alcohol. You may also offer places to sleep for those who have been drinking and should not drive home. Remember to eat when you drink and to provide food at your parties.

There is no evidence to indicate that total abstinence from alcohol is necessary for health and wellness. On the other hand, there is a great deal of evidence showing that excessive alcohol use can destroy personal health and family relationships, can cause traffic deaths and suicides, and can produce birth defects in newborns. We believe that you can significantly improve your health and happiness by developing responsible drinking habits while you are young and maintaining moderate drinking habits throughout life.

HEALTH IN REVIEW

- Alcohol abuse is the major drug problem in the United States. Consumption of alcohol is responsible for almost half of all highway fatalities and for numerous social, family, and health problems.
- Alcoholic beverages contain ethyl alcohol, which is produced by the action of yeast on sugar (fermentation) in the juices of grains, berries, and fruits. Beer and wine are direct products of fermentation; "hard" liquor, such as whiskey, vodka, rum, and brandy, is made from distilled fermented liquids. Most standard portions of alcoholic beverages contain ½ ounce of ethyl alcohol.
- Social and normative influences on drinking behavior are evident in specific drinking patterns among college students. Drinking on campus increases the risk for violence including sexual assault.
- Alcohol enters the bloodstream within minutes after ingestion. The physical and behavioral effects of alcohol depend on the blood alcohol content (BAC). A BAC of 0.02 produces a "loosening up" effect. A BAC of 0.10 seriously impairs motor coordination and judgment; in most states it is illegal to drive with a BAC of 0.10.

- Frequent and constant use of alcohol can lead to physical dependence and tolerance for the drug (alcoholism). Alcoholism develops in stages, starting with the inability to control drinking and advancing to complete physical dependence.

- Alcoholics may encounter severe health problems and their personal lives, family relationships, and friendships may be disrupted. Millions of children who grew up in families where one or both parents were alcoholics experience personal problems as adults stemming from their childhoods.

- Organizations such as Alcoholics Anonymous and individual or group psychotherapy can help people

recover from problem drinking and alcoholism. Alcohol abuse can be prevented by taking responsibility for one's drinking behavior.

REFERENCES

Abbey, A. (1991). "Acquaintance Rape and Alcohol Consumption on College Campuses." *Journal of American College Health,* 39: 165–169.

Baer, J. S., A. Stacy, and M. Larimer (1991). "Biases in the Perception of Drinking Norms among College Students." *Journal of Studies of Alcohol,* 52(6): 580–586.

"Campus Searches of Bags of Alcohol are Discontinued" (1990). *New York Times,* September 23: 50.

Flynn, C. A., and W. E. Brown (1991). "The Effects of a Mandatory Alcohol Education Program on College Student Problem Drinkers." *Journal of Alcohol and Drug Education,* 37(1): 15–24.

Johnston, L. D., P. O'Malley, and J. G. Bachman (1991). *Drug Use among American High School Seniors, College Students and Young Adults, 1975–1990.* National Institute of Drug Abuse, DHHS Pub (ADM) 91-1835.

Klein, H. (1992). "Prevention and Treatment of Alcohol Problems on a College Campus." *Journal of Alcohol and Drug Education,* 37(3): 35–52.

Lo, C. C., and G. Globetti (1993). "A Partial Analysis of the Campus Influence on Drinking Behaviors: Students Who Enter College as Non-drinkers." *Journal of Drug Issues,* 23(4): 715–725.

Meilman, P. W. (1993). "Alcohol-induced Sexual Behavior on Campus." *Journal of the American College Health,* 42(1): 27–31.

National Clearinghouse for Alcohol and Drug Information (1992). "The Fact Is . . . Alcoholism Tends to Run in Families." OSAP Prevention Resource Guide. Rockville, Md.

National Institute on Alcohol Abuse and Alcoholism (1990). *Seventh Special Report to the U.S. Congress on Alcohol and Health from the Secretary of Health and Human Services.* DHHS Publication (ADM) 281-88-0002.

National Institute on Alcohol Abuse and Alcoholism (1987). *Alcohol and Health: Sixth Special Report to Congress.* DHHS Publication (ADM) 87-1519.

National Institute on Drug Abuse (1988). *National Household Survey on Drug Abuse: Main Findings.* DHHS Publication (ADM) 88–1586.

Peele, S. (1990). "Second Thoughts about a Gene for Alcoholism." *The Atlantic Monthly,* August.

Scheel, K. R. (1994). *Alcohol Chemistry and Culture.* Waco, Texas: WRS Publishing.

United States Department of Health and Human Services (USDHHS) (1991). *Alcohol Practices, Policies, and Potentials of American Colleges and Universities.* DHHS Publications (ADM) 91-1842.

SUGGESTED READINGS

Adler, J. (1994). "The Endless Binge." *Newsweek,* December 19. Discusses the ongoing problem of excessive drinking on campus.

Beckman, L. J. (1994). "Treatment Needs of Women with Alcohol Problems." *Alcohol Health & Research World,* 18(3): 206–211. Provides specific risk factors and consequences of women's drinking and suggests "women-sensitive" treatment components.

Chiauzzi, E. J., and S. Liljegren (1993). "Taboo Topics in Addiction Treatment: An Empirical Review of Clinical Folklore." *Journal of Substance Abuse Treatment,* 10: 303–316. An excellent, nonstatistical review article that provides evidence that calls into serious question eleven basic assumptions and teachings of traditional addiction treatment (including the AA approach).

Goode, S. (1994). "Are America's College Students Majoring in Booze?" *Insight,* August 8. A look at the alcohol consumption of college students.

Holden, C. (1991). "Probing the Complex Genetics of Alco-

holism." *Science,* January 11. Examines the question of whether or not alcoholism is inherited.

Kaskutas, L. A. (1989). "Women for Sobriety: A Qualitative Analysis." *Contemporary Drug Problems,* 16: 177–200. Describes the workings of Women for Sobriety (WFS), focusing on what women get from WFS that they do not get from AA.

Peele, S. (1990). "Second Thoughts about a Gene for Alcoholism." *The Atlantic Monthly,* August. Discusses the controversy over whether alcoholism is caused by learned behavior or inherited genes.

Rorabaugh, W. J. (1991). "Alcohol in America." *Organization of American Historians Magazine of History,* Fall. In 1830, Americans drank three times the quantity of alcohol they do today. Article gives a history of alcohol use and abuse.

Wechsler, H., and N. Isaac (1992). "'Binge' Drinkers at Massachusetts Colleges." *Journal of the American Medical Association,* June 3. Shows that today's college students get drunk more often than in the past.

P A R T

six

Making Healthy Choices

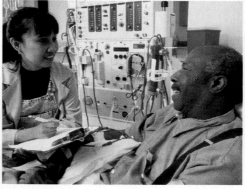

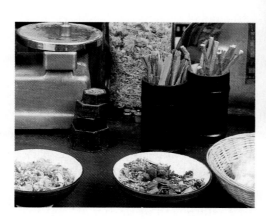

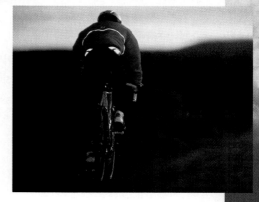

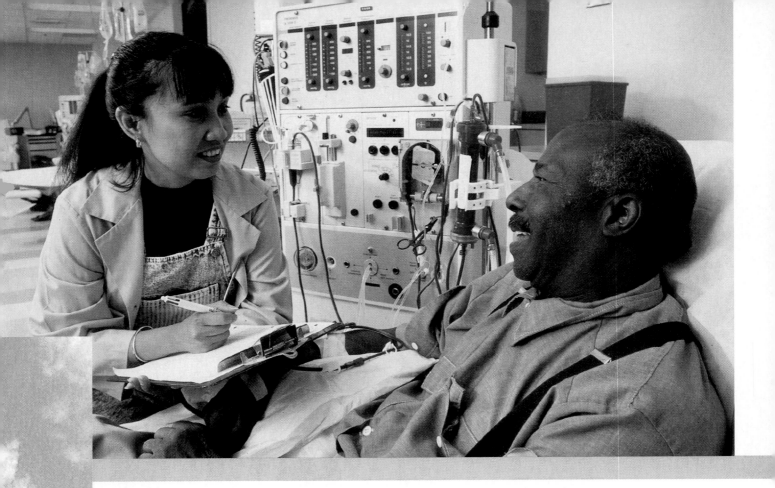

LEARNING OBJECTIVES

After reading this chapter you should be able to:

1. Describe what you need to know to be an intelligent health care consumer.
2. Distinguish between different types of health care professionals.
3. Compare and contrast private health insurance, preferred provider organizations, and health maintenance organizations.
4. Explain why health care costs have escalated.
5. Discuss health care reform and its impact on personal health care.
6. Discuss what you believe should be the essential elements of health care for all Americans.

Making Decisions about Health Care

*E*veryone will need health care at some time. People need to go to health care professionals for vaccinations, physical exams, diagnostic tests, and for assistance when they are not feeling well. Occasionally people need to be hospitalized for serious illness, injury, or surgery. Health care and the cost of medical services are among people's most important concerns. Both state and federal governments have been trying to ensure that all citizens have some form of health insurance and can receive health care when needed, but many people in this country still do not have access to health care services or cannot afford health care.

Modern medicine has become highly technical and expensive. The consumer of health care services needs to be able to evaluate the risks and benefits of diagnostic tests, treatments, recommended drugs, or surgery if he or she is to maintain control of decisions that affect health. Understanding your rights as a patient and knowing how to communicate your concerns and needs to health professionals will help you stay healthy and help in the healing process when you become sick.

BEING A WISE HEALTH CARE CONSUMER

Making wise decisions about your health is part of self-care and self-responsibility. As health care consumers, we make important decisions about the health products we purchase, the health services we select, and the information we receive.

Cornacchia and Barrett (1993) describe six behaviors that can help protect you from health frauds and unnecessary medical procedures. The wise health consumer:

1. Is well informed and knows how to make sound decisions.
2. Seeks reliable sources of information.
3. Is appropriately skeptical about health information and does not accept statements appearing in the news media or advertising at face value.
4. Is wary of unlicensed practitioners and undocumented claims by health practitioners.
5. Selects practitioners with great care and questions fees, diagnoses, treatments, and alternative treatments.
6. Reports health care fraud and wrongdoing to government regulating agencies.

Good health care should be a partnership between you and the health care provider. The quality and cost of health care can depend more on you than your doctor. Being a wise health care consumer starts with three basic principles: 1) working in partnership with your health care provider; 2) sharing in health care decision making; and 3) becoming skilled at obtaining health care (Healthwise Handbook, 1995).

Communication is extremely important in partnering with your health care provider. To work well with your health care provider you need to take care of yourself by exercising self-care and self-responsibility. One report states that one-fourth to one-half of all patients now seek active partnerships with their doctors (Consumer Reports, 1995). As a partner in your own health you are responsible for managing minor health care problems at home. At the first sign of a health problem, you should observe and record symptoms to share with your health care provider. By doing this you and your health care provider can better manage problems. When visiting your health care provider be prepared; you only have a limited time with them. Prepare a checklist of questions you want to ask, as well as a list of your signs and symptoms. During your visit state your concerns, signs, and symptoms, and ask questions regarding drugs prescribed, diagnosis, and treatment recommendations.

The second principle in being a wise health care consumer is shared decision making. In partnership with your health care provider you should actively participate in every medical decision. You have this right except in the emergency room, where informed consent is not necessary. There are eight ways to share in health care decisions with your health care provider (Healthwise Handbook, 1995): 1) letting your doctor know what you want; 2) doing your own research; 3) asking why; 4) asking about alternatives; 5) considering watchful waiting; 6) stating your health care preferences; 7) comparing expectations; and 8) accepting responsibility.

Being skilled at obtaining health care is the third principle. By communicating and partnering with your health care provider, you can become skilled in purchasing health care services. As a wise health consumer there are nine ways to cut the cost of health care without affecting the quality: 1) staying healthy; 2) exercising self-care and self-responsibility; 3) getting health care from a primary health care provider; 4) reducing your medical test costs; 5) reducing your drug costs; 6) using

Health Update

Sometimes Doing Nothing Is the Best Treatment

Back pain, especially acute pain in the lower back, is one of the most common disorders for which people seek medical help. Back pain can be caused by many different problems ranging from damaged discs in the spine to muscle strain. Diagnosing the cause of the pain is crucial for recommending the appropriate treatment. If the spine is not damaged and no disease can be detected, then the pain is probably due to muscle strain or tension.

The two recommended treatments for acute lower back pain due to strain are either bed rest for several days or back extension exercises. Among military recruits with acute lower back pain, bed rest proved the best treatment. However, among patients with lower back pain seen by family practice physicians, neither approach was beneficial. The most recent study compared bed rest, back exercises, and continuing with one's daily activities as normally as possible (Malmivaara et al., 1995). This study showed that people who did nothing and continued living as usual recovered faster than patients who rested or did exercises.

Wellness Guide

How to Have a Successful Interaction with Your Physician

- You should choose a physician you trust and in whose medical skills you have complete confidence. Take the time to find a primary care physician who can satisfy your medical needs. He or she should be someone with whom you can openly express your health concerns.

- Clear and open communication between you and your physician is essential. You should understand the nature of your medical problems and the reasons for any tests that are ordered. You should feel free to ask about different treatment options. You are entitled to all the information pertaining to your condition in language you can understand.

- You should feel confident enough to share with your physician any emotional problems you may have or any stress in your life. This information may be important in arriving at an accurate diagnosis and treatment recommendation. If you are upset in your interaction with a physician, the art of healing is not being practiced.

- Before going to a physician's office, try to relax your mind and body by practicing a meditation or image visualization exercise. This will help calm you when you are discussing your problems with the physician.

- Always remember how suggestible your mind is during a medical consultation. What the physician says about your condition can be as important in the healing process as the treatment. If the physician is positive and encouraging, the likelihood of a cure is increased.

- While negative statements made by the physician cannot be ignored, try not to let your mind be unduly influenced by them. Statements regarding complications, adverse effects, chance of permanent disability, probable duration of the sickness are general comments derived from statistical data collected from thousands of patients. You are not a statistic but an individual, and averages need not apply to you. Negative statements that are believed tend to produce negative effects on the body.

specialists for special problems; 7) using emergency services wisely; 8) using hospitals only when you need them; and 9) getting smart about your health care needs.

SELECTING A HEALTH CARE PRACTITIONER

The self-care movement became strong in the United States in the 1970s when health care costs began increasing and Americans became more interested in wellness and healthier life-styles. However, self-care is not always appropriate and can be dangerous in some situations. Today's health care system is extremely complex with numerous medical, dental, and allied health professionals addressing consumers' health care needs. Deciding which health care professional to choose can be confusing. Some health care professionals practice orthodox medicine, sometimes referred to as traditional, Western, or modern medicine. This traditional type of medicine is based on principles of modern science and validated clinical experiments. Practitioners of alternative medicine include chiropractors, homeopaths, and naturopaths,

> As to disease, make a habit of two things—to help, or at least to do no harm.
> Hippocrates

who rely on alternative methods of healing (Chapter 20). People often use alternative medicines to complement the treatments they receive from their physicians.

Medical Doctors

Physicians must have at least three years of undergraduate work and four years of training at an accredited medical school or osteopathic school. To be licensed to practice medicine one must pass a national or state examination. Because medical information is so broad, many medical school graduates choose to become specialists, requiring three or more years of specialty training (Table 19.1). Medical specialty boards have high standards of performance and training. Successful specialty training applicants are board certified. Many states and specialty boards require physicians to participate in continuing education programs to maintain their license and specialty license, respectively.

The doctor of medicine (M.D.) and the doctor of osteopathy (D.O.) provide both primary and specialty care. Many states have a single licensing board for doctors of medicine and doctors of osteopathy; others have separate boards for each profession. The training of these two physician groups are sim-

TABLE 19.1   Selected Medical Specialties

Specialty	Specializes in
Anesthesiology	Administration of drugs to prevent pain or to induce unconsciousness during surgical operations or diagnostic procedures
Dermatology	Diagnosis and treatment of skin diseases
Family practice	General medical services for patients and their families
Geriatrics	Concerned with problems of the elderly
Internal medicine	Diagnosis and nonsurgical treatment of internal organs of the body
Neurology	Diagnosis and nonsurgical treatment of diseases of the brain, spinal cord, and nerves
Obstetrics and gynecology	Care of pregnant women and treatment of disorders of the female reproductive system
Ophthalmology	Medical and surgical care of the eye, including prescription glasses
Pathology	Examination and diagnosis of organs, tissues, body fluids, and excrement
Preventive medicine	Prevention of disease through immunization, good health care, and concern with environmental factors
Psychiatry	Treatment of mental and emotional problems
Public health	Subspecialty of preventive medicine that deals with promoting the general health of the community
Radiology	Use of radiation for the diagnosis and treatment of disease
Urology	Treatment of male reproductive system and urinary tract, and treatment of female urinary tract

ilar, except doctors of osteopathy place greater emphasis on musculoskeletal diagnosis and treatment. The American Medical Association (AMA) estimates that there are over 670,000 physicians practicing in the United States, of whom about 34 percent belong to the AMA.

Dentists

Dentists are licensed in every state and hold either a doctor of dental surgery (D.D.S.) or a doctor of medical dentistry (D.M.D.) degree. Dental schools require at least two years of college; however, most entering dental students have a baccalaureate degree. Dental school takes four years with at least two or more years of training if entering a dental specialty (Table 19.2). The American Dental Association (ADA) estimates that over 196,000 dentists are practicing in the United States; approximately 71 percent belong to the ADA.

Podiatrists

Doctors of podiatric medicine (D.P.M.) are engaged in the diagnosis, prevention, and treatment of foot problems. Education includes at least three years of under-

graduate work and four years of study at one of seven accredited colleges of podiatric medicine in the United States. The American Podiatric Medical Association (APMA) estimates that there are approximately 13,800 practicing podiatrists in the United States, treating corns, bunions, calluses, and malformations.

SEEING THE DOCTOR

The majority of people who go to a doctor have minor complaints, have come for a routine follow-up of some chronic problem, or may simply need some kind of reassurance. In general, patients fall into three categories: 1) those who think they are sick and are; 2) those who think they are well but are actually sick; and 3) the "worried well" who come for reassurance that they are not sick. This last group may account for as many as half of all patients that are seen by family practice physicians.

Although some physicians encourage annual checkups, most studies show that frequent medical exams for people who are basically healthy are unnecessary. How often you see a physician depends on your personal needs, but many people go to a physician for minor

TABLE 19.2 Dental Specialties

Specialty	Specializes in
Endodontics	Prevention and treatment of diseases of the root pulp and related structures
Oral and maxillofacial surgery	Tooth extraction; surgical treatment of diseases, injuries, and defects of the mouth, jaw, and face
Oral pathology	Diagnosis of tumors, other diseases, and injuries of the head and neck
Orthodontics	Diagnosis and correction of tooth irregularities and facial deformities
Pediatric dentistry	Dental care of infants and children
Periodontics	Treatment of diseases of the gums and related structures
Prosthodontics	Treatment of oral dysfunction through the use of prosthetic devices such as crowns, bridges, and dentures
Public health dentistry	Prevention and control of dental disease and promotion of community dental health

complaints and illnesses that usually do not require medical attention (Table 19.3). Often people are asking more from their doctors than just medicine.

Patient satisfaction with health care usually depends on what occurs in the physician's office. The quality of health care depends to a great degree on the interaction between the physician and the patient. Often anxiety about what may be wrong, long waits to see the physician, and a seemingly endless number of tests can contribute to patients' stress. You can increase the chance of a successful encounter with your health care provider or hospital if you have a clear understanding of what you want to accomplish in the office visit or hospital.

The medical profession recognizes that medical education needs to be about more than biomedical facts. Learning to listen, asking questions, and expressing empathy also need to be part of medical education. A few medical schools have tried to help medical students understand what the patient is going through. Communication skills, like other skills, can be learned. As wise health care consumers you need to select physicians who

HEALTHY PEOPLE 2000

Increase the proportion of all degrees in the health professions and allied and associated health professions fields awarded to members of underrepresented racial and ethnic minority groups.

Minority and disadvantaged communities lag behind the U.S. population on virtually all health status indicators (e.g., infant mortality, overall mortality, morbidity). Furthermore, among the poor, minorities, and the uninsured, access to medical care has been deteriorating. Increasing the number of minority health professionals may offer a partial solution to this public health crisis.

TABLE 19.3 The 20 Most Common Complaints, Problems, or Symptoms for Doctor Visits Note that 1 in 8 persons go to the doctor without any complaint or symptom.

	Complaint
1	Progress visits
2	Physical exam
3	Pain, etc.—lower extremity
4	Pregnancy exam
5	Throat soreness
6	Pain, etc.—upper extremity
7	Pain, etc.—back region
8	Cough
9	Abdominal pain
10	Cold
11	Gynecological exam
12	Visit for medication
13	None
14	Headache
15	Fatigue
16	Pain in chest
17	Well-baby exam
18	Fever
19	Allergic skin reaction
20	All other symptoms

meet not only your health care needs, but your communication needs as well.

Diagnosis is separate and distinct from any agreement you make about treatment. In any illness there are two important choices: first, admitting that you are sick and finding out what is wrong, which is the process of the **diagnosis;** and second, deciding what is the best course of treatment based on the diagnosis.

For example, suppose you have had a slight pain in your chest and the diagnostic tests indicate that you have partial blockage of a coronary artery. One physician might recommend dietary changes, exercises, and a drug to control the pain. Another physician might insist on immediate surgery to correct the condition. Only by obtaining as much information as possible can you make a decision that feels right to you.

HOSPITALS

At some time in your life you will need to use a health care facility, whether a hospital for planned surgery, an emergency room, or as you, your parents, or friends become older, nursing home facilities. To make wise decisions concerning health care facilities, it is important to understand the types of facilities available and whether they meet your needs.

Most Americans will be admitted to a hospital at some time during their lives. For many people the hospital experience is confusing and frightening. To cope with this unpleasant reality, one should understand a hospital patient's rights.

On admission to a hospital, a patient is required to sign a consent form delegating all decisions regarding his or her care to the hospital and physicians. In most instances, physicians obtain informed consent for any invasive procedure, either diagnostic or therapeutic, before proceeding. But the amount of information that is given to the patient and how well a patient understands the proposed treatment usually depend on many factors affecting communication between the patient and the physician. The American Hospital Association publishes a Patient's Bill of Rights covering the situations and questions most often encountered by hospital patients. You are entitled to ask for a list of patients' rights in that hospital.

The most frustrating and anxiety-producing situations for a patient are not understanding what is going to happen and, even worse, not knowing what is happening while being subjected to unfamiliar and uncomfortable procedures. Except in the case of a life-threatening emergency that demands immediate action, you have the right to be fully informed of all medical procedures and the reasons for them. As a patient, you have the responsibility for deciding what you want done. Once you have made that decision, you should understand how to cooperate fully to gain the most benefit.

UNDERSTANDING HEALTH CARE FINANCING

In various ways the United States has attempted to make health care available to Americans. Some employers have provided health care for their employees and dependents; the federal government has provided health care for members of the armed services, and their dependents, war veterans, and government employees; and with assistance from local and state governments the federal government has provided health care for poor families. Nevertheless, a program to ensure universal access and equity in health care services has never materialized.

Health Update

Silicone Breast Implants Are Judged Unsafe

Prior to 1992 approximately 150,000 women annually received silicone breast implants, which have been available in the U.S. for more than 30 years. At least 80 percent of these breast implants were for breast enlargement to improve appearance; the other 20 percent were to repair the effects of mastectomy. A significant number of the implants rupture, allowing silicone to leak into the body. Due to persistent complaints of medical problems stemming from the implants and the failure of the manufacturers to demonstrate safety and effectiveness, the Food and Drug Administration (FDA) ordered the breast implants removed from the market in 1992.

The decision to ban silicone breast implants was, and still is, controversial. As a result of the FDA's decision, many women with breast implants became angry that they had not been told of potential risks and became anxious about their health. Many women sought to have their implants removed. Despite the concerns of many women, others felt that they should still have the right to obtain breast implants if they desired to have them. In 1994, legal proceedings for damages against the manufacturers of silicone breast implants was settled for $90 *billion*.

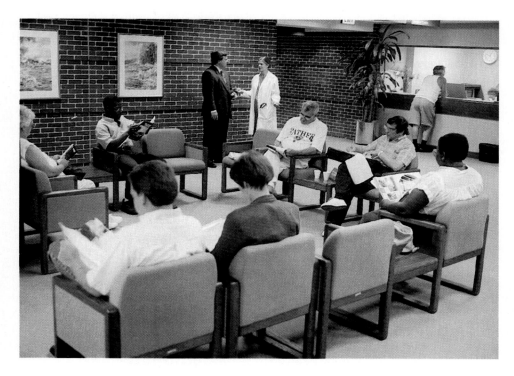

For many people, the hospital is an impersonal and confusing place. Developing good communication with health care providers and knowing your rights as a consumer can help combat those feelings.

There are three basic types of health insurance plans available: private insurance, health maintenance organizations (HMOs), and preferred provider organizations (PPOs).

Private Insurance

Fee-for-service or private health insurance is the traditional type of health care plan in the United States. Fee-for-service plans generally have a deductible the insured person pays before receiving benefits. Most plans pay some physician and hospital expenses; most do not cover preventive health care such as annual physicals or immunizations. In 1991 there were 670 million visits made to physicians' offices; 36 percent were paid for by private insurance (Green and Ottoson, 1994).

Health Maintenance Organizations (HMOs)

Health maintenance organizations (HMOs) are prepaid health insurance plans that are an alternative to private insurance. HMOs have almost tripled during the last two decades. HMOs are characterized by four principles defined and described by Congress in the Health Maintenance Organization Assistance Act of 1973: 1) an organized system of health care that accepts the responsibility to provide health care; 2) an agreed-upon set of comprehensive health maintenance and treatment services; 3) a voluntarily enrolled group of people in a specific geographic region; and 4) reimbursement through a prenegotiated and fixed payment schedule on behalf of

the enrollee. An example of a large, successful HMO is Kaiser-Permanente Medical Care Program, in which physicians emphasize early detection and disease prevention.

Preferred Provider Organizations (PPOs)

Preferred provider organizations (PPOs) are a combination of the traditional fee-for-service health care plan and an HMO. Employers or insurance companies negotiate low fee-for-service rates with selected hospitals and health care providers in a specific geographic region. Participants in PPOs must use one of the "preferred" providers for the majority of their medical bills to be paid. If a participant opts for care from a nonprovider, he or she will be charged a substantial fee. Group health insurance costs are reduced for both an HMO and PPO in exchange for a guaranteed pool of patients.

> ### T E R M S
> *diagnosis:* the cause of a disease or illness as determined by a physician
>
> *health maintenance organization (HMO):* an organization (either nonprofit or for-profit) of physicians, hospitals, and support staff that provides medical services to members
>
> *preferred provider organization (PPO):* physicians who belong to the organization provide medical care at reduced costs that are negotiated by the organization

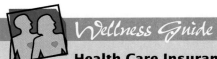
Wellness Guide

Health Care Insurance Terminology

Terminology to be familiar with when purchasing health insurance.

Coinsurance	Arrangements by which the insurer and the insured share, in a specific ratio, payment for losses covered by the policy after the deductible is met.
Comprehensive medical expense insurance	Form of health insurance that in one policy provides protection for both basic hospital expenses and major medical expense coverage.
Coordination of benefits (COB)	Method of integrating benefits payable under more than one health insurance plan so that the insured's benefits from all sources do not exceed 100 percent of allowable medical expenses or eliminate appropriate patient incentives to contain costs.
Deductible	Amount of covered expenses that must be incurred by the insured before benefits become payable by the insurer.
Health insurance	Coverage providing for payment of benefits as a result of sickness or injury. Includes insurance for losses from accident, disability, medical expense, or accidental death and dismemberment.
Managed care	Those systems that integrate the financing and delivery of appropriate health care services to covered individuals by means of:

- arrangements with selected providers to furnish a comprehensive set of health care services to members;
- explicit criteria for the selection of health care providers;
- formal programs for ongoing quality assurance and utilization review; and
- significant financial incentives for members to use providers and procedures associated with the plan

Maximum benefit	Highest amount an individual may receive under an insurance contract.
Reasonable and customary charges (R&C)	Amounts charged by health care providers that are consistent with charges from similar providers for identical or similar services in a given locale.
Utilization	Patterns of usage for a single medical service or type of service (hospital care, prescription drugs, physician visits). Measurement of utilization of all medical services in combination usually is done in terms of dollar expenditures. Use is expressed in rates per unit of population at risk for a given period, such as the number of annual admissions to a hospital per 1000 persons over age 65.
Utilization review	Program designed to reduce unnecessary hospital admissions and to control the length of stay for inpatients through the use of preliminary evaluations, concurrent inpatient evaluations, or discharge planning.

Federal Government Support: Medicare and Medicaid

It was not until the mid-1960s that the federal government played a substantial role in providing health care coverage. Resulting from a concern for the social conditions of the economically disadvantaged and the elderly, Congress passed legislation in 1965 establishing Medicare and Medicaid.

Medicare is a federal health insurance program for Americans over 65, for certain disabled Americans under the age of 65, and people of any age with permanent kidney failure. The basic purpose of Medicare is to make available health care for those who are eligible. In 1991 approximately 35 million people were covered by Medicare.

Medicaid provides health insurance for certain poor people in the United States. To be eligible for Medicaid benefits, an individual must be on welfare, have dependent children, or receive supplementary security income for the aged, blind, or disabled. In addition, Medicaid covers nursing home care for many elderly Americans. Approximately 31 million Americans received Medicaid benefits in 1992.

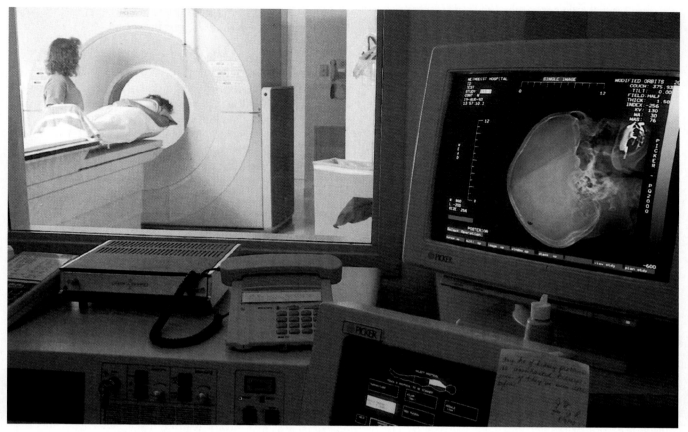

CAT scans help physicians make the correct diagnosis of an injury or disease.

HEALTH CARE ISSUES TODAY

Rising Health Care Costs

Anyone who has been to a physician, filled a prescription, paid a health insurance premium, or been admitted to a hospital realizes how expensive medical care in the United States has become. From the early 1980s to 1994, the costs of medical care more than doubled, exceeding $1 trillion in 1994 (Figure 19.1). These increases have occurred in all areas—physician fees, prescription costs, hospital rooms, emergency services, and health insurance. No single factor explains why our health care costs are increasing.

In 1995 approximately 14 percent of the U.S. gross domestic product was spent on medical care, more than in any other country. One reason may be our fascination with medicine, health, and wellness. Every day both print and visual media inform us of new medical technologies, medical science breakthroughs, and promising hopes of the cures for AIDS and cancer.

Two issues often surface in analyzing why health care costs are increasing so dramatically: malpractice and

health insurance (Robert Wood Johnson Foundation, 1995). Malpractice insurance does cost more for physicians in the United States compared to those in other countries, and it is not uncommon for an individual

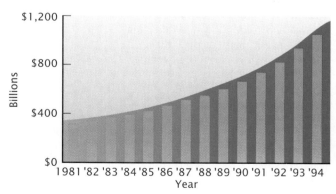

FIGURE 19.1 Skyrocketing Costs of Health Care in the United States Between 1981 and 1994 spending on health care has more than doubled and is now over $1 trillion a year.
Source: U.S. Department of Health and Human Services.

izens of other countries. Americans pay over 20 percent of their health care costs, not including health insurance premiums.

Another factor affecting health care costs is that more Americans are living longer. As the population ages so does its risk increase for chronic and acute illnesses. The elderly population also predominates in hospitals, intensive care units, and nursing homes.

Life-style behaviors are another factor contributing to high health care costs. Many health conditions that strain our health care system are preventable. Cancer due to smoking, heart disease due to smoking, automobile accidents due to drinking and driving—all are behaviors that we choose and are responsible for. They cost us millions of dollars each year. Other factors include greed, inefficiency, and fraud. Fraud occurs when an individual files false medical disability claims or dishonest health care providers submit false insurance forms for reimbursement.

Some believe the greatest factor in health care costs is the United States' overdeveloped medical capacity. The medical community has invested heavily in people, facilities, and equipment. For example, Orange County, California, has more magnetic resonance imaging machines for its 2.4 million population than Canada has for 27 million people (Robert Wood Johnson Foundation, 1995). Medical technology in the United States often translates into short waiting times for care, whether

physician in a high-risk specialty (obstetrics, neurology, or anesthesiology) to pay premiums of over $100,000 per year. However, it is estimated that malpractice, including insurance premiums, costs only 3.5 percent of the projected $1 trillion spent on health care in 1994. Health insurance costs have increased and Americans are paying more out-of-pocket for their health care than cit-

Health Update

Diagnostic Imaging Techniques

The development of X-ray imaging techniques in the early part of the century helped medical diagnosis in countless ways by allowing physicians to visualize the internal skeleton and organs. X-rays assist in setting broken bones, in locating swallowed objects, and in detecting tumors. For many medical diagnoses, an X-ray is still the imaging technique of choice. However, new, sophisticated imaging techniques are now used in addition to X-rays.

An imaging technique called **computerized tomography scan** (CAT scan) also uses X-rays but uses a computer to calculate a detailed, three-dimensional image of the diseased or damaged body part. Because a CAT scan provides the physician with a detailed image of

an organ from several different perspectives, it makes the diagnosis more accurate and surgical procedures safer.

CAT scans of the head are the most common imaging procedure. These are performed for any head injury, for migraine headaches, for possible stroke diagnosis, and for suspected tumors or brain damage of any kind. Some brain abnormalities that may go undetected by a CAT scan may show up in an image obtained from an MRI scan, so sometimes both imaging techniques are used.

Magnetic resonance imaging scans (MRI scans) are valuable in viewing soft tissues, especially in the brain, spine, and joints, for damage that is not visible with X-rays or CAT scans. MRI requires that a person

remain immobilized in a small chamber for a considerable length of time. This experience often produces anxiety and claustrophobia that can be relieved by communicating with the technician via an intercom. MRI is particularly useful in detecting injuries to soft tissues, which is why it is widely used to diagnose sports injuries.

Ultrasound scans are most frequently used in pregnancy, primarily in the second or third trimester, to detect abnormalities in the developing fetus (Chapter 15). However, ultrasound scans also are used to detect tumors and skeletal abnormalities. Because ultrasound scans use sound energy rather than electromagnetic energy, they are considered to be safer than other imaging techniques.

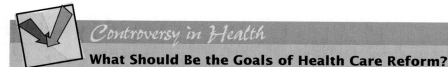

Controversy in Health

What Should Be the Goals of Health Care Reform?

The American Medical Association (AMA) has proposed ten criteria that it believes must be met in any health care reform legislation. Because the AMA and other health-related industries felt that these goals were not met in the health care reform bills introduced in Congress, they lobbied against their passage. The ten criteria proposed by the AMA state that a reformed health care system should:

- Provide accesses for everyone to basic medical care
- Produce real control of costs
- Ensure quality of medical care
- Reduce administrative costs and hassles

- Promote disease prevention
- Encourage primary care
- Provide for long-term care
- Maintain patient autonomy
- Maintain physician autonomy
- Limit physicians' liability
- Work now and into the foreseeable future

STUDENT REFLECTION

- Do you agree with these goals or would you formulate a different set for health care reform?

Source: Adapted from *The Journal of the American Medical Association*, May 18, 1994.

---

urgent or elective, compared to other countries where one is placed on a waiting list for coronary artery surgery or for a CAT scan.

Overtrained, overspecialized physicians may also be another source of increasing health care costs. It is estimated that by the year 2000 the United States will have an excess of 139,000 specialty physicians, almost one-third of the total supply of physicians (Robert Wood Johnson Foundation, 1995). This oversupply adds to the cost of health care.

The administrative overhead for health care is enormous. Overhead costs include insurance paperwork as well as internal and external paperwork for hospitals. Processing all this paperwork requires large numbers of workers. "Many experts estimate that these administrative costs account for at least 10 percent of the nation's total health bill. Based on the 1994 estimated expenditure of $1 trillion, administrative costs could amount to some $100 billion—enough to provide health insurance coverage for every one of the 40 million Americans who are currently uninsured" (Robert Wood Johnson Foundation, 1995, p. 13).

The health care system in the United States has reached a state of crisis in terms of costs and services. In a survey on consumer satisfaction with health care, almost 90 percent of Americans believed our health care system needed a major change, higher than any other country's perception of its health care needs (Blendon et al., 1990). Everyone agrees that change must come, but so far it has been impossible to reach consensus on how to change the health care system and its financing.

Inequities in Health Care

Socioeconomic status plays a crucial role in health (Angell, 1993). Level of education, amount of income, and type of job all contribute to a person's health. One study showed that people earning less than $9,000 a year died at a rate three to seven times greater than those earning more than $25,000 a year. Black and Hispanic Americans generally have lower incomes than white Americans, experience more health problems, and are less likely to receive medical care. Poor people smoke more cigarettes, drink more alcohol, use more illegal drugs, and are exposed to violence more than people with good incomes and good education; these factors contribute to their increased health risks.

In the past twenty years, the health of economically and educationally disadvantaged Americans has declined steadily. A major challenge facing American society is reversing this trend and raising the level of health of its poorest citizens. More health education is necessary, along with universal health insurance that will guarantee basic medical services for all.

T E R M S

computerized tomography scan: use of multiple X-ray images to construct a three-dimensional image of a diseased organ or body part

magnetic resonance imaging scan: use of a strong magnetic field to produce images of internal parts of the body; especially useful for soft tissues

Health Care Reform

The United States spends more on health care than any other industrialized country (Fein, 1992). For example, Japan spends about half as much per capita on health care and Great Britain spends about one-third as much per capita as the United States. Yet some analysts regard health care in these countries as satisfactory and, in some cases, superior to health care in the United States. Despite enormous outlays of money, in 1994 approximately 40 million Americans, including 10 million children, lacked health insurance and access to essential health care.

Currently, Washington is taking on health care reform and moving cautiously toward solutions to the escalating costs of health care and the inequities in access to quality health care for all. Health care reform will be difficult. It will require all Americans to make many decisions. How much are they are willing to pay for assured, quality health care? Do Americans want assured quality health care for all? Is health care a right or privilege? The outcome of the health care reform initiatives are unknown at this time.

HEALTH IN REVIEW

- Everyone needs medical care at some time in his or her life. Knowing what to ask and what to expect from your physician is essential.
- The physician's responsibility is to diagnose the cause of illness. The patient's responsibility is working in partnership with your health care provider, sharing in health care decision making, and becoming skilled at obtaining health care.
- Admission to a hospital is often an unsettling experience. Patients should be aware of their rights and ask questions that will ease their concerns.

- Health care is increasingly provided by large organizations of physicians and hospitals called preferred provider organizations or health maintenance organizations.
- The costs of medical care in the United States have grown so rapidly that some form of health care reform is needed. Millions of citizens lack health insurance and access to health care.

REFERENCES

Angell, M. (1993). "Privileged and Health—What Is the Connection?" *New England Journal of Medicine*, July 8.

Blendon, R. J., et al. (1994). "The Beliefs and Values Shaping Today's Health Reform Debate." *Health Affairs*, 13(1): 274–284.

Cornacchia, H. J., and S. Barrett (1993). *Consumer Health: A Guide to Intelligent Decisions*, 5th ed. St. Louis: Mosby-Year Book.

Fein, R. (1992). "Health Care Reform." *Scientific American*, November.

Green, L. W., and J. M. Ottoson (1994). *Community Health*, 7th ed. St. Louis: Mosby-Year Book.

Healthwise Handbook (1995). Boise, Id.: Health Alliance.

"How Is Your Doctor Treating You?" (1995). *Consumer Reports*, February: 81–88.

Malmivaara, A., et al. (1995). "The Treatment of Acute Lower Back Pain—Bed Rest, Exercises, or Ordinary Activity?" *New England Journal of Medicine*: 1245.

The Robert Wood Johnson Foundation Annual Report, 1994: Cost Containment (1995). Princeton, N.J.: Robert Wood Johnson Foundation.

SUGGESTED READINGS

Cundiff, D., and M. E. McCarthy (1994). *The Right Medicine*. Totowa, N.J.: Humana Press. Discusses the major health care problems in America and how to cure them.

Fein, R. (1992). "Health Care Reform." *Scientific American*, November. An analysis of why universal health insurance is needed.

Lewis, J. (1990). *So Your Doctor Recommended Surgery*. New York: December Books. A good book to read before deciding to undergo surgery.

Pinckney, E. R., and C. Pinckney (1989). "Unnecessary Measures." *The Sciences*, January/February. A discussion of the overuse and reliability of medical diagnostic tests.

Roberts, M. J. (1993). *Your Money or Your Life: The Health Care Crisis Explained*. New York: Doubleday. Explains clearly what is wrong with health care in this country.

Rosenfeld, I. (1991). *The Best Treatment*. New York: Simon and Schuster. A physician explains almost all disorders so that the average person can understand what is wrong and what treatment options are available.

Russell, L. B. (1994). *Educated Guesses.: Making Policy about Medical Screening Tests*. Berkeley: University of California Press. Documents clearly why many medical screening tests, particularly for cholesterol and some cancers, are unnecessary and a waste of money.

Snow, L. F. (1993). *Walkin' Over Medicine*. Boulder, Col.: Westview Press. A detailed examination of African-American cultural beliefs and how they influence disease prevention and treatment among African-Americans using Western medicine.

West, S., and P. Dranov (1995). *The Hysterectomy Hoax*. New York: Doubleday. Explains why up to 90 percent of hysterectomies are medically unnecessary and provides other options.

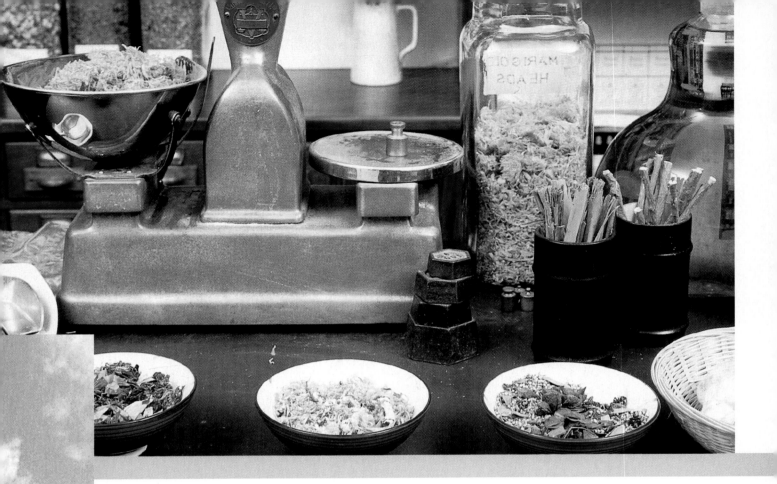

LEARNING OBJECTIVES

After reading this chapter you should be able to:

1. Describe the main differences between modern medical care and alternative medicines.

2. Define the four categories of alternative medicines.

3. Discuss the philosophy and method of treatment in acupuncture, chiropractic, osteopathy, herbal medicine, and homeopathy.

4. Discuss the reasons some people choose an alternative medicine in addition to, or instead of, modern medicine.

5. List some diseases that can be treated successfully by alternative medicines.

6. Describe an alternative medicine that you regard as fraudulent and explain your reasons.

7. Explain how you can protect yourself from being victimized by quackery.

Exploring Alternative Medicines

Although most people elect to visit a physician when they are sick, many seek alternatives to modern medicine for a variety of reasons. One reason may be cultural: persons raised in cultures that rely on herbal remedies and tribal healers to treat sickness often continue to use their own remedies even if they live in a foreign country.

Another large group that seeks healing alternatives are those persons for whom modern medicine has little to offer to relieve their suffering or to cure their disease. People suffering from terminal cancer for which no further treatments are available will often seek any help that offers hope. People with chronic diseases, such as arthritis or allergies that do not respond satisfactorily to medical care or drugs, often find relief in alternative therapies.

The medical profession is just beginning to acknowledge the importance of alternative therapies, often referred to as **alternative medicine,** in the lives of many of their patients. Some people prefer the term *complementary medicine* to emphasize that both approaches facilitate healing. A recent survey found that at least one-third of patients with serious medical problems were using some form of alternative medicine (Eisenberg et al., 1993). The conditions most often treated by alternative medicine are cancer, arthritis, chronic back pain, AIDS, gastrointestinal problems, and eating disorders.

Some investigators of alternative medicine as practiced today find that it actually has been part of American culture for many years.

> Alternative medicine has long played an important role in the care of people with health problems in this country. Although there has been no comprehensive assessment of its use, there are good reasons to believe that alternative medicine has many adherents among all social classes. Most physicians are unaware of its popularity, much less that many of their own patients are also being cared for by practitioners of alternative medicine.
>
> —Murray and Rubel, 1992

Confirming the popularity of alternative medicine, *USA Weekend,* a Sunday newspaper supplement read by almost 40 million people, devoted an entire issue to alternative medicine on January 1, 1995.

In recognition of the growing use of alternative medicine, Congress established the Office of Alternative

> *The art of medicine consists of amusing the patient while nature cures the disease.*
> Voltaire

Medicine (OAM) in 1992. The task of OAM is to explore the validity of the many alternative health practices that many Americans already utilize extensively. The OAM funds studies of massage, hypnosis, biofeedback, acupuncture, yoga, macrobiotic diets, and other alternative treatments for various illnesses.

DEFINING ALTERNATIVE MEDICINE

Alternative medicine can be divided into four broad categories based on the method of healing or intervention: 1) spiritual, psychic, or mental approaches, including prayer, meditation, hypnotherapy, and faith healing; 2) nutritional therapies including change in diet, fasting, and the use of supplements; 3) therapies using herbs or other substances derived from natural sources such as

Exploring Your Health

Intelligent Health Consumer Profile

This exercise can help determine the extent to which consumers act intelligently when exposed to misleading and inaccurate information, to health fraud, and to health quackery. Place an X in the column to the right that best represents your answer:

Are you sufficiently informed to be able to make sound decisions?
Where do you go for information when needed?
  Professional health organizations/individuals
  Health books, magazines, newsletters
  Government health agencies
  Advertisements
  Newspapers/magazines
  Radio/television
  People you know
To what extent do you accept statements appearing in news reports or advertisements at face value?
To what extent can you identify quacks, quackery, fraudulent schemes, and hucksters?
When selecting health practitioners to what extent do you:
  Talk with or visit before first appointment
  Check/inquire regarding qualifications/credentials
  Ask friend/neighbor about reputation
  Inquire about fees and payment procedures
When you have been exposed to a fraudulent practice, quack, quackery, or a poor product or service, to what extent do you report your experience?

VM	M	S	L	N

Key: VM = very much; M = much; S = some; L = little; N = none.
Source: H. J. Cornacchia and S. Barrett, *Consumer Health: A Guide to Intelligent Decisions,* 5th ed. (St. Louis, Mo.: Mosby, 1993), p. 11.

TABLE 20.1 A Partial List of Alternative Medicine Healing Methods

Physical and nutritional	Mental and spiritual
Rolfing	Hypnosis
Massage	Autosuggestion
Feldenkrais technique	Progressive relaxation
Alexander technique	Meditation
Reflexology	Biofeedback
Kinesiology (Touch for Health)	Cocounseling
Acupressure	Psychodrama
Shiatsu	Rebirthing
Yoga	Primal scream therapy
T'ai chi ch'uan	Psychic healing
	Psychic surgery
	Past lives therapy
	Christian Science
	Encounter groups

homeopathy, herbal medicine, or immune system boosters; and 4) physical therapies such as chiropractic, acupuncture, massage, and yoga. Table 20.1 presents a partial list of the hundreds of different kinds of alternative medicine.

Some alternative medicines, such as acupuncture and herbal remedies, have been used for thousands of years and would not have survived if people had not benefited. Other alternative medicines, such as homeopathy and chiropractic, are of recent origin and emerged partly as a response to the extraordinary harsh practices of conventional medicine in the eighteenth and nineteenth centuries. (Some would argue that certain modern medical practices, such as bone marrow transplants, spinal surgeries, and chemotherapy, are still extremely harsh and only marginally successful.)

Before this century, irritants of all kinds were used to purge the body of unknown causes of illness. Bleedings, cuppings, leechings, enemas, and emetics (vomiting inducers) were all commonly used by doctors to treat diseases of which they had no understanding. These treatments generally weakened the patient and usually interfered with the processes of healing. Today, patients with chronic, painful problems still seek treatments that offer the promise of help, and which do little harm. The

T E R M S

alternative medicine: any form of therapy or healing performed by someone other than a physician

homeopathy: an alternative medicine that administers very dilute solutions of substances that mimic the patient's symptoms

problem for the consumer is knowing what alternative medicines might be of help and which also are safe. To help you understand how to choose an alternative medicine should you so desire, some of the more widely used alternative medicines are described below.

Homeopathy

Homeopathy emerged in the early 1800s in reaction to the ineffective and abusive treatments of conventional medicine—cuppings, leechings, bleedings, forced vomitings, and so on. The principles of homeopathy were developed by Samuel Hahnemann, a doctor and pharmacologist who was born in Saxony in 1775. Hahnemann believed that tiny doses of a substance (a drug) that evoked disease-like symptoms could somehow stimulate the body's natural defenses and promote healing. According to Hahnemann, homeopathy is based on four principles:

- Substances that produce the same symptoms in an individual as the disease does will cure him (Law of Similiars).
- Substances are tested by giving them to healthy subjects and observing the symptoms (Law of Proving).
- Smaller doses are more potent than undiluted solutions (Law of Potentization).
- Vital forces must be released in the individual that will result in reestablishing body harmony or homeostasis.

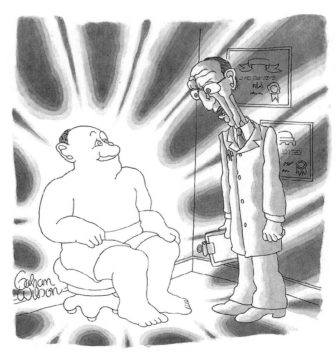

"You've been fooling around with alternative medicines, haven't you?"
Drawing by Gahan Wilson; © 1994 The New Yorker Magazine, Inc.

Introducing Nine Popular Alternatives

Chiropractic Treatment usually involves direct spinal manipulation. Chiropractors contend that the spine is literally the backbone of health, and misalignment sabotages it. Practitioners diagnose with palpation and X-rays.
Information: American Chiropractic Assoc., 1701 Clarendon Boulevard, Arlington, Va., 22209, 1-800-637-6244.

Homeopathy Treatments aim to stimulate the body's defenses with tiny doses of substances that, in larger amounts, would cause the disease's symptoms.
Information: National Center for Homeopathy, 801 North Fairfax Street, Suite 306, Alexandria, Va., 22314, 1-703-548-7790.

Wellness A combination of very low-fat diet, moderate exercise, and relaxation is thought to reduce stress and reverse heart disease.
Information: Lifechoice catalog, 1-800-328-3738.

Aromatherapy "Essential oils" distilled from plants and herbs are massaged into the skin, inhaled, or placed in baths in an attempt to treat stress, anxiety, and other conditions.
Information: Ann Berwick, Aromatherapy, P.O. Box 4996, Boulder, Col., 80306.

Massage Therapy The muscles and soft tissues are kneaded and manipulated with the aim of alleviating pain and improving well-being.
Information: American Massage Therapy Association, 820 Davis Street, Suite 100, Evanston, Ill., 60201, 1-708-864-0123.

Ayurveda Disease, says this ancient practice from India, is caused by an imbalance of movement, structure, and metabolism. Herbs, diet, meditation, and yoga are treatments.
Information: Center for Mind and Body Medicine, 1110 Camino del Mar, Suite G, Del Mar, Calif., 92014, 1-619-794-2425.

Herbal Medicine Plants or plant-based substances are used to treat a wide range of illnesses and enhance physical functions.
Information: American Botanical Council, P.O. Box 201660, Austin, Tex., 78720; fax 512-331-1924.

Mind and Body Connection Negative effects of stress are treated with exercise, meditation, concentration.
Information: Center for Mind-Body Medicine, 5225 Connecticut Avenue, N.W., Suite 414, Washington, D.C., 20015, 1-202-966-7338.

Chinese Medicine Ancient healing says an imbalance of vital force, *qi,* causes disease. Diet, herbs, and acupuncture are preventive treatments.
Information: American Foundation of Traditional Chinese Medicine, 505 Beach Street, San Francisco, Calif., 94133, 1-415-776-0502.

Source: Adapted from *USA Weekend,* January 1, 1995.

Homeopathic practitioners are trained to attend to the patient's physical, mental, and emotional state—in other words, to treat holistically. In addition to dispensing a substance that the homeopath determines is specific for the disease, the practitioner will also recommend exercise, nutritional changes, relaxation techniques, and so on.

The most controversial scientific aspect of homeopathy is its reliance on doses of drugs that frequently are so dilute that the solutions contain little or none of the active substance that is supposed to mimic the symptoms and produce a cure. Certainly administering such dilute solutions may do the patient no harm; on the other hand, how can they do any good? One explanation

for homeopathic cures is that they result from placebo effects. However, homeopaths staunchly maintain that their dilute drug solutions do produce a real effect and are responsible for curing many different diseases.

Since it was founded in 1846, the American Medical Association (AMA) has vigorously opposed homeopathy. According to the AMA's code of ethics, physicians are prohibited from consulting with "practitioners whose practice is based upon a specific dogma." This particular edict was specifically designed to isolate homeopaths. By 1855 the AMA directed state affiliates to expel all homeopaths from their membership. (In 1878 a physician was expelled from the AMA for consulting with a homeopath—his wife.) Despite persistent AMA attacks between 1850 and 1900, homeopathic practitioners increased in number. In 1900 there were about 15,000 homeopaths in the United States and twenty-two homeopathic colleges (Hahnemann founded the first homeopathic college in Philadelphia in 1836).

Today, homeopathy is experiencing a resurgence of interest both in the United States and the rest of the

T E R M

chiropractic: an alternative medicine that uses manipulation of the spine and joints for healing

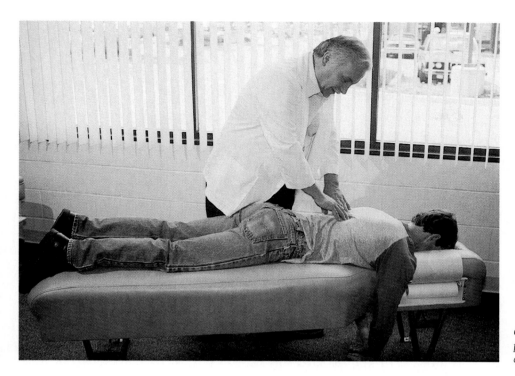

Chiropractic manipulations help many people who suffer from back pain and other musculoskeletal disorders.

Western world. While this rebound seems to fly in the face of scientific evidence, which consistently fails to demonstrate the effectiveness of homeopathic remedies, many people find that homeopathic practitioners help them with their health problems.

> *He is the best physician who is the most ingenious inspirer of hope.*
> Samuel Taylor Coleridge

Chiropractic

Chiropractic was founded by Daniel David Palmer (1845–1913), who had no scientific training but who believed throughout his life that he had a "calling" to heal people. At age 50, Palmer cured a man of deafness by manipulating his spine. After several other cures by spinal manipulation, Palmer concluded that virtually all diseases are caused by subluxed (misaligned) vertebrae. Palmer coined the name "chiropractic" (literally, "done by hand") to describe his new healing technique, and he opened the Palmer School for Chiropractic in Davenport, Iowa, in 1895. In 1906, father and son (Bartlett Joshua, better known as B. J.) were arrested for practicing medicine without a license. The father was tried and jailed; the son's case never came to trial.

B. J. Palmer took over chiropractic and turned it into a multimillion-dollar business. B. J. was a genius at commercializing chiropractic; he invented the concept of mail-order diplomas and he advertised widely and effec-

Health Update

Homeopathy Helps Asthmatics

A recurrent criticism of homeopathy charges that the drug doses recommended are so dilute that they contain little or no active chemical that could benefit the patient. As a result, any benefit that experienced from a homeopathic treatment is usually ascribed by critics to a placebo effect. To test this notion, a group of physicians in Scotland treated 28 patients who suffered from allergic asthma with either a homeopathic remedy or with a placebo in a double blind experiment (Reilly et al., 1994). This is the kind of rigorous study generally performed to test the efficacy of a drug.

Analysis of the results based on several criteria showed that patients given the homeopathic remedy improved substantially more than patients who received the placebo. This study demonstrates that homeopathic remedies *do* have an effect that is not the result of a placebo effect. The challenge to science now is to discover how homeopathic remedies work.

Consulting a Chiropractor

Chiropractic treatments use "adjustments," specific manipulations of the spine or joints with pressure applied directly to a vertebra or joint. A visit to chiropractor usually involves the following:

- The chiropractor takes a case history, performs a physical and other exams, and takes X-rays to identify the problems that are causing the symptoms.
- With the body twisted, the chiropractor palpates each spinal joint to determine the degree of "fixation," the lack of movement, or excessive movement in that part of the spine.
- Using a small rubber hammer, various reflexes are checked.
- Pressure on the sciatic nerve in the leg and flexibility of the hip joint are tested by manipulation of each leg.
- Following the tests, the chiropractor explains the problem to the patient, then treats the patient by manipulation of the spine and joints.

---

tively. His philosophy of chiropractic was summed up in his description of the spine: "The principal functions of the spine are to support the head, to support the ribs, and to support the chiropractor."

Eventually, chiropractic split into two groups with different philosophies about chiropractic. One group, "the straights," adhere to the original ideas that almost all diseases are caused by subluxation of the vertebrae and that diseases can be cured by spinal manipulation. The other group, "the mixers," take a more holistic approach and, while practicing spinal manipulations to correct subluxations, also dispense advice on nutrition, relaxation, exercise, and other techniques.

The spine consists of twenty-four movable vertebrae (disks) that should flex and move freely. Chiropractors define a **subluxation** as a vertebra that is partly dis-

> The human body is the universe in miniature. It follows, therefore, that if our knowledge of our own body could be perfect, we would know the universe.
>
> Mahatma Gandhi

placed from its correct position and a **fixation** as the restricted movement of one or more vertebrae. Chiropractors are trained to diagnose subluxations and fixations of the spine by studying a person's posture, by touching the spine, and by X-ray exams. The purpose of chiropractic is to realign the vertebrae so that normal nervous system functions are restored, which, in turn, should alleviate the symptoms and cure the disease.

The American Association of Chiropractors defines chiropractic as "that science and art which utilizes the inherent recuperative powers of the body, and deals with the relationship between the nervous system and the spinal column, including its immediate articulations and the role of this relationship in the restoration and maintenance of health." Today, chiropractors receive extensive scientific training that is comparable to medical school education in many respects. Musculoskeletal disorders, which include not only backaches, pains, and muscle spasms and arthritis but also headaches, allergies, and digestive disorders, are often cured or relieved by chiropractic. Chiropractors are licensed to administer any therapy except surgery and prescription drugs.

Osteopathy

Osteopathy, like chiropractic, is basically treatment by manipulation of the spine and other structural parts of the body. Osteopathic physicians, called doctors of osteopathy or D.O.'s, undergo training that is as rigorous as the education of physicians, and generally osteopaths have the same medical privileges of prescribing drugs and performing surgery as do physicians. However, most practitioners of osteopathy rely primarily on physical manipulation and exercises for their patients' conditions.

Osteopathic medicine was founded in the United States by Andrew Taylor Still, who was born in Virginia

---

T E R M S

subluxation: partial displacement of a vertebra from its correct position

fixation: the restricted movement of one or more vertebrae

osteopathy: an alternative medicine that uses manipulation and medicines for healing; osteopaths receive training comparable to that of physicians and can prescribe drugs

acupuncture: an ancient Chinese alternative medicine that uses thin needles inserted into specific points on the body to produce healing energy

meridians: the channels along the body where energy flows and where acupuncture points are located

Ayurvedic medicine: a form of medicine that has its roots in the Hindu religion and is practiced widely in India

prana: the life force in the body that is derived from cosmic consciousness

in 1828. His father was a preacher-physician, and Andrew grew up observing his father treat patients. He eventually developed his own methods of healing, which depended heavily on manipulation. Today, there are hundreds of osteopathic hospitals in the United States and thousands of doctors of osteopathy.

Acupuncture

Acupuncture is an ancient Chinese healing art that is described in books dating to 2500 B.C. According to Chinese medical philosophy, disease results from disruption of the harmonious balance of vital energy called *ch'i* in the human body. The balance of energy is maintained by the forces of Yin and Yang (Chapter 2) and can be adjusted by inserting thin needles (called acupuncture needles) into specific points on the body that correspond to specific energy points associated with specific organs.

Usually many needles are inserted at a number of different acupuncture points that lie along **meridians**, invisible channels of energy that traverse the body. The acupuncturist inserts the needles into those points that are related to the health problem. The needles are left in place for a period. While in place, the needles may be twirled, heated, or used to pass small electrical currents into the body to help restore the correct balance of energy (Figure 20.1).

In the United States, an estimated 90 million acupuncture treatments are performed annually, and the use of acupuncture continues to rise (Holden, 1994). While acupuncture is used to treat almost every conceivable illness, it seems most effective in relief of chronic

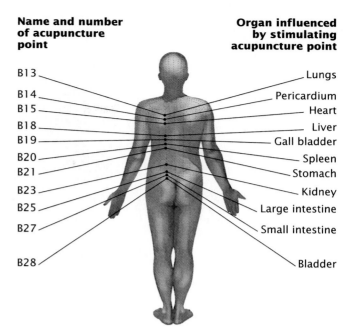

Name and number of acupuncture point	Organ influenced by stimulating acupuncture point
B13	Lungs
B14	Pericardium
B15	Heart
B18	Liver
B19	Gall bladder
B20	Spleen
B21	Stomach
B23	Kidney
B25	Large intestine
B27	Small intestine
B28	Bladder

FIGURE 20.1 Acupuncture points supposedly influence the functions of internal organs.

pain, in reducing stress, and, quite remarkably, in curing drug and smoking addictions.

As with other alternative medicines, the biological mechanisms that underlie curing with acupuncture are unknown. It may be that the autonomic nervous system (Chapter 2) is affected by the inserted needles or, as some studies have shown, hormone levels may be altered. Because there is no scientific theory that

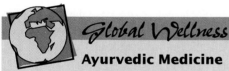

Global Wellness

Ayurvedic Medicine

Ayurvedic medicine, which has been practiced for at least 2500 years, is an integral part of the Hindu religion. According to Hindu mythology, "cosmic consciousness" manifests itself in the life force called **prana,** which provides the vitality and endurance of each living being. Prana also is the source of healing. According to the teachings of ayurvedic medicine, two forces emerge from the cosmic consciousness. One of these forces is male (Shiva) and the other female (Shakti).

The body itself is composed of five elements: earth, water, fire, air, and ether. The function or dysfunction of various organs are described in ayurvedic medicine in terms of these five elements. For example, digestion is a fire function because food is consumed in the digestive system. Bone and muscle are earth elements because they are composed of minerals. Forces within the body act on the five elements to maintain a harmonious balance among the different functions of the body. When the forces are out of balance, disease and sickness result.

Ayurvedic medicine and Chinese medicine share many of the same principles. Diseases are diagnosed by taking the pulse and by studying the person's physiognomy. Both systems believe that the life force flows through the body along fixed channels called meridians. Treatments include change of diet, use of herbs as medicines, and other treatments whose purpose is to restore harmony. Ayurvedic medicine, like Chinese medicine, involves spiritual healing as well as physical treatments.

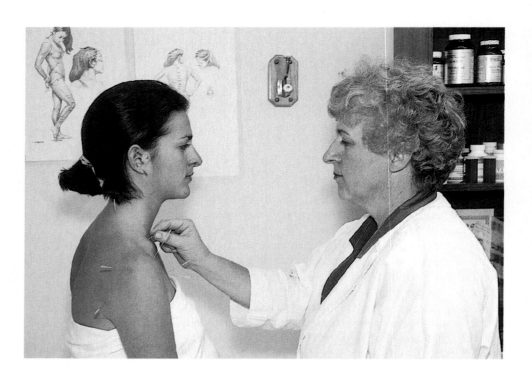

Acupuncture is one of the more frequently used treatments in complementary medicine.

accounts for the effects of acupuncture, it is not accepted as a medically reimbursable treatment in the U.S., although many physicians have learned to perform acupuncture and incorporate it into their practices.

Herbal Medicine

Herbs in various forms have been used as medicines for centuries to treat every conceivable form of ailment. Ancient Chinese, Greek, and Roman societies compiled extensive *Pharmacopoeia* describing the uses and preparation of herbal remedies. One herbal compilation published by Nicholas Culpepper in the seventeenth century has gone through countless printings and lists over 3000 herbal remedies.

Herbal medicines consist of materials derived from plants and can be prepared in the form of pills, teas, extracts, tinctures, salves, and other forms. In the 1780s, an English physician noted that one of his patients was cured of dropsy by drinking tea made from dried, powdered foxglove leaves. The physician, William Withering, made the connection between dropsy and heart disease. Subsequently, the chemical digitoxin in foxglove leaves was identified as the ingredient that helps heart functions.

Herbs have been the source for extracting and purifying modern drugs such as ephedrine, digitalis, atropine, reserpine, quinine, and most recently taxol, used to treat cancer. Herbal medicines often contain a mixture of herbs, so it is difficult to know what component is involved in alleviating symptoms or in healing. Only with the advent of modern chemistry could herbs be broken down into individual chemical components that can be tested for medicinal properties.

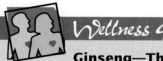

Wellness Guide

Ginseng—The Magical Herb

Ginseng (pronounced gin-sing) is an Asian plant whose roots have been used for centuries to treat a wide range of symptoms. When investigated by modern scientific methods, extracts of ginseng have been effective in treating infections and in reducing fatigue and stress.

In ancient Chinese herbal texts, ginseng is described as a preventive for headache, exhaustion, depression, and as a remedy for diseases of the blood, kidneys, and nervous system.

Ginseng is a mildly psychoactive. As a consequence of its complex chemistry, its specific effects on symptoms are difficult to document. Since it appears to influence the body's response to stress, it is not surprising that it can have a positive effect on stress-related symptoms such as fatigue and headaches.

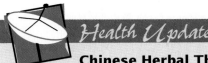
Chinese Herbal Therapy Helps Heal Eczema

Eczema, also referred to medically as atopic dermatitis, often is resistant to most drugs and treatments. Even when it does clear up temporarily, it usually reoccurs. Many people find relief in herbal medicines. To test the usefulness of Chinese herbs for eczema, a group of physicians performed a standard placebo controlled, double blind experiment to determine if an herbal tea taken daily was effective in treating symptoms of eczema (Sheehan et al., 1992).

By analyzing the patients' conditions in a number of ways, the study concluded that the herbal tea was effective. However, some patients found the tea hard to swallow because of its taste, a factor that limits the usefulness of the herbal medicine. Also, it is impossible to know if other batches of tea would be just as effective, since each mixture of Chinese herbs is concocted a little differently by each herbalist. The herbal teas sold in stores in the United States generally have acceptable tastes; however, herbal teas concocted by herbalists in China or Chinese Americans in this country usually have a taste that is unacceptable to most Western palates.

Herbal medicines possess the same potential for healing and the same potential for side effects and harm as do prescription drugs (Table 20.2). Many plants contain toxic chemicals in addition to beneficial substances. Also the amount of chemicals in plants varies from plant to plant and season to season. The herbalist can only guess how much to recommend and patients may find one batch of herbs quite effective and another useless.

Like other alternative medicines, herbal medicine is widely used in many countries of the world, especially among people who cannot afford expensive drugs. And even in Western industrialized countries including the United States, more and more people consult herbologists for their aches and illnesses. More research is being conducted to test the efficacy of herbal medicines, and some studies show that they do help patients with specific conditions (Wu, 1995).

TABLE 20.2 Herbs and Their Use in Common Ailments

Herb	Use
Aloe	Burns, skin irritations
Chamomile	Digestion
Feverfew	Reduces fever, helps migraine
Foxglove	Control heart rhythm, angina
Garlic	Digestion, protects against high blood pressure
Ginger root	Motion sickness, cough
Peppermint	Indigestion
Senna	Strong laxative
Valerian root	Mild sedative
Willow bark	Headache

Naturopathy

Naturopathy comprises a potpourri of healing strategies that include nutrition therapy, hydrotherapy, color therapy, herbalism, acupuncture, and massage. Naturopaths are trained to deal with all aspects of health and to tailor their treatments to the individual's needs. The basic principles of naturopathy are 1) all diseases have the same fundamental cause—namely, accumulation of toxic waste substances in the body; 2) disease is caused by the body's attempt to rid itself of these toxic substances; and 3) the body contains the power to heal itself.

Naturopaths teach their patients how to detoxify themselves by fasting, by restricted diets, and by other purifying techniques. Patients are also taught how to rejuvenate their body's vital energies. Many naturopaths work at health resorts that include mineral baths and saunas as part of their treatments. At present only a few states license naturopaths, so the consumer has to be knowledgeable and careful in choosing one. Since most naturopathic techniques are gentle and self-administered, there is little danger to the patient. Most persons will experience some benefit from an occasional fast, a soak in a warm bath, or a massage to relax tense muscles.

A fad among some naturopaths is the use of hair shaft analyses to diagnose biochemical abnormalities in the person's body. A strand of hair can be analyzed for many nutrients and minerals that, in principle, might

T E R M S

herbal medicines: materials derived from plants and other organisms that are made into teas, powders, and salves to treat diseases and injuries

ginseng: an Asian plant whose roots are used in herbal medicines and teas

naturopathy: an alternative medicine that uses nutrition, herbs, massage, and other techniques to promote healing

TABLE 20.3 Some Common Health Frauds

Claims for	Schemes
Arthritis	Arthritis affects about 40 million Americans, many of whom seek help from alternative medicine. Arthritis often goes into remission, so what seems like a cure is actually a temporary, natural reduction of symptoms.
Overweight	One out of four Americans is overweight and some may be searching for magic weight-loss therapy. Weight-loss gimmicks include patches, elastic belts, herbs, and "wonder" diets. There is no easy way to lose weight except by reducing eating and increasing exercise.
Sexual aids	Products to increase breast and penis size and to enhance sexual prowess are worthless. Some chemicals and herbs are sold as aphrodisiacs. Most are useless, but some can be harmful to health.
Chelation therapy	Promoters of this therapy claim that a chemical substance called EDTA can help purify the blood and clear arteries of fatty deposits. No scientific evidence for these claims exists and EDTA can harm the kidneys and cause other health problems.

indicate biochemical abnormalities. Computer printouts that may appear scientific and impressive to naturopathic practitioners and patients actually contain little or no useful health information. First, there is no evidence to indicate that hair chemistry reflects body chemistry to any significant degree. For example, a high level of lead in hair does not mean that blood serum levels of lead are also high. In addition, analyses of hair samples vary markedly from hair to hair and from laboratory to laboratory. Generally speaking, hair shaft analyses produce income for laboratories and practitioners that use them; no other benefits have been documented.

CHOOSING AN ALTERNATIVE MEDICINE

In the broadest sense, the use of any medicine or therapy that is scientifically unproved is called quackery (Consumers' Research, 1990). Various federal agencies such as the Federal Drug Administration, the Federal Trade Commission, and the U.S. Postal Service try to protect the public by exposing false claims and useless health products. Deceptive advertising entices millions of people to buy products or services that promise to improve health or cure an illness. Some conditions are more susceptible to fraudulent practices than others (Table 20.3).

Anything that sounds "too good to be true" most likely is not true. Don't let your vanity or your hopes for health lure you into undergoing unproved procedures or into buying worthless products. Remedies based on "secret formulas" or the promise of quick, painless cures for serious diseases such as cancer are invariably fraudulent. Learn to recognize frauds and quacks. Seek help from qualified professionals in whom you feel you can trust regardless of the therapy you seek.

Many people are satisfied with the care they receive from modern medicine and the physicians who treat them. However, many Americans also seek alternative medicines to supplement conventional treatments. And some persons choose to rely on alternative medicines exclusively. For many kinds of sickness, alternative medicines may provide relief and even a cure.

It often is wise to begin with the least harsh form of treatment before undergoing surgery or taking drugs that can also do harm. Our society is gradually coming to the view that healing can be accomplished by both modern and alternative medicine. And, as we have pointed out repeatedly, the belief of the patient in a particular treatment, physician, acupuncturist, or chiropractor may be what heals.

HEALTH IN REVIEW

- Alternative medicine consists of hundreds of methods for dealing with sickness and disease in ways that are different from modern medical care performed by physicians.

- The broad categories of alternative medicine include spiritual and mental therapies, nutritional therapies, herbal remedies, and physical therapies.
- Homeopathy administers very dilute solutions of sub-

stances that are supposed to mimic the symptoms of sick persons and help the body cure itself of the disease.

- Chiropractic and osteopathy use manipulation of the spine and joints to treat musculoskeletal disorders and other diseases.
- Acupuncture involves inserting very thin needles into specific points on the body to restore harmony to the functioning of tissues and organs.

- Herbal medicine uses mixtures of herbs in the form of pills, powders, teas, and elixers to help the healing process.
- Consumers of alternative medicine need to guard against fraudulent claims and unscrupulous persons who advertise therapies of unproved safety and of dubious value.

REFERENCES

Eisenberg, D. M., et al. (1993). "Unconventional Medicine in the United States." *New England Journal of Medicine,* January 28, 328(4): 246–252.

Holden, C. (1994). "Acupuncture: Stuck on the Fringe." *Science,* May 6: 264, 770.

Murray, R. H., and A. J. Rubel (1992). "Physicians and Healers—Unwitting Partners in Health Care." *New England Journal of Medicine,* January 2, 326 (1): 61–64.

Reilly, D., et al. (1994) "Is Evidence for Homeopathy Reproducible?" *The Lancet,* December 10, 344: 1601–1606.

Sheehan, M. P. (1992). "Efficacy of Traditional Chinese Herbal Therapy in Adult Atopic Dermatitis." *The Lancet,* July 4, 340: 13–17.

"Top Ten Health Frauds" (1990). *Consumers' Research,* February: 34–36.

Wu, C. (1995). "Yin and Yang—Western Medicine Makes Room for Chinese Herbal Medicine." *Science News,* September 9, 148: 172–173.

SUGGESTED READINGS

Borysenko, J., and M. Borysenko (1994). *The Power of the Mind to Heal.* Carson, Calif.: Hay House. Two researchers explain how to use the mind for self-healing.

Heyn, B. (1990). *Ayurveda: The Indian Art of Natural Medicine and Life Extension.* Rochester, Vt.: Healing Arts Press. Explains Hindu views of health and healing.

"Homeopathy: Keeping an Open Mind" (1994). *The Lancet,* September 16. A brief discussion of research into homeopathy and how it might work.

Martin, J. E. (1995). *Alternative Health Medicine Encyclopedia.* Detroit, Mich.: Visible Ink Press. Just what the title says.

Tyler, V. E. (1993). *The Honest Herbal: A Sensible Guide to the Use of Herbs and Related Remedies.* Binghamton, N.Y.: Haworth Press. A practical guide to using plant remedies.

Ulett, G. A. (1992). *Beyond Yin and Yang: How Acupuncture Really Works.* New York: Warren H. Green. An American physician demystifies acupuncture.

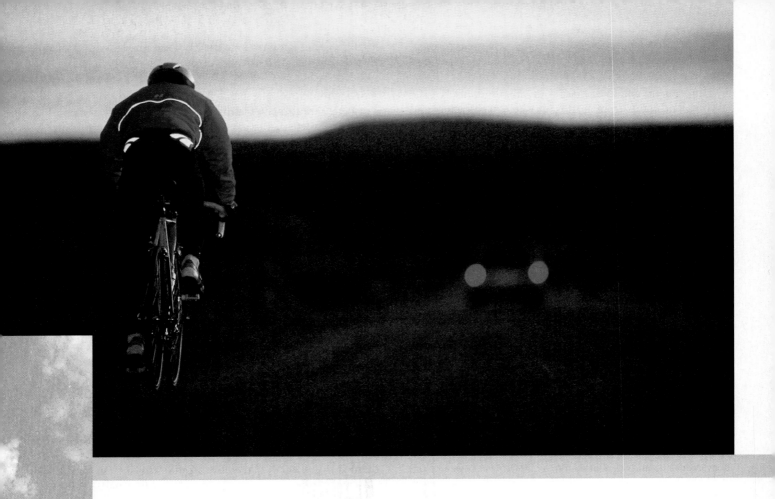

LEARNING OBJECTIVES

After reading this chapter you should be able to:

1. Describe safety, accidents, and unintentional injuries.
2. Describe various strategies to prevent unintentional injuries.
3. Describe the Haddon Matrix and explain why it was developed.
4. Discuss various ways to prevent motor vehicle crashes, motorcycle accidents, bicycle accidents, and pedestrian accidents.
5. Describe various strategies to improve home and work safety.

Preventing Accidents
What You Can Do

*I*njuries affect the health and well-being of millions of Americans every year. Accidents of various kinds are a far greater source of ill health and death than most people realize. Safety warnings and increased public awareness measures have reduced the number of accidental injuries and deaths in recent years (Figure 21.1). In 1993, the number of accidental deaths from all causes in the United States was 90,000. Despite the encouraging reduction in accidental deaths, the adverse health consequences of accidental injuries are still serious and can be reduced. For example, accidental deaths in Canada are 16 percent less than in the United States and in the United Kingdom 40 percent less.

SAFETY AND UNINTENTIONAL INJURIES

Safety

What is **safety?** The word safety is used in a wide context with various meanings to different individuals. Few individuals or agencies can agree on one universal definition. "Is this a safe part of town to be this late at night?" "He is not a very safe motorcycle driver." "My daughter's safety has been a concern of mine since she obtained her driver's license." "Is that old ladder safe to use?" As you can see, the word "safe" or "safety" may be used in a variety of situations.

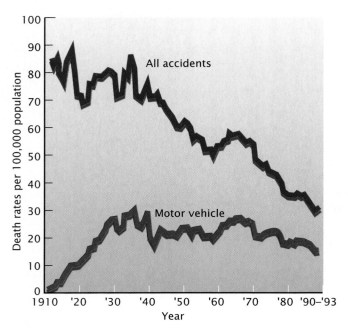

FIGURE 21.1 Trends in Unintentional-Injury Death Rates Between 1912 and 1993, unintentional injury deaths per 100,000 population were reduced 57 percent from 82 to 35. The reduction in the overall rate during a period when the nation's population more than doubled has resulted in 3,600,000 fewer people being killed by unintentional injuries than would have occurred if the rate had not been reduced.
Source: Accident Facts, 1994 Edition (Itasca, Ill.: National Safety Council, 1994).

One common tie to all these different scenarios is the word **accident**. As defined by the National Safety Council, an accident "is that occurrence in a sequence of events which produces unintended injury, death, or property damage. Accident refers to the event, not the result of the event" (National Safety Council, 1994). Each year one in four individuals will sustain some type of serious injury that requires medical attention and that is a result of an accident. Injuries are a serious problem, but many individuals lack the necessary knowledge and skills to provide assistance if an emergency were to occur. Injuries are the leading cause of disability in young people today, and cause more deaths in children than all the infectious diseases combined.

Unintentional injury is a term often used interchangeably with the term accident and we also will use both terms. Unintentional injury is the term preferred by public health officials and refers to the result of an accident (National Safety Council, 1994). Some classic examples of unintentional injuries are motor vehicle accidents, home accidents (falls, poisonings, fires), workplace accidents, unintentional and intentional discharge of firearms, and pedestrian accidents with motor vehicles (Table 21.1).

Unintentional injuries are the leading cause of death among persons ages 1 to 37. Among persons of all ages, unintentional injuries are the fifth leading cause of death. For youths ages 15 to 24, unintentional injuries claim almost twice as many lives as the next leading cause of death (pneumonia). More than 3 out of 4 victims in the 15- to 24-year-old age group are males (National Safety Council, 1994). The cost of unintentional injuries in 1994 alone was approximately $400 billion.

Total costs incurred for unintentional injuries in 1994 are estimated at $410.6 billion. Besides this economic loss, an additional $788.6 billion were spent on lost quality of life. The comprehensive cost of unintentional injuries in 1993 was $1,196.1 billion (Figure 21.2).

The causes of unintentional injury death change with age. Factors such as poor diet, sedentary life-style, arthritis, decreased mobility, poverty, chronic diseases, or lack of access to primary medical care may contribute to injuries and accidental death as people get older.

Determinants of Safety

Safety experts traditionally have focused on two areas: 1) accident mitigation—methods to reduce damage caused

HEALTHY PEOPLE 2000

Reduce deaths causes by unintentional injuries to no more than 29.3 per 100,000 people.

Nearly two-thirds of all injury deaths involve unintentional injuries. Males are more likely to experience unintentional injuries than females and are 2.5 times more likely to die from them. Higher death rates from unintentional injury occur among blacks than among whites over the entire age range with black males generally having the highest death rates. Reduction in deaths caused by unintentional injuries requires interventions directed at preventing the leading causes of those injuries, each of which is the topic of objectives in this area.

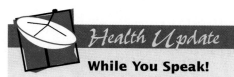

Health Update

While You Speak!

While you make a 10-minute safety speech, 2 persons will be killed and about 350 will suffer a disabling injury. Costs will amount to $7,800,000. On the average, there are 10 unintentional-injury deaths and about 2,080 disabling injuries every hour during the year. Deaths and disabling injuries in the nation by class occurred at the following rates in 1993:

Class of accident	Severity	One every—	No. per hour	No. per day	No. per week	Total 1993
All classes	Deaths	6 minutes	10	247	1,730	90,000
	Injuries	2 seconds	2,080	49,900	350,000	18,200,000
Motor-vehicle	Deaths	13 minutes	5	115	810	42,000
	Injuries	16 seconds	230	5,500	38,500	2,000,000
Work	Deaths	58 minutes	1	25	180	9,100
	Injuries	10 seconds	370	8,800	61,500	3,200,000
Workers off-the-job	Deaths	16 minutes	4	91	640	33,300
	Injuries	6 seconds	590	14,200	100,000	5,200,000
Home	Deaths	23 minutes	3	62	430	22,500
	Injuries	5 seconds	750	18,100	126,900	6,600,000
Public nonmotor-vehicle	Deaths	26 minutes	2	55	380	20,000
	Injuries	5 seconds	750	18,100	126,900	6,600,000

Source: Accident Facts, 1994 Edition (Itasca, Ill.: National Safety Council, 1994).

by unplanned events; and 2) accident prevention—ways to eliminate the occurrence of unintentional injuries (Bever, 1992). Safety can be viewed in two contexts: 1) individual or personal safety and security; and 2) environmental or community safety and security. Many factors are involved in unintentional injury: knowledge, attitudes, beliefs and behaviors; economic and social conditions; ability level of the performer of tasks; conditions of the environment; and alcohol and other drugs. Positive changes in these factors will reduce injuries, but more attention needs to be directed to prevention strategies. Even though unintentional injuries have

TABLE 21.1 The Leading Causes of Unintentional Deaths in the U.S. in 1993 The cause of death is ascribed to a single category although many factors contribute to all kinds of accidents.

Cause of death	Number of deaths
Motor vehicle crashes	42,000
Falls	13,500
Poisoning by solids/liquids	6,500
Drowning	4,800
Fires and burns	4,000
Suffocation by ingested object	2,900
Firearm	1,600
All others (air, water, and land transport, machinery, falling object, etc.)	14,000

Source: Accident Facts, 1994 Edition (Itasca, Ill.: National Safety Council, 1994).

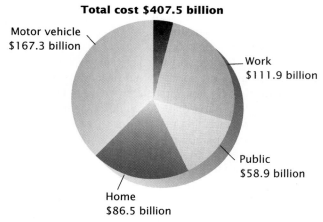

Total cost $407.5 billion

Motor vehicle $167.3 billion

Work $111.9 billion

Public $58.9 billion

Home $86.5 billion

*Duplication between motor vehicle and work was $17.1 billion.

FIGURE 21.2 Costs of Unintentional Injuries by Classification, 1993 The total cost of unintentional injuries was over $4 billion, with the majority of the costs from motor-vehicle accidents.

Source: Accident Facts, 1994 Edition (Itasca, Ill.: National Safety Council, 1994).

What's Your Accident IQ?

What Is Considered an Accident or Unintentional Injury?

What criteria must an event meet to be considered an accident or unintentional injury? Take this short self-assessment test to determine if you can differentiate between an event that is an accident and one that is not.

Directions: Check the items you believe are considered an accident.

_____ 1. A 3-year-old child drowned after falling into the fountain in the garden.

_____ 2. A junior high student contracted mono from her girlfriend at school.

_____ 3. The veterinarian was bitten unexpectedly while giving a dog a rabies vaccine.

_____ 4. A depressed college student died from an overdose of sleeping pills.

_____ 5. A patient became angered while waiting nearly two hours to see the doctor.

_____ 6. Due to practicing dental hygiene for over twenty years, the hygienist has developed carpal tunnel syndrome.

_____ 7. An elderly man with Alzheimer's disease nearly died from hypothermia when he wandered from the nursing home and became lost.

_____ 8. A carpenter received second-degree burns after being struck by lightning while working on a roof.

_____ 9. A 4-year-old died after swallowing a bottle of aspirins she found in the family medicine cabinet.

_____10. A college student became angry when he forgot the mid-term exam was today.

(Statements 1, 3, 7, 8, and 9 should have been checked; these meet the criteria of an accident.)

---

decreased 73 percent from 1912 to 1993, the cost is still staggering.

Attitudes and beliefs may be the greatest factor involved in unintentional injuries. Your individual attitude toward safety precautions will greatly influence the likelihood of an injury. You may believe that safety precautions are a waste of time, that you have no control over the situation (what will happen, will happen), or you may have a reckless attitude (you like to take risks).

Lack of knowledge and skills also play a role in unintentional injury. In special circumstances, especially when performing a new procedure or task, lacking the proper knowledge and/or skills could result in unintentional injury (operating a new power tool before reading the instructions, operating a motorcycle the first time, or using a new kitchen appliance).

Socioeconomic factors also play a role in unintentional injury. Some individuals may lack the necessary funds to replace unsafe or old equipment. Some may even lack the necessary funds to obtain proper training in safety related matters. Safety training can be received through a local National Safety Council office on such topics as proper storage of household cleaning items, tool safety, and safety tips for the babysitter. Local health departments may also provide educational workshops on safety issues as well.

> *There is no such thing as an accident. What we call by that name is the effect of some cause which we do not see.*
> Voltaire

Some social settings may lend themselves to accidents. Attitudes and beliefs as well as the social setting can raise or lower the probability of an intentional injury. For example, alcohol and drug abuse definitely affect the frequency of unintentional injuries. Prescribed medications, especially ones with a sedative effect, can increase the likelihood of an accident while operating a motor vehicle, motorcycle, or power tool.

The ability of the individual performing a task or activity may affect the probability of an unintentional injury. The person may be a child who is too young to perform a task competently. At the other end of the spectrum, an elderly individual may not be strong enough or steady enough to perform a simple task like carving the Thanksgiving turkey with an electric knife.

Your environment can be the most unpredictable risk factor in unintentional injuries. Natural disasters such as floods, hurricanes, earthquakes, or tornadoes have caused numerous and tragic unintentional injuries and

T E R M

injury epidemiology: the study of the occurrence, causes, and prevention of injury

deaths. The devastation caused by natural disasters has, or will, affect every one of us at some point in our lifetime.

Stress and fatigue contribute greatly to higher rates of unintentional injuries. Stress may interfere with your concentration when performing even a simple task or may distract you while engaged in an activity. Fatigue causes you to be less alert or have slower reaction times; fatigue affects your coordination, and, at worst, can cause you to fall asleep. It is not wise to attempt difficult tasks while you are fatigued or under stress.

Unintentional Injury Analysis

Scientific study of unintentional injury uncovers why injuries occur, what determinants play a role, and who or what age group is the most susceptible. Analysis of unintentional injury provides us with necessary assessments before effective educational, preventive, or enforcement strategies can be implemented.

Injury epidemiology, used to investigate risk factors that cause unintentional injuries, is analogous to the disease epidemiologic model. For injuries to result, three factors are involved: 1) the agent or source of energy exchange: mechanical, chemical, electrical, or thermal; 2) the vehicle for the transmission of mechanical energy: a car, truck, or motorcycle, powerline, poison; and 3) a host or object: a person, school building, or house (Figure 21.3).

Most unintentional injuries are complex and many factors can be involved. Also, interactions among risk factors affect the likelihood of an accident. For example, cutting trees with a chain saw on a windy or rainy day may increase the risk of accident, whereas choosing a dry, calm day might reduce the chance of an accident (Lawson, 1992).

One of the most famous scientific models used in unintentional injury analysis is the Haddon Matrix.

> *The best way to avoid something is to cause that which is to be avoided to avoid you of its own accord.*
>
> Sufi saying

Developed by William Haddon, Jr., in the 1960s, this model was used originally to investigate motor vehicle risk factors and to develop and implement programs to prevent or reduce the occurrence of car accidents. The Haddon Matrix analyzed accidents in three phases:

- *Phase 1: the pre-event phase.* Includes factors that may determine if an accident will happen; lack of knowledge or skills or alcohol use are the most significant factors.
- *Phase 2: the event phase.* Occurs when the host comes into contact with forces of energy. Many preventive measures, such as the use of helmets, safety belts, or protective goggles, are associated with this phase.
- *Phase 3: the post-event phase.* Includes emergency procedures provided after the injury has occurred. Preventive signaling devices, smoke and carbon monoxide detectors, or fire alarms will facilitate the speed with which an injury is attended to. Emergency transportation and care of an injured or sick person occurs in this phase (Lawson, 1992).

All approaches to unintentional injury reduction include: 1) educational and prevention strategies; 2) stricter laws and regulations to prevent unintentional injuries (mandates to enforce safety belt and helmet compliance); and 3) better product design and automatic protection devices (air bags, child-proof car door locks, child-proof safety caps on medicines) to help prevent unintentional injuries.

MOTOR VEHICLE SAFETY

Even though motor vehicle death rates have been declining since 1962, the number of deaths is still a major concern. In 1994 there were 41,300 motor vehicle deaths (National Safety Council, 1995), a decrease of 2 percent from 1993. In 1994 Americans spent $169 billion for

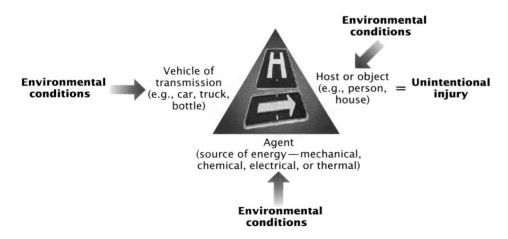

FIGURE 21.3 Epidemiologic Model for Unintentional Injuries

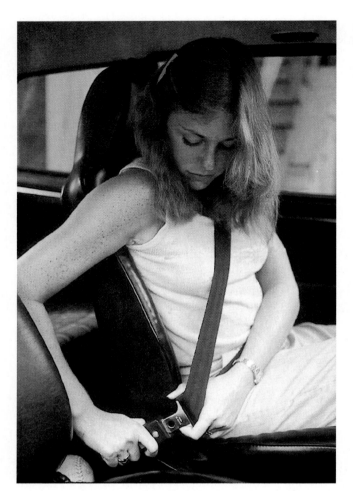

Using a seatbelt helps prevent injuries and fatalities in automobile accidents.

insurance claims and property damage. This amount includes related costs: productivity and wage loss, administrative costs, medical expenses, property damage, and employer costs for lost work productivity.

Although alcohol involvement in fatal motor vehicle accidents has declined since 1962, over 45 percent of all motor vehicle fatalities still involve an alcohol impaired or intoxicated driver or nonmotorist (Chapter 18), an average of one alcohol-related death every half hour. During the year-end holiday season, 50 percent of all motor vehicle fatalities are alcohol related. Although states outlaw sale of alcohol to youths under 21, alcohol-related deaths and injuries among underage youth is still high (National Safety Council, 1994).

All drivers are at risk for accidents, but teenagers and young adults injure and kill themselves and others in car accidents more often than all other drivers under age 60 (National Safety Council, 1994). Many accidents involving youth occur after dark, after parties, and after drinking. Alcohol in the blood and brain impairs a driver's judgment, coordination, and reaction time. The effects of alcohol vary considerably from one person to another, so

even small amounts of alcohol may impair driving skills and cause an accident. New laws have been proposed that set a zero tolerance for alcohol in blood for persons under 21 (Chapter 18).

Many factors other than alcohol are also involved in motor vehicle fatalities and injuries. The condition of the vehicle itself or the road, the speed at which the vehicle was traveling, and the interaction between these factors will affect the probability of an accident. In all severe accidents, rural and urban, exceeding the posted speed limit was the most common factor. Table 21.2 lists other unsafe driver practices.

The conditions of the road, vehicle, or environment are also important when assessing these statistics. In 1993, vehicle defects contributed to approximately 1.6 percent of all police-reported motor vehicle accidents. Among the numerous vehicle defects that contribute to accidents are faulty tires, brakes, headlights, steering system, body, doors, and hood (National Safety Council, 1994).

An estimated 39,794 lives were saved by seatbelts from 1983 through 1992. According to the National Safety Council, safety belts saved an estimated 5,226 lives in 1992 among front-seat vehicle occupants, while an estimated additional 8,912 lives could have been saved if *all* front-seat occupants were wearing safety belts. Governmental regulations, and safety belt and child safety seats which were initially opposed by many individuals, have greatly reduced the number of motor vehicle fatalities and injuries.

MOTORCYCLE SAFETY

Motorcycles appeal to many individuals for various reasons: lower cost to purchase, repair, and operate; the exciting feeling of open-air riding; and association with fellow motorcycle riders. However, risks include inclement weather, less crash protection than an automobile, and less visibility by other drivers. Motorcycle operators can ensure a safer ride by securing proper training in operational procedures and by using a helmet

Mindfulness Meditation

Ninety percent of all accidents are the result of human error. This fact, cited by the National Safety Council, suggests what those in the field of stress management already know: the mind can focus on only one or two thoughts at a time. When the mind is overwhelmed with thoughts, something always drops. When you are just sitting at your desk studying for an exam and your mind wanders, your life isn't in jeopardy. But when you are engaged in an activity like driving your car, and you have got one hand on the cellular phone, the other grabbing your eye liner, electric razor, or radio dial, and your mind is focused on the news broadcast of the latest disaster, an accident is waiting to happen.

Nine times out of ten accidents occur because your mind is somewhere other than where it is supposed to be. Drifting attention, unfocused thoughts, and mental distractions are normal in the course of a typical day, but the mind *can* be trained to stay focused. Training the mind in this fashion is called "mindfulness meditation," a type of meditation used to domesticate your thoughts and gain control of your awareness. Athletes, surgeons, and actors practice this technique to improve their performance. It is a technique that everyone should master, in this context, specifically to avoid the risk of accidents.

Mindfulness meditation can take many forms and with repeated practice, the effects of one experience (like eating an apple) can transfer to virtually any activity. Mindfulness meditation is a great way to keep focused on whatever task you are engaged in. Try this exercise.

1. Take an apple and hold it in your hand.

2. Sit comfortably with your back straight. You may choose to sit against a wall for support.

3. Hold the apple and feel its weight in your hand. Feel the apple. Feel the texture of the apple's skin. Feel the curves. Feel the stem if there is one. Notice all the nuances of the apple with your fingers.

4. Look at the apple. What color(s) is it? Look at it carefully. Study it. Know this apple so well, that if it was put back in a barrel of apples, you could easily find it.

5. Now smell the apple. Close your eyes and focus your sense of smell on the apple. What does it smell like?

6. Bite into the apple. Savor its taste, flavor, and texture. Feel your tongue and jaws move as you chew.

Now, sensing and eating an apple may seem far removed from preventing an accident at home, work, or on the road, but the truth is that the skills of concentration and focusing are important in every activity you do. Mindfulness meditation will help you stay focused and attentive to details that require your undivided attention.

TABLE 21.2 Improper Driving Reported in Accidents, 1993 Driving too fast or unsafely and right of way violations were the two most common improper driving habits reported in motor vehicle accidents.

	Percent of all accidents		
	Total	Urban	Rural
Improper driving	**68.6**	**69.8**	**66.1**
Speed too fast or unsafe	12.2	11.1	15.4
Right of way	20.6	23.2	13.7
Failed to yield	15.1	16.6	11.3
Passed stop sign	2.0	2.1	1.4
Disregarded signal	3.5	4.5	1.0
Drove left of center	1.8	1.1	3.4
Improper overtaking	1.3	1.1	1.7
Made improper turn	4.5	4.6	4.2
Followed too closely	5.5	6.2	3.6
Other improper driving	22.7	22.5	24.1
No improper driving stated	**31.4**	**30.2**	**33.9**
Total	**100.00**	**100.00**	**100.00**

Source: Accident Facts, 1994 Edition (Itasca, Ill.: National Safety Council).

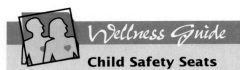
Child Safety Seats

The type of child safety seat to buy and how you position it depend on the child's age, weight, and size. Every state requires that infants and children ride buckled up in child safety seats or safety belts. A few pointers:

- Always check the labels to make sure they meet current federal safety standards. Don't buy a seat if it was made before January 1, 1981.

- If your car has a passenger-side air bag, always put your child in the back seat (when they are in a child safety seat).

Infants under 26 inches tall and weighing less than 20 pounds must ride rear-facing in an infant or convertible safety seat. An infant, with its less than fully developed skeletal system, needs spinal support. Only rear-facing seats can provide this support, Jeff Michael with NHTSA says. Without it, the infant can be severely injured in even a moderate crash.

When your children are 26 inches tall, weigh at least 17-20 pounds, and can sit up by themselves, you can move them to forward-facing convertible safety seats. If you put toddlers in safety belts

alone, the belts will probably not fit correctly and may allow the child to be seriously injured in a crash.

When your children are 40 inches tall and weigh 40 pounds, you can move them into booster seats. Or they can use safety belts if they fit correctly. A safety belt fits correctly if the lap belt stays low and tight on the hips; it does not ride up over the stomach; and the shoulder belt does not cross in front of the face or neck. It should fit across the shoulder and chest.

Source: Family Safety and Health (Itasca, Ill.: National Safety Council, Fall, 1993).

and proper protective clothing. Less than 10 percent of all motorcycle operators receive any formal training. The wearing of a motorcycle helmet may reduce the likelihood of fatal injuries by 29 percent. Protective clothing, long sleeves and pants, jackets, and boots, may lessen the chance for abrasions should an accident occur, or protect from the unpredictable elements of weather (Bever, 1992).

In 1966, Congress mandated that motorcycle riders and passengers use helmets in all states. If states did not enforce this mandate, they would lose federal highway funds, but only three states at first adopted helmet laws. However by 1975, 47 states had helmet laws in force. During this ten-year period (1966–1975), fatal motorcycle accidents declined from 12.8 to 6.5 deaths per 100,000. Nevertheless, the American Motorcycle Association and A Brotherhood Against Totalitarian Enactment

(ABATE) have opposed helmet regulations. They argue that riders should not be forced to wear protective equipment, a sentiment also held by many who opposed auto safety belt mandates (Bever, 1992). Nonetheless safety belts and helmets *do* reduce motor vehicle injuries and deaths.

PEDESTRIAN SAFETY

In urban areas, nearly one-fourth of all accident victims were pedestrians (National Safety Council, 1994). Nearly 51 percent of all pedestrian deaths and injuries involve children 5 to 9 years old when they either cross or enter a street. Among young children, implementation of preventive strategies and educational efforts addressing safety procedures in traffic areas may reduce accidents. Many young children don't know what traffic signals or signs mean. Young children are also unable to judge the distance and speed of vehicles, which puts them in danger when trying to cross a busy intersection. Closer supervision by adults helps. Safety education of child-care workers at school and elsewhere is another preventive strategy.

The elderly are also at risk for pedestrian injuries, due to failing eyesight and hearing and mobility problems. Some pedestrian injuries occur when individuals dart into a busy street, or are unable to see oncoming traffic because their view is blocked by a parked vehicle. Many pedestrian injuries involve joggers, runners, and walkers. Bright-colored clothes, especially reflective clothes, offer protection for pedestrians during both day

HEALTHY PEOPLE 2000

Increase use of helmets to at least 80 percent of motorcyclists and at least 50 percent of bicyclists.

Head injury is the leading cause of death in motorcycle and bicycle crashes. Compared with motorcycle riders wearing helmets, unhelmeted riders are two times more likely to incur a fatal head injury and three times more likely to incur a nonfatal head injury. The risk of head injury for unhelmeted bicyclists is more than $6\frac{1}{2}$ times greater than for helmeted bicyclists.

and night. Just as alcohol impairs the judgment of motor vehicle operators, it also impairs the judgment of pedestrians.

Other preventive strategies help reduce the number of pedestrian injuries and deaths. Underpasses and overpasses in high traffic areas, well-marked crosswalks, and pedestrian guardrails all offer greater protection for the pedestrian. Limiting traffic during peak hours of pedestrian traffic—for instance, before and after school or church—might also be beneficial.

BICYCLE SAFETY

Safety concerns have been increasing as more bicycles and pedalcycles are used for exercise and recreation. According to a 1991 survey by the U.S. Consumer Product Safety Commission, an estimated 66.9 million people ride bicycles annually. Seventy-six percent of these individuals rarely or never wore helmets, while 17.6 percent of the respondents wore helmets most or all of the time (Bever, 1992). In 1992, 649,536 injured bicycle riders were treated in hospital emergency rooms; of those, 75,816 suffered head injuries. Since 1940, the use of bicycles has increased 15 times, but the death rate from bicycle accidents is one-fourteenth that of 1940. The single most important factor in reducing bicycle deaths is the use of protective helmets (National Safety Council, 1994).

Bicycle riders are required to follow the same rules of the road as automobile operators. But many bicycle riders lack knowledge of these rules, do not use proper hand signals, or ride on the wrong side of the street, contributing to bicycle injuries and fatalities. Also, lack of skill in handling a bicycle increases the risk of an acci-

dent. Individuals who purchase a new bicycle should be familiar with all its devices before riding it. Also, many young bicycle riders are unaware of the rules of the road or are too small to see over motor vehicles.

Just as pedestrians need to wear bright, reflective clothing the same holds true for bicycle riders, and the bicycle itself should be properly equipped with reflectors and lights. A recent and dangerous phenomenon is wearing headphones while riding. Inability to hear the sounds of traffic, the honk of a horn, or a shout of warning may contribute to an accident. Construction of more bicycle paths, underpasses, overpasses, and guardrails, combined with defensive riding skills, can reduce bicycle injuries and deaths.

HOME SAFETY

Accidental deaths in the home are gradually declining, but are still a major source of concern. Accidents in the home take a special toll on both the young and elderly. As the elderly population continues to grow, accidents in the home will threaten more individuals. The main categories of home accidents include: falls, poisonings, drowning, choking and suffocation, and fires. Although not all falls, drowning, or poisonings occur in the home, they are classified as home accidents.

Falls

People of all ages fall, but most injuries occur among persons under age 15 and the elderly. Children often fall because of their strenuous activities, but usually the injuries are minor and heal rapidly. Children fall down stairs, out of trees, from open windows, and the backs of

Take a Walk on the Safe Side

Despite media attention to violence in schools, far more children die or are seriously injured while they walk to or from school.

Pedestrian injuries are the leading cause of preventable death for children ages 4 to 8; they kill about 1,300 children under age 15 annually. Boys up to age 9 or 10 are at the greatest risk of pedestrian injury, especially during after-school hours.

"Even 10- and 11-year-olds can't always make accurate judgments about speed and distance," says Johns Hopkins Medical Institutions pediatrician Modena Wilson, who is coauthor of the book *Saving Children*. Wilson urges parents to plan safe-walking routes to school that avoid busy highways. If possible, children should use routes and streets with crossing guards. Even with school-zone signals and crossing guards, children should always stop, look left, right and left again for approaching traffic. Children age 7 and younger should always walk to and from school with an adult.

Adults should supervise students as they exit school buses. Handrails can snag clothing or book bags and drag children as buses pull away. Also, teach your children never to fetch a book or other dropped objects after they leave the school bus.

Source: Family Safety and Health (Itasca, Ill.: National Safety Council, Fall, 1993).

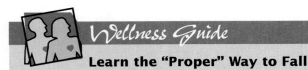
trucks. They fall while climbing, jumping, or running. People responsible for watching children at play need to be alert to the danger of a fall.

Falls are a more serious problem for the elderly, who often fracture hip or head bones. For people over 79 years, falls were the leading cause of unintentional injury deaths. Bone breaks in the elderly heal slowly and often lead to complications and death. If hospitalized, the elderly person may suffer nosocomial infections (Chapter 9) and die from infectious disease acquired in the hospital. Being careful and in good physical condition are the best deterrents to being seriously injured in a fall.

HEALTHY PEOPLE 2000

Reduce deaths from falls and fall-related injuries to no more than 2.3 per 100,000 people.

Falls and fall-related injuries occur at every age, but the greater severity of injuries in old age combined with longer recovery periods makes falls particularly serious threats to older people. Falls are the leading cause of death from injury for people ages 65 and older and are particularly common among those over age 85. Although 11,733 deaths were attributed to falls and fall-related injuries in 1987, the actual number of deaths in which a fall was a contributing factor may be much higher. While most falls do not result in serious physical injuries or death, they are often associated with loss of confidence in ability to function independently; restriction of physical and social activities; speech, language, and cognitive disorders; increased dependence; and increased need for long-term care.

Certain areas in the home are hazardous for falls. The kitchen, bathroom, and laundry room are dangerous because they often have wet floors. Stairs are also hazardous; a person may stumble while walking up or down, particularly if he or she is distracted, or if the stairs are not well lit. Bumping into furniture or tripping over the legs of tables, chairs, or loose rugs are also common causes of falls. Climbing ladders may be an invitation for a fall if a person is careless or the ladder is weak or unstable. When performing any activity in which a fall is possible, extra safety measures should be taken, such as having someone hold the ladder that you are climbing. After motor vehicle accidents, falls cause the greatest number of unintentional injury deaths.

Poisonings

A **poison** is any chemical substance that causes illness, injury, or death. Poisons enter the body by being ingested (food, medicines, illegal drugs, chemicals), inhaled (carbon monoxide, hydrogen sulfide), injected (bee sting, snake bite), or by contact with the skin (poison ivy, solutions that burn). Chemical poisons such as pesticides disturb essential biological reactions in the body and cause a variety of symptoms, even death. Some poisons cause only transitory symptoms; the body returns to normal once the poison is eliminated. How-

T E R M S

poison: any chemical substance that causes illness, injury, or death

laryngospasm: spasm of the larynx

ever, some poisons that do not kill can cause permanent and irreversible damage to body functions.

Many cultivated and wild plants, trees, and bushes contain poisonous compounds. Eating the berries, seeds, and roots, or leaves of many plants can produce mild symptoms, severe symptoms, or death (Table 21.3). Many common household plants are also poisonous, even the Christmas poinsettia. Collecting and eating wild mushrooms can be dangerous unless you are knowledgeable about what species are edible.

Young children, especially once they have learned to crawl or walk, are particularly susceptible to poisoning accidents. Children are curious, active, and adventurous, and it is natural for young children to put things in their mouths, including nonfood items such as paint chips, dirt, marbles, and almost any small object. When children are hungry, thirsty, or just curious, they are likely to ingest whatever is closest to hand—medicines, pills, household products, pesticides, as well as food. Children between one and five suffer the greatest number of accidental poisonings.

Precautions by manufacturers of drugs, solvents, paints, and other products have markedly reduced the number of accidental childhood poisonings. Child-resistant lids, tamper-proof caps, and internal seals help to prevent children from ingesting harmful substances. Precautions by parents and other child caregivers are essential to reduce the risk further. All household products and medicines should be kept out of reach of small children. Dangerous substances should be kept in locked cabinets. Small children should not be left unsupervised in areas like bathrooms, kitchens, and garages, where dangerous household products are stored.

There are several hundred poison control centers across the country. Should a poisoning accident occur, someone at a poison control center can give you immediate expert advice. Keep the number of a poison control center near the phone in case of emergency.

Death rates for poisonings have doubled from 1961 to 1991. Individuals ages 25–44 had the greatest increase, which may be due to recent increased cocaine and other illicit drug use. The poisoning death rates for children 4 years and under has dropped since 1961, and this decrease is believed to be associated with child-proof medicine caps, safety locks for cabinets, and better labeling procedures (including procedures to take if a child ingests a poisonous substance) (National Safety Council, 1994).

Carbon monoxide fatalities also have decreased since 1984. Most deaths are the result of suicide, but many are accidental. The largest number of carbon monoxide fatalities occurred in the 15- to 24-year age group; males die three times as often as females of the same age. Most carbon monoxide deaths occurred in stationary motor vehicles, although fireplaces, stoves, and appliances using natural or liquid propane gas also were responsible

TABLE 21.3 Substances That Most Frequently Poison Children under 5

Rank	Substance
1.	Plants
2.	Soaps, detergents, cleaners
3.	Perfume, cologne, toilet water
4.	Antihistamines, cold medications
5.	Vitamins, minerals
6.	Aspirin
7.	Household disinfectants, deodorizers
8.	Insecticides
9.	Miscellaneous analgesics
10.	Miscellaneous internal medicines
11.	Fingernail preparations
12.	Liniments
13.	Household bleach
14.	Miscellaneous external medicines
15.	Cosmetic lotions, creams

Source: National Clearinghouse for Poison Control Centers.

for 10 percent of all unintentional carbon monoxide fatalities. Regulations that have lowered carbon monoxide emissions have contributed significantly to reducing the rates of unintentional carbon monoxide fatalities (National Safety Council, 1994).

Drowning

Drowning accounts for many unintentional injuries and fatalities in the home; young children are especially vulnerable. Young children can drown even in five-gallon buckets or in toilet bowls. Drownings were the fifth leading cause of deaths from unintentional injuries in 1993. Included are drownings from boating accidents, playing in water, swimming, falling into water, or even taking a bath. About half of all drownings occur during June, July, and August when many people are engaged in summer water activities. Recreation in large bodies of water, rivers, and streams provides the opportunities for accidental drowning (statistics exclude drowning from natural disasters, such as floods).

When a person is under water and inhales water instead of air, an automatic muscular contraction of the larynx occurs that is called **laryngospasm.** This muscular reflex closes the body's main airway in an attempt to keep water from entering the lungs. The spasm continues as long as the person is under water and within a few minutes can lead to death by suffocation. Once the laryngospasm relaxes, water enters the lungs. Only about 10 percent of people survive not breathing under water

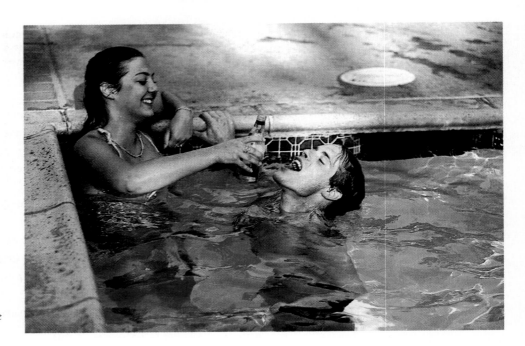

Many swimming accidents are associated with drinking alcohol while having fun in the water.

for as long as six minutes and these victims will survive only if artificial respiration is applied immediately. Few people recover if breathing has stopped for as long as ten minutes.

Scientific evidence does not support the widely held belief that swimming shortly after eating induces stomach cramps, thereby increasing the risk of drowning. However, it is true that after eating, blood is diverted to the stomach to assist digestion and consequently less oxygen may be available for muscles, which can lead to muscle spasms. This sequence poses no problem for a healthy person, but if a person is in poor health, is overweight, or has existing heart disease, the risk of drowning may be increased.

Knowing your swimming ability and avoiding swimming in dangerous waters are ways to reduce the risk of accidental drowning. Using a personal floatation device (commonly called a life-jacket) while you engage in water sports can also reduce the risk of drowning.

Alcohol and other drugs may be the biggest predisposing factor in drowning for individuals ages 15 or older. Impairment of the individual's judgment may lead to the death of others as well, for example, operating a boat with passengers while intoxicated or supervising children who are in or near the water while drinking.

Choking and Suffocation

Choking to death as a result of an object lodged in the airway passage occurs more often than one might expect. Each year in the United States several thousand people die because a piece of food or a foreign object became stuck in their throats and caused them to stop breathing.

Food that is swallowed without being chewed sufficiently is a common cause of choking and blockage of the air passage. Small bones from fish or chicken also can be swallowed inadvertently and become stuck in the airway. Sometimes dentures, fillings, or crowns become loose, are accidentally swallowed, and may cause the person to choke. Being intoxicated also increases the risk of swallowing improperly.

When the airway is completely blocked, a choking victim is unable to speak, breathe, or cough. A choking person often clutches his or her throat. If the object is not removed quickly, the victim may become unconscious and death can follow rapidly due to lack of oxygen.

Mechanical suffocation of young children is another type of unintentional injury occurring most frequently in the 0- to 4-year age group. A small child can get into tight spaces and become trapped or wedged, resulting in suffocation. As infants become more mobile and inquisitive, the risk of entrapment and suffocation increases. Long cords dangling from appliances, draperies, or blinds need to be placed well out of the way of a curious infant or toddler. Bulky bedding materials have been responsible for the suffocation of young children, especially fluffy comforters or infant bean bag cushions, and some household items such as the bean bag cushion have been recalled because of suffocation risks (Bever, 1992).

Prevention and education strategies reduce the risk of suffocation of young children. Eliminate products and access to dangerous areas in the house by using a safety gate or closing doors. Child-care providers should know what steps to take to prevent unintentional injuries of young children in the home.

Fires

Household fires rank sixth in causing unintentional injuries. Again, the very young (0- to 4-years of age) and the elderly (75 years and older) are at greatest risk of injury or fatality from fires and burns (excluding burns from hot objects or liquids). Fires in the home may be attributed to many factors: fireplaces, woodstoves, kerosene or space heaters, improper placement of appliances, faulty wiring of the house and/or appliances, grease fires in the kitchen (loose sleeves dangling over open flames), improper storage of combustible materials, or a careless smoker in the house (National Safety Council, 1994).

Death rates due to fires or burns have markedly decreased since the 1950s. Modern technology and fire detection devices have contributed significantly to this reduction. Smoke and fire detectors, portable ladders, and fire extinguishers have helped reduce fatalities. Also, many elementary school students are receiving annual training from local fire departments concerning fire safety and many children are now better prepared for escape when a fire occurs than many adults. Prevention and education are, once again, the best strategies to eliminate unintentional injuries from fires and burns in the home. Each household should have a planned escape route, smoke and fire detectors placed at key locations throughout the home, and posted emergency phone numbers. Everyone should know how to operate a fire extinguisher and know exactly where it is kept, and in two-story houses, a portable ladder should be readily accessible.

WORK SAFETY

Work-related unintentional injuries cost Americans approximately $111.9 billion in 1993, even though work-related injuries have declined 23 percent since 1984. In 1993 the death rate per 100,000 was 4, the lowest work-related death rate on record (National

Wellness Guide

Smoke Detectors Give You a Chance

Most deaths and injuries in fires result from inhalation of smoke and toxic gases that reach victims before the flames do. Survival depends on an early warning system that gives you time to vacate the premises at once. The best warning system available is a smoke detector.

According to *Consumer Reports,* installation of a smoke detector in your home cuts in half your risk of dying in a fire. The U.S. Consumer Product Safety Commission offers these suggestions about smoke detectors:

- Many localities require that you have a smoke detector in your home, so buy one—at least one. They're inexpensive and are available at most hardware stores and supermarkets. Check your local codes and regulations; they may require you to purchase a specific kind.

- Read the instructions that come with the detector for advice on where to install it. You should purchase at least one for every floor in your house. Preferably you should place one outside every bedroom.

- Manufacturers know what is best for their products and tell you how to care for them. Follow their instructions. Detectors can save lives, but only if you install and maintain them properly.

- Never disconnect a fire detector. If it goes off at wrong times because of heat from a stove or steam from a bathroom, move it to another location.

- Replace the battery annually (January 1 is an easy day to remember) or when you hear a "chirping" sound. (*Consumer Reports* estimates that one-third of all detectors would not respond to a fire because of dead or missing batteries.) And press the test button regularly to be sure the batteries work.

- Keep your detector clean. Dust, grease or other materials can interfere with efficient operation. You may want to vacuum the grill work on the detector.

Source: Safety and Health (Itasca, Ill.: National Safety Council, February, 1995).

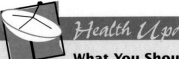
What You Should Know about Fire Extinguishers

A fire extinguisher is a valuable home-safety tool—if you know how to use it and maintain it, says Norbert Makowka, technical director for the National Association of Fire Equipment.

Check your extinguishers once a month to make sure the pressure is within the fully charged margin on the gauge. If your extinguisher is rusting or corroded, get a new one. Typically, nonrechargeable extinguishers last for 12 years. You should service rechargeable extinguishers after six years. The contents of your typical home fire extinguisher discharge in approximately 8-10 seconds.

The most common home extinguishers use dry chemicals, such as sodium bicarbonate, to suffocate blazes. They are usually rated *ABC* or *BC*. The *A* rating is suitable to douse fires that involve household materials, such as wood, paper and cloth. The *B* rating is for flammable liquids, such as grease and gasoline. The *C* rating means that you can use the extinguisher in an energized electrical current fire without causing a short.

Keep extinguishers in the kitchen, utility room, the garage, and near fireplaces. Makowka stresses that an extinguisher is not a substitute for calling the fire department. Before you fight a blaze, get everyone else out of the building. Call firefighters for help and make sure you keep your back to an accessible exit. If you're with someone, one person can use an extinguisher while the other person makes the phone call. It is important for the fire department to inspect your home after any fire, even though the flames may appear to be out. Fires can smolder in walls and furniture and ignite later. If you have the slightest doubt about whether to fight a small fire—don't. Get out!

The acronym PASS might help you remember how to use a fire extinguisher:

P—Pull the pin that acts as a safety.

A—Aim at the base of the flame.

S—Squeeze the handle.

S—Sweep back and forth.

Source: Family Safety and Health (Itasca, Ill.: National Safety Council, Fall, 1993).

Safety Council, 1994). Nearly half of all fatal occupational injuries in 1992 were to those aged 25 to 44. Injuries to the back are the most frequent, followed by those of legs, arms, and trunk (Figure 21.4).

A recent phenomenon of work-related injury and illness is **sick building syndrome**, a variety of symptoms reported by workers in modern office buildings. Recent investigations have found a correlation between pollutants in or near the building or a poor ventilation system and sick building syndrome. Much of the evidence of these symptoms is self-reported by the workers or documented by physicians. Symptoms include asthma, lung infections, dizziness, nausea, throat and eye irritations, fatigue, cough, and shortness of breath (Figure 21.5). Based on limited research to date on sick building syndrome, ventilation alone was not a significant factor. Possibly the combination of the ventilation system and

T E R M S

sick building syndrome: collection of symptoms reported by workers in some modern buildings

cumulative trauma disorders: disorders caused by repeated stress to a body part; carpal tunnel syndrome is considered a cumulative trauma disorder

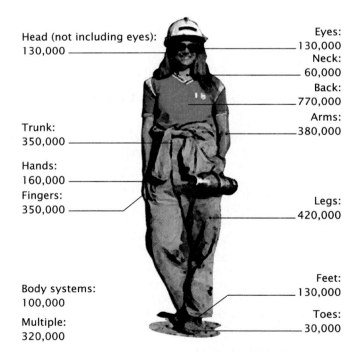

Head (not including eyes): 130,000
Eyes: 130,000
Neck: 60,000
Back: 770,000
Arms: 380,000
Trunk: 350,000
Hands: 160,000
Fingers: 350,000
Legs: 420,000
Body systems: 100,000
Multiple: 320,000
Feet: 130,000
Toes: 30,000

FIGURE 21.4 Parts of Body Where Work-Related Injuries Occur The majority of injuries occur to the back, with the least number of injuries occurring to the toes.
Source: Adapted from *Accident Facts, 1994,* National Safety Council.

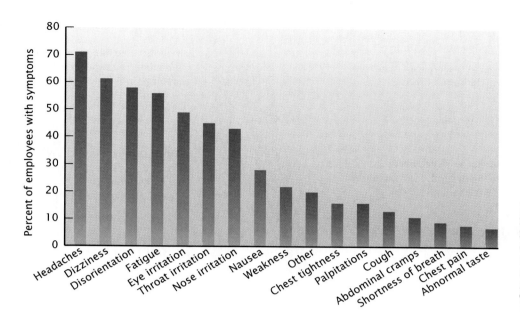

FIGURE 21.5 Most Common Sick Building Syndrome Symptoms Headaches and dizziness account for most of reported sick building syndrome symptoms.
Source: Accident Facts, 1994 Edition (Itasca, Ill.: National Safety Council, 1994).

volatile organic substances used in many new building products may be the determinants (National Safety Council, 1994).

The overall incidence rate for occupational illnesses and injuries is 59.8 per 100,000. In 1992, manufacturing industries had the highest rate of 165 per 100,000. Agriculture had the second highest rate, 61.7 per 100,000. Agriculture had the highest incidence of skin diseases, which may be attributed to agricultural workers' close contact with many chemicals. Common occupational illnesses include skin disorders, respiratory conditions due to inhalation of toxic substances, disorders

associated with repeated trauma, poisonings, and dust-related diseases of the lungs. These incidence rates are suspected to be actually higher than reported, as many workers do not seek medical attention for their illnesses and/or injuries (National Safety Council, 1994).

Carpal tunnel syndrome is one of a group of injuries known as **cumulative trauma disorders,** caused by repeated stress of a body part resulting from repetitive motion for long periods (Figure 21.6). Symptoms of carpal tunnel syndrome are burning, numbness, tingling, and stiffness of the hand, fingers, or wrist. Dentists, dental hygienists, supermarket cashiers, seamstresses, musicians, factory workers, computer keyboard operators, and surgeons are at risk for carpal tunnel syndrome. Better product design, correct positioning of the operator and the tool, and limiting time spent at the same task are being investigated as possible solutions to the rising incidence of cumulative trauma disorders (National Safety Council, 1994).

HEALTHY PEOPLE 2000

Reduce cumulative trauma disorders to an incidence of no more than 60 cases per 100,000 full-time workers.

Cumulative trauma disorders result from repetitive motion, repeated pressure, or repeated exposure to noise. Repetitive motion may lead to disorders such as carpal tunnel syndrome, tendonitis, ganglionitis, tenosynovistis, bursitis, and epicondylitis. Repetitive wrist flexing or arm-wrist-finger movement may lead to damage of the muscles, tendons, and ligaments in the wrist that becomes noticeable only after months or years of routine work. Carpal tunnel syndrome and other cumulative trauma disorders affecting the wrist are often associated with work on the assembly lines, such as in the automotive, electronics, and meat processing industries. It also affects musicians, waitresses, and office workers.

FIRST AID AND EMERGENCIES

First aid and medical emergencies can be handled appropriately if you take a deep breath and tell yourself you can handle the situation until a qualified medical professional arrives to take over. First aid is defined as the immediate care given to an injured or ill person. First aid is temporary assistance given until a person has recovered or until a qualified medical person can provide assistance.

Knowledge about first aid and medical emergencies can literally mean the difference between life, death, disability, or permanent injury. Knowledge of first aid skills

Cervical radiculopathy: People who look up to a computer screen or who balance a phone on their shoulder are at risk.

Thoracic outlet syndrome: Violinists and other musicians are at risk.

Pronator syndrome: Mechanics, baseball pitchers, and barbers are at risk.

Cubital tunnel syndrome: Truck drivers or other persons who keep their arms in fixed, flexed positions are at risk.

Carpal tunnel syndrome: Typists, computer programmers, and potters are at risk.

FIGURE 21.6 Cumulative Trauma Injuries Cumulative trauma injuries affect muscles, tendons, and nerves.

Distal ulnar neuropathy: Meat packers, assembly-line workers, and machine operators are at risk.

will increase your confidence in dealing with both minor and major emergencies, and be reassuring to an injured person.

TAKING RISKS AND PREVENTING ACCIDENTS

Risks cannot be avoided in life; accidents and injuries are a consequence of the risks we take. As soon as a child learns to crawl, he or she begins to take risks to explore and understand the environment. At each stage of life we take risks to learn and to expand our capabilities and experiences. We take a risk when we cross the street in traffic, run to catch a bus, or swing from the branch of a tree. When we go hiking, climbing, or engage in sport activities, we are taking risks.

The important question YOU need to ask is: "What risks are necessary and acceptable for me to live the way I want to?" The answer will also, to some extent, determine your risk of unintentional injury. People differ enormously in their need for risk-taking behaviors. Some people thrive on high-risk endeavors, such as

Health Update

Legal Aspects of First Aid

- No one is duty bound to act by giving aid when no legal duty to do so exists.
- You do have a duty to administer first aid when there is a pre-existing contractual relationship (e.g., parent-child, teacher-student, driver-passenger, and so forth).
- If you do choose to administer first aid, obtain the victim's oral, informed consent prior to giving care, or risk possible charges of technical assault. Consent will be implied if the victim is unconscious.

- Once you begin to administer first aid, you cannot legally stop; you must not abandon the victim after administering first aid until competent or professional help arrives.
- When oral consent to receive first aid is refused by a conscious, rational adult victim, you may not give care. For your own protection, however, attempt to document the interaction and obtain the victim's signature.
- A few states offer protection to the first aid provider under a

Good Samaritan law which protects those acting in good faith, without gross negligence, or willful misconduct. Some legal experts believe this law may create a false sense of security for the person administering first aid.

Source: S. F. Smith and C. M. Smith, *Personal Health Choices.* Boston: Jones and Bartlett, 1990.

playing polo, racing cars, or climbing mountains. However, even people who live more sedate lives may be at risk for unintentional injuries because of destructive behaviors or unhealthy mental attitudes.

Whatever your personal beliefs, a commitment to safe living can be made at any time. Why not make the commitment now? Eliminating or reducing the use of alcohol can reduce the risk of many kinds of injuries, especially motor vehicle accidents. Lowering your stress level will also contribute significantly to reducing unintentional injuries. Not keeping a loaded firearm in the house can eliminate the risk of an unintentional firearm injury. Reading and following the manufacturer's instructions and warnings before operating a new product will

> *God does not play dice.*
> Albert Einstein

also help to reduce the risk of unintentional injury. Before undertaking any sport activity, climbing a ladder, or riding a bike, take a moment to consider essential safety measures. Observe posted safety rules and warning signs. Keep in good physical condition and have a positive mental attitude when undertaking a potentially dangerous activity.

Although unintentional injuries are usually not a laughing matter, one accident statistic does sound a humorous note. Saturday and Sunday are the two most dangerous days of the week for fatal accidents. Going out on the weekends just to have fun increases the risks of serious injuries. Maybe studying or reading on weekends is a good idea after all.

HEALTH IN REVIEW

- Accidents cause many injuries and deaths each year, and cost Americans billions of dollars in medical costs as well as costs due to loss of work. Accidents are preventable!
- Many factors contribute to unintentional injuries: knowledge, attitudes, beliefs, and behaviors; economic and social factors; competence; environmental conditions; and alcohol and other drugs.
- The Haddon Matrix was developed to assess motor vehicle risk factors and is used to develop prevention programs.
- A multidimensional approach to injury prevention includes education, prevention strategies, stricter laws and regulations, and better product design.
- Motor vehicle deaths are decreasing; however, almost $200 billion are spent each year on insurance claims and property damage. Over 45 percent of all motor

vehicle fatalities involve an alcohol-impaired or intoxicated driver or nonmotorist.
- Pedestrian and bicycle safety rules and equipment are keys to preventing accidents. Wear reflective clothing and obey the rules of the road.
- Safety in the home includes preventing falls, poisonings, drownings, choking, and fires.
- Work-related injuries have decreased since 1984; however, they still cost employers and employees large amounts of time and money. Injuries to the back are most frequent, followed by legs, arms, and trunk. Proper work safety procedures can prevent the majority of work-related injuries.
- Accidents and injuries are a consequence of the many risks we take. Although most of what we do has some degree of risk, we can decrease that risk by increasing safety knowledge and taking the necessary precautions.

REFERENCES

Accident Facts, 1994 Edition. Itasca, Ill.: National Safety Council.

Accident Facts Up-to-Date (April 1995). Itasca, Ill.: National Safety Council.

Bever, D. L. (1992). *Safety: A Personal Focus.* St. Louis, Mo.: Mosby-Year Book.

Family Safety and Health (Fall 1993). Itasca, Ill.: National Safety Council.

Lawson, D. C. (1992). *Wellness: Safety and Accident Prevention.* Guilford, Conn.: The Dushkin Publishing Group.

Safety and Health (February, 1995). "Smoke Detectors Give You a Chance." Itasca, Ill.: National Safety Council.

SUGGESTED READINGS

Baker, S. P., B. O'Neill, M. J. Ginsburg, and G. Li (1992). *The Injury Fact Book,* 2nd edition. New York: Oxford University Press. More facts than you need to know about all kinds of accidental injuries.

Graham, J. D. (1993). "Injuries from Traffic Crashes: Meeting the Challenge." *Annual Review of Public Health,* 14: 515–543. Discusses ways to further reduce traffic fatalities.

Lescohier, I., S. S. Gallagher, and B. Guyer (1990). "Not by Accident." *Issues in Science and Technology,* Summer. Explains why most accidental injuries and deaths are largely preventable.

Thygerson, A. (1989). *First Aid Essentials.* Boston: Jones and Bartlett. Provides clear and concise instructions for responding to a wide variety of injuries. Endorsed by the National Safety Council.

Turkington, C. (1994). *Poisons and Antidotes.* New York: Facts on File. Describes more than 600 toxic substances, symptoms, and treatments for poisoning.

Overcoming Obstacles

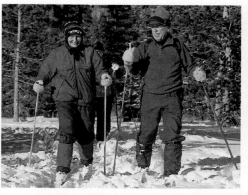

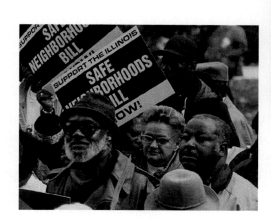

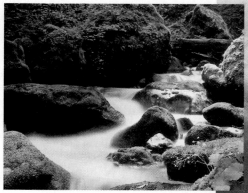

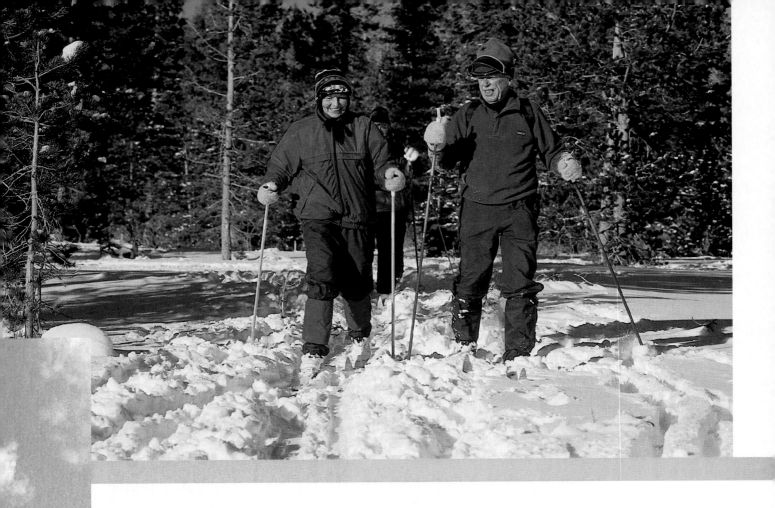

LEARNING OBJECTIVES

After reading this chapter you should be able to:

1. Describe some biological changes that occur with aging.
2. Define aging, maximum life span, average life span, life expectancy, ageism, and gerontology.
3. Discuss some of the implications of the average increase in age of the U.S. population.
4. Briefly explain two theories of aging.
5. Discuss the impact of undernutrition on the aging process.
6. Compare and contrast Alzheimer's disease and senile dementia.
7. Describe several ways to help prevent osteoporosis.
8. Identify the stages of dying as defined by Elizabeth Kubler-Ross.
9. Discuss the implications of active euthanasia.

Understanding Aging and Dying

For centuries people have tried to slow down aging and to postpone the inevitability of death. Almost everything has been tried, from magic spells to modern drugs. In the sixteenth century, Spanish explorer Ponce de Leon sought a legendary "fountain of youth," which was supposed to restore the health and youth of anyone who drank its waters. Today some people try to cheat death by having their bodies frozen immediately after dying in the hope that they can be revived and returned to health sometime in the future when science has learned how to cure all diseases and prevent aging.

Everything in the universe—plants, animals, mountains, planets, and stars—change over time and eventually die (plants and animals) or disintegrate and disappear (planets and stars). Our planet is aging in the sense that its resources are being used up and the environment is changing. The nuclear reactions that fuel the sun will eventually slow down, and the sun is expected to explode about five billion years from now.

Many people associate aging with sickness, disability, loneliness, and increased inactivity. However, such negative views of aging are false; many older persons today are sexually and physically active and continue to work well into their 80s or even 90s. George Burns, comedian and movie star, performed on stage and in movies until he was nearly 100 years old.

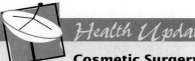
Cosmetic Surgery to Hide the Effects of Aging

Some people worry about wrinkles as they get older. The cosmetic surgery industry does a booming business removing wrinkles and other skin flaws from the face. Here are some of the more popular procedures.

Facelift Under general anesthesia, incisions are made along the hairline, along the temples and around the ears, and down into the lower back scalp. Tissue and fat are removed from the neck and the skin is pulled tight and sewn back into place. A facelift may last five to seven years. Infections and hematomas (blood under the skin) are possible side effects.

Blepharoplasty (eyelid surgery) This is used to remove eyelid wrinkles and bags under the eyes. An incision is made on the upper and/or lower eyelids. Excess skin and tissues are removed and the incision is sutured. Swelling and bruising persist for several weeks and a long-term possible complication is inability to close the upper eyelid completely for up to a year.

Chemical Peel Surgery that removes wrinkles around the mouth, forehead, and eyes. A chemical solution is applied on the skin, destroying the top layer. New skin appears after several weeks. This process risks infection or scarring and sometimes the pigmentation of the new skin is different from the old skin.

In America, negative views about aging are still prominent in movies, television, and especially in advertising. The ideal American is portrayed as eternally young, active, attractive, and wrinkle-free. Advertisements exhort people to retard the noticeable signs of aging by using face and body creams that restore youth, dyes for the hair, special herbs or vitamins that stop aging, or by resorting to various kinds of cosmetic surgery.

The normal processes of aging are not caused by disease, so aging cannot be cured. The noticeable effects of aging result from wear and tear on essential functions in the body that change and become less efficient over the years. Even the healthiest body wears out slowly. However, by developing healthy habits while young and by understanding the aging processes, one can remain vigorous and healthy until the very end of life.

AMERICA'S AGING POPULATION

Aging refers to the normal changes in body functions that occur after sexual maturity and continue until death. In an idealized situation, everyone would survive close to the **maximum life span** for the species; for human beings maximum longevity is about 110 to 115 years (for mice maximum longevity is only about two years) (Figure 22.1). The **average life span** is defined as the age at which half of the members of a population have died. Insurance companies use data based on actual populations to determine what insurance premiums are necessary to pay survivor benefits. **Life expectancy** is the average length of time that members of a population

Many elderly people continue to enjoy work long after the "normal" retirement age.

T E R M S

aging: normal changes in body functions that begin after sexual maturity and continue until death

maximum life span: the theoretical maximum number of years that individuals of a species can live

average life span: the age at which half the members of a population have died

life expectancy: average number of years a person can expect to live

ageism: prejudice against older people

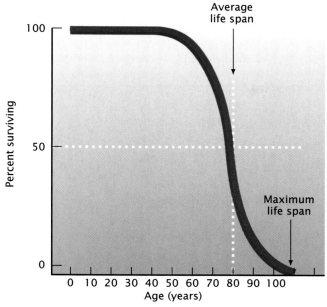

FIGURE 22.1 Survival as a Function of Years in an Idealized Aging Human Population

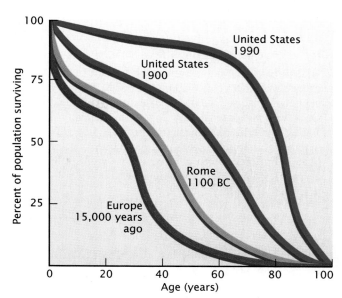

FIGURE 22.2 Approximate Survival Curves for Various Populations The U.S. population is beginning to approximate the idealized curve.

can expect to live. The average life expectancy at birth increased by almost two years during the past decade and is now 75.7 years of age. Males born in 1991 can expect to live 72.2 years, and females, 79.1 years. In 1900, life expectancy was only 46.3 years for men and 48.2 years for women.

Because of disease, accidents, and other factors, populations in the real world do not survive according to the idealized situation but have followed various curves throughout history (Figure 22.2). The average U.S. life span has increased dramatically in the last century. Because of this increase in the average life span, the U.S. population is becoming increasingly older. By the year 2040 it is estimated that there will be approximately 70 million Americans over age 65 and 12 million over age 85 (Figure 22.3).

This "graying" of America will create a broad range of social, medical, and economic problems. First and most important is the ability of the federal government to sustain Social Security payments. At the present rate, the government has estimated that the Social Security system will run out of money within ten to twenty years. To avoid this, Congress has begun to discuss ways to reform Social Security so that future retirees will receive some benefits. Another problem is the extra medical care required by this group of older people. Although many older people are vigorous and healthy, a large number of people over 65 have chronic illnesses and disabilities that require ongoing medical care and some need expensive, long-term care. The costs of health care for the elderly are going to rise in the years ahead. These rising costs will be a burden to the government and the general public, which is why there is an urgent need for health care reform (Chapter 19).

Age-related prejudice is called **ageism**, systematic stereotyping and discrimination against people because they are old (just as racism and sexism is discrimination based on race and gender). Ageism is based on the misconceptions that older people cannot work efficiently,

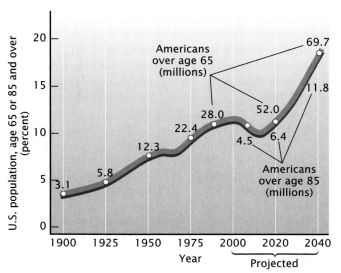

FIGURE 22.3 Percentage of the American Population Age 65 and Older from 1900 to 1984, with Projected Percentages over Age 65 and over Age 85 to the Year 2040
Source: Social Security Area Projections, Actuarial Study No. 102, 1988.

TABLE 22.1 Life Expectancy for Men and Women in Various Countries Countries at the top of the list have populations that may be approaching the maximum average human life expectancy. Life expectancy in poor, undeveloped countries still is not much more than 50 years.

Country	Life expectancy at birth	
	Female	Male
Japan	82	77
Iceland	81	76
Spain	82	75
France	84	72
Italy	81	74
Australia	80	74
United Kingdom	79	73
United States	79	72
Mexico	76	69
China	72	69
Brazil	68	62
Iran	66	64
Bangladesh	55	54
Haiti	55	53
Guinea	48	45
Afghanistan	45	43

Source: World Almanac, 1994. Rank is based on sum of male and female life expectancy.

are sickly, and are mentally less competent than younger people. Older people are asserting themselves more and demanding the same opportunities for work as younger people.

HOW LONG CAN HUMAN BEINGS LIVE?

Some experts in **gerontology** (the science that studies the causes and mechanisms of aging) believe that populations in many countries are approaching the current maximum average life span, estimated at 85-90 years, although a few exceptional individuals may live longer. One bit of evidence for a maximum average life span of 85 to 90 years comes from government estimates that show differences in the life expectancies of people in their countries (Table 22.1). Japan tops the list with an average life expectancy of 82.4 years for Japanese women. Two other small countries, Iceland and Italy, with vastly different cultures and climates, are also close to the top of the list. At the bottom are countries where life expectancy is still less than 50 years.

Americans' life expectancy is about three years less for women and five years less for men compared with Japan. This difference is primarily due to the lower life expectancy of African-American women (75.6 years) and African-American men (67.8 years). The United States also has about twice the infant mortality rate as Japan.

Another line of evidence suggests that the maximum average life span cannot be increased significantly above 85 to 90 years of age. Statistical studies can estimate how much average human life expectancy would increase if major diseases were eliminated. For example, if *all* cancers could be cured or prevented, only about three years of life would be added to the average baby born today. If *all* heart disease was eliminated, average life expectancy at birth would increase by about fourteen years

> *Every man desires to live long; but no man would be old.*
> Jonathan Swift

(Hayflick, 1994). Even with remarkable (and unexpected) breakthroughs in medical care, most people still would die under 100 years of age.

A slightly different picture of aging emerges from studies of people between the ages of 85 to 100—a group known as the "oldest old." Statistical studies of oldest old Scandinavians suggest that, in the absence of disease, senescent death (death due to old age) could occur as late as 110 years of age (Barinaga, 1991). However, whether the maximum life expectancy for most people in the absence of disease is 85, 100, or 110 years, nobody is going to live to be as old as Methuselah, the biblical patriarch who lived for 967 years.

T E R M S

gerontology: science that studies the causes and mechanisms of aging

specific metabolic rate: the amount of energy per gram of body weight consumed per day by mammals of different species

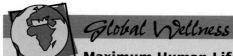
Maximum Human Life Span in Pakistan

The Hunza people live in a remote mountain region of Pakistan and have been romanticized for years as a population whose members routinely live to be 100 years or older. However, in a recent visit to the region an investigative reporter found the myth of Hunza longevity to be just that—a myth (Tierney, 1990). Hunzas have an exceptionally high rate of infant mortality, and many suffer from mental retardation, goiter, and dwarfism due to iodine deficiency in the diet. Medical researchers in Pakistan who studied the Hunzas found that their average life expectancy was about 60 years, although some Hunzas claimed to be over 100 years old. Birth certificates do not exist in the region, so it is difficult to document anyone's age. At present, there is no living person whose age can be proved to be more than 110 to 115 years.

THEORIES OF AGING

Biological Clocks Regulate Aging

Theories of aging fall into two categories. One ascribes aging to biological and genetic mechanisms that are specific for each species of animal and determine its maximum life span and rate of aging. The other category focuses on environmental factors that affect aging, such as nutrition, susceptibility to diseases, and exercise. Evidence for a "biological clock" that determines the maximum life span comes from measuring the amount of energy per gram of body weight consumed per day by mammals of different species. This energy consumption per day, called the **specific metabolic rate,** shows a striking correlation with the maximum life span of different species (Figure 22.4). Mammals that have the highest specific metabolic rate have the shortest life span; human beings have the slowest metabolic rate and the longest life span.

Further evidence for a biological clock related to aging comes from studying cell growth in the laboratory. Conditions have been established in which cells from various tissues of different animals can be grown under fixed laboratory conditions. The surprising result of these experiments is that cells grow and divide in a laboratory medium for a fixed number of generations and then die (Hayflick, 1994). The number of generations of

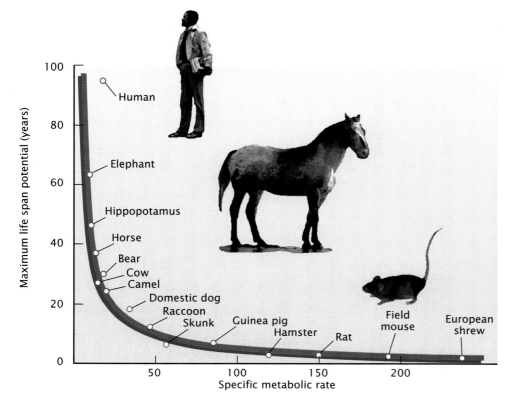

FIGURE 22.4 Correlation between the Rate of Energy Consumed (per Gram of Body Weight per Day) and the Maximum Life Span Potential of Different Species of Mammals The correlation suggests that the maximum human life span is a function of human biology and ultimately of human genes.

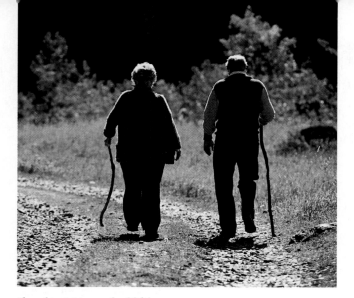
Shared activities are healthful at any age.

Another effect of exposure to radiation and chemicals is the production of very reactive molecules in cells called free radicals (Chapter 14). These substances are normally inactivated in cells, but as we age our cells may be less able to cope with the damaging effects of free radicals (Stadtman, 1992). In addition, the immune system's functions become less efficient with age so that we become more susceptible to infections and autoimmune diseases. Overall, aging is a complicated process more than likely brought on by a combination of genetic and environmental factors.

Does Undernutrition Slow Aging?

A recurrent idea about aging is that it can be slowed by staying as lean as possible. This notion is not true and is one of the myths disproved by the findings of the Baltimore Longitudinal Study of Aging that has been ongoing since 1958. However, there is a large body of evidence from experimental laboratory animals that **undernutrition** does allow them to live longer (Raloff, 1992). Laboratory rats and mice on restricted calorie diets live longer than animals that are allowed to eat as much as they want. Undernutrition does not mean malnutrition; the animals are not starved or deprived of essential nutrients, but are restricted in the amount of food that they are provided. Repeated studies show that calorie-restricted laboratory animals invariably live longer.

One criticism of these experiments is that laboratory animals are not typical of animals in nature. It is likely that rats and mice in nature often have difficulty finding food and have restricted diets. We really do not know how long mice and rats live in nature and it may be that the undernourished experimental animals are merely living as long as their brothers and sisters in nature.

One respected researcher on aging, Roy L. Walford, has been studying the effects of undernutrition on aging for many years (Weindruch and Walford, 1989). In 1987, he became convinced that the effects of undernutrition were so real and important that he chose to be the subject of his own experiment. Since then he has been living on a calorie-restricted diet. If Walford lives to be 80 or 90 years old, nothing will be proved because many

growth is related to the maximum life span of the animal from which the cells were taken. Mouse cells only divide a few times, but human cells divide many times before dying. The inescapable conclusion from these experiments is that built into the cells of every animal is a genetically controlled clock that determines how many times cells can grow and divide before a signal tells them to stop.

A distinguishing feature of cancer cells is that they are immortal when grown under the same laboratory conditions used for growing normal cells. Cancer cells grow and divide indefinitely; cells taken from human tumors more than 30 years ago are still kept growing in the laboratory. Thus, cancer cells have lost the ability to regulate normal growth and aging both in people and in the laboratory (Chapter 13). As a result of these experiments, researchers on aging are searching for the genes that control the aging processes (Horgan, 1992). Perhaps in the future therapeutic manipulation of aging genes will slow the aging processes.

> *How old would you be if you didn't know how old you was?*
> Satchel Paige,
> baseball pitcher

Environmental Factors Affect Aging

Although genetic factors contribute to aging, environmental factors also play a role. The longer we live, the more we are exposed to radiation and chemicals that can damage DNA in cells and, over time, may cause the death of essential cells in the body. For example, most cells possess enzymes that repair damage to their DNA; loss of these cellular repair enzymes with age could lead to widespread cell death. This has been called the "error catastrophe" theory of aging. Accumulated mutations in cells may be responsible for development of cancer and also for aging changes.

T E R M S

undernutrition: restricting the daily caloric intake of an animal or person without causing malnutrition

senile dementia: loss of cognitive functions in elderly people

Alzheimer's disease: a common cause of senile dementia and other symptoms, eventually leading to death

amyloid protein: accumulation of an abnormal protein in the brain of patients with Alzheimer's disease

Some Facts about Biological Changes That Occur with Aging

The Baltimore Longitudinal Study of Aging (BLSA) has been going on since 1958. The goal of this study is to measure physical, mental, and emotional changes in healthy people as they become older. Some of the findings of the BLSA are:

- **Height**   Persons of both sexes lose about one-sixteenth of an inch in height each year beginning around age 30.
- **Teeth**   Cavities and gum disease increase with age.

- **Weight**   Weight increases until about age 55 and then begins to fall. Longevity does not favor the very lean person, but is greatest for those in the middle or slightly above the "ideal" weight category in life insurance tables.
- **Cognitive changes**   Most loss occurs after age 70 in short-term memory and ability to solve logic and verbal problems.
- **Personality**   In the absence of disease, no changes in personality

are observed.
- **Sexual activity**   Activity decreases with age even if the level of sex hormones does not decrease appreciably.
- **Strength**   Physical activity and maximum exercise performance decrease with age.
- **Senses**   There is loss of visual acuity, hearing, and smell. The ability to taste sweet and sour does not change.

---

people live to this age. But if he lives to the maximum age of 115 years, he may have proved his point. However, few people will elect to live their lives in a perpetual state of caloric undernutrition.

ALZHEIMER'S DISEASE AND SENILE DEMENTIA

In the absence of disease, normal mental functions can be maintained to age 100 or longer. However, approximately 20 percent of people over age 85 have some loss of normal cognitive functions that are readily determined by asking a few simple questions. The medical term for impairment or loss of mental functions in elderly people

is **senile dementia.** Many diseases and conditions can result in senile dementia but the most common cause is **Alzheimer's disease**, which is characterized by memory loss, reduced ability to use language, losses in perception and problem-solving abilities, and reduced mobility. Ultimately, Alzheimer's disease causes death.

The disease is named for Alois Alzheimer, a German physician who in 1907 described the abnormal brain structures he observed under the microscope in tissues obtained from patients who died from senile dementia. Alzheimer's findings at autopsy revealed what are still the diagnostic criteria for the disease: 1) the presence of bundles of tangled nerve fibrils in certain areas of the brain; and 2) the presence of a specific protein called the **amyloid protein,** which is localized in certain areas and

Exploring Your Health

A Simple Test for Loss of Cognitive Functions

Forgetting a person's name or an appointment is not a sign that you are "losing your mind." Loss of cognitive functions due to disease or injury can prevent a person from answering even simple questions.

Below is a simple test to determine loss of some cognitive functions. Score 1 point for each correct answer. Most older persons score at least 17 points.

	Total points
▪ Name the season, year, date, month, and day.	5
▪ Name three objects that you see.	3
▪ Name the last five letters of the alphabet backwards.	5
▪ Repeat the sentence: "No ifs, ands, or buts."	3
▪ Repeat the three objects that you mentioned before.	3

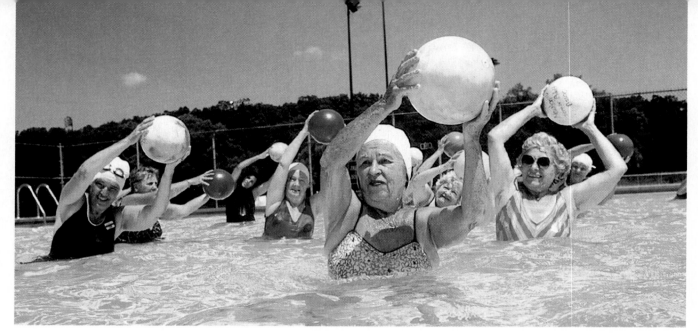

Water exercises can be enjoyed by people who may find other activities too strenuous.

blood vessels of the brain. How all these changes affect the brain to produce loss of cognitive functions is still not understood.

No definitive cause for Alzheimer's disease is known, although it seems to develop as a result of both genetic and environmental factors. In some families, Alzheimer's disease occurs over several generations and family members often die at an early age. In these families inherited genes must contribute to disease susceptibility. However, Alzheimer's disease also occurs in individuals whose families have never had a prior case. Most cases of Alzheimer's disease fall into this category and probably are due to unknown environmental factors.

At present, no cure or effective treatment for Alzheimer's disease exists. The care of a person with Alzheimer's disease is arduous, stressful, and financially draining. Patients usually are placed in long-term care facilities; about one-fourth of all patients in nursing homes suffer from Alzheimer's disease. As the American population grows older in the future, the number of Alzheimer patients will also increase.

Researchers have discovered at least four genes so far that contribute to the development of Alzheimer's disease. Understanding how these genes function in causing abnormal brain functions may provide clues to developing drugs to combat the development of the disease (Freundlich, 1993). Also, simple chemical tests are being developed that can tell if a person has Alzheimer's disease while it is still in its early stages, although nothing can be done now to slow the progression of the disease.

Health Update

First Alzheimer's Drug Approved

The first drug specifically for treating symptoms of Alzheimer's disease was approved by the FDA in September 1993. The drug is Cognex (tacrine hydrochloride).

Alzheimer's disease, which affects an estimated 4 million Americans, causes progressive loss of memory, judgment, and ability to reason.

In two controlled trials, Cognex provided a small but clinically meaningful benefit for some patients with mild to moderate Alzheimer's disease. The trials showed that the drug is superior to a placebo, based on results of tests designed to assess memory and reasoning ability, and on an overall assessment of function by a trained clinician.

Cognex can cause mild liver toxicity that is reversible if treatment is withdrawn promptly. The drug's labeling recommends an escalating dosing regimen with frequent blood tests to identify patients sensitive to the drug. Patients who have mild liver toxicity can often continue taking a lower dose, or stop and then resume therapy at a lower dose. Other side effects include nausea, vomiting, diarrhea, and rash.

Source: FDA Consumer (November, 1993).

A curious fact concerning Alzheimer's disease may be of particular interest to students. Many epidemiological studies in the United States and Europe show that people with more education are much less likely to develop Alzheimer's disease than are people with little or no education (Schardt, 1994). The reason is unclear. It could be that "mental exercise" is good for the brain, just as physical exercise is good for the body. Or it may be that uneducated people are more likely to be poor and, as a consequence, have a poor diet and smoke more cigarettes. However, the message of these studies is clear: Don't drop out of school.

OSTEOPOROSIS

The bone density that we build up during our growing years is important in later life to prevent life-threatening fractures. **Osteoporosis** is a condition in older persons, particularly women, that results from loss of bone material, causing bones to become thin, porous, and brittle. The brittleness of bones make them extremely vulnerable to fractures with even a minimal amount of stress. Fracture of the hip is the most frequent result of osteoporosis and approximately one quarter of older people who suffer a hip fracture die within six months (Mundy, 1994).

Osteoporosis affects 20 to 25 million women in the United States over age 45 and is responsible for 1.5 million bone fractures each year. Medical costs related to caring for people with bone fractures due to osteoporosis amount to $10 billion each year and will rise sharply as the American population ages.

Osteoporosis occurs because the rate of bone breakdown exceeds the rate of bone renewal; many factors contribute to this. In older women, estrogen loss due to menopause contributes to loss of bone material. In both older men and women, aging results in bone loss and increases the risk of fracture depending on how much bone mass is reduced (Figure 22.5). Generally, the bone loss in women due to low estrogen levels following menopause is significantly greater than the bone loss due to normal aging processes.

The risk of osteoporosis in older women can be lessened by replacing the lost hormone with **estrogen replacement therapy (ERT)**. For most women ERT is

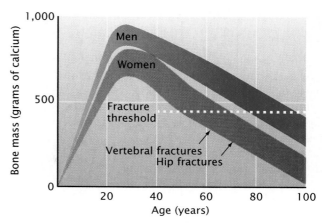

FIGURE 22.5 Changes in Bone Mass in Men and Women That Occur with Age The risk of bone fracture due to osteoporosis occurs when bone mass falls below a theoretical threshold and even a slight strain can cause a fracture.

beneficial because it reduces the risk of osteoporosis (and heart disease, to some degree) but for other women ERT may increase the risk of breast and uterine cancer. Thus, the use of ERT must be carefully weighed by each post-menopausal woman. Women whose families have a history of breast cancer or blood clotting problems are not good risks for estrogen supplementation.

The best way to avoid osteoporosis is to build up as much bone mass as possible while young through calcium consumption and exercise. After maturity, calcium is still needed to maintain bone density. Nearly half of all Americans do not consume enough calcium to maintain bone mass. Consuming at least a gram of calcium a day throughout life can reduce the risk of osteoporosis and bone fractures later in life. In addition, adequate vitamin D in the diet is essential in the assimilation of calcium. The best sources of calcium are dairy products and green vegetables. Calcium also can be obtained in supplements such as calcium lactate or calcium citrate.

Exercise, especially weightlifting, running, hiking, and walking briskly, reduces the risk of osteoporosis because bone is renewed with exercise. A sedentary lifestyle contributes to the risk of osteoporosis. Regular exercise throughout life will help keep bones strong and prevent fractures later. Not smoking and not consuming alcohol excessively also help prevent osteoporosis.

Some people are genetically more susceptible to osteoporosis than others. Some people, because of an inherited gene that produces the vitamin D receptor protein, are more efficient in utilizing vitamin D and calcium. These people are at lower risk for osteoporosis than those who have inherited a different form of the vitamin D receptor protein gene. Regardless of one's vitamin D receptor gene, adequate calcium in the diet and regular exercise are the keys to preventing osteoporosis.

T E R M S

osteoporosis: a condition in older people, particularly women, in which bones lose density and become porous and brittle

estrogen replacement therapy (ERT): administration of estrogen to menopausal and postmenopausal women to help prevent symptoms of menopause, osteoporosis, and heart disease

FEAR OF AGING AND DYING

Nobody wants to grow old or die. When we are young, we never think about becoming old, nor can we imagine what it is like not to be strong, vigorous, and active. With few exceptions, the media in the United States and elsewhere portray aging as a time of life beset with sickness, inactivity, and slow deterioration of physical and mental functions. These negative views of aging are used to sell products and do not truthfully portray the experiences of most older Americans.

Fear of aging and death may lead to anxiety and stress that may hasten aging processes. A few of the many fears that people associate with aging are illness, poverty, being attacked or victimized, falling and being injured while alone, loss of responsibility for one's life, memory loss, and sexual inadequacy. Most of these fears are unfounded, but may turn out to be self-fulfilling prophesies. However, chronological age often does not correlate with biological age. Some people lose very little in biological functions as they get older, and look and act young almost until the time of death. Generally, older people have about half as many acute illnesses as younger people, although they do suffer more from chronic health problems.

> I used to believe in reincarnation, but that was in a past life.
>
> Paul Krassner,
> humorist

APPROACHING DEATH WITH DIGNITY

Death can strike without warning in the form of an accident or an unexpected heart attack. However, for most people thoughts of death do not occupy their daily lives until old age. People in their 20s are too busy living to think about dying. But people in their 70s and 80s realize the inevitability of death and may modify their lives and affairs accordingly. Younger people who acquire a life-threatening disease such as cancer also are forced to face the possibility of dying.

Most people would prefer to die peacefully in their sleep after living a full, satisfying life. Some may be fortunate to die like this but others may have to endure considerable pain and suffering. In addition to wondering how they are going to die, people usually wonder what will happen to them after death. Christianity provides a heaven where one's "soul" can exist in the grace of God for all eternity. Buddhism embraces a belief in reincarnation; after a series of deaths and rebirths a person can attain "Buddhahood," a perpetual state of enlightenment.

Whatever one's fears or beliefs about death, understanding the process of dying and the preparations that can be made for it can help ensure experiencing a death with peace and dignity (Table 22.2).

 Global Wellness

Can Beliefs Influence Disease Susceptibility?

Just how powerful are thoughts and feelings in influencing health? Can beliefs affect the duration of a person's life? A recent survey of the causes and ages of death among Chinese-Americans shows that strongly held beliefs can affect the cause of death and how long a person lives (Phillips et al., 1993).

In Chinese astrology a particular phase—metal, water, wood, fire, or earth—is associated with the year of a person's birth. Also associated with each phase is susceptibility to partic-

ular diseases (see table below). According to Chinese astrology and medicine, being born in a particular year make a person more likely than usual to succumb to diseases associated with the phase of their birth year. An analysis of almost 30,000 death certificates of Chinese-Americans showed that people with the predicted combination of birth year and disease susceptibility died one to five years younger than white Americans with the same diseases and phases.

The more traditional the Chinese life-style of the person, the shorter their life was once they contracted the disease associated with their birth year. The most plausible explanation of the findings is that Chinese-Americans who believe in the predictions of Chinese astrology are the most likely to succumb to the disease that they expect will kill them. It appears that beliefs not only affect health through the onset and progression of disease, but beliefs even affect life span.

Association between phases of a person's birth year with susceptibility to certain diseases according to Chinese astrology and medicine. Persons born in years corresponding to a particular phase are more susceptible to certain diseases.

Birth year ends in	Phase	Susceptibility to
0 or 1	Metal	Pulmonary diseases
2 or 3	Water	Kidney disease
4 or 5	Wood	Cirrhosis of liver
6 or 7	Fire	Heart attack
8 or 9	Earth	Cancer, diabetes, ulcers

Facing the Fear of Death

Of all human fears, perhaps none is greater than the fear of death. At a young age, thoughts of death and dying are usually absent. Instead we are occupied with life, learning, and daily activities. We can't imagine that someday we will die. As we grow older and see parents, relatives, and friends die, we become more aware of our own mortality. We may begin to wonder about our own death. In the United States, death is not discussed widely or openly. We isolate the dying in hospitals and leave their care to physicians. In the past, people died with dignity in the comfort of their homes surrounded by loving family members. Sterile, impersonal death in a hospital has accentuated many people's fears of death and the process of dying.

Fear is a crippling emotion. It paralyzes thoughts and actions and stifles spiritual growth. Psychologists suggest that the best way to overcome fear is by confronting small pieces of the larger fear. In psychology this technique is called *systematic desensitization*. Here are some suggestions for beginning to rid yourself of fears associated with death.

- Become a volunteer with the American Cancer Society or American Hospice Centers. Spend time with cancer or AIDS patients who are dying and may be willing to share their thoughts with you.
- Familiarize yourself with stories about people who have had near-death experiences. Study how they felt and what the experience was like for them. Ask yourself if these experiences make you feel more comfortable about the idea of death.
- Write down your feelings about death and dying. Record any experiences you have had with death, funerals, or being with someone who is dying. Write down your fears and how you coped with them.
- A powerful technique for dealing with fear is through humor therapy and comic relief. Humor associated with death and dying is called black humor because it deals with the dark side of our thoughts and feelings. Black humor was used to portray the dead and dying in the long-running TV show *M*A*S*H**. Many movies also portray death and dying in a humorous way. The *Far Side* cartoons are another example of comic relief of frightening topics. See if you can confront your fears by drawing cartoons or writing a humorous story about dying.

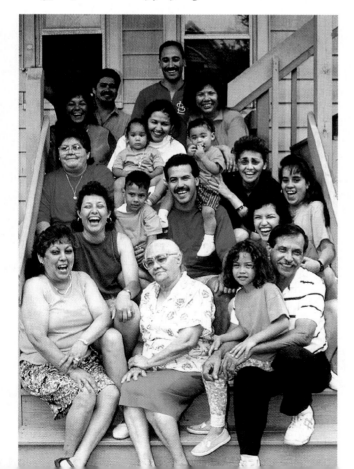

Strong family ties are healthy for young and old alike.

TABLE 22.2 Chronic Conditions among Persons Aged 65 and Over

	Persons with condition (%)
Arthritis	46.5
Hypertensive disease	37.9
Hearing impairments	28.4
Heart conditions	27.7
Chronic sinusitis	18.4
Visual impairments	13.7
Orthopedic impairments (back/extremities/other)	12.8
Arteriosclerosis	9.7
Diabetes	8.3
Varicose veins	8.3
Hemorrhoids	6.6
Frequent constipation	5.9
Urinary system disease	5.6
Corns and callosities	5.2
Hay fever	5.2
Hernia of abdominal cavity	4.9

Source: U.S. National Center for Health Statistics.

Stages of Dying

People have different attitudes toward death and dying. In conversations with many persons who were facing death, Elisabeth Kubler-Ross (1975) identified five distinct stages in the process of dying. Not all persons experienced all stages, but most experienced some of them. These stages of dying are: 1) denial and isolation, 2) anger, 3) bargaining, 4) depression, and 5) acceptance.

> *I don't mind dying. I just don't want to be there when it happens.*
> Woody Allen

The work of Kubler-Ross has found both widespread acceptance, especially among counselors and those who help dying patients, but also received much criticism (Fulton and Metress, 1995). The leading criticism is the fact that the studies were not conducted scientifically, but were based on personal observation and interpretation. Another criticism is that because the stages of dying that Kubler-Ross proposed have been widely accepted and publicized, some dying patients may feel obliged to follow the stages she described.

More and more it is recognized that dying like living is an individual, personal matter. People can do as poet Dylan Thomas recommended and "Rage, rage against the dying of the light." Or they can quickly come to a place of inner peace and accept the idea that the soul will soon be free of its body.

Living Wills

Some people are more concerned about the quality of life than about its duration. For them, the issue is not how long they live but *how* they live. These people do not want to lose control of their life due to a serious accident or unforeseen, serious illness. They do not want to delegate to their physicians or others the right to make decisions about treatments in case they are unable to make the decisions themselves. A **living will** or a similar document can spell out what your wishes are with respect to medical care should you be incapacitated (Figure 22.6). A living will should be given to your primary physician and close relatives so that they can follow your wishes should the occasion arise.

Euthanasia

Almost everyone would like to live a full, active, satisfying life right up to the moment of death. But some peo-

---

A LIVING WILL

TO MY FAMILY, MY PHYSICIAN, MY LAWYER, MY CLERGYMAN
TO ANY MEDICAL FACILITY IN WHOSE CARE I HAPPEN TO BE
TO ANY INDIVIDUAL WHO MAY BECOME RESPONSIBLE FOR MY HEALTH, WELFARE OR AFFAIRS

Death is as much a reality as birth, growth, maturity and old age—it is the one certainty of life. If the time comes when I, _____, can no longer take part in decisions for my own future, let this statement stand as an expression of my wishes, while I am still of sound mind.

If the situation should arise in which there is no reasonable expectation of my recovery from physical or mental disability, I request that I be allowed to die and not be kept alive by artificial means or "heroic measures." I do not fear death itself as much as the indignities of deterioration, dependence, and hopeless pain. I, therefore, ask that medication be mercifully administered to me to alleviate suffering even though this may hasten the moment of death.

This request is made after careful consideration. I hope you who care for me will be morally bound to follow its mandate. I recognize that this appears to place a heavy responsibility on you, but it is with the intention of relieving you of such responsibility and of placing it upon myself in accordance with my strong convictions, that this statement is made.

Date_____   Signed _____
Witness_____   Witness_____

Copies of this request have been given to:

_____   _____
_____   _____

FIGURE 22.6 An Example of a Living Will A copy should be given to your physician and relatives so that they will understand your wishes. Many states have passed laws upholding the legality of living wills.

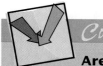

Are Terminally Ill Patients Entitled to Physician-Assisted Suicide?

Most physicians are uncomfortable in dealing with dying patients. What do you say to someone who is terminally ill and has only a short time left to live? It is difficult for any physician to talk candidly to a patient who has no hope of recovery, who is in constant pain, and who may be completely helpless in a hospital bed.

Dr. Jack Kevorkian is a physician who believes passionately that terminally ill patients should have the right to end their lives painlessly and comfortably, and that physicians have an obligation to help them do so if that is the patient's wish.

To this end, Dr. Kevorkian developed a "suicide machine" to help terminally ill patients who requested

his help (Annas, 1993). The machine consists of three bottles connected to an intravenous line. When connected to a patient's vein, the first bottle delivers a harmless saline solution. When the patient decides to press a button, the line switches to the second bottle containing a sedative. Later, the line automatically switches to a cylinder of carbon monoxide, which causes death within minutes.

As of 1993, Dr. Kevorkian had helped fifteen terminally ill patients commit suicide in Michigan. He chose Michigan because the Michigan Supreme Court had ruled that suicide is not a crime, so he concluded that assisting in a suicide cannot be a crime either. However,

Dr. Kevorkian was charged with murder by Michigan authorities in the deaths of several patients who used his machine. The charges were later dismissed. To stop his activities, Michigan revoked his license to practice medicine and also passed a law making physician-assisted suicide a crime.

While many physicians and ethicists reject Dr. Kevorkian's solution for terminally ill patients, the issue he raised will not disappear. American physicians and society together must find a way to help dying patients meet their final needs in a manner that is both compassionate and correct for each individual who is trying to manage the final stage of his or her life.

STUDENT REFLECTIONS

- If a member of your family were terminally ill and in constant pain, would you suggest a physician-assisted suicide?
- Should a terminally ill patient be able to get assistance when requesting "please let me die peacefully" *or* should the health-care community make every effort possible to keep the patient alive?

ple will experience illnesses that bring on a prolonged period of disability, suffering, and pain that cannot be relieved by medical care. Modern medical technology often has the means to prolong life beyond the point where the dying person wishes to live. Given the choice, some terminally ill patients would elect **euthanasia,** which is defined as the act of helping a person experience a peaceful, painless death. In recent years **physician-assisted suicide** has become a controversial form of active euthanasia.

Thousands of people in the United States are kept alive in hospitals in a permanent vegetative state. They are fed artificially and maintained by machines and medical technology. There is no hope of recovery for these persons and most would die if they were unhooked from the machines that keep them alive. There is intense legal and ethical controversy about proper choices regarding these individuals, as well as those who want the option of active euthanasia.

Physicians are trained to prolong human life as long as possible and it is illegal in most instances to help a person die in any way or to remove the life-support system from a person in a vegetative state. However, support for the right to choose active euthanasia has been gaining among Americans; surveys show that in many areas of the country it has majority support. Although most American physicians still oppose the idea, active euthanasia has been practiced in the Netherlands for many years.

Many advocates of active euthanasia believe that it eventually will be adopted in some form in many countries, including the United States (Benrubi, 1992). The

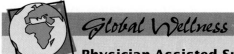
Hemlock Society publishes materials for persons who may be contemplating euthanasia. As a society with an increasing number of terminally ill older persons, we all will have to address the issues of living wills and active euthanasia at some time or other in our lives.

The Hospice

The term **hospice** originally applied to medieval Christian hospitals caring for the poor, the aged, and the sick. Hospices also provided refuge for people on religious pilgrimages. Providing physical necessities, medical care, and spiritual comfort was the primary purpose of the early religious hospices. In the United States today there are over 2000 hospices offering comprehensive care for terminally ill patients. The goal of a hospice is to meet the total health needs—physical, psychological, and spiritual—of patients who have weeks or months to live. Medications are given to ease pain, but heroic treatments are not attempted. Family and friends are free to visit with the patient in a comfortable setting, whether it is in a patient's home or a hospital with a hospice attached.

The hospice philosophy is that dying is part of living and should not be resisted with every weapon in the modern medical arsenal. Hospice care is designed to control pain and make patients comfortable, but staff also are trained to discuss emotional and spiritual issues relevant to death. Counseling and social services are available in hospices and close family members are encouraged to participate in daily activities. About two-thirds of hospices in the United States are certified for Medicare reimbursement.

More than 200,000 patients each year in the United States elect to spend their final weeks or months in hospice care. As the population in this country becomes older, more and more families and individuals will have to face the issues raised by terminal illness and death. Although hospices do everything possible to make patients comfortable, they do not permit active euthanasia.

THINKING ABOUT DEATH

There is no way of knowing how or when we are going to die or what we will do or think when confronted with death. Most of us only think about death when someone close to us dies, or if we ourselves become seriously sick or injured. However, if thoughts of death do arise often, of if you feel that you are unreasonably afraid of death, then it is advisable to seek help to overcome fears.

Every age of life provides opportunities for growth and satisfaction. Even though we have no way of knowing when serious illness or death will confront us, we do have control of how we live each day and the satisfactions we find in life. The way we choose to live when we are young will greatly affect our health later on. For example, smoking while young increases the likelihood of developing cancer and heart disease later. Drinking alcohol to excess and taking unnecessary chances invite accidents that can cause death or permanent disability. While each person's life span is partly determined by genes, environmental factors such as nutrition, exercise, and life-style are also important not only in determining how long we live, but how well we live.

T E R M

hospice: usually a place for terminally ill patients to spend the time before death in an environment that attends to their physical, emotional, and spiritual needs, but where no further treatments are administered; hospice care also can be given in a patient's home

---

HEALTH IN REVIEW

- Aging and dying are natural stages of life. People should strive to remain physically, emotionally, mentally, and spiritually active at all stages of life regardless of chronological age.

- The maximum human life span is approximately 115 years; the average life span is about 85 years. In many countries, people born now can expect to live the average human life span or more.

- The average age of the population in the United States is increasing, causing increasing health care costs as well as financing problems for the Social Security system.

- Aging is partly determined by genes and partly by environmental factors that cause cellular changes with age. Undernutrition slows aging in laboratory animals and may slow down aging processes in people.

- Loss of cognitive mental functions in older people is called senile dementia; the most common cause of this is Alzheimer's disease. Bone loss with age is called osteoporosis and occurs most frequently in post-menopausal women.

- Active euthanasia refers to helping someone die without pain or suffering. Physician-assisted suicide is a form of active euthanasia that is presently illegal in the United States, although some states have attempted to enact laws legalizing these activities by physicians. Hospice care provides terminally ill patients with medical, emotional, and spiritual support during the final weeks or months of their lives.

REFERENCES

Annas, G. J. (1993). "Physician-Assisted Suicide—Michigan's Temporary Solution." *New England Journal of Medicine,* May 27, 328(21): 1573–1576.

Barinaga, M. (1991). "How Long Is the Human Life-span?" *Science,* November 15, 254: 936–938.

Benrubi, G. I. (1992). "Euthanasia—The Need for Procedural Safeguards." *New England Journal of Medicine,* January 16, 326(3): 197–198.

Freundlich, N. (1993). "Quietly Closing In on Alzheimer's." *Business Week,* May 3: 112–113.

Fulton, G. B., and E. K. Metress (1995). *Perspectives on Death and Dying.* Boston: Jones and Bartlett.

Hayflick, L. (1994). *How and Why We Age.* New York: Ballantine.

Horgan, J. (1992). "How Long Can We Live?" *Scientific American,* December: 131–141.

Kubler-Ross, E. (1975). *Death: The Final Stage of Growth.* New York: Prentice-Hall.

Mundy, G. R. (1994). "Boning Up on Genes." *Nature,* January 20.

Phillips, D. P., T. E. Ruth, and L. M. Wagner (1993). "Psychology and Survival." *The Lancet,* November 6.

Raloff, J. (1992). "Paring Protein: Low Protein Cuisines May Slow Aging." *Science News,* November 21, 142: 346–347.

Schardt, D. (1994). "Alzheimer's in the Family." *Nutrition Action Healthletter,* June: 10–14.

Stadtman, E. R. (1992). "Protein Oxidation and Aging." *Science,* August 28, 257: 1220–1224.

Tierney, J. (1990). "Lost Horizon." *In Health,* July/August: 39–48.

Weindruch, R., and R. L. Walford (1989). *The Retardation of Aging and Disease by Dietary Restriction.* Springfield, Ill.: Charles C. Thomas.

SUGGESTED READINGS

Beresford, L. (1993). *The Hospice Handbook.* Boston: Little, Brown. A complete guide to hospice care.

"Despite New Clues, Alzheimer's Mystery Remains Unsolved." *FDA Consumer,* March. Describes current research on Alzheimer's disease.

Evans, W., and I. H. Rosenberg (1992). *Biomarkers: The 10 Keys to Prolonging Vitality.* New York: Fireside Books. Increasing longevity through nutrition and exercise.

Fulton, G. B., and E. K. Metress (1995). *Perspectives on Death and Dying.* Boston: Jones and Bartlett. A textbook covering dying and death in detail.

Hayflick, L. (1994). *How and Why We Age.* New York: Ballantine Books. Excellent discussion of all aspects of aging by an eminent researcher.

Humphrey, D. (1991). *Final Exit: The Practicalities of Self-Deliverance and Assisted Suicide for the Dying.* Eugene, Ore.: The Hemlock Society. A controversial book that explains euthanasia and how it can be done with or without assistance.

Moore, T. J. (1994). *Lifespan: New Perspectives on Extending Human Longevity.* New York: Touchstone Books. Information on all aspects of longevity.

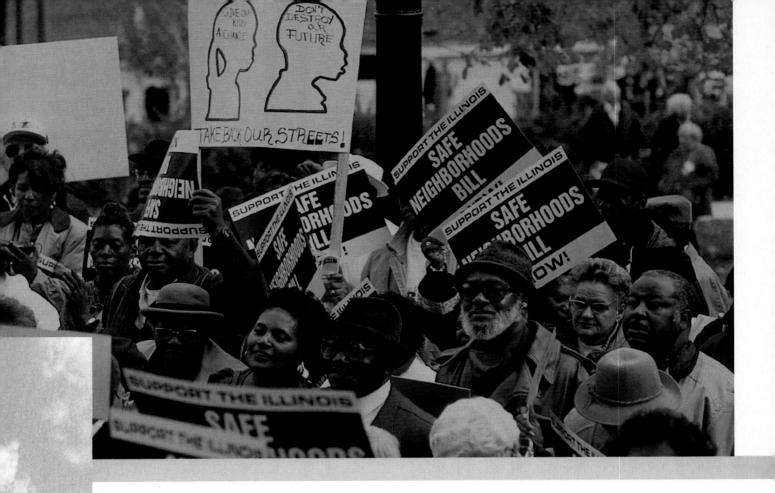

LEARNING OBJECTIVES

After reading this chapter you should be able to:

1. Describe the incidence of guns in schools.
2. Discuss how violence can affect your health.
3. Describe post-traumatic stress disorder.
4. Describe different determinants of domestic violence.
5. Define sexual assault, forcible rape, and acquaintance rape.
6. Describe the impact of acquaintance rape in your college community.
7. Discuss child abuse and factors that may contribute to it.
8. Describe child abuse prevention strategies.

Violence in Our Society

iolence in the United States is an important health problem; it occurs every day and in many forms. Violence is a major killer of young people today. More than 20,000 people die every year from homicide and more than 2.2 million people suffer injuries due to violent conflicts. Among industrialized nations the United States ranks first in violent death rates (USDHHS, 1991). **Violence** refers to the use of force or power that can result in injury or death. The definition implies more than the physical aspects of violence, and includes social norms, values, and political and economic policies. Homicide is the second leading cause of death among 15- to 24-year-olds, and suicide is the third leading cause of death among the same age group (Chapters 1 and 4). Forty percent of unintentional injury deaths are homicides.

Our culture has come to believe that violence is an inevitable part of life. By age 16 the average person has seen 200,000 acts of violence on television alone (Cohen, 1993). Violence is pervasive, is glamorized through the media, and is real—when the child accidentally shoots his playmate, when a neighborhood is terrorized by gangs, or when a city is devastated by a single act of terrorism. Former U.S. Surgeon General Antonia Novello said, "prevention of violence is ultimately our only road to success."

Adolescence

between thirteen and nineteen they exist
traveling the bridge to adulthood
their parents wishing to be psychiatrists
just to understand, if they could

the journey is long and hard
with many paths to choose
some let down their guard
and turn to drugs or booze

some stay on the yellow brick road
responsible and mature they try to be
increasing the weight on an already heavy load
locking emotions up and throwing away the key

living for the here and now
consequences are seldom thought about
it won't happen to me, they vow
besides the scientists will figure it out

living in a world of violence
desensitized to it all
no longer a time of innocence
roaming around a mini-mall

killing each other with ease
drugs and guns as the source
making violence an age-specific disease
ravaging this population with such force

becoming parents way too fast
dropping out of school to support a child
taking a job and putting fun in the past
no more nights partying and being wild

kids raising kids
violence and gangs and guns and knives
no longer seeing friends because of coffin lids
consuming their everyday lives

being an adolescent is not so simple
too young for this, too old for that
dealing with sex to drugs to violence to pimples
surviving deserves a tip of the hat

thirteen to nineteen, an adolescent
the time flies by, keeping busy
developing an identity and becoming independent
being an adolescent is not so easy

—*Stepanie Vahle*

Printed with permission of author.

T E R M
violence: use of force and power

FIREARM VIOLENCE

Unintentional and intentional discharge of firearms was the second leading cause of fatal injuries in 1991. Firearm fatalities have been increasing since 1980. Overall for persons ages 15 to 24, they have increased 40 percent; for African-American males ages 15 to 34, the death rates are even higher. Native Americans and Hispanics also have higher firearm death rates than do white males (National Safety Council, 1994).

Social scientists and others ask why these figures continue to rise. Is our society becoming more violent, and more accepting of violence? Why have firearms become the choice for conflict resolution among many young persons? Why are certain age groups and ethnic groups more susceptible to firearm fatalities? Should there be stricter regulations concerning the sale and ownership of firearms? These questions need to be addressed before we can reduce firearm injury and fatality.

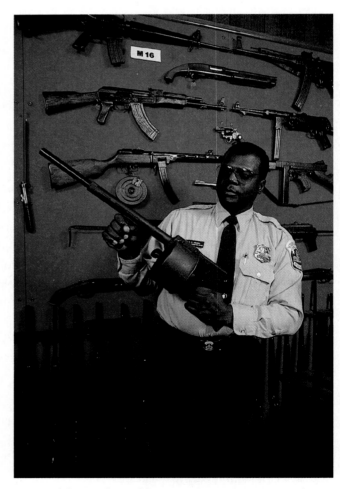

Because of the prevalence of firearms in our society, some cities have implemented buy-back programs, in which illegal guns can be anonymously exchanged for cash with no questions asked.

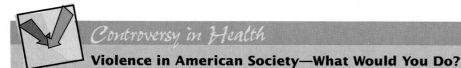
Violence in American Society—What Would You Do?

Year after year the use of pistols, rifles, and other firearms causes thousands of deaths in the United States, both accidental and deliberate. In 1987 almost 33,000 deaths were caused by firearms—about half of these were suicides, about 13,000 were homicides, and the rest were unintentional accidents or involved shootings by police officers. Every year more than 60,000 injuries result from firearms. Numerous studies come to the same conclusion; ready availability of firearms in the United States is associated with increased risk of suicide and homicide (Kellerman et al., 1992).

Americans have a longstanding love-hate relationship with firearms and many people believe strongly in the constitutionally guaranteed right to carry and use firearms. Their views are defended with money and lobbying by the National Rifle Association (NRA) which works to prevent passage of laws limiting or regulating the purchase and use of

guns by civilians. The NRA is opposed by physicians, health organizations, and law enforcement agencies including the Federal Bureau of Investigation (FBI), which supports stricter gun control laws.

In 1993 in response to the escalating number of homicides, suicides, and assaults, eleven states including New York, New Jersey, and California passed gun control laws. In addition, the U.S. Congress passed a gun control law known as the Brady bill. (Jim Brady was permanently disabled in the assassination attempt on President Reagan in 1981.) The Brady bill imposes a five-day waiting period for the purchase of handguns and requires local police agencies to determine if the prospective buyer has a criminal record.

Violence and the use of firearms in the United States has become one of society's most pressing concerns (Kassirer, 1991). Juveniles under 21 now account for 20 percent of all

arrests for the possession or use of a gun. African-American youths are three times more likely to be arrested for a gun violation than are white American youths (Kantrowitz, 1993). Even more disturbing is the fact that of the 23,760 murders recorded in 1992, about half of the victims were black Americans. The motives are not racial since 94 percent of the victims were killed by members of their own race; 83 percent of white American murder victims also were killed by other whites.

The majority of homicides involve juveniles, many of whom are in gangs and involved in selling and using illegal drugs. While law enforcement can be increased in some ways, laws cannot solve the problems of violence and murder. Solutions to the social problems that underlie the violence must come from parents, clergy, teachers, and the youths involved.

STUDENT REFLECTIONS

- Do you believe all individuals should be allowed to own a firearm?
- From your perspective, what can America do to decrease the amount of violence among youth?

Many risk factors are associated with firearm use, resulting in both unintentional and intentional injuries and fatalities. Most states have laws prohibiting the sale

HEALTHY PEOPLE 2000

Reduce deaths caused by unintentional injuries to no more than 29.3 per 100,000 people.

Nearly two-thirds of all injury deaths involve unintentional injuries. Males are more likely to experience unintentional injuries than females and are 2.5 times more likely to die from them. Higher death rates from unintentional injury occur among blacks than among whites over the entire age range with black males generally having the highest death rates.

of firearms to persons under 18 and controversial federal bills have been proposed to further limit the sale of certain types of weapons and ammunition. These bills are strongly opposed by the National Rifle Association and other organized groups. Opponents believe these bills are unconstitutional violations of the right to bear arms under the Fourth Amendment. Others argue that rapid-fire automatic weapons were not envisioned by the founding fathers in drafting the Constitution. Arguments over firearm laws are highly acrimonious and controversial and have divided voters sharply. In 1994 Congress passed the Brady bill, which prohibits the sale of certain weapons and requires police checks of all persons seeking to purchase a gun.

Many young people under 18 already know how to make their own firearms, commonly referred to as "Saturday Night Specials." The black market for firearms is a large illegal industry that continues to flourish despite strict laws. Many individuals who are not legally able to purchase a firearm because of age or previous criminal history resort to the black market to purchase firearms.

Among environmental factors that increase the likelihood of a firearm injury are easy access to firearms and poverty (use of firearms in theft). The use of alcohol and other drugs also increases the likelihood of a firearm injury or fatality.

Guns in Schools

Schools are mirror images of their communities. From 1986 to 1990, at least 65 students were shot to death and 186 were wounded on school grounds. Overall, 10,052 children ages 15 to 19 were murdered with guns in America, and an additional 9,213 deaths from firearm-related suicides or unintentional shootings took place during the same time period (Duker, 1994). Some of this violence is affecting our schools and students.

Teenagers carry guns and bring them to school because they think they offer protection, to intimidate others, or to be liked by their peers. Today, an argument between students may be resolved in a shooting rather than a fistfight. Teachers and students alike indicate that the presence of guns in the schools generates fear and impedes learning.

In 1987 a national survey revealed the following:

- One out of every 36 tenth-grade boys reported carrying a handgun to school in the past year.
- One in every 100 boys brought a gun to school nearly every day.

The odds are that on any given day, in any urban high-school classroom, at least one student is carrying a handgun (Duker, 1994).

INTERPERSONAL VIOLENCE

Domestic violence, which includes relationship abuse and child abuse, is just one type of violence occurring today in our society. Interpersonal violence can exist in both criminal and intimate forms. Criminal violence includes robbery, burglary, aggravated assault, forcible rape, and homicide. Intimate violence, which in many cases is also a criminal act, includes behaviors such as child abuse, incest, courtship violence, date rape, battering, marital rape, and elder abuse (Alexander and LaRosa, 1994). Historically, intimate violence within the family setting has been condoned, despite the fact that it is a crime. And most often women are the victims, as shown by the following statistics (American Public Health Association, 1993):

- 12 percent of couples report that in the prior year the wife had been physically assaulted by her husband one or more times.
- 25 to 30 percent of women are physically and/or sexually assaulted at some time by their intimate partners.
- 52 percent of women homicide victims are killed by their husbands, boyfriends, or ex-spouses.
- 30 percent of all emergency room visits are made by women victims of battering, making battering the most common cause of emergency care.

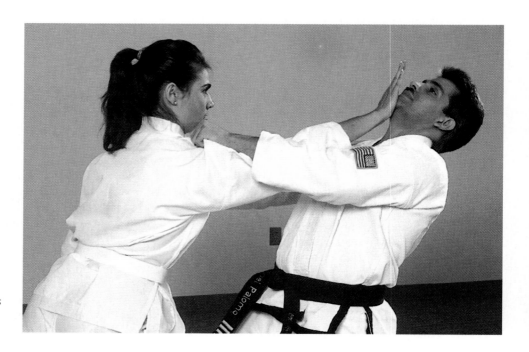

Many women take self-defense classes in order to prepare themselves in the event of a physical attack.

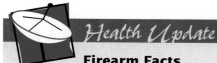

Firearm Facts

- In 1990, 4,941 children in the United States under the age of 19 died from gunshot wounds; 538 of these children were shot unintentionally.
- Guns are used in approximately 60 percent of all teenage suicides.
- In 1990, 3,165 youths ages 15–24 killed themselves with guns.
- In 1990, 2,861 children 19 and under were murdered with guns, an increase of 114 percent since 1985.
- In 1987, 1,300 males under the age of 19 were murdered with guns in the United States. In the same time period, in Canada, Japan, France, West Germany, Australia, England, Wales, and Sweden combined, fewer than 80 males under the age of 19 were murdered with guns.
- A gun in the home is 43 times more likely to be used to kill a family member or friend than it is to kill in self-defense.
- In 1992, approximately 78 percent of murder victims were killed by someone they knew.
- In 1990, 4,371,000 guns were produced for the American market. That is 12,000 new guns every day.
- In 1991, nearly 92,000 Americans applied to get or renew a federal firearms license; only 52 were denied.
- In 1992, the cost of direct medical spending, emergency services, and claims processing for the victims of gun violence nationwide totaled approximately $3 billion.

Adapted from: L. Duker, *Firearm Facts* (McLean, Va.: National Maternal and Child Health Clearinghouse, 1994).

- 90 percent of rape victims are female.
- 20 percent of women are raped at some time in their lives.
- 40 percent of rapes are committed by spouses, partners, or relatives of the victim.

A public opinion research poll conducted for the Project of the Family Violence Prevention Fund found that:

- The FBI estimates a women is beaten by her husband or boyfriend every 15 seconds.
- Americans of every age group and race agree that violence against women is not just physical assault, but also an attack on women's dignity and freedom.
- 81 percent of respondents agreed something can be done to reduce the amount of violence against women, but 26 percent stated they did not know what action to take.
- 90 percent of respondents stated they would call police if they witnessed a man beating a woman.

RELATIONSHIP VIOLENCE

As described by one expert, "violence is a learned behavior. The basic values, attitudes, and interpersonal skills acquired early in life are likely to be pivotal in developing predisposition for violent behavior later in life" (Fenley et al., 1993, p. 7). Many American women are victims of relationship violence, including physical assault (slapping, kicking, punching, threatening with a weapon), forced sexual activity, and childhood sexual abuse (molestation and incest). Recognizing that relationship violence is the greatest cause of injury to women and children in the United States, the federal government has declared it a public health emergency. Former Surgeon General C. Everett Koop regarded domestic violence as a major public health problem in America, as serious as communicable diseases were in the last century. To lessen its prevalence through public awareness education, October has been designated National Domestic Violence Month.

Women who experience partner-battering and/or rape have medical problems and may also suffer from anxiety, depression, chronic pelvic pain, gastrointestinal upset, substance abuse, obesity, and/or headaches. Assaulted women may also develop symptoms of **post-traumatic stress disorder (PTSD)** and its variants, battered women's syndrome or rape trauma syndrome. Many long-term health consequences of battering, rape, and sexual abuse are associated with PTSD. For example, traumatized individuals tend to be more susceptible to arousal by stimuli that makes it difficult for them to differentiate normal aches, pains, and sensations from signals of disease, leading to increased incidence of seeking help from health professionals. Also, emotional tension and guardedness can produce painful muscle tension and skeletal misalignment. Chronic anxiety can lead to

T E R M

post-traumatic stress disorder (PTSD): reactions following an event that is outside the range of usual human experience and would be distressing to almost anyone

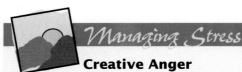

Creative Anger

Anger. The word itself brings to mind images of pounding fists, yelling, and smoke pouring out of ears and nose. But anger is as natural a human emotion as love. It is universal among human beings. Anger is a survival emotion; it's the fight component of the fight or flight response. We use anger to communicate our feelings, from impatience to rage. We employ anger to communicate boundaries and defend values. Studies show that the average person has between 14-15 anger episodes a day, which often occur when our expectations are not met upon demand. Although feeling angry is within the normal limits of human emotions, anger is often mismanaged and misdirected. Unfortunately, we have been socialized to suppress our feelings of anger. As a result, it either tears us apart from the inside or promotes intermittent eruptions of verbal or physical violence, which we see played out in local and national headlines. In most cases we do not deal with our anger wisely.

Research reveals four very distinct ways in which people mismanage their anger. They include:

1. **Somatizers:** People who never show any signs of anger and internalize their feelings until eventually there is major bodily damage (i.e., temporomandibular joint, colitis, migraines).

2. **Exploders:** Individuals who erupt like a volcano and spread their temper like hot lava, destroying anyone and anything in their path with either verbal or physical abuse. This type of mismanaged anger style is what makes the news headlines.

3. **Self-Punishers:** People who neither repress their anger nor explode, but rather deny themselves a proper outlet of anger because of feelings of guilt. Examples of their behavior include excessive sleeping, eating, and shopping.

4. **Underhanders:** Individuals who sabotage or seek revenge against someone through barely socially acceptable behavior (e.g., sarcasm, tardiness, not returning phone calls).

When anger is mismanaged and left unresolved it becomes a control issue, if not a control drama. Although we tend to employ all of these styles at one time or another, we also tend to rely on one dominant style of mismanaged anger. Of the four mismanaged anger styles described, what is your most dominant style? When do situations arise that you get angry? How do you deal with these feelings of anger?

There are some ways to deal with anger sensibly or perhaps even creatively. For example:

1. Take "time-out" from the situation, followed by a "time-in" to resolve the issue.
2. Communicate your feelings diplomatically.
3. Learn to outthink your anger.
4. Plan several options to a situation.
5. Lower personal expectations.
6. Most important, learn to forgive—"make past anger pass."

What are some ways you can vent your anger creatively?

Although anger is an emotion we all experience and should recognize when it arises, it is crucial to manage anger. Sometimes just writing down what frustrates you can be the beginning of the resolution process. And anger must be resolved. Above all, make a habit to resolve your anger feelings once they arise. Learn to let go of your feelings of anger before they become toxic to your mind, body, and spirit.

---

gastrointestinal upsets. Alcohol, nicotine, and other drugs may be used to block out memories of abuse and to alleviate uncomfortable emotions and physical sensations that accompany memories of the assault or abuse.

Recovering from the trauma of relationship violence requires patience and support. Victims are encouraged to seek psychological counseling from professionals who specialize in helping victims of relationship violence and to join support groups of other assaulted individuals. Support can hasten healing and recovery and help restore the trust that is shattered by assault. Support groups can also provide a place to stay if the victim needs to escape the abuser or the group can offer companionship if the victim is afraid to be alone.

Determinants of Domestic Violence

There is no single cause of domestic violence, but contributing factors include:

- A high level of conflict and stress in the family.
- Male dominance and the view that women and children are men's property.

T E R M S

sexual assault: violent actions that include rape, incest, attempted rape, and unwanted sexual touching

forcible rape: sexual assault using force or threat of force, and involving sexual penetration of the victim's vagina, mouth, or rectum

Symptoms of Post-Traumatic Stress Disorder

- Re-experiencing the traumatic event(s) via recurrent intrusive images, thoughts, dreams of the trauma, and "flashbacks"—having a sense of reliving the trauma, including re-experiencing the disturbing accompanying emotions.

- Intense reactions to things that symbolize the traumatic experience. For example, in recovering from a rape, victims may intensely fear being in locales that resemble the scene of the assault.

They may experience nausea when thinking of the rape. Many have difficulties with sexual relations.

- Persistent avoidance of stimuli associated with the event. Victims may be unable to recall the trauma (denial), or they may engage in a mild form of self-hypnosis to "make the mind go somewhere else" to avoid the intensity of the pain associated with the memory of the trauma (dissociation). They may feel detached or estranged.

- Control seeking. Victims may manipulate others and the environment as a way to keep things calm and under control. They may become compliant as a way to avoid real or imagined abuse.

- Persistent arousal symptoms, such as difficulty falling or staying asleep, being edgy, jumpy, irritable, and sometimes irrationally angry. Victims may have difficulty concentrating, be hypervigilant to their surroundings, and have an exaggerated startle response.

- Cultural norms that permit family violence.
- Displays of violence on TV and other media.
- Being raised in a violent family.
- Alcohol and drug abuse.
- Victim-blaming ("people get what they deserve").
- Denying the existence of physical violence or sexual abuse.

Ways to prevent domestic violence include providing shelters, safe houses, and other protective environments for abused women; reducing contributing social and economic factors (unemployment, poverty, and racism); holding the abusers accountable for their actions; training law enforcement and health-care professionals to recognize and intervene in cases of domestic violence; training everyone in nonviolent conflict resolution; and reducing the amount of violent imagery on TV, in films, and in popular music.

SEXUAL ASSAULT

Rape, incest, attempted rape, and unwanted sexual touching are often called **sexual assault.** There has been a significant increase recently in public recognition of sexual crimes against women, including intense media scrutiny of rape issues in high profile rape trials. The legal definition of **forcible rape** varies from state to state. However, rape is generally viewed as penetration by force or threat of force of a body orifice, including the mouth, rectum, or vagina. Penetration includes the use of objects or other

> For a while we pondered whether to take a vacation or get a divorce. We decided that a trip to Bermuda is over in two weeks, but a divorce is something you always have.
> Woody Allen

body parts, such as fingers. Forced sexual activity can occur between men and women, men and men, women and women, and married and unmarried people. Regardless of the identity of the victims and perpetrators, sexual assault is a criminal activity; it is not sex and has nothing to do with sex. Sexual assault is an act of power, an attempt to humiliate a victim. Whether the term is sexual assault or forcible rape, the end result is physical violence to the victim.

Some men try to deny the fact of sexual assault with statements such as "women enjoy being raped," "she asked for it," and "I didn't think she meant no." These

HEALTHY PEOPLE 2000

Reduce rape and attempted rape of women ages 12 and older to no more than 108 per 100,000 women.

Young, unmarried, and low-income women are the most common victims of rape and rape attempts. Women between the ages of 12 and 34 are particularly vulnerable, with victimization rates more than twice as high as women in other age categories. Most rapists are unarmed and operate alone. Reported offenders are usually strangers to the victim, but this may reflect the reluctance of victims of acquaintance and date rape to report their experiences. Most sexual assaults occur at night and are attempts rather than completed rapes.

kinds of statements are heard repeatedly; however, the facts of sexual assault are plain:

- Sexual assault is an act of power and control—*not* an act of sex or passion.
- Most sexual assaults go unreported.
- Most sexual assaults do not occur on impulse or in remote areas.
- In 80 percent of all sexual assaults, according to some estimates, the assailant was a casual acquaintance, friend, or relative of the victim.

- Sexual assailants come from *all* socioeconomic and ethnic backgrounds.
- Rapists are not sexually deprived people.
- Women do not secretly want to be raped.
- Forced intimacy in a dating situation is sexual assault.

Incidence of Sexual Assault

In 1990, the FBI found that 102,555 women were victims of forcible rape. This number includes only sexual

Health Update

Time/CNN Rape Attitude Survey

Would you classify the following as rape or not?		Rape	Not rape
A man has sex with a woman who has passed out after drinking too much	Female	88%	9%
	Male	77%	17%
A married man has sex with his wife even though she does not want him to	Female	61%	30%
	Male	56%	38%
A man argues with a woman who does not want to have sex until she agrees to have sex	Female	42%	53%
	Male	33%	59%
A man uses emotional pressure, but no physical force, to get a woman to have sex	Female	39%	55%
	Male	33%	59%
		Yes	No
Do you believe that some women like to be talked into having sex?	Female	54%	33%
	Male	69%	20%

From a telephone poll of 500 American adults taken for TIME/CNN on May 8 by Yankslovich Clancy Shulman. Sampling error is plus or minus 4.5%. "Not sures" omitted.

Do you believe a woman who is raped is partly to blame if:	Age	Yes	No
She is under the influence of drugs or alcohol	18–34	31%	66%
	35–49	35%	58%
	50+	57%	36%
She initially says yes to having sex and then changes her mind	18–34	34%	60%
	35–49	43%	53%
	50+	43%	46%
She dresses provocatively	18–34	28%	70%
	35–49	31%	67%
	50+	53%	42%
She agrees to go to the man's room or home	18–34	20%	76%
	35–49	29%	70%
	50+	53%	41%
		Yes	No
Have you ever been in a situation with a man in which you said no but ended up having sex anyway?	Asked of females	18%	80%

Source: Time, June 3, 1991. Copyright 1991, Time, Inc. Reprinted by permission.

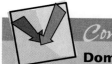

Domestic Violence Is No Longer Silent

From the middle of 1994 through 1995, there was extraordinarily heavy media coverage of the murders of football hero O. J. Simpson's ex-wife, Nicole Brown Simpson, and her friend Ronald Goldman. Television newscasts and newspaper articles included discussions of O. J. Simpson's celebrity as well as his possible guilt or innocence of the murders. One upsetting aspect of the case was that despite Simpson's history of battering, the problem of domestic violence was shoved into the background. Many would say that it was taken less seriously than it should have been. Some jurors, after O. J. was found not guilty of murder, said that the claims of battering had no effect on their verdict. The awful facts are that 2–4 million women each year are battered by their husbands or boyfriends, and 1,500 women are murdered each year by their intimate partners. The American Medical Association has developed guidelines to help the medical community better identify, treat, and report cases of domestic violence and sexual assault.

The numbers are staggering yet most abusers get away with battering and domestic violence. For instance, in 1989 after O. J. Simpson beat his then-wife Nicole Brown Simpson, he received a small fine, limited community service, and psychiatric counseling by phone. Many battered women never call 911 or others for help, due to fear of being battered again. This crime has been silenced because of unfair social myths and biases that incriminate victims rather than offenders.

STUDENT REFLECTIONS

- What services are available in your community to help battered women?
- In your opinion, why don't battered women immediately leave their spouse or partner after being abused?
- In your opinion, why are our laws lenient toward the battering spouse?

assaults reported to police and complaints which law enforcement officers considered legitimate. The FBI defines forcible rape as vaginal penetration by a penis. It does not include other forms of rape as defined under most state statutes, such as oral or anal sex and penetration by fingers or objects (U.S. Department of Justice, 1990). The National Crime Survey found that 207,610 sexual assaults and attempted sexual assaults were reported in 1991, an increase of 59 percent from 1990, but a number considered low by the Department of Justice (1991). Other data indicate that 20 percent of all adult women are sexually assaulted in their lifetimes (Koss and Harvey, 1991).

In August 1995, the Department of Justice Bureau of Statistics estimated that there are 500,000 sexual assaults on women annually, including 170,000 rapes and 140,000 attempted rapes (*Chicago Sun-Times,* August 17, 1995). These data come from the annual National Crime Victimization Survey, which interviews 100,000 Americans over age 12. The survey is used to determine the incidence of crimes not reported to the police. Before 1993 the survey did not have a specific question on rape or sexual assault; questions asked only about attacks of any kind without mentioning sexual

assault or rape. The survey now asks if you were raped or sexually assaulted. This survey does not necessarily mean that the number of rapes or sexual assaults has increased; it does indicate that, when asked specific questions about rape and sexual assault, affirmative responses increased. However, overall data indicate that sexual assault is clearly a growing national problem.

Acquaintance Rape

Acquaintance rape, or date rape, occurs when a person known to the victim uses force to coerce the victim into having sex. Warsaw (1988) reports that 84 percent of all sexual assaults are committed by an acquaintance of the victim, 57 percent of all sexual assaults occur during a date, and 60 percent of men raped by other men knew their attacker. Acquaintance rape carries the same legal penalties as sexual assault committed by a stranger.

High school and college-age women are the most vulnerable to acquaintance rape. A survey of 6,000 students from 32 colleges found that one in six female students had been a victim of rape or attempted rape within the preceding year, and one of fifteen male students reported committing sexual assaults within the preceding year (Koss and Harvey, 1991).

Cultural views on sexual relationships between men and women play a significant role in acquaintance rape. Many young women who are victims of attacks that meet the legal definition of rape do not know that what happened to them was sexual assault. Victims may believe that a sexual assault can only be committed by a

---

T E R M

acquaintance rape: (also known as "date rape") sexual assault occurring when the victim and the rapist are known to each other and may have previously interacted in some socially appropriate manner

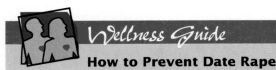
stranger, or they may blame themselves for the act. An offender may not realize that the victim's refusal really means NO. Sex—especially with aggressive males—is often an inherently adversarial relationship. These men believe that when women say no, men should insist. The result is miscommunication, aggression, and sometimes acquaintance rape (Illinois Coalition Against Sexual Assault [ICASA], 1993). Usually, the assailant is someone the victim trusts enough to accept a ride home from or to let into his or her apartment or office.

In a survey conducted by *MS.* magazine, 84 percent of men whose actions came under the legal definition of sexual assault believed they had not committed sexual assault. This reinforces the myth that women really do not mean NO when they say no. Another study found that 43 percent of college-age men admitted using coercion to have sex, including ignoring a women's protest, using physical aggression, and forcing intercourse. Fifteen percent of the same group acknowledged they had committed acquaintance rape, and 11 percent admitted using physical restraint to force a woman to have sex (Rapaport and Posey, 1991).

Victims of acquaintance rape often suffer serious, long-term psychological effects. Compared with victims of stranger rapes, acquaintance rape victims often blame themselves for what happened. They often have difficulty trusting people in later relationships. It may take acquaintance rape victims longer to recover, particularly if the rape involved physical violence. Acquaintance rape victims are less likely than other rape victims to seek crisis services, tell someone, report the incident to the police, or seek counseling. Family and friends may not provide the same support for acquaintance rape victims as they might offer victims of stranger rape. If victims tell friends or family, the severity of the attack may be minimized or the victim may be blamed for the sexual assault (Gidycz and Koss, 1991).

> *No one can make you feel inferior without your consent.*
> Eleanor Roosevelt

Styles of Behavioral Reaction

Victims usually have two types of behavioral reactions, expressed or controlled. Those who express their feelings usually manifest fear, anger, and anxiety. They may display these emotions through crying, tension, nervousness, restlessness, and hysteria. Those who control their feelings may appear calm or quiet, but either reaction indicates that the victim is in a state of shock (Table 23.1). Expressed or controlled feelings may occur at any time and often come and go more than once after the incident. Acknowledging or recognizing these feelings are a normal part of the healing process.

Family members and significant others have also been victimized when someone they know, love, and care for has been sexually assaulted. Significant others may also have expressed or controlled reactions that indicate a state of shock from the incident. Some common feelings felt by the sexual assault victim's family members and significant others are listed in Table 23.2.

What to Do after a Sexual Assault

A person who has been sexually assaulted is advised to do the following:

- Contact a rape-crisis hotline.
- DO NOT shower, bathe, douche, change or destroy clothing, or straighten up the area where the sexual assault occurred (if indoors), because these actions would destroy important evidence.
- Go to the nearest hospital emergency room.
- Notify the police.
- Seek professional counseling.

Each person's reaction to being sexually assaulted is different. It is natural that each victim's pain and needs

TABLE 23.1   Feelings Reported by Sexual Assault Victims

Fear of rapist	Embarrassment	Shame	Guilt	Anxiety
• Fear of death	• Embarrassed to discuss details	• Destruction of self-esteem, self-worth, self-respect	• Feelings of shame as though s/he provoked the rape	• Shaking
• Fear of rapist	• Embarrassed about his/her body	• Ashamed at having the medical exam	• Feeling s/he is to blame for the assault	• Nightmares
		• Ashamed at having to perform a sexual act in order to stay alive		• Difficulty sleeping or sleeping all the time
				• Constantly reminds self what s/he "should or shouldn't have" done

Stupidity	Vulnerability	Concern for rapist	Anger	Loss of control
• Feels stupid for engaging in risk-taking behavior(s)	• General fear of people	• Will the rapist get psychiatric help?	• Toward assailant	• Small decisions seem monumental
• Feels stupid for being too trusting	• Feels paranoid	• What will happen to offender if s/he reports?	• Toward self	• Unsure about self or actions
	• Intense heightened awareness of environment		• Toward men and women in general, especially if they resemble assailant	

Source: Adapted from Illinois Coalition against Sexual Assault, Springfield, Ill.: 1993.

also will be unique. The following are guidelines to help in the recovery process (ICASA, 1993):

• Let your friends or relatives take the lead in their own recovery.
• Recognize that nothing you can do will erase the sexual assault.
• Face your own fears and prejudices about sexual assault.
• Seek counseling.

CHILD ABUSE

Child abuse is a form of domestic violence and has received increased attention as a public health issue. It is a widespread and serious problem that reaches across all social, economic, racial, ethnic, geographic, and educational groups. According to one expert, "Its prevalence

and annual incidence in the population have reached epidemic proportions" (Donnelly, 1992). Child abuse is defined as intentional harm or threat of harm to a child by parent, friend, or caregiver. The abuse generally is divided in four categories: physical abuse, sexual abuse, emotional abuse, and neglect (Wissow, 1995). Approximately 1000 children die of child abuse each year in the United States (Devlin and Reynolds, 1994).

Many factors account for or play a role in child abuse. There is a strong relationship between being

T E R M

child abuse: physical or mental injury, sexual abuse or exploitation, maltreatment, or neglect of a child by a person who is responsible for the child's welfare; circumstances in which a child's health or welfare is harmed or threatened

TABLE 23.2 Reactions and Feelings of Significant Others of Sexual Assault Victims

Anger	Concern	Guilt	Embarrassment	Vulnerability
• At assailant for committing crime	• For the survivor's well-being and safety	• Feel guilty for not having prevented assault ("I should have been with them" OR "I should have given her/him a ride home")	• Worry about gossip (myth/stigma holds strong effect)	• Realization that it can happen to them as well
• At system for letting "those kinds of people" run the streets	• About how the relationship between survivor and significant other will change	• Feel guilty for not having been there to protect survivor	• Embarrassed for survivor	• Intense heightened awareness of environment
• Survivor for engaging in "risky behavior"	• For the survivor's rights			

Source: Adapted from Illinois Coalition against Sexual Assault, Springfield, Ill.: 1993.

abused as a child and later abusing one's own children. There is also strong evidence that children who witness child abuse regularly, even though they are not physically abused themselves, have a higher risk of abusing their own children in the future. Parents who had been abused or witnessed abuse as children tend to regard child abuse as a normal disciplinary behavior. They perceive their attitudes toward child abuse to be normal and socially acceptable because they do not understand nonabusive adult and child relationships (Miller, 1992).

Child abuse affects children not only physically (broken bones, burns, or even death), but emotionally as well (they may become abusive themselves, suicidal, or withdrawn). Effects are both short- and long-term and invariably devastating to all victims. As the abused child reaches the age of 10 years and older and becomes more independent, he or she may feel in a hopeless situation and many will run away from home. The consequences for many runaways are dismal: teenage prostitution, illicit drug and alcohol use, higher rates of juvenile crimes, and higher school dropout rates (Donnelly, 1992). Child abuse is costly to society and directly or indirectly affects everyone.

Social Dimensions of Child Abuse

Because many cases of child abuse go unreported, reliable data are difficult to obtain; also, abusers and the abused usually do not offer information freely. As a result, much information on child abuse has been incorrect or misleading (Allen and Epperson, 1993).

As more women enter the work force, more males assume greater responsibility for child care. For whatever reasons males tend to abuse their children at a higher rate than females. However, no unique factors have been found that distinguish male abusers of children from female abusers. Male children are abused more frequently and seen by parents as more deserving of harsh treatment than female children. Male children even blamed themselves more than female children for their maltreatment.

Two-thirds of all abused children are between the ages of 5 and 17. Younger children are abused more frequently because they lack both physical strength to resist child abuse and knowledge about what is normal and abnormal behavior. Infants are attacked less frequently than older children by abusive parents, but are at greater

---

HEALTHY PEOPLE 2000

Reduce to less than 25.2 per 1,000 children the rising incidence of maltreatment of children younger than age 18.

The Child Abuse Prevention, Adoption, and Family Services Act of 1988 defines child abuse and neglect as physical or mental injury, sexual abuse or exploitation, negligent treatment, or maltreatment of a child by a person responsible for the child's welfare. In 1986, an estimated 1.6 million children nationwide experienced some form of abuse or neglect. Physical abuse accounted for the greatest portion of abuse incidents, followed by emotional and then sexual abuse. Educational neglect was the most frequent category of neglect, followed by physical and then emotional neglect.

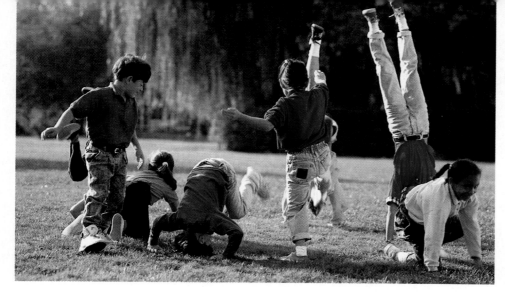

Child abuse is a particularly tragic consequence of the stresses of modern life.

risk of death than older children, especially when shaken. As children pass the age of 15 they are more likely to be abused by peers than by family members.

Children with physical or mental handicaps such as blindness, deafness, mental retardation, or cerebral palsy are at a greater risk for child abuse than others. It is unclear if the physical handicap itself provokes the abuse or if stress created by caring for such a child is the underlying cause of the abuse. Children who are temperamental, impulsive, aggressive, depressed, or hyperactive are also at a higher risk for child abuse. As with physical and mental handicaps, it is unclear if these behaviors create stress that contributes to parental child abuse.

Physical Dimensions of Child Abuse

The underlying causes of child abuse usually vary from one social environment or community to another. In particular, parents who are isolated because of frequent moves or the inability to make friends tend to abuse their children more than others (Devlin and Reynolds, 1994). Many of these parents feel there is nowhere to go for advice on parenting skills and have no close friends or relatives to confide in.

If the family lives in an unsafe neighborhood, members may feel afraid to venture out to seek help for their problems. This fear results in even more isolation and may exacerbate family conflicts and abuse. If the family lives in an area of limited public transportation or owns no car, these factors also contribute to the risk of child abuse. Contributing reasons for child abuse seem to be social isolation, lack of friends, dangerous neighborhoods, or lack of access to transportation (Finkelhor and Dziuba-Leatherman, 1994).

> *Loneliness and the feeling of being unwanted is the most terrible poverty.*
> Mother Teresa

Cultural Dimensions of Child Abuse

Different cultural beliefs play a role in the risk of child abuse. Latino men tend to regard themselves as *macho* (masculine), which may be used to justify abusive behavior towards their families and children. Their society has accepted macho behavior as the social norm, although as Latino families become acculturated to the value system of middle-class Americans, child abuse shows a decline. However, it should be noted that *machismo* (the need for males to appear powerful) manifests itself in all ethnic groups. Child abuse occurs among all socioeconomic classes.

In the past, physical punishment by fathers was viewed as necessary discipline and was not regarded as child abuse. Abuse by mothers was more the focus of attention, as mothers were expected to be supportive of their children and not physically violent. However, beliefs and attitudes regarding child abuse are slowly changing and males and females are now regarded as equally responsible.

Lack of knowledge and skills about child care predispose parents to child abuse, possibly due to frustration and stress created by the needs of a child and its apparent lack of cooperation. Males who are primary care givers usually have received little or no training regarding child care.

The same holds true for adolescent mothers and mothers with low educational levels, for example, high school dropouts. They, too, lack the knowledge and skills necessary for adequate child care. This lack places them in a stressful situation in which abuse is more likely to occur. These mothers feel they have no one to turn to for help and they may not even know where to obtain help. In frustration, they abuse their children.

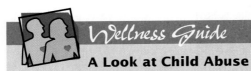

A Look at Child Abuse

Incidence and Prevalence

- Nearly 3 million cases of child abuse and neglect were reported in 1992.
- Approximately 1,000 children will die as a result of child abuse each year.

Facts about Child Abuse

- More males are abused as children.
- Average age of abused child—7 years of age.
- Special children at higher risk for abuse (hyperactive, handicapped, impulsive).
- Fathers' rates of child abuse are rising.
- Younger mothers higher risk for child abuse.

Definition

- Four types of abuse: physical, sexual, emotional, and neglect.
- "An injury or pattern of nonaccidental injuries to a child or some type of damage for which there is no reasonable explanation" (National Committee for Prevention of Child Abuse).

Environmental Determinants

- Social isolation—higher risk.
- Unsafe neighborhood.
- Lack of transportation.

Internal Determinants (factors one may have control of)

- Violence is a learned behavior.
- Parents previously abused as children or witnessed abused—higher risk.
- Cultural beliefs—males are dominant.
- Lack of knowledge and skills— parenting and child care.

External Determinants (factors one may not have control of)

- Financial difficulties.
- Marital conflict.
- Step-parents or significant others.
- Family cohesiveness.
- Work-related stress.
- Peer and sibling abuse.

Recommendations for Programming

- Birth control education.
- Stress management.
- Conflict resolution.
- Anger mediation.
- Life and social skills training.
- Alternatives to foster care.
- Provide transportation.
- Increase funding to treat and prevent child abuse.
- Empowerment programs.
- Training of health care providers and educators.

Child Abuse Prevention Strategies

There are child abuse prevention programs that can help parents reduce the stress that is a risk factor in child abuse. These programs emphasize educating parents on how to care for their children and to avoid abuse. Different stress reduction programs have been developed for adolescent mothers, young parents, fathers who have never been in charge of child care before, working mothers, single parents, step-parents, and siblings who are in charge of child care. Stress management programs are particularly important in communities where unemployment rates are high (Fenley et al., 1993).

Conflict resolution programs also can help prevent child abuse. If people are able to manage conflict without using physical force, the risk of child abuse is lower.

Both anger mediation programs and conflict resolution programs have been shown to help lower rates of child abuse (Fenley et al., 1993).

Training in life and social skills for all individuals involved with child abuse is recommended. Training in parenting skills for both males and females of all ages is also strongly suggested. This training also educates them about resources for assistance.

Violence, no matter what form it takes, is harmful to children, adults, families, and communities. We all need to become more aware of how to prevent acquaintance rape and child abuse. Reducing all forms of physical and emotional violence in our society will make it a healthier place for everyone.

HEALTH IN REVIEW

- Domestic violence includes relationship abuse and child abuse. Violence refers to use of force and power.
- Women who have been assaulted may experience anxiety, depression, substance abuse, headaches, and other medical problems. These symptoms are diagnostic of post-traumatic stress disorder (PTSD). Many long-term consequences of sexual abuse are associated with PTSD.

- Acquaintance rape or date rape occurs when a person known to the victim uses force or power to coerce the victim into having sex. High school and college-age women are most vulnerable to acquaintance rape.
- Child abuse is a form of domestic violence that reaches across all social, economic, racial, ethnic, geographic, and educational groups.
- Education is the key to all forms of violence prevention, including firearm violence, relationship abuse, acquaintance rape, and child abuse.
- Violence in the United States is an important health problem, with more than 20,000 annual victims of homicide.
- Violence and the presence of handguns in schools mirror our communities. Violence is generating fear in our schools, not learning.

REFERENCES

Accident Facts, 1994 Edition (1994). Itasca, Ill.: National Safety Council.

Alexander, L. L., and J. H. LaRosa (1994). *New Dimensions in Women's Health.* Boston: Jones and Bartlett.

Allen, C. M., and D. L. Epperson (1993). "Perpetrator Gender and Type of Child Maltreatment: Overcoming Limited Conceptualizations and Obtaining Representative Samples." *Child Welfare,* 72(6): 543–554.

American Public Health Association (1993). "Policy Statement on Domestic Violence." *American Journal of Public Health,* 83(3): 458–463.

Cohen, L. (1993). "Together We Can Stop the Violence," in *Violence as a Public Health Problem.* Proceedings of the Annual Public Health Social Work, Maternal, and Child Health Institute. Maternal and Child Health Bureau Health Resources and Services Administration, Public Health Service, Washington, D.C.

Devlin, B. K., and E. Reynolds (1994). "Child Abuse: How to Recognize It, How to Intervene." *American Journal of Nursing,* 94(3): 26–32.

Donnelly, D. (1992). "Healthy Families America." *Child Today,* 21(2): 25–28.

Duker, L. (ed.) (1994). *Firearm Facts.* McLean, Va.: National Maternal and Child Health Clearinghouse.

Fenley, M. A., J. L. Gaiter, M. Hammet, L. C. Liburd, J. A. Mercy, P. W. O'Carroll, C. Onwuachi-Saunders, K. E. Powell, and T. N. Thornton (1993). *The Prevention of Youth Violence: A Framework for Community Action.* Atlanta, Ga.: Centers for Disease Control and Prevention.

Finkelhor, D., and J. Dziuba-Leatherman (1994). "Victimization of Children." *The American Psychologist,* 49(3): 173–184.

Gidycz, C. A., and M. P. Koss (1991). "The Effects of Acquaintance Rape on the Female Victim." in A. Parrot, ed., *Acquaintance Rape: The Hidden Crime.* New York: John Wiley.

Illinois Coalition against Sexual Assault [ICASA] (1993). Springfield, Ill.

Kantrowitz, B. (1993). "Teen Violence: Wild in the Streets." *Newsweek,* August 2.

Kassirer, J. P. (1991). "Firearms and the Killing Threshold." *New England Journal of Medicine,* 325(23): 1647–1650.

Kellerman, A. L., et al. (1992). "Suicide in the Home in Relation to Gun Ownership." *New England Journal of Medicine,* 327(7): 467.

Koss, M. P., and M. R. Harvey (1991). *The Rape Victim: Clinical and Community Interventions.* Newbury Park, Calif.: Sage Library of Social Research, Sage Publications.

Miller, T. R. (1992). "The Relationship of Abuse and Witnessing Violence on the Child Abuse Potential Inventory with Black Adolescents." *Journal of the American Medical Association,* 267(23): 3142.

Rapaport, K., and C. D. Posey (1991). "Sexually Coercive College Males," in A. Parrot, ed., *Acquaintance Rape: The Hidden Crime.* New York: John Wiley.

Sniffen, M. J. (1995). "New Survey Method Doubles Reports of Rapes." *Chicago Sun-Times,* August 17.

United States Department of Health and Human Services (1991). *Healthy People 2000: National Health Promotion and Disease Prevention Objectives.* (USDHHS Pub. No. [PHS] 91-50212). Washington, D.C.: U.S. Government Printing Office.

United States Department of Justice, Bureau of Statistics (1991). *Female Victims of Violent Crime.* Washington, D.C.: U.S. Government Printing Office.

United States Department of Justice (1990). *Uniform Crime Reports, 1990: Crime in the United States.* Washington, D.C.: U.S. Government Printing Office.

Warsaw, R. (1988). *I Never Called It Rape.* New York: Harper and Row.

Wissow, L. S. (1995). "Current Concepts: Child Abuse and Neglect." *New England Journal of Medicine,* 332(21): 1425.

SUGGESTED READINGS

Alexander, L. L., and J. H. LaRosa (1994). *New Dimensions in Women's Health.* Boston: Jones and Bartlett. The chapter on violence goes into detail about violence issues including rape, relationship abuse, elder abuse, child abuse, and sexual harassment.

Peden, L. D. (1992). "What Every Woman Needs to Know about Personal Safety." *McCall's,* May. This article discusses safety measures women can take to reduce their risk of becoming victims of date rape or other violent crimes.

Wissow, L. (1995). "Current Concepts: Child Abuse and Neglect." *New England Journal of Medicine,* 332(21): 1425. Defines the various kinds of child abuse and treatment strategies.

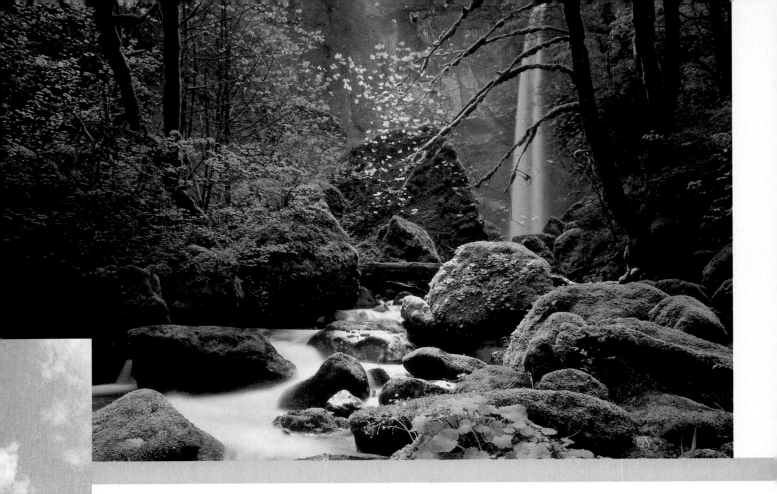

LEARNING OBJECTIVES

After reading this chapter you should be able to:

1. Discuss the relationship between environment and optimal health.
2. Describe the effects of air pollution, including smog, acid rain, the greenhouse effect, and the ozone layer.
3. Describe the effects of radon.
4. Describe the effects of lead.
5. Explain how water is polluted in the United States and the potential consequences of this pollution.
6. Discuss the impact of land pollution.
7. Explain how pesticides contaminate our soil, water, and food.
8. Identify the potential health problems associated with noise pollution.
9. Discuss how human population growth will impact global health and environmental issues.

Working toward a Healthy Environment

*T*he term **environment** refers to all external physical factors that affect us. In order to survive, all animals including human beings require a certain amount and quality of air, water, food, and shelter. If people are deprived of any essential environmental factors, or if factors in the environment are toxic, their health and lives are adversely affected. Anyone who has experienced difficulty breathing smoggy, dusty, or smoke-filled air realizes the unhealthy effects of polluted air. Anyone who has become sick from consuming contaminated food or water knows the importance of uncontaminated food and water in maintaining health.

To achieve optimal health, we must live in a high quality environment. Unfortunately, the quality of many aspects of the environment is deteriorating from pollution, degradation, and depletion of environmental resources. The effects of environmental pollution are long lasting and often irreversible. People and nations are just beginning to appreciate the serious consequences of ongoing air, water, and land pollution that adversely affect health. Dramatic changes in personal life-styles and economic goals are required to reduce existing pollution and prevent future pollution.

Environmental problems are not restricted to the United States or even to industrialized countries; environmental problems are now of global concern. Worldwide problems are: 1) the threat of nuclear war that could affect the environment (this concern has been significantly reduced with the breakup of the former Soviet Union); 2) depletion of the ozone layer due to emissions of certain synthetic chemicals released into the atmosphere; since stratospheric ozone protects earthly life from harmful ultraviolet radiation, its destruction may result in a higher incidence of skin cancer, mutations, and immune system problems; 3) global warming from increased levels of carbon dioxide in the atmosphere; global warming could damage crops and raise the level of the oceans causing flooding of coastlines; 4) land degradation caused by deforestation, desertification, and soil erosion is undermining the ability of many local environments to support their current populations, let alone sustain the increases projected for the years ahead; and 5) loss of biodiversity; the rate of species extinction is increasing due to overhunting, habitat destruction, and the introduction of non-native species into new environments which undermines and impoverishes the stability of natural biotic communities.

Environmental health hazards stem from many different causes, which is why environmental problems are not easily solved. However, underlying all environmental problems is human overpopulation and the consequent overuse of environmental and natural resources. The United States is making progress in reducing environmental pollution and in preserving natural resources, but the government can only do so much. All of us need to

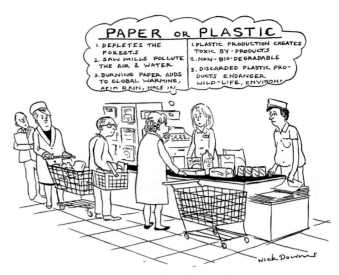

pay more attention to protecting the environment if future generations are to have a safe and healthy environment. As the comic strip character Pogo declared years ago, *"We have met the enemy and he is us."* People's activities are at the root of almost *all* environmental pollution.

Managing Stress

Honoring Mother Earth

"All things connect. Man did not weave the web of life. He is merely a strand in it. Whatever he does to the web, he does to himself." These prophetic words were written by Chief Seattle over a century ago and still ring true today. The neglect and abuse that human beings have inflicted on the planet, primarily in the last few centuries, are beginning to take their toll. Water and air pollution, nuclear and chemical wastes, depletion of the ozone layer, deforestation, and the increased rate of extinction of plant and animal life are all signs of a sick planet.

It may seem hard to believe that the earth is a living entity. Western thought, heavily grounded in science and technology, tends to regard such an idea as foolish or more suitable to myths. But if you really pay

attention to the words of Native Americans and tribal elders around the world, you begin to see the wisdom of viewing the earth as a living entity. But human beings have grown distant and separate from nature and these attitudes have caused major harm to the planet that nourishes all of us.

Whether we realize it or not, we are all connected to the earth like threads of a web. Despite all the advances of technology, we still depend on Mother Earth for the air, water, and food that keeps us alive. Wellness means living in an environment that is healthy, not one that is sick. We can begin to interact with the environment in less harmful ways; even small actions are important as the slogan "Think globally, act locally" points out.

Here are some questions you can reflect on to become more environmentally aware and proactive.

1. How would you best describe your relationship with the earth?

2. Do you see the earth as a rock spinning in space, or as a living entity that provides sustenance in one form or another to all her species of flora and fauna?

3. Getting back to nature can take many forms, from gardening to exotic vacations. What do you do to get back to nature when the urge strikes?

4. Any good relationship takes work. What steps do you feel you can take to enhance your relationship with the earth?

TABLE 24.1   The Six Major Air Pollutants

Substance	Description	Symptoms
Carbon monoxide	Poisonous gas	Large amounts can kill; small amounts can cause dizziness, headaches, and fatigue. Often present in tunnels, garages, and heavy traffic. Especially dangerous for people with heart disease, asthma, anemia, and so on.
Hydrocarbons	Chemicals	Unburned chemicals in combustion, such as car exhaust, which react in air to produce smog. Hydrocarbons have produced cancer in animals.
Sulfur oxides	Poisonous gases	Poisonous gases that come from factories and power plants burning coal or oil containing sulfur. Forms sulfur dioxide, a poison that irritates the eyes, nose, and throat, damages the lungs, kills plants, rusts metals, and reduces visibility.
Nitrogen oxides	Poisonous gases	A result of burning fuels that convert the nitrogen and oxygen in the air to nitrogen dioxide. Can cause a stinking brown haze that irritates the eyes and nose and shuts out sunlight.
Particulates	Small particles	Solid and liquid matter in air such as smoke, fly ash, dust, and fumes. They may settle to the ground or stay suspended. They soil clothes, dirty window sills, scatter light, and carry poisonous gases to lungs. They come from autos, fuels, smelters, building materials, fertilizers, and so on.
Photochemical oxidants	Toxic gases	A mixture of gases and particles oxidized by the sun from products of gasoline and other burned fuels. They irritate the eyes, nose, and throat, make breathing difficult, and damage crops.

OUTDOOR POLLUTION

Smog

Each of us breathes about 35 pounds of air per day—more than 6 tons over the course of a year. Pure, unpolluted air is essential for body functions and for health. Fresh, clean air consists of about 21 percent oxygen, 78 percent nitrogen, and trace amounts of 7 other gases. It is the oxygen in air that is essential for life. If the oxygen content of air drops below 16 percent, body and brain functions are affected. If breathing stops for even a few minutes, a person becomes unconscious and will die unless breathing is restored.

Everybody has heard of **smog**, a term first used in England to describe a hazardous combination of *smoke* and *fog*. Smog causes breathing problems, coughs, bronchitis, asthma, and can even result in death among people with lung diseases. In most U.S. cities, smog is not associated with fog but results from the action of sun-light on various chemicals and particles in the air that come from automobiles, oil refineries, electricity generating plants, and other industrial sources (Table 24.1).

Smoggy, polluted air not only irritates eyes and lungs, but also contributes to health problems such as allergies, lung infections, and heart disease. Carbon monoxide, one of the most common pollutants in urban air, interferes with oxygen utilization in the body. If the air contains 80 ppm (parts per million) of carbon monoxide, the oxygen supplied to the body is reduced by 15 percent. In heavy freeway traffic, the levels of carbon monoxide may reach levels of 400 ppm. It is no surprise that many commuters in large cities who get stuck in traffic jams arrive home with headaches. Car mechan-

> **T E R M S**
>
> **environment:** all external physical factors that affect us
>
> **smog:** air polluted by chemicals, smoke, particles, dust, and so on

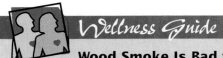

Wood Smoke Is Bad for the Lungs

Everyone likes to sit around a campfire or in front of a fireplace with a roaring fire on a cold winter night. Campfires are both useful and cozy. Fireplaces warm the house and also are romantic. While wood fires may be useful and emotionally satisfying, breathing wood smoke for any length of time can be unhealthy. New studies with laboratory mice that were exposed to wood smoke showed increased susceptibility to lung infections (Stone, 1995).

Of mice exposed to air containing wood smoke, more than 20 percent died after being exposed to bacteria that cause lung infections. Only 5 percent of the mice that breathed unpolluted air succumbed to the infection. The smoke-breathing mice also were more susceptible to infections by a flu virus.

If you get a lot of colds in winter, you might look at your exposure to smoky air. All wood-burning stoves in homes should be airtight and rooms should be ventilated to admit some fresh air. Fireplaces should draw well so that very little smoke escapes into the room. Don't give up the stove or fireplace; just be sure the air you breathe is not smoky.

---

ics and parking garage attendants also are exposed to high levels of carbon monoxide for long periods, and may develop health problems.

The world's automobile population is exploding along with its human population. In 1950, there were

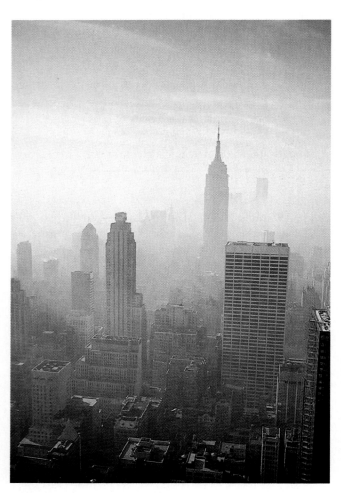

Polluted, "smoggy" air over many large cities contributes to respiratory problems and other diseases.

about 50 million cars worldwide; by 1990, the number had increased to at least 400 million. As nations such as India and China, which together have 38 percent of the world's population, continue to progress economically, the car population in these and other less developed countries also will increase. Car manufacturers will rejoice, but the effects on air and land pollution will be devastating.

A modern U.S. car with a catalytic converter to reduce emissions still produces about 20 pounds of carbon dioxide for every gallon of gas that is burned; this is a significant factor in global warming. Over an average 10-year life, each American car spews 50 tons of carbon dioxide into the atmosphere. If mileage standards were increased and cars were made still more fuel efficient, CO_2 emissions could be reduced significantly.

One major victory in the battle of air pollution was the elimination of lead in gasoline in the United States. There is evidence that the phaseout of leaded gasoline, which began in 1984, has markedly reduced the blood levels of lead in the U.S. population (Figure 24.1). This battle to eliminate lead in gasoline took over ten years to accomplish, which shows the amount of time and effort that goes into changing just one factor in air pollution. Efforts are ongoing to develop less polluting fuels.

Sulfur oxides are produced when coal or oil, which contain sulfur, is burned in industrial or home furnaces. If the air is damp, sulfuric acid is formed, which is a corrosive substance either as a gas or a liquid. Air containing sulfur oxides can erode stone, pit metal, and harm

T E R M S

acid rain: rain, snow, fog, mist, etc., with a pH lower than 5.6

greenhouse effect: the ability of atmospheric carbon dioxide to reflect heat radiated from the earth back to the earth and to thereby raise the earth's temperature globally

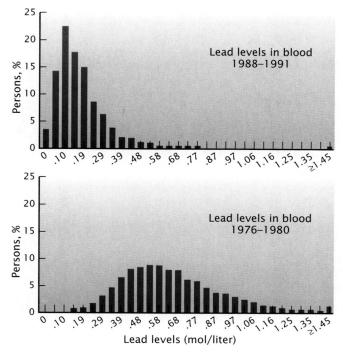

FIGURE 24.1 Reduction in Blood Lead Levels as a Result of the Elimination of Leaded Gasoline
Source: Data from the National Health and Nutrition Examination Survey.

FIGURE 24.2 The Greenhouse Effect Carbon dioxide (CO_2) in the Earth's atmosphere acts like the glass roof in a greenhouse. Carbon dioxide is transparent to the radiation from the sun and lets it pass to the ground, which warms up.

lungs. Sulfur oxides can also combine with water vapor in the air to form acid precipitation, a phenomenon responsible for widespread damage to aquatic ecosystems and forests in many parts of the world.

Nitrogen oxides, which come primarily from automobile exhausts, also interfere with the body's use of oxygen. Photochemical smog, common over Los Angeles and other cities, is due to nitrogen gases produced by sunlight acting on pollutants from automobiles. Cities that have many smoggy days have higher-than-expected death rates and admissions to hospitals for emergency lung conditions (Dockery et al., 1993).

Acid Rain

Acid rain is rainwater containing large amounts of sulfur dioxide and nitrogen oxides, gases that have been released into the atmosphere. When these gases combine with water, they produce sulfuric acid and nitric acid that are dispersed in the rain. Acid rain harms forests, and raises the acidity of lakes and rivers to levels that kill fish and vegetation. Acid rain is a global problem.

Canada began to monitor the acidity of rain in 1976 and the United States began monitoring in 1978. How-

> *Men stumble over the truth from time to time, but most pick themselves up and hurry off as if nothing happened.*
> Winston Churchill

ever, despite the evidence that acid rain harms the environment, the problem persists.

Solutions to the acid rain problem involve difficult economic and political decisions. Acid rain can fall hundreds of miles from the source of the sulfur dioxide emission, making it difficult to determine the exact source and responsibility. Acid rain does not observe national boundaries, so countries need to cooperate if the problem is to be solved. Like other atmospheric pollution problems, acid rain is likely to fall far into the future.

The Greenhouse Effect

Greenhouses came into widespread use in seventeenth-century Europe to prevent plants from freezing in winter. The glass roofs over a greenhouse allow heat to build up inside because the sun's rays penetrate the glass and warm the air. However, heat does not radiate back through the glass very efficiently. Carbon dioxide (CO_2) in the earth's atmosphere acts much like the glass in a greenhouse, hence the term **greenhouse effect** (Figure 24.2).

The greenhouse effect was first described in 1861 by an English scientist who pointed out that carbon dioxide is a good absorber of infrared (heat) radiation. As the

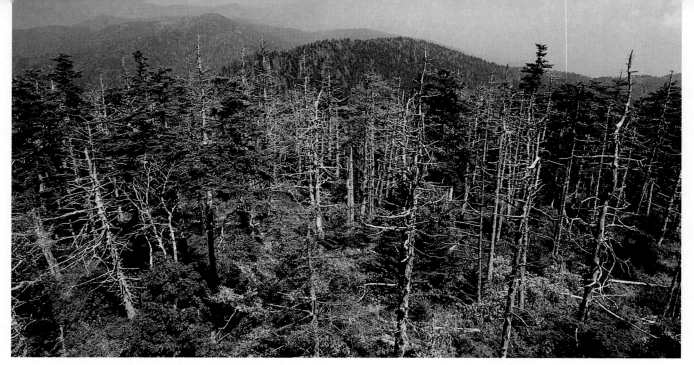

Acid rain can reduce a forest to a graveyard of trees.

sun's rays warm the earth, heat is radiated back into the atmosphere. But some of the radiated heat is absorbed by carbon dioxide in the atmosphere and radiated back to earth. As the amount of carbon dioxide in the atmosphere increases, the temperature of the earth tends to rise slightly because more of the sun's heat is absorbed by the atmosphere.

Until the recent widespread industrialization, the carbon dioxide content of the atmosphere was relatively constant because plants and trees use the carbon dioxide in the atmosphere and give off oxygen. Carbon dioxide also is washed from the air by rain and is absorbed into the oceans and into the formation of carbonate-containing rocks. However, with the great increase in the burning of wood, coal, and oil for transportation, for cooking and

heating, and for industrial uses, the carbon dioxide in the atmosphere has been rising steadily.

Around the world, billions of tons of carbon dioxide are spewed into the atmosphere annually, most of it from human activities. The United States accounts for about 22 percent of total carbon dioxide emissions, but because of the economic impact the United States has been reluctant to pass laws that would reduce carbon dioxide emissions. So far, the global greenhouse effect is small. However, if the average temperature of the earth continues to rise, nations may decide to take actions that will reduce carbon dioxide emissions. The global temperature has risen by 1° F in the last 100 years.

The Ozone Layer

The **ozone layer** consists of ozone molecules (3 atoms of oxygen bonded together, O_3) that form a layer in the outermost region of the earth's atmosphere. The ozone layer absorbs much of the dangerous ultraviolet (UV) light that is radiated from the sun, and protects us from excessive exposure to UV radiation that can increase the risk of skin cancer and cataracts in the lens of the eye.

A class of chemicals called **chlorofluorocarbons (CFCs)** have been widely used as refrigerant gases and as propellant gases in cans during the past 30 years. These CFCs escape into the atmosphere and rise to the ozone layer where they destroy ozone molecules. In the 1970s it was discovered that the ozone layer was thinning; over the Antarctic an **ozone hole** appears during the Antarctic spring (September–October) during which ozone disappears completely in that region. The ozone

> ### T E R M S
>
> ***ozone layer:*** a layer of ozone molecules located in the stratosphere in a diffuse band extending from 10 to 30 miles above the earth's surface
>
> ***chlorofluorocarbons (CFCs):*** chemicals formerly used as coolants that are released into the atmosphere and are responsible for destroying stratospheric ozone
>
> ***ozone hole:*** an ozone-deficient portion of the atmosphere above Antarctica that has been steadily growing since the problem was first reported in 1985
>
> ***emission:*** amount of substance that is released into the atmosphere
>
> ***exposure:*** actual amount of the substance people are exposed to

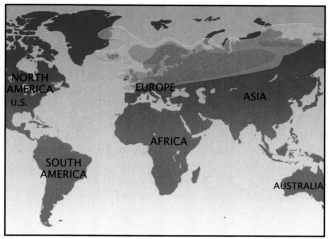

Source: NASA

FIGURE 24.3 The "Ozone Hole" Since its discovery in 1985, the ozone hole has spread dramatically. The lighter color shows the area of most damage to the ozone layer; the darker color shows somewhat less damage.

hole has now spread over populated areas of Asia and northern Europe (Figure 24.3). The intensity of UV radiation in these areas is increasing, exposing people to a higher risk of skin cancer and cataracts.

When the seriousness of the thinning of the ozone layer was realized, 31 industrialized countries agreed in 1987 to phase out the use of CFCs. Even though CFC use has now dropped significantly, due to the large amounts of these chemicals already in the atmosphere, the ozone layer will continue to thin well into the next century and will cause health problems for millions of people (Leaf, 1994).

Evaluating the Risks of Air Pollution

In evaluating the health hazards of toxic air pollutants, two important factors must be evaluated separately. **Emission** refers to the amount of a substance that is released into the atmosphere from an automobile or other source of air pollution. **Exposure** refers to the actual amount of the substance people are exposed to. Frequently, emission can be high, but exposure can be low. Alternatively, emission can be low, but exposure can be high (Smith, 1988).

For many air pollutants such as carbon monoxide, benzene, and chloroform, the major sources of emissions are automobiles, industry, and sewage treatment plants, respectively. However, the major health risks from these substances are *not* from the sources of highest emission, but from gas stoves, cigarettes, and chloroform in shower water, respectively (Table 24.2).

To regulate all of the possible pollutants of the air is impossible, so it is important to identify both the sources of greatest emission and the sources of greatest exposure. For example, benzene is an important chemical used in many industrial processes; it also can cause leukemia in people who are exposed to it. Of all the benzene released into the air, 50 percent comes from automobiles. However, although cigarettes emit only a tiny amount of benzene compared to automobiles, at least half of the total population's exposure to benzene comes from smoking cigarettes (Figure 24.4). Even nonsmokers get most of their exposure to benzene from second-hand cigarette smoke compared to benzene from automobile exhausts. The most serious indoor air pollutant is cigarette smoke.

INDOOR POLLUTION

Cigarette smoke is not only harmful to the person who smokes, but the "second-hand smoke" that is produced is harmful to others who breathe it (Chapter 17). The carbon monoxide levels in smoke-filled rooms can rise to hazardous levels. For example, in bars and conference rooms where many people are smoking, the air may contain levels of carbon monoxide as high as 50 ppm. This

TABLE 24.2 Major Sources of Emission of a Pollutant versus Major Sources of Exposure to It*

Pollutant	Major emission sources	Major exposure sources
Benzene	Industry; automobiles	Smoking
Tetrachloroethylene	Dry-cleaning shops	Dry-cleaned clothes
Chloroform	Sewage treatment plants	Showers
p-Dichlorobenzene	Chemical manufacturing	Air deodorizers
Particulates	Industry; automobiles; home heating	Smoker at home
Carbon monoxide	Automobiles	Driving; gas stoves
Nitrogen dioxide	Industry; automobiles	Gas stoves

*For many hazardous airborne pollutants, the health risk is not related significantly to the major source of emission.

Source: Kirk Smith, "Air Pollution," *Environment* (October 1988): 34.

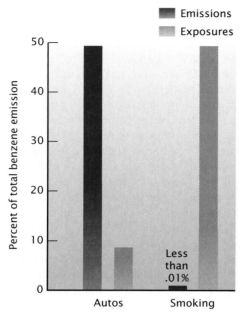

FIGURE 24.4   Benzene Emissions   Automobiles emit the greatest amount of benzene into the air—about 50 percent of the total. However, in terms of the amount of benzene that people inhale, most exposure comes from cigarette smoking.

level is sufficient to produce headache, nausea, impaired judgment, and other symptoms (Table 24.3).

Radon

Another form of indoor air pollution is **radon**, a radioactive gas that is invisible and odorless. Radon is naturally produced in the ground in areas that contain uranium ore. In New Jersey, for example, some homes built on top of rocks that contain uranium ore have over one hundred times the safe level of radon in air inside the

Increase to at least 40 percent the proportion of homes in which homeowners/occupants have tested for radon concentrations and that have either been found to pose minimal risk or have been modified to reduce risk to health.

Radon is a unique environmental problem because it occurs naturally. Most indoor radon comes from the rock and soil beneath buildings and enters structures through cracks or openings in foundations or basements. When inhaled, radon decay products release ionizing radiation that can damage lung tissue and lead to lung cancer.

house. Homes also may be constructed from bricks or building materials that contain radioactive minerals, one of the decay products of which is radon gas. The radon is slowly released into the house over many years.

Long-term exposure to radon increases the risk of lung cancer. Uranium miners exposed to radon for years have a much higher risk of lung cancer than average people not occupationally exposed to the gas. Cigarette smoking seems to act synergistically with radon; smokers who also are exposed to radon get lung cancer at rates much higher than individuals whose exposure is limited solely to cigarette smoke or solely to radon.

The extent of danger from radon exposure in the home is controversial. In 1988, the EPA estimated that as many as 20,000 lung cancer deaths a year might be caused by radon in homes. In reaction to these findings, the media covered the dangers of radon in article after article, creating widespread public concern. As a result of the publicity, millions of people had their homes tested for radon levels.

TABLE 24.3   Symptoms of Carbon Monoxide (CO) Poisoning

Percentage of CO in blood	Symptoms
0–2	No symptoms.
2–5	No symptoms in most people, but sensitive tests reveal slight impairment of arithmetic and other cognitive abilities. Levels of 2–5% are found in light or moderate smokers.
5–10	Slight breathlessness on severe exertion. Levels of 5–10% are found in smokers who inhale one or more packs of cigarettes per day.
10–20	Mild headache, breathlessness on moderate exertion. These levels are sometimes seen in smokers who are exposed to additional CO from other sources.
20–30	Throbbing headache, irritability, impaired judgment, defective memory, rapid fatigue.
30–40	Severe headache, weakness, nausea, dimness of vision, confusion.
40–50	Confusion, hallucinations, ataxia, hyperventilation, and collapse.
50–60	Deep coma with possible convulsions.
Above 60	Usually results in death.

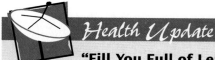
"Fill You Full of Lead" Is No Joke

More than 15,000 indoor firing ranges operate in the United States. Gun enthusiasts who like to spend time at the shooting range and law enforcement personnel are at high risk for elevated levels of lead in their blood. Lead accumulates in the air of firing ranges from the many rounds that are fired from pistols. (Jacketed ammunition used in rifles releases much less lead.) In some firing ranges the level of lead in the air has been measured and found to be forty times above the level that is considered safe. Persons using this range were tested and found to have elevated levels of lead in their blood.

If you fire pistols frequently at an indoor range, you might want to have the lead level in your blood tested.

Lead Pollution

Lead is a heavy metal that is a serious threat to the health of millions of Americans, especially children. Lead contaminates air, land, water, and houses that still contain lead-based paints. Early symptoms of **plumbism** (lead poisoning) are loss of appetite, weakness, and anemia. Lead poisoning also causes brain damage and is responsible for an enormous number of learning disabilities among children (Table 24.4).

Federal guidelines currently permit a level of 10 micrograms of lead per deciliter of blood. Even this low level puts 17 percent of American preschool children of all social classes at risk for some degree of intellectual impairment (Needleman, 1991). Prior to the banning of leaded gasoline, much of the lead ingested by people came from lead-contaminated air. Land and water are still contaminated with lead that finds its way into the body.

A source of lead poisoning among children, especially those living in old, decrepit inner-city housing, is ingestion of lead paints. In old houses paint flakes off, and as children crawl around they are apt to pick up and eat paint flakes. A main source of childhood lead poisoning is now believed to be ingestion of lead-containing house dust. The lead ingested is often sufficient to hinder brain development causing mental deficits later on. Medical authorities on the effects of lead poisoning

HEALTHY PEOPLE 2000

Reduce the prevalence of blood lead levels exceeding 15 μg/dl and 25 μg/dl among children aged 6 months through 5 years to no more than 500,000 and zero, respectively.

High blood lead levels are among the most prevalent childhood conditions and the most prevalent environmental health threat to children in the United States. Childhood lead poisoning is totally preventable. Decreased levels of lead in gasoline, air, food, and releases from industrial sources have resulted in lower mean blood lead levels. However, lead in paint, dust, and soil in the inner-city urban areas has been reduced only to a limited extent. Lead in the home environment is the major remaining source of human lead exposure in the United States.

believe that almost all American children are at risk for some degree of lead poisoning from all sources, and should be tested and treated if necessary (Chao and Kikano, 1993).

Lead is important to many industries, particularly the battery industry, so it is still an uphill battle to reduce the amount of lead released into the environment and to clean up all sources of lead poisoning. Most of the children who suffer from lead poisoning come from poor families with little political power, so the government has not conducted an all-out effort to further reduce the lead in the environment. And it is not only children who are at risk of lead poisoning, but even gun enthusiasts may be exposed to lead poisoning without being aware of it.

TABLE 24.4 The Effects of Lead in People

Amount of lead in blood (micrograms/100 ml)	Observable effects
10	Enzyme inhibition, learning disabilities
15–40	Red blood cells affected
40–50	Anemia, infertility (men)
50–60	Central nervous system affected, cognitive disabilities
60–100	Permanent brain damage, death

T E R M S

radon: a radioactive gas found in some homes that can increase the risk of cancer

plumbism: disease caused by lead poisoning

WATER POLLUTION

After air, water is probably the body's most essential requirement. We can survive without air for only a few minutes and without water perhaps several days. The human body is composed of about 60 percent water, which is essential to every function carried out by the body, including digestion, blood circulation, and excretion.

Agriculture, cities, and industry in this country are enormous consumers of water. For example, producing a gallon of gasoline requires five gallons of water; brewing a barrel of beer consumes a thousand gallons; a ton of newspaper takes about 50,000 gallons; a ton of steel requires 25,000 gallons; and irrigating an acre of orange trees requires almost a million gallons of water a year. A family of four uses about 600 gallons of water daily. Water is as vital to the maintenance of our life-style as it is to the body's continued health.

Water is continuously recycled in the environment by evaporation and rain. However, as more and more water becomes polluted from pesticides, chemicals, oil spills, and sewage, less and less water is suitable for human consumption and agricultural use. Of special concern is the chemical contamination of rivers, lakes, and underground water supplies, which provide most of our water needs.

Waterborne diseases such as cholera, typhoid fever, and dysentery have been virtually eliminated in North America through sanitation and water treatment methods. In many communities the water supplied to homes is purified by sedimentation, filtration, and/or chlorination. The addition of chlorine to water to kill dangerous bacteria, however, may create other health hazards. Interaction of chlorine with other chemicals in the water produces toxic substances such as chloroform and chloramines, which are cancer-causing

> *Your daily life is nothing but an expression of your spiritual condition.*
> *Thaddeus Golas,*
> *The Lazy Man's Guide to Enlightenment*

agents. The widespread use of detergents, herbicides, pesticides, fertilizers, and other chemicals also has contributed to increased water pollution.

In the early 1970s, the Environmental Protection Agency found that the water supplies of many towns and cities were dangerously contaminated with pathogenic organisms and toxic chemicals. As a result of these findings, Congress passed the Safe Drinking Water Act of 1974, which covers 58,000 community water supply systems and another 160,000 private systems. The Act requires that these systems meet federal drinking water safety standards. But it is one thing to pass such a law and another thing to enforce it.

HEALTHY PEOPLE 2000

Increase from 80 to at least 85 percent the proportion of people who receive a supply of drinking water that meets the safe drinking water standards established by the Environmental Protection Agency.

Drinking water is supplied to 200 million Americans (about 80 percent of the population) by 58,000 community water systems and to nonresidential locations such as campgrounds, schools, and factories by 160,000 small suppliers. The remainder of the population is served by private wells, surface water, cisterns, and springs. The most acute and severe public health effects from contaminated water, such as cholera and typhoid, have been eliminated in the United States. However, hazards do remain in our drinking water supply.

HEALTHY PEOPLE 2000

Reduce the outbreaks of waterborne disease from infectious agents and chemical poisoning to no more than 11 per year.

Between 1971 and 1988, a total of 564 waterborne disease outbreaks, affecting approximately 140,000 people, were reported in the United States. A waterborne disease outbreak is an incident in which 1) two or more people experience similar illness after drinking or using water intended for drinking and 2) epidemiologic evidence implicates water as the source of illness.

LAND POLLUTION

Until relatively recently, little attention was paid to the disposal of garbage and solid wastes in landfills around the country. Now, however, we are beginning to run out of space to dump the stuff we want to get rid of. Each year in the U.S., we junk about 8 million cars and trucks, 100 billion cans, bottles, and jars, and more than 200 million tons of garbage. The average American generates more than twice as much garbage as citizens of other industrialized countries. The United States produces 1,584 pounds of trash per person annually, Japan 902 pounds, and the European Union only 660 pounds.

Many old, abandoned solid waste disposal sites are dangerous to health because they contain hazardous materials that may be corrosive, flammable, or contain toxic chemicals (Table 24.5). In 1980, Congress passed

CASE STUDY

Most of us assume that drinking water from the tap is safe anywhere in the United States. Recent events show that drinking city water can be dangerous. A protozoan parasite that can infect the human intestines goes by the exotic name of *cryptosporidium*. This parasite and its eggs are passed in feces and find their way into municipal water supplies. If eggs are ingested with drinking water, the eggs hatch in the intestines and the parasites cause fever, vomiting, and watery diarrhea.

Milwaukee obtains its drinking water from Lake Michigan and uses several water treatment plants to filter and purify the water dispensed to citizens of the city. In April 1993 one treatment plant was shut down, and as a result of inadequate filtration massive amounts of cryptosporidium eggs entered the city's

water supply. A study by the Environmental Protection Agency (EPA) subsequently estimated that 403,000 people became sick to varying degrees from the contaminated water (MacKenzie, 1994). Many communities in the U.S. do not have safe drinking water supplies due to chemical or microbial contamination.

STUDENT REFLECTIONS

• The quality of drinking water in some U.S. communities is threatened by contamination with toxic chemicals or microbial pathogens; what precautions will you now take when drinking water?
• How safe do you believe your community's water supply to be?

the Superfund Act which was supposed to provide for the clean-up of the most dangerous waste sites. Despite spending many billions of dollars, the Superfund Act has only made a small dent in cleaning up hazardous waste sites. By 1993, only 217 of almost 1,300 hazardous sites on the Superfund list had been cleaned up (Stix, 1993). The average cost to clean up a site has been $27 million. These high costs prompt many people to believe we should be looking for more environmentally safe ways of

manufacturing what we need and of recycling what we discard.

For example, discarded automobile tires are a major problem for landfills. Americans throw away about 250 million tires a year; one Connecticut landfill contains 15 million tires and is half full (McPhee, 1993). Some recycling experts have suggested that the government should investigate environmentally safe ways to use the scrapped tires to generate electricity. Each automobile

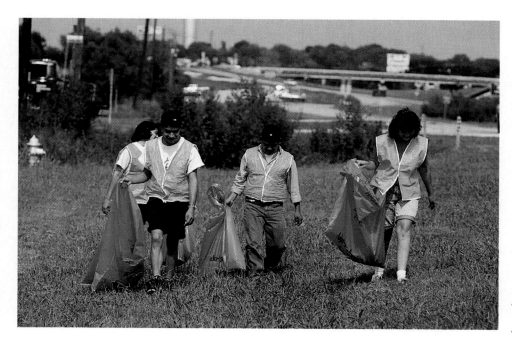

Getting involved in community programs to clean up trash is a great way to help the environment and to feel good about yourself.

TABLE 24.5 Disposal of Hazardous Wastes That Escape into the Environment Causes a Variety of Health Problems Millions of tons of these substances are discarded every year in the U.S.

Substance	Source	Health effects
Mercury	Sludge from chloralkali plants; electrical equipment, fluorescent lights	Tremors, mental retardation, loss of teeth, kidney damage, neurological damage
Arsenic	Arsenic trioxide from coal combustion and from metal smelters	Diarrhea, vomiting, paralysis, skin cancers
Cadmium	Waste from electroplating industry; paint containers, nickel-cadmium batteries	Lung diseases
Cyanide	Electroplating industry waste	Poisoning, interferes with cellular energy metabolism
Pesticides	Solid wastes and wastes in solutions	Multiple effects including rashes, respiratory and gastrointestinal symptoms, neurological disorders, hemorrhages

tire is the equivalent of about 2.5 gallons of oil. Stacked up in landfills around the country are tires that add up to about 178 million barrels of oil. But political and economic pressures force the U.S. to import foreign oil, rather than explore new ways to clean up the environment and produce energy.

PESTICIDES

Soil, water, and some foods have become increasingly contaminated with chemicals used to control weeds, insects, and plant diseases in the environment. Any chemical capable of killing is called a **pesticide**. Specific kinds of chemicals that destroy certain kinds of organisms are **insecticides** (kills insects), **fungicides** (kills molds and fungi), **herbicides** (kills weeds), and **rodenticides** (kills rats and mice). Pesticides are important to the agriculture industry, which has

claimed over the years that the abundance and quality of food grown in the United States depend on the use of chemicals to destroy crop pests. While pesticides may contribute to agricultural productivity (although this is contested by people who practice organic farming), widespread dissemination of pesticides in the environment has created health and pollution problems for people and animals.

The evidence over the safety of pesticide use is both confusing and controversial. Pesticide manufacturers claim that their products are perfectly safe when used as directed. Monitoring of pesticide residues on food shows that the levels are not dangerous. However, consumer groups and many scientists argue that pesticides cause much more harm than good both to people and to the environment, and are responsible for many serious health problems.

Many pesticides have been found to be so dangerous that their use has been banned by EPA, the federal agency that regulates pesticide use. One of the most widely used pesticides, DDT, was found to be carcinogenic and was banned by the EPA more than 20 years ago. However, DDT residues persist in soil and water.

In 1989 a report on pesticides in food by the National Resource Defense Council forced the EPA to ban the pesticide Alar, which was being sprayed on apples. It was felt that the pesticide residues that wound up in applesauce and apple juice would put children at risk for health problems. The ban on the use of Alar was fought unsuccessfully by the apple-growing industry. The use of other pesticides such as heptachlor, kepone, dieldrin, mirex, and toxophene has been banned and off the market in the United States for a number of years. The quandary faced by EPA is balancing the necessary use of chemicals by agriculture and other industries while safeguarding the public's health.

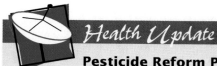

Pesticide Reform Proposed

Reforms to update and improve U.S. food safety and pesticide laws to reduce pesticide risks, especially to infants and children, were proposed during the fall 1993 by the Food and Drug Administration, U.S. Department of Agriculture, and the Environmental Protection Agency. The reforms would extend the strict FDA health-based food additives standard of a "reasonable certainty of no harm" to all pesticide-treated foods, including raw fruits and vegetables. Proposals also contain specific provisions to protect infants and children from pesticide risks. These proposals are the first reforms of pesticide laws since the 1970s.

Source: Adapted from *FDA Consumer* (January-February, 1994).

For example, millions of homes in the United States have been treated for termite control. Until recently, the two most commonly used chemicals for killing termites were chlordane and heptachlor, both related in chemical structure to DDT. These chemicals do not break down and persist in houses and the environment for at least 25 years. Exposure to these pesticides is claimed by some to cause headaches, breathing problems, fatigue, nervous system disorders, liver and kidney damage, and possibly cancer. Some people have had to abandon their homes because of health problems resulting from the pesticides used to kill termites.

Generally, the health effects of pesticides on people and other animals are subtle. For the most part, pesticides do not cause sudden, severe sickness or death unless the amount of exposure is extremely high. The amount of pesticide capable of causing death varies widely depending on the specific chemical in question as well as on individual susceptibility to these poisons. For some insecticides and rodenticides, a very small amount can kill a full-grown person. However, there is growing concern over pesticide residues in the environment that may be responsible for the increase in breast and uterine cancer (Davis et al., 1993).

Year after year, thousands of tons of various pesticides are released into the environment (Table 24.6). Most of these chemicals do not degrade easily and accumulate in soil, lakes, and rivers. Plants and animals in the environment absorb chemicals, which become more and more concentrated as they move up the food chain.

Many large animals, birds, and fish now have high levels of pesticides in their tissues. For example, in a lake in Florida, 80 to 95 percent of alligator eggs have failed to hatch in recent years, a mortality rate ten times normal. The alligator eggs contain abnormal levels of estrogen and testosterone, which are essential reproductive hormones in all animals (Begley and Glick, 1994). The few male and female alligators that do survive are reproductively abnormal and males have abnormally small penises. A pesticide called **dicofol**, similar to

TERMS

pesticide: a chemical that kills insects and other unwanted organisms

insecticide: a pesticide that kills insects

fungicide: a chemical that kills fungi

herbicide: a chemical that kills weeds

rodenticide: a chemical that kills mice and rats

dicofol: a pesticide that mimics the action of estrogen and causes reproductive abnormalities

TABLE 24.6   Amounts of Pesticides Released into the Environment Each Year in the U.S.
Environmental Protection Agency estimates for 1990.

Pesticide	Usage (1000 lb)
Alachlor	100,000
Atrazine	100,000
2,4-D	67,000
Butylate	58,000
Metolachlor	55,000
Trifluralin	35,000
Cyanazine	25,000
Carbaryl	25,000
Malathion	20,000
Metribuzin	17,000
Glyphosate	15,000
Captan	11,000
Mancozeb	12,000
Chlorpyrifos	11,000
Methyl Parathion	10,000
Maneb	6,000

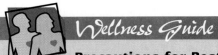

Wellness Guide

Precautions for Pesticide Use

- Before you buy a pesticide product, read the instructions for use and any health and safety warnings. When mixing, do not increase the concentration of the pesticide above the label-recommended amount. Do not purchase the product if you can't use the pesticide properly (you may not have the right equipment). If you don't understand, or feel completely comfortable with, the health and safety information provided, get more information before you buy the product. Also, consider whether you have adequate storage space for the pesticide. A bigger bottle may be cheaper, but can you store it safely?

- Use the least toxic pesticide available for your pest control problem. Try to strike a balance between effective pest control and the safety of people, pets, and other nontarget organisms. Minimize skin and respiratory contact with pesticides. Wear rubber gloves. When you select gloves, consider both the solvent used in the pesticide formulation and the possibility that the pesticide itself can penetrate skin. You may want to use a respirator to guard against inhaling pesticide spray or dust.

- Use pesticides only for the uses for which they are intended. For instance, some wood preservatives are meant for outside use only, so don't use them inside the house!

- Don't leave seemingly empty pesticide containers where children can get them. Children have been poisoned by drinking from "empty" containers that actually contained leftover pesticide.

- Never smoke, eat, or drink while using pesticides.

DDT in structure, is present in the lake as a result of dumping by a chemical company that used to operate on its shore. Dicofol mimics the action of estrogen and causes abnormalities in reproduction and in sexual development.

As a society, we are not ready to abandon the use of pesticides. However, as individuals we should restrict our use of pesticides as much as possible to protect ourselves and the environment. To achieve this goal, many people now grow their own vegetables without the use of pesticides. Others shop at stores that sell fruits and vegetables grown without the use of pesticides and herbicides.

POLYCHLORINATED BIPHENYLS (PCBs)

Polychlorinated biphenyls (PCBs) belong to a family of more than 200 structurally related chemicals that were widely used from 1930 until the late 1970s as industrial coolants, especially in power transformers. PCBs were found to cause cancer in laboratory animals and have been banned for more than 20 years in the United States. However, they persist in the environment and may have contributed to the death of seals and other animals in water contaminated with PCBs. Now scientists have found that PCBs mimic the action of **thyroxin,** a hormone produced by the thyroid gland that causes abnormal development of the thyroid (Stone, 1995).

Thyroxin controls many essential functions in the body and is involved in regulating sperm production. Based on studies of laboratory rats exposed to PCBs, scientists speculate that PCBs may be contributing to the decline in sperm production in men that has been observed in many countries. PCBs and some pesticides share similar chemical structures and may affect human hormones in ways that are just beginning to be discovered. In the future, we may pay a price in health for the past and continuing use of pesticides and other chemicals released into the environment.

ELECTROMAGNETIC FIELDS (EMFs)

Electric power lines, appliances, motors, TV sets, microwave ovens, and power tools all emit very low frequency **electromagnetic fields (EMFs)**. Except for the earth's electromagnetic field, all EMFs come from electricity that is generated by electrical devices of all kinds.

T E R M S

polychlorinated biphenyls (PCBs): a family of banned synthetic, organic chemicals that affect the human thyroid gland and reproductive systems of animals

thyroxin: a hormone produced by the thyroid gland

electromagnetic fields (EMFs): a form of radiation produced by electrical power lines and appliances that may increase the risk of cancer

Only in the past few generations have people been exposed to the magnetic fields that are produced by every sort of electrical device. Until recently, these EMFs were thought to be too weak to affect living organisms, so their impact on health was ignored. Largely as a result of a book by an investigative reporter (Brodeur, 1993), the biological effects of EMFs are now being investigated intensely.

Some epidemiological studies have found an association between the incidence of childhood leukemia and brain tumors and exposure to EMFs (Pool, 1990). Families that live close to high voltage power lines or electrical distribution boxes tend to experience more sickness and more cancers. But the association between EMFs and cancer is very weak, and not every study has found a harmful effect.

All of us are exposed to EMFs every day. An electric shaver or hair dryer puts out a strong EMF, although users are exposed for only a few minutes a day (Figure 24.5). If a person lives near a high voltage transmission line, exposure to EMFs may be considerable depending on the distance between the house and the wires. And the exposure goes on day and night. Calculating EMF exposure, at best, yields crude approximations, one reason why the evidence regarding EMFs and harmful health effects is conflicting.

Despite extensive research on the biological and health effects of EMFs, the only conclusions that can be drawn are that EMFs *may* increase the risk of certain cancers and *may* contribute to ill health, for example, by diminishing the functions of the immune system. Despite ongoing uncertainty about the health effects of EMFs, certain precautions can be taken that will reduce exposure.

Based on current research, the risk to health from exposure to EMFs must be regarded as small when compared to the risks of chemical pollutants in air, soil, water, and food. Moreover, our lives are so dependent on electricity and the gadgets that make life more comfortable, that major changes in electrical use are not anticipated.

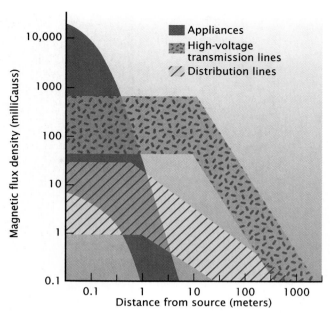

FIGURE 24.5 The Strength of the Magnetic Fields from Sources of Electromagnetic Fields (EMFs) Small appliances produce strong fields, but the strength disappears within a few feet. High voltage lines produce less dense magnetic fields but they cover a large area. *Source:* Adapted from Keith Florig.

NOISE POLLUTION

Have you ever been kept awake at night by a dripping faucet or a neighbor's party? Does the sound of sirens and horns put you on edge? Have you ever found yourself thinking, "If that noise doesn't stop, I'm going to scream." Everyone is sensitive to noise, and excessive noise produces stress and can cause health problems. Noise interferes with sleep and over periods of time can cause fatigue, irritability, tension, and anxiety.

Sound activates the nervous system thereby affecting functions of the endocrine, cardiovascular, and reproductive systems. Noise is a "stressor" and can increase

Wellness Guide

Ways to Reduce Your Exposure to EMFs

- Don't use an electric blanket or water bed heater unless it is a newer model with reduced EMFs.
- Use battery-operated shavers and hair dryers. Battery-operated appliances and toys do not put out EMFs.

- Don't sit too close to computers, TVs, fans, or light fixtures.
- If your work requires long exposure to EMFs, look for ways to reduce it. Do not sit too close to computer screens for long periods.

- If you rent or buy a house, choose one that is not near a high voltage line or distribution transformer.

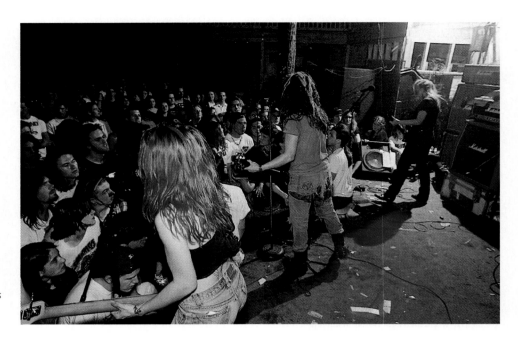

The sound level at many rock concerts is high enough to cause permanent hearing loss.

blood pressure, alter hormone levels, constrict blood vessels, and cause intense pain at high levels.

Sound levels are measured in **decibels** (dB). The danger zone for hearing loss begins at about 85 dB, a level present on schoolbuses crowded with kids or driving in freeway traffic with the window open (Table 24.7). Many daily activities expose us to sound levels that can permanently damage hearing; this level begins at

approximately 85 dB. An estimated 20 million men, women, and children in the United States are exposed to dangerous levels of sound every day that can cause hearing loss (Flodin, 1992).

Rock musicians and people who listen to loud rock music are particularly at risk for hearing loss. Members of many famous rock bands suffer from **tinnitus**, a persistent ringing in the ears, or have lost a significant amount of their hearing. Children are especially prone to turning up the volume and to listening to music with earphones at dangerously high sound levels.

Many people live and work amidst the din of urban life, and have forgotten the rest and peacefulness that come with silence. If you have the good fortune to spend time at isolated spots in the woods or at the ocean, you become aware of the beneficial effects of quiet. The human need for stillness was expressed eloquently in 1854 by Chief Seattle, after whom the modern city in Washington is named:

> There is no quiet place in the white man's cities. No place to hear the unfurling of leaves in spring or the rustle of insects' wings. But perhaps it is because I am a savage and do not understand. The clatter only seems to insult the ears. And what is there to life if a man cannot hear the lonely cry of the whippoorwill or the arguments of the frogs around a pond at night?

TABLE 24.7 Noise Levels Produced by Daily Activities and Machines A noise level above 85 dB can damage hearing and cause hearing loss over time.

Source of noise	Sound level in decibels
Firearms	140 to 170 dB
Jet engines	140 dB
Rock concerts	90 to 130 dB
Amplified car stereos	140 dB at full volume
Portable stereos (e.g., Sony Walkman)	115 dB at full volume
Power mowers	105 dB
Jackhammers	100 dB
Subway trains	100 dB
Video arcades	100 dB
Freeway driving in a convertible	95 dB
Power saws	95 dB
Electric razors	85 dB
Crowded school buses	85 dB
School recesses/assemblies	85 dB

T E R M S

decibel: a measure of noise level

tinnitus: a persistent ringing in the ears often caused by repeated or sudden exposure to loud noises

HOW HUMAN POPULATION GROWTH AFFECTS US

In 1995, the world's population was estimated at 5.7 billion people. By 2050, the world's population is expected to increase to 11.5 billion, assuming fertility continues to fall and that the average family produces just 2.6 children (Figure 24.6). India, with one of the fastest growing populations, is expected to reach 1 billion people by the year 2000. What do these numbers mean with respect to environmental degradation and to human health? One unresolved question of a rapidly growing population is whether the world can produce enough food to feed its people (Bongaarts, 1994). In addition, crowding and poverty lead to disease epidemics and increased crime, conditions that are already appearing in some areas of this country and around the world.

All of the world's environmental problems stem, in one way or another, from human activities and human overpopulation. Deforestation, loss of native species of plants and animals, depletion of natural resources, air, water, and land pollution are all related to too many people needing too many scarce resources. The demand for modern life-styles and products adds to the destruction and pollution of the environment. Indeed, as one close observer of nature has observed, we already may be witnessing the "end of nature," a process that progressed for billions of years before the emergence of human beings a few million years ago (McKibben, 1989).

The actions, needs, and goals of people are at the root of all environmental problems and the ongoing destruction of nature. As the economies and aspirations of people around the globe increase, so does the rate of environmental destruction. Political and economic solutions to the population problem are discussed, but many nations are unable or unwilling to undertake the measures that might curb population growth. Some countries have family planning programs, but the success of these programs depends on educating people and in raising their standard of living so that they understand that large families are not in their interest. Most of the

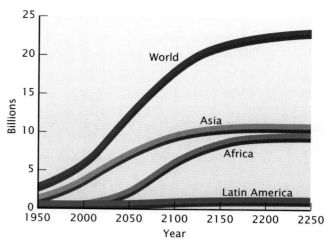

FIGURE 24.6 Estimated Population Increases A global population of more than 20 billion is predicted before growth levels off.

world's population is opposed to any form of birth control, so the world's population is expected to continue to increase for at least the next 50 years.

The United States has made progress in reducing environmental pollution and in slowing population growth (the goal of most industrialized nations is zero population growth). Thanks to legislation, environmental lawsuits, and improved technology, air quality has improved, many waterways are cleaner than they were 20 years ago, and disposal of hazardous wastes has declined dramatically (Easterbrook, 1995). While all this is good news, we have a long way to go in solving environmental and population problems before we can say we have learned to live in harmony with nature. Anytime is a good time to begin to help the environment.

> What we call the beginning is the end
> And to make an end is to make a beginning.
> The end is where we start from.
>
> —T.S. Eliot
> *Four Quartets*

HEALTH IN REVIEW

- To maintain good health, people require adequate unpolluted air, water, food, and shelter.
- The air we breathe is often polluted with ozone, carbon monoxide, hydrocarbons, nitrogen and sulfur oxides, lead, cigarette smoke, and other contaminants.
- Drinking water may be contaminated with particulates or microorganisms that can cause disease. Pesticides in land, water, and food that have hormone-like prop-

erties may be damaging human endocrine and reproductive systems.
- The greenhouse effect and the ozone hole are examples of global environmental problems caused by human tampering and the composition of the atmosphere.
- Pollution of air, land, and water from heavy metals such as lead is particularly hazardous to health. Chil-

dren with even small amounts of lead in their bodies may suffer from learning deficits.

- Noise pollution can cause a wide range of health problems including tinnitus and hearing loss.

- World population is expected to double in the next 50 years, severely taxing an already depleted environment and creating more health and environmental problems.

REFERENCES

Begley, S., and D. Glick (1994). "The Estrogen Complex." *Newsweek*, March 21: 76–77.

Bongaarts, J. (1994). "Can the Growing Human Population Feed Itself?" *Scientific American*, March: 36–42.

Brodeur, P. (1993). *The Great Power Line Coverup*. Boston: Little, Brown.

Chao, J., and G. E. Kikano (1993). "Lead Poisoning in Children." *American Family Physician*, January: 113–120.

Davis, D. L., et al. (1993). "Medical Hypothesis: Xenoestrogens as Preventable Causes of Breast Cancer." *Environmental Health Perspectives*, 101 (5): 372–377.

Dockery, D. W., et al. (1993). "An Association between Air Pollution and Mortality in Six U.S. Cities." *New England Journal of Medicine*, 329 (24): 1753–1759.

Easterbrook, G. (1995). "Here Comes the Sun." *The New Yorker*, April 10: 38–43.

Flodin, K. C. (1992). "Now Hear This." *American Health*, January/February: 59–62.

Gorham, E. (1994). "Neutralizing Acid Rain." *Nature*, January 27.

Leaf, A. (1994). "Ozone Depletion and Public Health." *Hospital Practice*, June 15: 9–10.

MacKenzie, W. R., et al. (1994). "A Massive Outbreak in Milwaukee of Cryptosporidium Infection Transmitted through the Public Water Supply." *New England Journal of Medicine*, 331: 161.

McKibben, B. (1989). *The End of Nature*. New York: Random House.

McPhee, J. (1993). "Duty of Care." *The New Yorker*, June 28: 72–80.

Needleman, H. L. (1991). "Childhood Lead Poisoning: A Disease for the History Texts." *American Journal of Public Health*, 81 (6): 685–687.

Peto, J., and S. Darby (1994). "Radon Risk Assessment." *Nature*, 368: 97–98.

Poole, R. (1990). "Electromagnetic Fields: The Biological Evidence." *Science*, 249: 1348.

Smith, K. R. (1988). "Air Pollution: Assessing Total Exposure in the United States." *Environment*, October.

Stix, G. (1993). "Clean Definitions: The Nation Contemplates What to Do with Superfund." *Scientific American*, December: 26–27.

Stone, R. (1995). "PCBs Pack a Hormonal Punch." *Science*, March 24: 1770–1771.

SUGGESTED READINGS

Bongaarts, J. (1994). "Can the Growing Human Population Feed Itself?" *Scientic American*, March. Discusses the options for feeding a population of ten billion people.

50 Simple Things You Can Do to Save the Earth (1989). Berkeley, Calif.: The Earthworks Group. Simple, practical things each person can do to help heal the environment.

McKibben, B. (1989). *The End of Nature*. New York: Random House. Discusses why we may have gone too far in conquering nature.

Moffet, G. D. (1994). *Critical Masses: The Global Population Challenge*. New York: Viking Press. Examines the impact of human population growth, particularly in the developing world, in terms of the exploding size of cities, pressures on world food supply, impact of population growth, and environmental degradation.

Nadakavukaren, A. (1995). *Our Global Environment*, 4th edition. Prospect Heights, Ill.: Waveland. A broad, up-to-date survey of the environmental issues facing the world today.

Needleman, H. L., and P. J. Landrigan (1994). *Raising Children: Toxic Free*. New York: Farrar, Straus, and Giroux. Two physicians concerned with environmental hazards to health explain how to protect children from the most dangerous ones.

Raloff, J. (1993). "EMFs Run Aground." *Science News*, August 21. Discusses what is being done to reduce exposure to electromagnetic fields.

Raloff, J. (1994). "Gender Benders: Are Environmental 'Hormones' Emasculating Wildlife?" *Science News*, January 8 and 22. Discusses why certain environmental chemical pollutants may be affecting the reproductive systems of animals and people.

Relaxation Exercises and Stress Management Techniques

This appendix contains several relaxation exercises and stress management techniques that you may find useful. As noted throughout this book, the association between stress and adverse health consequences is well documented. By incorporating relaxation and stress reduction exercises into our daily lives, we help maintain our physical, mental, and spiritual health.

You may want to try one or more of the physical and mental relaxation exercises described in this appendix. The techniques include mental imagery (Experiencing the Peacefulness of a Mountain Lake), muscular stress reduction (Progressive Muscular Relaxation), and mind-body harmony exercises (Yoga and T'ai chi). You may want to record the instructions on an audiotape so that you can listen to the instructions while focusing on the exercise. A selection of relaxation exercises on audiotape is available from Jones and Bartlett Publishers, at 1 (800) 832-0034.

EXERCISE 1
EXPERIENCING THE PEACEFULNESS OF A MOUNTAIN LAKE

Imagine yourself walking alone in the early morning along a path leading to some nearby mountains. All around you are trees rustling in the breeze; the path is covered with soft leaves and pine needles. The air is cool but not cold; your body feels relaxed as you walk slowly through the woods. You become aware of the quietness of the surroundings, how different from the constant noise of city life. As you stroll along you hear the calls of different songbirds announcing your arrival. You breathe in the cool air tinged with the fragrance of pine and eucalyptus. You walk through patches of sunlight and see the shadows of the mountain peaks in the distance.

As you gradually move higher, you notice the faint sound of water cascading over rocks and the sound mixes with the wind moving through the branches of the tall trees. Up ahead, a chipmunk is perched on an old stump of a tree, frozen in time in the moment before it decides which way to jump. Suddenly it is gone and you notice the colored insects that are buzzing around the flowers on the bushes. As the path begins to level off, your pace quickens and the air turns slightly cooler. Now the path is more rocky and, as you come around a bend a deep blue mountain lake abruptly comes into view. You climb up onto a boulder to get a better vantage point from which to view the entire lake. You sit down on the boulder weathered smooth by water, wind, and time.

Near the shore of the lake are tall green grasses and spreading back from the shore are clusters of spruce, pine, aspen, and birch. On top of one tree off in the distance a large bird is perched, possibly an eagle. As you watch, the bird spreads its wings and swoops down over the lake, soars up again, and is gone. The peaks of the mountains surrounding the lake are a mixture of grays and white, snow left over from the winter's snowfall. As your eyes move from the lake to the peaks and back to the lake again, you become aware of the harmony of nature, how each part seems to be in balance with the other parts of the scene.

The sky is cloudless except for small puffs of white clouds that circle the peaks and vanish into the endless blue. The rock you are sitting on radiates back the heat it absorbed from the sun, and you feel your body relaxing, melting into the comfortable saddle of the rock. Your eyes return to the surface of the lake and now you notice the evenly spaced ripples moving across its surface.

As your attention becomes more aware of the wind-induced ripples on the otherwise still surface of the lake, you make the symbolic association between the ripples on the lake and the tensions that move through your body. You would like your body to become as quiet and relaxed as the stillest part of the lake. As the cessation of the breeze causes the ripples to cease, so the cessation of thoughts in your mind causes the tension to disappear. As you watch the surface of the lake, all of your attention is focused on the ripples as they form, move toward the shore, and disappear.

Breathe slowly and deeply from your diaphragm and continue to focus on the stillness of the beautiful, clear mountain lake that you have created in your mind. Notice that you can make the surface of the lake as smooth as a mirror; as you do this all of your tensions, thoughts, and worries also disappear and your mind and body become fully relaxed. Hold onto this feeling of calm and relaxation for as long as your mind desires. Remind yourself that this is a place you can come back to in your mind time and time again whenever you feel tense, stressed, or angry. It's your personal safe haven that will always induce a feeling of calmness and relaxation.

Note: You can record this image-visualization exercise yourself or have a friend read it into a tape recorder so that you can simply listen to the instructions whenever you feel the need for some mental and physical relaxation. Also, the details of the image can be changed to suit your own experiences or imagination.

EXERCISE 2
OPEN HEART AND COMPASSION MEDITATION

The heart is vital to life, and heart disease is still the number one cause of death in most industrialized countries. The heart is a pump; it circulates blood through the body. But symbolically, we think of the heart as the center of feeling; love flows from the heart. However, we also think of a *hardened heart,* one that may express mean, hateful, destructive, indifferent, and inconsiderate sentiments. What we feel in our heart symbolically can be manifested as stress and in physiological changes that may eventually produce illness. Feelings of anger, hate, or fear directed toward others may contribute to heart disease as well as other ailments. A healthy goal is to rid the heart of acrimonious, destructive feelings and to develop feelings of love and compassion for others, even

those that hurt us either deliberately or unwittingly. The following suggestions are designed to help you open your heart to feeling love and compassion for others.

- Sit quietly for a few minutes in a comfortable position on a chair or on the floor, and pay attention to your breathing. Feel the air come in through your nose and flow down into your lungs as the lungs expand and your diaphragm moves outward. Breathe in slowly and exhale slowly to a count of ten. Repeat this a number of times while noticing your body becoming more relaxed with each breath. It may help to repeat silently in your mind, "My body is calm and relaxed."

- After your breathing has become slow and even, focus your attention on the left side of your chest where your heart is located. Picture in your mind a symbol of your heart, such as a flower or some other object you associate with love. If you visualize a flower, imagine it starting out as a bud and opening up into a full blossom just as a rosebud opens up.

- As you breathe in and out, see the flower or other object symbolic of your heart radiating love outward through your chest.

- Bring into your mind the image of some person to whom you want to send your love or deep feeling of compassion. Use your imagination to surround that person with the rays of your love and caring.

- Make the feeling of love or compassion as profound as your mind can imagine it to be. Feel the warmth of it in your chest.

- Realize that this love can be sent both to people whom you truly love as well as to people with whom you feel angry or frustrated. Use your imagination to beam your love and caring feelings to the person whose image you have in your mind. You may want to visualize the person at work or at home and see how the person responds to the feelings you are sending.

- Feeling and sharing love and compassion with others helps to keep you emotionally and spiritually well.

EXERCISE 3
PROGRESSIVE MUSCULAR RELAXATION

The following is a slight variation of a stress reduction technique developed by a physician, Edmund Jacobson, in 1929 in Chicago. Our technique involves deliberately tensing various muscles in the body to varying degrees. For each area of the body listed below, tense the muscles for about 5 seconds 1) as hard as you can, 2) about half as hard as the first time, and 3) just the slightest tension. In so doing, you train your mind to recognize varying degrees of tension in different parts of the body and, more importantly, how to relax the tension. After performing these exercises for a while, your mind automatically recognizes tension building up in different parts of your body and that awareness leads to relaxation of the tension.

Below we describe how to tense and relax various parts of the body that most commonly accumulate tension. After you have practiced progressive muscle relaxation exercises for a while, you can apply the same principles to any area of your body that needs to learn how to relax.

Jaws

Take a moment to feel the muscles of your jaws. Notice any tension, even the slightest amount. The jaw muscles can harbor a lot of undetected muscle tension. Now consciously tense the muscles of your jaws really tight, as tight as you can and hold it, even tighter, hold it. Now relax these muscles, exhale, and sense the tension disappear completely. You may even feel your mouth begin to open a little. Feel the difference between how these muscles feel now, compared with what you just experienced at 100 percent contraction. Feel the absence of tension. Now, contract these same muscles, but at half the full intensity, a 50 percent contraction. Hold the tension, keep holding, and now relax again. Feel how relaxed these muscles are. Compare this feeling of relaxation with what you felt before. By comparing the difference in tension levels, a greater sense of relaxation will surface. Once again, contract these same muscles, but with only a 5 percent contraction. A 5 percent contraction is a very slight twinge, with no motion whatsoever, just the acknowledgment that these muscles can contract. Now hold it, keep holding, and relax. Release any remaining tension so that these muscles are completely loose and relaxed. And sense just how relaxed these muscles are. To enhance this feeling of relaxation, take a comfortably slow, deep breath and sense how relaxed your jaw muscles have become.

Shoulders

Concentrate on the muscles of your shoulders and isolate these from the surrounding neck and upper arm muscles. Take a moment to sense these muscles. The shoulder muscles can also harbor a lot of undetected muscle tension resulting in stiffness. Symbolically, your shoulders carry the weight of all your thoughts, the weight of your worries and concerns. Now, consciously tense the muscles of your shoulder really tight, as tight as you can and hold it, even tighter, hold it. Now relax these muscles and sense the tension disappear completely. Sense the difference between how these muscles feel now compared with what you just experienced at 100 percent contraction. Once again, contract these same muscles, but this time only half as tight, a 50 per-

cent contraction. Hold the tension, keep holding, and now completely relax these muscles. Sense how relaxed your shoulder muscles are. Compare this feeling of relaxation with what you felt before. By comparing the difference in tension levels, a greater sense of relaxation will surface. Finally, contract these same muscles at only 5 percent. A 5 percent contraction is a very slight twinge, with no motion whatsoever—just the acknowledgment that these muscles can contract, just a sense of the clothing touching the shoulder muscles. Now hold it, keep holding, and relax. Release any remaining tension so that these muscles are completely loose and relaxed. To enhance this feeling of relaxation, take a slow, deep breath and sense how relaxed your shoulder muscles have become.

Hands and Forearms

Concentrate on the muscles of your hands and forearms. Take a moment to feel these muscles including your fingers, palms, wrists, and forearms. Notice the slightest bit of tension. Now consciously tense the muscles of each hand and forearm really tight by making a fist, as tight as you can and hold it, like you're going to punch something. Now release the fist and relax these muscles. Sense the tension disappear completely. Open the palm of each hand slowly, extend your fingers, and let them recoil just a bit. Sense the difference between how relaxed these muscles feel now compared with what you just experienced at 100 percent contraction. They should feel very relaxed. Now contract these same muscles at half the intensity, a 50 percent contraction. Hold the tension, keep holding, and now relax again. Sense how relaxed these muscles are. Compare this feeling of relaxation with what you felt before. By comparing the difference between tension and relaxation, a more profound sense of relaxation will surface. Now, barely contract these same muscles. A slight contraction is like holding an empty, delicate eggshell in the palm of your hand. Try to imagine that. Now hold it, keep holding, and relax. Release any remaining tension so that hand and arm muscles are completely relaxed. To enhance this feeling of relaxation, take a slow, deep breath and sense how relaxed your forearm and hand muscles have become.

Abdominals

Really focus your attention on your abdominal muscles. Take a moment to sense any residual tension in either the muscles or organs of the abdomen. Now consciously tense your abdominal muscles really tight as if someone is about to punch you in the stomach and you want to block that punch. Contract as tight as you can and hold it, even tighter, hold it. Now relax these muscles and sense the tension disappear completely. Feel the complete absence of tension. Compare the difference between how these muscles feel now with what you just experienced at 100 percent contraction. Once again contract these same muscles, this time at half the full intensity. A 50 percent contraction is like preparing for a false stomach punch. You know they won't make contact, but just in case you want to be ready. Hold the tension, keep holding, and now relax again. Feel how relaxed these muscles are. Compare this feeling of relaxation with what you felt before. When you compare the difference between tension levels and this current state of relaxation, a greater sense of relaxation will follow. Finally, contract these same muscles so slightly you barely feel the clothing over your stomach area. Now hold it, keep holding, and relax. Release any remaining tension so that these muscles are completely relaxed. Sense just how relaxed these muscles have become. To enhance this feeling of relaxation, take a slow, deep breath and feel how relaxed your abdominal region has become.

Feet

Focus your attention on the muscles of your feet. Typically the muscles of the feet are not tense, but standing can produce a lot of tension. In addition, in the confinement of shoes, feet muscles become tense. Now consciously contract the muscles of your feet by scrunching your toes really tight, as tight as you can. Hold it, even tighter, hold it. Now relax these muscles and sense the tension disappear completely. You may even feel your feet become warm as they relax. Feel the difference between how these muscles feel now as compared with when they were tense. Once again contract these same muscles at half the tension. Hold the tension, keep holding, and now relax again. Compare this feeling of relaxation with the tension you felt at full tension. By comparing the difference in tension levels, a greater sense of relaxation will surface. Now, contract these same muscles only slightly. Now hold it, keep holding, and relax. Release any remaining tension so that these muscles are completely relaxed. Sense just how completely relaxed these muscles are. To enhance this feeling of relaxation, take a slow, deep breath and feel how relaxed your feet and whole body are now. Your whole body feels completely relaxed and calm.

Now lie still, and enjoy the complete feeling of relaxation.

EXERCISE 4
HATHA YOGA POSTURES (ASANAS)

Hatha yoga has been used for centuries as a way to relax the mind and body and to promote health and spiritual well-being. The following Hatha yoga postures are arranged from standing to sitting to lying down positions. Each position should be done slowly and held for about 10 seconds. Always remember that these should be done without experiencing any pain. These postures should be done gently and without strain or excess effort. The postures (asanas) described below are some of the more basic exercises. If you find these enjoyable and helpful in reducing tension, you may want to enroll in a yoga class, as it is very helpful to have an instructor. Also, videotapes are available that allow you to follow a course of instruction in your own home at your own convenience.

1. Mountain Pose (Tadasana) Stand with your feet about shoulder width apart, spine completely straight, eyes straight ahead. Raise your arms completely over your head, palms facing inward and inhale. Hold comfortably for 10 seconds, and exhale as arms slowly return to sides.

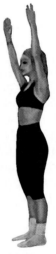

2. Head of Cow (Gomukhasana) Stand with your feet shoulder width apart, spine straight. Reach under and behind your back with your left arm as if to scratch between the shoulder blades. Reach over and behind with your right arm. Try to meet and reach hands behind the shoulders and hold for 10 seconds. If hands cannot touch, you may use a handkerchief. Relax. Then reverse arm positions and try to meet and reach hands. Hold for 10 seconds. Breathe normally throughout this exercise.

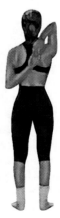

3. Fist over Head (Araha Chakrasana) Begin with the mountain pose. Place arms behind waist grasping hands (fist) together. Lean forward while slowly raising hands over head. Hold for 10 seconds. Then slowly release hands, and let them hang to the floor. Slowly straighten spine to full erect position. Exhale as you raise fist over head, inhale as you release and return to mountain pose.

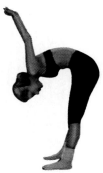

4. Human Triangle (Trikonasana) Begin with the mountain pose and slowly move stance to a three-foot space between feet. Raise right arm and hand straight above head. Rotate head to look at right hand. Slightly bend at the waist and extend left arm and hand down to left ankle, palm open and facing out. As you reach down, rotate left foot out to protect knee joint. Hold for 10 seconds. Inhale as your right hand reaches up, then exhale. Inhale as you return to mountain pose. Exhale upon completion.

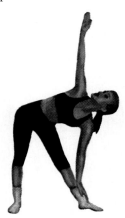

5. Thigh Stretch (Bandha Konasana) Assume a comfortable sitting position with knees bent, soles of feet facing each other. Gently apply pressure on the knees toward the floor until tension is felt, hold for 10 sec-

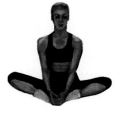

onds. Allow the thighs to relax and repeat again. Breathe normally.

6. One Knee to Chest Lying on your back, keeping the back flat, bring right knee to chest by holding back of right leg at knee joint and hold for 10 seconds. Relax by extending right leg on the floor, and bring left leg to chest and hold for 10 seconds. Exhale as each leg is brought to chest, inhale as leg is returned to full extension.

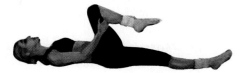

7. Two Knees to Chest Lying on your back keeping the back flat, bring both legs to the chest by holding the legs with your hands behind the knees. "Hug" the knees to the chest for 10 seconds. Breathe normally.

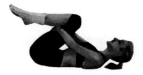

8. Cobra (Bhujanghasana) Begin lying on your stomach, legs fully extended, and feet curled. Place your hands directly under your shoulders. Slowly raise your chest and head off the floor by contracting the lower back muscles. Try not to push with your hands. Hold for 10 seconds, then slowly return chest to the floor. Inhale as chest rises off the floor, and exhale as you return to starting position.

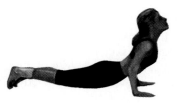

9. Sit and Reach (Paschimottasana) In a sitting position, extend legs straight in front of hips, spine straight. Lean chest comfortably toward knees, ankles, or feet, reaching with hands. Keep back straight. Hold for 10 seconds, then relax by slightly bending knees, sitting upright. Exhale as you lean toward feet, inhale as you relax. Repeat three times.

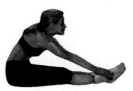

10. Spinal Twist (Ardha Matsyendrasana) In a sitting position, with spine erect, place left leg over right knee, foot flat on floor. Extend right arm with hand placed on left ankle. Extend left arm behind waist, palm on floor for balance. Turn head and trunk to left side, keep chin up. Hold for 10 seconds. Breathe normally.

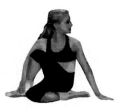

11. The Fish (Matsyasana)   Lying on back, legs fully extended, place hands palm down underneath lower back. Raise chest by arching lower back. Arch neck as well. Hold for 10 seconds. Relax and repeat three times. Breathe normally.

12. Back Arch* (Dhanurasana)   Lying on stomach, grab feet with respective hands. Slowly arch back by pulling feet over buttocks. Hold for 10 seconds, and relax with hands on floor by shoulders, legs fully extended. Repeat three times. Inhale as back is arched. Exhale as the body comes to full extension.

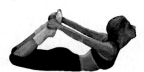

13. Corpse Pose (Shavasana)   Lie symmetrically on your back. Rotate your legs in and out to find a comfortable position. Rotate your arms from the shoulders and rest comfortably palms facing up. Rotate your spine turning your head side to side and then let it rest in complete alignment with your body. Breathe with emphasis on the diaphragm. The end of a yoga session should always conclude with this position.

EXERCISE 5
T'AI CHI MOVEMENTS

The first eight positions of t'ai chi or "moving meditation," as it is sometimes called, are described below. The orientation of the body is described in terms of north, south, east, and west directions. When starting, you should be facing north. T'ai chi movements should be

*Should be avoided if lower back problems exist.

done barefoot or in socks as the feet play an important role in the body movements.

Position 1. Starting Posture   Stand erect with feet shoulder width apart, arms by your side, palms facing back. Chin up, eyes looking directly ahead.

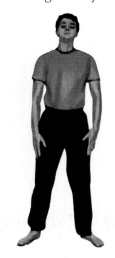

Position 2. Beginning Position   Raise your arms directly in front to about shoulder level, leading with the wrists. Elbows should be slightly bent, shoulders relaxed. Slowly allow the arms and hands to return to starting position below waist level, leading with the elbows.

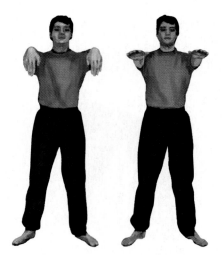

Position 3. Right Hand Ward-off   The body's weight first shifts to left foot allowing left knee to bend slightly. Next, pivoting on right foot, slowly rotate body clockwise about 90 degrees. As you turn east, slowly raise *right hand* to mid-chest level, palm facing down while at the same time raise left hand to your waist level, palm facing up, as if you are carrying a beach ball between both hands. With the completion of the pivot, the majority of your body's weight now rests on the right foot. The left heel leaves the ground and the body then

begins to rotate back (counterclockwise) with the weight returning to left foot. Right foot remains pointed in the eastward direction. Right arm returns to side while left arm slowly raises up to mid-chest level, palm facing in. Hips should remain directly under shoulders.

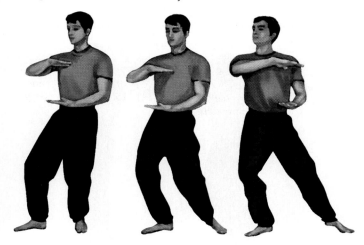

Position 4. Left Hand Ward-off With the majority of weight on your left foot, raise your right heel off the ground and turn your body clockwise, to the east. Raise *left hand* to mid-chest level, palm facing down, while right palm turns upward remaining just below the waist. Again, hold the imaginary beach ball between your palms. With your weight on your left foot, raise the heel of your right foot and direct it to the place where the right toe was previously facing east. As you rotate your body east, shift 70 percent of your body weight from the left foot to the right, knees slightly bent, hips directly parallel to shoulders, the left foot pivoting east. As your body turns east, the right hand rises to shoulder level, palm facing toward the chest. The left hand moves with the body, remaining at mid-chest level.

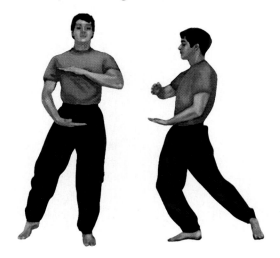

Position 5. Grasp the Bird's Tail (Rollback and Press) Your body weight now shifts (70–30 percent)

from right to left foot. With this shift, body begins to turn slightly north. The left hand, palm facing in, swings slowly down past waist and circles back, up, and over left shoulder. Right hand, palm facing toward chest, moves in toward chest. As left hand comes back to mid-chest level, body continues to rotate east and your body weight transfers back to right foot. Left palm makes light contact with right wrist in a brushing motion.

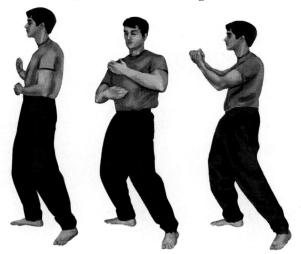

Position 6. Grasp the Bird's Tail (Push) Facing east, the hands begin to separate and descend slowly to upper abdominal level, palms facing out. Your weight shifts from right to left foot, as if you are slowly backing away. Then reverse your weight back to right foot and extend your hands out slowly as if you are pushing an object away from your face. As you push, become conscious of directing energy in that direction.

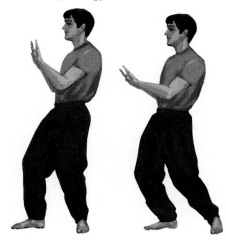

Position 7. The Single Whip Shift your body weight from right foot to left and rotate your body counterclockwise to the north, northwest direction. Arms and hands swing slowly in the same direction, hands directly in front, at mid-chest level. Right heel lifts and is placed where right toe was, now pointing north. As right foot

becomes placed, the body's weight shifts to right foot, and a slight rotation to the northeast follows. Left hand slowly swings to waist level by the right hip, palm facing up. Right arm draws back to right hip, leading with the elbow. Right hand draws to a close with the fingers as if it is going to drop a coin into palm of left hand. Next, slowly rotate your body west, shifting weight from right foot to left. To do this, take a step with the left foot. Right hand rises to about shoulder level. Left hand slowly sweeps in an upward arc from right to left, the wrist twisting to allow the palm to face out as the hand comes to about shoulder level.

Position 8. Lift Hands Slowly lift your right heel off the floor and place it where the right toe was pointing north once again. As the heel makes contact, begin to shift your weight from the left foot to the right, coming back to face north. The hands, loosely extended to make a cross, are drawn close together palms facing inward, with left hand positioned near right elbow.

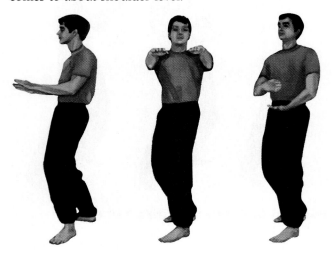

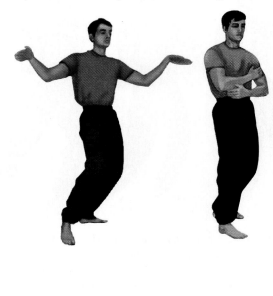

Calendar of Events and Health Organizations

JANUARY

National Volunteer Blood Donor Month

American Association of Blood Banks
8101 Glenbrook Road
Bethesda, MD 20814
301-907-6977
Contact: Public Relations

FEBRUARY

American Heart Month

American Heart Association
7272 Greenville Avenue
Dallas, TX 75231
800-AHA-USA1
Contact: Local chapters

National Children's Dental Health Month

American Dental Association
211 E. Chicago Avenue
Chicago, IL 60611
312-440-2593

National Child Passenger Safety Awareness Week

U.S. Dept. of Transportation
National Highway Traffic Safety Administration
400 Seventh Street, SW
Washington, DC 20590
202-366-9550

MARCH

Hemophilia Month

National Hemophilia Foundation
Soho Building
110 Greene Street
Suite 303
New York, NY 10012
800-42-HANDI

National Kidney Month

National Kidney Foundation
30 E. 33rd Street
New York, NY 10016
800-622-9010
Contact: Local chapters

National Chronic Fatigue Syndrome Awareness Month

National Chronic Fatigue Syndrome Awareness
    Association
3521 Broadway
Suite 222
Kansas City, MO 64111
816-931-4777

National Nutrition Month

American Dietetic Association
216 W. Jackson Blvd.
Suite 800
Chicago, IL 60606-6995
312-899-0040

Red Cross Month

American Red Cross
431 18th Street, NW
Washington, DC 20006
202-737-8300
Contact: Public Inquiries

National Poison Prevention Week

Poison Prevention Week Council
P.O. Box 1543
Washington, DC 20013
301-504-0580
Third full week in March

APRIL

National Alcohol Awareness Month

National Council on Alcoholism and Drug Dependence
12 West 21st Street
New York, NY 10010
212-206-6770

National Cancer Control Month

American Cancer Society
1599 Clifton Road, NE
Atlanta, GA 30329-4251
800-ACS-2345
Contact: Local chapters

National Child Abuse Prevention Month

National Committee for Prevention of Child Abuse
332 Michigan Avenue
Suite 1600
Chicago, IL 60604
312-663-3520
Contact: Public Awareness

Alcohol-Free Weekend

Rhode Island Council on Alcoholism and Drug
    Dependence
500 Prospect Street
Pawtucket, RI 02860
401-725-0410

World Health Day

American Association for World Health
1129 20th Street, NW
Suite 400
Washington, DC 20036
202-466-5883
April 7

Minority Cancer Awareness Week

National Cancer Institute
Building 31, Room 10A03
9000 Rockville Pike
Bethesda, MD 20892
800-4-CANCER
April 16–22

MAY

Clean Air Month

American Lung Association
1740 Broadway
New York, NY 10019-4374
212-315-8700

Mental Health Month

National Mental Health Association
1021 Prince Street
Alexandria, VA 22314-7971
703-684-7722

National High Blood Pressure Month

National High Blood Pressure Education Program
    Center
P.O. Box 30105
Bethesda, MD 20824-0105
301-251-1222

National Physical Fitness and Sports Month

President's Council on Physical Fitness and Sports
701 Pennsylvania Avenue, NW
Suite 250
Washington, DC 20004
202-272-3424

Older Americans Month

Administration on Aging
330 Independence Avenue, SW
Washington, DC 20201
202-401-4547

National Employee Health and Fitness Day

National Association of Governor's Councils on
    Physical Fitness and Sports
201 South Capitol Avenue
Suite 560
Indianapolis, IN 46225-1072
317-237-5630
Third Wednesday in May

World No Tobacco Day

American Association for World Health
1129 20th Street, NW
Suite 400
Washington, DC 20036
202-466-5883

Dairy Month

American Dairy Association
O'Hare International Center
10255 W. Higgins
Suite 900
Rosemont, IL 60018-5615
708-803-2000

National Safety Week

American Society of Safety Engineers
1800 E. Oakton Street
Des Plains, IL 60018-2187
708-692-4121
First full week in June

National Therapeutic Recreation Week

National Therapeutic Recreation Society
2775 S. Quincy Street
Suite 300
Arlington, VA 22206
703-578-5548
Second full week in July

National Water Quality Month

Culligan International
One Culligan Parkway
Northbrook, IL 60062
708-205-6000

National Cholesterol Education Month

National Cholesterol Education
Program Information Center
P.O. Box 30105
Bethesda, MD 20824-0105
301-251-1222
Contact: Information Center

National Sickle Cell Month

National Association for Sickle Cell Disease
200 Corporate Pointe
Suite 495
Culver City, CA 90230-7633
800-421-8453

Treatment Works Month

National Association of Alcoholism and Drug
    Dependence
1511 K Street, NW
Washington, DC 20005
202-737-8122

Family Health Month

American Academy of Family Physicians
8880 Ward Parkway
Kansas City, MO 64114
800-274-2237

National Breast Cancer Awareness Month

National Breast Cancer Awareness Month
Foresight Communications
P.O. Box 57424
Washington, DC 20036
212-581-2200

National Dental Hygiene Month

American Dental Hygienists' Association
444 N. Michigan Avenue
Suite 3400
Chicago, IL 60611
312-440-8900
Contact: Public Relations

National Disability Employment Awareness Month

President's Committee on Employment of People
    with Disabilities
1331 F Street, NW
Suite 300
Washington, DC 20004
202-376-6200

Talk About Prescriptions Month

National Council on Patient Information and
    Education
666 11th Street, NW
Suite 810
Washington, DC 20001
202-347-6711

National Collegiate Alcohol Awareness Week

Interassociation Task Force on Campus Alcohol and
    Other Substance Abuse Issues
P.O. Box 100430
Denver, CO 80250
Starts the third Sunday in October

World Food Day

National Committee for World Food Day
1001 22nd Street, NW
Washington, DC 20437
202-653-2404
October 16

American Heart Association's Heartfest

American Heart Association
7272 Greenville Avenue
Dallas, TX 75231
800-141-8721
Contact: Local chapters

National Red Ribbon Week

National Family Partnership
111590-B, S. Towne Square
St. Louis, MO 63123
314-845-1933
Dates through the year 2000 are October 23–October 31

National Adult Immunization Awareness Week

National Coalition for Adult Immunization and
    National Foundation for Infectious Diseases
4733 Bethesda Avenue
Suite 750
Bethesda, MD 20814-5228
301-656-0003
Last full week in October

NOVEMBER

National Alzheimer's Awareness Month

Alzheimer's Disease and Related Disorders
    Association
919 N. Michigan Avenue
Suite 1000
Chicago, IL 60611-1676
800-272-3900

Great American Smokeout

American Cancer Society
1599 Clifton Road NE
Atlanta, GA 30329-4251
800-227-2345
Contact: Local chapters
Third Thursday in November

DECEMBER

National Drunk and Drugged Driving Prevention Month

Office of Occupant Protection
U.S. Department of Transportation
National Highway Traffic Safety Administration
400 Seventh Street, SW
Washington, DC 20590
202-366-6976

World AIDS Day

American Association for World Health
1129 20th Street, NW
Suite 400
Washington, DC 20036
202-466-5883
December 1

Health and Wellness on the Internet

The Internet has much to offer with regard to resources and information on health and wellness issues. New resources are appearing daily. Major medical centers have discovered the usefulness of the Internet in organizing and communicating medical information to patients, students, and other health care professionals. Resources such as Virtual Hospital and OncoLink have led the way in presenting solid health information to a wide variety of audiences.

The U.S. government has been in the forefront of electronic communication and has made significant strides in making documents and resources in U.S. health agencies available on-line. The U.S. health agencies have always generated health information for consumers, and now the Internet has made this information available to everyone, anywhere.

This appendix contains a short list of Internet health and wellness sites on both the World Wide Web and Gopher. This list is by no means exhaustive; it is just the beginning to finding out what's out there on the Internet. Some suggested sites if you've never "surfed" the net: Go Ask Alice, CDC AIDS/HIV Information Page, Health and Medicine in the News, and, my favorite, Safer Sex Homepage.

When surfing the Internet you will need some time, so sit back, and enjoy all the health and wellness information that is at your fingertips!

WHERE CAN I FIND MORE INFORMATION ABOUT THE INTERNET?

Dern, D. (1994). *The Internet Guide for New Users*. New York: McGraw-Hill.

Gilster, P. (1993). *The Internet Navigator*. New York: John Wiley and Sons.

Gilster, P. (1995). *The Mosaic Navigator*. New York: John Wiley and Sons.

LaQuey, T., and Ryer, J. C. (1993). *The Internet Companion: A Beginner's Guide to Global Networking*. Sebastopol, CA: O'Reilly and Associates.

Levine, J. R., and Baroudi, C. (1993). *The Internet for Dummies*. San Mateo, CA: IDG Books Worldwide, Inc.

Levine, J. R., and Young, M. L. (1994). *More Internet for Dummies*. San Mateo, CA: IDG Books Worldwide, Inc.

Minatel, J. (1995). *World Wide Web with Netscape*. Carmel, IN: Que Corporation.

Ryer, J. C. (1995). *Health & Fitness on the Internet*. San Francisco: Sybex.

Gopher Sites

Address	Topic
gopher://gopher.nlm.nih.gov	Agency for Health Care Policy and Research (AHCPR) Clinical Guidelines
gopher://gopher.niaid.nih.gov:70	AIDS Daily Summary; Daily clipping service published by CDC
gopher://inform.uchc.edu/11gopher_root%3a%5b_data04.data0401%5d	Biomedicine
gopher://tinman.mes.umn.edu	Children, Youth, and Family; a clearinghouse on family-life issues
gopher://gopher.nih.gov:70/00/clin/cancernet/instructions	Cancer; National Institutes of Health
gopher://gopher.niaid.nih.gov:70/11/aids/csr	CDC AIDS Surveillance Data
gopher://healthline.umt.edu:700/General Health Information	Common Illnesses Healthline; The University of Montana
gopher://gopher.health.state.ny.us:70	Consumer Health Information; New York State Department of Health
gopher://info.med.yale.edu:70	Consumer Health Information; Yale University
gopher://cyfer.esusda.gov:70/11/fnic	Food and Nutrition Information Center (FNIC)
gopher://lenti.med.umn.edu:71/11/news	Health and Medicine in the News
gopher://gopher.uiuc.edu/Campus Info/Campus Services/Health Services/Health Information	Health Information, University of Illinois at Urbana-Champaign
gopher://riceinfo.rice.edu:70/11/Safety/HealthInfo	Health Information, Rice University
gopher://healthline.umt.edu:70/11/UofM/hhp	Healthline, University of Montana
gopher://oasis.cc.purdue.edu	Mental Health Maintenance; fact sheets on maintaining positive emotional health
gopher://gopher.nhlbi.nih.gov	National Heart, Lung, and Blood Institute (NHLBI)
gopher://dewey.tis.inel.gov:2013/1	Safety and Health; The U.S. Department of Energy
gopher://enews.com/Health and Medical Center/Health & Medical Periodicals	The Wellness Letter, published by the School of Public Health at the University of California at Berkeley
gopher://mail.coin.missouri.edu:70/11/reference/census/us	United States Census Data
gopher://odie.niaid.nih.gov	U.S. Government AIDS Information; National Institute for Allergy and Infectious Diseases (NIAID)

World Wide Web

Address	Topic
http://www.cdc.gov/diseases/bacterial.html	Bacterial/Fungal Diseases
http://www.ualberta.ca/vjhancock/HealthEd.html	Basic health information
http://stats.bls.gov	Bureau of Labor Statistics
http://www.cdc.gov/diseases/aids.html	CDC AIDS/HIV Info Page
http://www.cdc.gov	CDC Home Page
http://www.netgen.com/cgi/comprehensive	Comprehensive List of Sites
http://www.biostat.wisc.edu/diaknow/index.htm	Diabetes
http://nuinfo.nwu.edu/research	Dissertation Sources for NorthWest U
http://www.interport.net/~asherman/dv.html	Domestic Violence
http://hyperreal.com/drugs/faqs/resources.html	Drug Related Network
http://h-devil-www.mc.duke.edu/h-devil	Duke University Health Devil
http://kuhttp.cc.ukans.edu/cwis/units/Lee/JOURNALS.HTML	Electronic Health Journals
http://www.pacificrim.net/~nature/	Environmental-Project NatureConnect
http://www.epa.gov/gumpo/emap-dat.html	EPA
http://www.columbia.edu/cu/healthwise	Go Ask Alice
http://www.yahoo.com/government/agencies	Government Agencies
http://www.perspective.com/health/index.html	Health in Perspective
http://osler.wustl.edu/~murphy/cardiology/compass.html	Heart Disease
http://www.ifrc.org/	International Red Cross
http://www.vix.com/pub/men/health/health.html	Men's health
http://www.crawford.com/cdc/mmwr/mmwr.html	Morbidity & Mortality Weekly Report
http://www.cdc.gov/nchswww/nchshome.htm	National Center for Health Statistics
http://www.niehs.nih.gov/	National Institute Environmental Health Sciences
http://www.gov/diseases/niosh.html	National Institute of Occupational Safety and Health
http://www.nlm.nih.gov/	National Library of Medicine
http://www.nih.gov	NIH Home page
http://www.yahoo.com/Health/Nutrition	Nutrition/Diet Analysis
http://www.osha-slc.gov	OSHA
http://www.cmpharm.ucsf.edu/~troyer/safesex	Safer Sex page
http://www.cts.com/~health/strssbus.html	Stress
http://cortex.uchc.edu/~libweb/libpg1.html	UCHC Library Page
http://healthline.umt.edu:700	University of Montana Student Health Services
http://www.os.dhhs.gov:80	U.S. Department Health and Human Services
http://www.cdc.gov/diseases/viral.html	Viral diseases
http://www.who.ch	WHO
http://www.who.ch/others/OtherHealthWeb.html	WHO
http://sfgate.com/examiner/womensweb.html	Women's Health

Glossary

A

abortion: the expulsion or extraction of the products of conception from the uterus before the embryo or fetus is capable of independent life; abortions may be spontaneous or induced

accident: sequence of events which produces unintended injury, death, or property damage; refers to the event, not the result

acetaldehyde: a toxic substance produced when liver breaks alcohol down

acid rain: rain, snow, fog, mist, etc., with a pH lower than 5.6

acquaintance rape: (also known as "date rape") sexual assault occurring when the victim and the rapist are known to each other and may have previously interacted in some socially appropriate manner

acrophobia: fear of heights

activators: potential stressors; occurrences, situations, or events one may perceive as stressful

actual effectiveness: how well a birth control method performs in actual use in a population

acupuncture: an ancient Chinese alternative medicine that uses thin needles inserted into specific points on the body to produce healing energy

acyclovir: an antiviral drug that is used to treat herpes virus infections

adipose tissue: type of connective tissue containing fat cells that forms a layer under the skin; serves as an insulating layer and as an energy reserve

adipsin: a protein made by fat cells and released into the bloodstream

aerobic training: exercise that increases the body's capacity to utilize oxygen

afterbirth: the third stage of labor, in which the placenta is discharged

ageism: prejudice against older people

aging: normal changes in body functions that begin after sexual maturity and continue until death

agoraphobia: fear of open spaces

AIDS (acquired immune deficiency syndrome): a syndrome of more than two dozen diseases caused by HIV

AIDS antibody test: detects antibodies in blood that are produced in response to infection by HIV

alcohol abuse: frequent, continued use of alcohol; binge drinking

alcoholic: a person dependent on alcohol

alcoholism: loss of control over drinking alcohol

allergens: foreign substances that trigger an allergic response by the immune system

alpha-one-protease inhibitor: a blood protein that inhibits destructive enzymes implicated in causing emphysema

alternative medicine: any form of therapy or healing performed by someone other than a physician

alveoli: air sacs in the lungs that exchange oxygen and carbon dioxide

Alzheimer's disease: a common cause of senile dementia and other symptoms, eventually leading to death

amino acids: compounds containing nitrogen, which are the building blocks of protein

amniocentesis: a procedure in which amniotic fluid is removed from the uterus and tested to determine if genetic or anatomical defects exist in the fetus

amnion: the inner membrane which forms a fluid-filled sac surrounding and protecting the embryo and fetus

amniotic fluid: fluid from the amnion

amphetamines: central nervous system stimulants used to decrease appetite and to treat hyperactivity in children; also used illegally as recreational drugs

amyloid protein: accumulation of an abnormal protein in the brain of patients with Alzheimer's disease

anabolic steroids: synthetic male hormones used to increase muscle size and strength

analgesics: drugs that relieve pain without affecting consciousness

anaphylactic shock: a severe allergic reaction involving the whole body that can cause death

anemia: a deficiency of red blood cells; often caused by insufficient iron

aneurysm: a ballooning out of a vein or artery

angina pectoris: medical term for chest pain due to coronary heart disease; a condition in which the heart muscle doesn't receive enough blood, resulting in chest pain

angiocardiography: an X-ray examination of the coronary arteries and heart

angiogram: the X-ray image that is obtained from angiocardiography

anorexia athletica: athletes who restrict their food intake to stay slim and/or lean

anorexia nervosa: emotional disorder occurring most commonly in adolescent females, characterized by abnormal body image, fear of obesity, and prolonged refusal to eat, sometimes resulting in death

antibodies: proteins that recognize and inactivate viruses, bacteria, and other organisms and toxic substances that enter the body

antigens: foreign proteins on infectious organisms that stimulate an antibody response

antioxidants: substances that in small amounts inhibit the oxidation of other compounds.

aorta: the large artery that transports blood from the heart to the body

appendicitis: an infection of the appendix

arteries: any one of a series of blood vessels that carry blood from the heart to all parts of the body

arteriosclerosis: hardening of the arteries

artificial insemination: introduction of semen into the uterus or oviduct by other than natural means

asyptomatic carotid bruit: an abnormal sound when a stethoscope is placed over the carotid artery

atherosclerosis: a disease process in which fatty deposits build up in the arteries and block the flow of blood

athletic amenorrhea: irregular or cessation of menstruation due to excessive participation in athletics

autoimmune diseases: mistakes in the functioning of the immune system that cause it to attack tissues in the body

autonomic nervous system: the special group of nerves that automatically control some of the body's organs and their functions

average life span: the age at which half the members of a population have died

Ayurvedic medicine: a form of medicine that has its roots in the Hindu religion and is practiced widely in India

B-cells: cells of the immune system that produce antibodies

balloon angioplasty: a procedure to open blocked arteries

basal body temperature (BBT): a method of contraception that uses daily temperature readings immediately after wakening to identify the time of ovulation; approximately 24 hours after ovulation the BBT increases

bender: several days of binge drinking

benign tumor: a tumor whose cells do not spread to other parts of the body

benzocaine: an anesthetic sometimes used in over-the-counter weight-control products to numb the sense of taste

biofeedback training: adjustment of a physiological process by using a monitor that feeds back information allowing the mind to move the response in the desired direction

biopsy: removal of cells from a tumor for examination under a microscope

bisexual: someone who is attracted to members of both genders

blackout: failure to recall normal or abnormal behavior or events that occurred while drinking

blood alcohol content (BAC): the percent of alcohol in the blood

body fat: essential fats and storage fats; needed for normal physiological functioning

body image: a person's mental image of his or her body

body mass index (BMI): a measure of overweight

Braxton-Hicks contractions: normal uterine contractions that occur periodically throughout pregnancy

breasts: secondary sex characteristics; a network of milk glands and ducts in fatty tissue

bronchitis: inflammation of the bronchi of the lungs as a result of irritation; often accompanied by a chronic cough

bulimia: serious disorder, especially common in adolescents and young women, marked by excessive eating, often followed by self-induced vomiting, purging, or fasting

bulk-producing agents: agents used to promote a sense of fullness in the gastrointestinal tract, thus suppressing appetite

caffeine: a natural stimulant found in a variety of plants; commonly found in tea, coffee, chocolate, and soft drinks

calendar rhythm: an estimate of fertile or unsafe days to have intercourse

calorie: the amount of energy required to raise one gram of water from 14.5 to 15.5 degrees Celsius. The energy released from food is too enormous to be described in these units, so nutritionists use the term kilocalorie

cancer: unregulated growth of cells in the body

cancer-susceptibility gene: gene responsible for familial breast cancer and genes which cause susceptibility to colon cancer; increases the risk of a person developing cancer in his or her lifetime

cannula: a hollow tube for insertion into the body cavity

capillaries: extremely small blood vessels that carry oxygenated blood to tissues

carbohydrates: the most economical and efficient source of energy; biological molecules consisting of one or more sugar molecules

carcinogens: any substances that can cause cancer in people and other animals

cardiologist: a physician who specializes in diseases of the heart

cardiovascular disease: any disease that causes damage to the heart or to arteries that carry blood to and from the heart

carotid endarterectomy: removal of fatty deposits in arteries in the neck to prevent a stroke

celibacy: sexual abstinence

cell-mediated immunity: the response of T-cells to infections

cellulose: a carbohydrate forming the skeleton of most plant structures and plant cells. It is the most abundant polysaccharide in nature and is the source of dietary fiber, preventing constipation by adding bulk to the bowels

cervical cap: small latex cap that covers the cervix, used with spermicidal jelly or cream inside the cap

cervix: the lower and narrow end of the uterus

cesarean section: delivery of the fetus through a surgical opening in the abdomen and uterus

chancre: the primary lesion of syphilis, which appears as a hard, painless sore or ulcer often on the penis or vaginal tissue

chemical carcinogen: a chemical that damages cells and causes cancer

chemotherapy: use of toxic chemicals to kill cancer cells and treat some forms of cancer

chewing tobacco: a form of smokeless tobacco; chewed or placed in mouth between lower lip and gum

ch'i: a Chinese term referring to the balance of energy in the body

child abuse: physical or mental injury, sexual abuse or exploitation, maltreatment, or neglect of a child by a person who is responsible for the child's welfare; circumstances in which a child's health or welfare is harmed or threatened

chiropractic: an alternative medicine that uses manipulation of the spine and joints for healing

chlamydia: a sexually transmitted disease caused by the bacterium *Chlamydia trachomatis*

chlorofluorocarbons (CFCs): chemicals formerly used as coolants that are released into the atmosphere and are responsible for destroying stratospheric ozone

cholesterol: a fatlike compound occurring in bile, blood, brain and nerve tissue, liver, and other parts of the body

chorionic villus analysis: a prenatal procedure used to determine if genetic or anatomical defects exist in a fetus; an alternative to amniocentesis

chronic fatigue syndrome (CFS): a debilitating disease associated with abnormalities in the immune system; the cause of the disease is not known

chronic obstructive pulmonary diseases (COPD): diseases that restrict the ability of the body to obtain oxygen through the respiratory structures (bronchi and lungs); these diseases include asthma, bronchitis, and emphysema

cilia: microscopic hairs in the lining of the bronchial tubes

circumcision: a surgical procedure to remove the foreskin from the penis

claustrophobia: fear of closed spaces

clitoris: small, sensitive organ located in front of the vaginal opening; center of sexual pleasuring

cocaine: a stimulant drug obtained from the leaves of the coca shrub that causes feelings of exhilaration, euphoria, and physical vigor

codependency: a relationship pattern in which the nonaddicted family members identify with the alcoholic

cognition: the act or process of knowing in the broadest sense

coitus interruptus: removing the penis from the vagina just prior to ejaculation; also called withdrawal or pulling out

colostrum: yellowish liquid secreted from the breasts; contains antibodies and protein

communicable disease: an infectious disease that is usually transmitted from person to person

complex carbohydrates: a class of carbohydrates called polysaccharides; foods composed of starch and cellulose

complex diseases and **complex traits:** diseases or traits determined by many genes as well as environmental factors

computerized tomography scan: use of multiple X-ray images to construct a three-dimensional image of a diseased organ or body part

condom: a latex or polyurethane sheath worn over the penis (male condom) or inside the vagina (female condom); can be both a barrier method and act as a prophylactic against sexually transmitted diseases

congeners: flavorings, colorings, and other chemicals present in alcoholic beverages

congenital defect: any physical or biological abnormality observed in a newborn

conscious: knowing or perceiving something within oneself

consequences: the effect of one's action; the effect of stress response

contact dermatitis: an allergic reaction of the skin to something that is touched

contraceptive sponge: a polyurethane sponge that contains one gram of the spermicide nonoxynol-9

contraindication: any medical reason for not taking a particular drug

cool-down: the period in which an individual performs light or mild exercise immediately following competition or a training session; the primary purpose is to speed the removal of lactic acid from the muscles and allow the body to gradually return to a resting state

coping: the ability to manage yourself in a difficult situation

coping strategies: ways people devise to prevent, avoid, or control emotional distress from unfulfilled needs

copulation: sexual intercourse

coronary arteries: two arteries arising from the aorta that supply blood to the heart muscle

coronary bypass surgery: surgery to improve blood supply to the heart muscle. Most often performed when narrowed coronary arteries reduce the flow of oxygenated blood to the heart.

cortisol: a steroid hormone secreted by the cortex (outer layer) of the adrenal gland

Cowper's glands: small glands secreting drops of alkalinizing fluid into the urethra

culpotomy: a female sterilization procedure

cumulative trauma disorders: disorders caused by repeated stress to a body part; carpal tunnel syndrome is considered a cumulative trauma disorder

cystitis: inflammation of the bladder

cytokines: small molecules that coordinate the activities of B-cells and T-cells

decibel: a measure of noise level

defense mechanisms: mental strategies for controlling anxiety

delirium tremens (DTs): hallucinations and uncontrollable shaking sometimes caused by withdrawal of alcohol in alcohol-dependent individuals

denial: refusal to admit you (or someone else) have a drinking problem

Depo-Provera: injectable form of medroxyprogesterone acetate

depression: a mental disorder characterized by sadness, feelings of inadequacy, and low self-esteem

diagnosis: the cause of a disease or illness as determined by a physician

diaphragm: a soft, rubber, dome-shaped contraceptive device worn over the cervix and used with spermicidal jelly or cream

diastole: the pressure in the arteries when the heart relaxes

dicofol: a pesticide that mimics the action of estrogen and causes reproductive abnormalities

dilation and curettage (D and C): dilation of the cervix with use of a wand or laminaria and scraping the uterine lining; this procedure is often used during abortion

dilation and evacuation (D and E): dilation of the cervix and evacuation of the uterine contents using vacuum techniques

distress: stress resulting from unpleasant stressors

diuretics: drugs that increase the urine production

DNA (deoxyribonucleic acid): the chemical substance in chromosomes that carries genetic information; DNA is present in virtually all body cells

dose: amount of drug that is administered

double blind: when neither the person receiving the drug nor the person administering the drug know whether it is a placebo or the real drug

douching: rinsing the vaginal canal with a liquid; not an effective means of birth control or STD prevention

drug: a single chemical substance in a medicine that alters the structure or function of one or more of the body's biological processes

drug abuse: persistent or excessive use of a drug without medical or health reasons

drug hypersensitivity: an allergic reaction to a drug

ectopic pregnancy: a pregnancy occurring outside the uterus, usually in the fallopian tubes

electromagnetic fields (EMFs): a form of radiation produced by electrical power lines and appliances that may increase the risk of cancer

embryo: the developing infant during the first two months of conception

emission: amount of substance that is released into the atmosphere

emotional wellness: understanding emotions and knowing how to cope with problems that arise in everyday life, and how to endure stress

emphysema: a progressive degeneration of the lung alveoli, causing breathing and oxygen assimilation to become more and more difficult

enabling: denial of, or excuses for, the excessive drinking by an alcoholic to whom one is close

endometrium: the inner lining of the uterus

endorphins and **enkephalins:** morphine-like substances that are secreted by the brain which mitigate pain; produced during strenuous exercise and childbirth

endurance: the ability to work out over a period of time without fatigue

environment: all external physical factors that affect us

environmental model: modern analyses of ecosystems and environmental risks to health, such as socioeconomic status, education, and various environmental factors that affect health

enzymes: proteins in cells that carry out and speed up chemical reactions

epidemiology: a branch of science that studies the causes and frequencies of diseases in human populations

epididymitis: inflammation of the epididymis (a structure that connects the vas deferens and the testes)

epinephrine: a hormone secreted by the medulla (inner core) of the adrenal gland; also called adrenaline

episiotomy: an incision in the perineum to facilitate passage of the baby's head during childbirth while minimizing injury to the woman

essential amino acids: amino acids that cannot be synthesized by the body and must be provided by food

essential fat: necessary and required fat in the diet; required for normal physiological functioning

essential hypertension: high blood pressure that is not caused by any observable disease

essential nutrients: chemical substances obtained from food and needed by the body for growth, maintenance, or repair of tissues. Essential nutrients are not made by the body; they must be obtained from food

estrogen replacement therapy (ERT): administration of estrogen to menopausal and postmenopausal women to help prevent symptoms of menopause, osteoporosis, and heart disease

ethyl alcohol (ethanol): the consumable type of alcohol that is the psychoactive ingredient in alcoholic beverages; often called grain alcohol

etiology: specific cause of disease

etopic pregnancy: implanting of the embryo outside the uterus, usually in the fallopian tubes

eugenics: the science of improving human beings by selective breeding of people with desirable traits

eustress: stress resulting from pleasant stressors

euthanasia: helping someone who is on the verge of death or in a coma to die without suffering

exposure: actual amount of the substance people are exposed to

failure rate: likelihood of becoming pregnant if using a birth control method for one year

fallopian tubes: a pair of tube-like structures that transport ova from the ovaries to the uterus and that are the usual site of fertilization

familial hyperlipidemia (FH): an inherited disease causing extremely high levels of cholesterol in the blood

fat-soluble: soluble in fat; there are four fat-soluble vitamins

fatty acids: naturally occurring in fats, either saturated or unsaturated (monounsaturated or polyunsaturated)

feedback: response of the receiver of a message letting the sender know he or she received the message and what the message was

fertility awareness methods: methods of birth control in which a couple charts the cyclic signs of the woman's fertility and ovulation, using basal body temperature, mucus changes, and other signs to determine fertile periods

fertilization: the fusion of a sperm cell and an ovum

fetal alcohol syndrome: birth defects caused by ingestion of alcohol during pregnancy

fetus: the developing infant during the second and third trimesters of pregnancy

fiber: a group of compounds that make up the framework of plants; fiber cannot be digested

fibrillation: rapid, erratic contraction of the heart

fight-or-flight response: a defensive reaction that prepares the organism for conflict or escape by triggering hormonal, cardiovascular, metabolic, and other changes

fitness: the extent to which the body can respond to the demands of physical effort

fixation: the restricted movement of one or more vertebrae

flavonoids: antioxidant substance that may reduce the risk of heart disease

flexibility: the ability of a joint to move through its range of motion

food allergies: allergic responses to something that is eaten

forcible rape: sexual assault using force or threat of force, and involving sexual penetration of the victim's vagina, mouth, or rectum

foreskin: a fold of skin over the end of the penis

free radicals: oxidizing substances in the body that can damage blood vessels and tissues

fructose: a simple sugar found in fruits and honey

fungicide: a chemical that kills fungi

galactose: a monosaccharide derived from lactose, found in many gums and seaweeds

galvanic skin response: changes in the skin's electrical resistance in response to changes in a person's emotional state or arousal level

gametes: sex cells, either sperm or ova, that fuse at fertilization; gametes carry a complete set of genetic information from each parent that is passed on to the child

gamma irradiation: nonchemical method of food preservation

gangrene: decay of tissue when the blood supply is restricted

gender identity: awareness of being male or female

gender role: gender specific behaviors

gene therapy: a technique for replacing defective genes with normal ones in certain tissues of a person affected with a hereditary disease

genetic counseling: information to help prospective parents evaluate the risks of having or delivering a genetically handicapped child

gerontology: science that studies the causes and mechanisms of aging

gestation period: 266 days of fetal development

ginseng: an Asian plant whose roots are used in herbal medicines and teas

glucose: the principal source of energy in all cells; also called dextrose

glycogen: polysaccharide that is the principal form in which carbohydrates are stored in the body

goiter: an enlargement of the thyroid gland resulting from lack of iodine, causing a swelling in the front part of the neck

gonadotropins: pituitary hormones; induce production of the hormones estrogen and progesterone in the ovary

gonorrhea: a sexually transmitted disease caused by gonococal bacteria (*Neisseria gonorrhea*)

greenhouse effect: the ability of atmospheric carbon dioxide to reflect heat radiated from the earth back to the earth and to thereby raise the earth's temperature globally

growth needs: a human need that includes social belonging, self-esteem, and spiritual growth

habituation: repeating certain patterns of behavior until they become established or habitual

hallucinogens: psychoactive substances that alter sensory processing in the brain; produce visual or auditory sensations that are not real (are hallucinatory)

hangover: unpleasant physical sensations resulting from excessive alcohol consumption

hashish: the sticky resin of the Cannabis plant

health: state of sound physical, mental, and social well-being

health maintenance organization (HMO): an organization (either nonprofit or for-profit) of physicians, hospitals, and support staff that provides medical services to members

heart attack: death of, or damage to, part of the heart muscle due to an insufficient blood supply

hemicellulose: substances found in plant cell walls that are composed of various sugars chemically linked together

hemophilia: a hereditary disease (primarily in men) caused by a lack of an essential blood clotting factor; results in excessive bleeding in response to any scratch or injury

hepatitis: inflammation of the liver

herbal medicines: materials derived from plants and other organisms that are made into teas, powders, and salves to treat diseases and injuries

herbicide: a chemical that kills weeds

hereditary (genetic) disease: any disease due to the inheritance of defective genes or chromosomes from one or both parents

herpes: a sexually transmitted disease caused by Herpes simplex virus, HSV

heterosexual: someone who is attracted to people of the opposite gender

hierarchy of needs: a progression of human requirements, including physiological needs, safety, love, self-esteem, and self-actualization

high-density lipoprotein (HDL): the carrier of cholesterol from tissues to the liver for removal from the circulation; carrier of "good" cholesterol

histamine: a chemical released by cells in an allergic response; causes inflammation

histocompatibility: the degree to which the antigens on cells of different persons are similar

HIV (human immunodeficiency virus): the virus defined as the cause of AIDS

HLA (human leukocyte antigens): antigens that are measured to determine the suitability of an organ for transplantation from donor to recipient

homeopathy: an alternative medicine that administers very dilute solutions of substances that mimic the patient's symptoms

homeostasis: the tendency for body systems to interact in ways that maintain a constant physiological state

homosexual: someone who is attracted to people of the same gender

hormones: chemicals produced in the body that regulate body functions

hospice: usually a place for terminally ill patients to spend the time before death in an environment that attends to their physical, emotional, and spiritual needs, but where no further treatments are administered; hospice care also can be given in a patient's home

Human Chorionic Gonadotropin (HCG): a hormone produced furing the first stages of pregnancy; it is used as a basis for pregnancy tests

human immunodeficiency virus (HIV): the virus that causes AIDS; it causes a defect in the body's immune system by invading and then multiplying within the white blood cells

human papillomavirus (HPV): a genus of viruses including those causing papillomas (small nipple-like protrusions of the skin or mucous membrane) and warts

humoral immunity: the response of B-cells to infections

hypertension: high blood pressure

hypnotherapy: the use of hypnosis to treat sickness

hypnotics: CNS depressants used to induce drowsiness and encourage sleep

hypothalamus: a part of the brain that activates, controls, and integrates the autonomic nervous system, the endocrine system, and other bodily functions

hysterectomy: surgical removal of the uterus

I-statements: statements beginning with "I"; positive communication skill

illegal recreational use: taking illicit drugs for fun or pleasure to experience euphoria

image visualization: use of mental images to promote healing and to change behaviors

immune system: an interacting system of organs and cells that protect the body from infectious organisms and harmful substances

immunizations: vaccinations to prevent a variety of serious diseases caused by both bacteria and viruses

immunosuppressive drugs: drugs to suppress the functions of the immune system, for example, following organ transplants

immunotherapy: an experimental cancer therapy using immune system cells to kill cancer cells

in vitro fertilization (IVF): a procedure in which an egg is removed from a ripe follicle and fertilized by a sperm cell outside the human body; the fertilized egg is allowed to divide in a protected environment for about two days and then is inserted back into the uterus

incidence: frequency of occurrence of particular diseases

infarction: death of heart cells due to a blocked blood supply

infertile: unable to become pregnant or to impregnate

inhalants: vaporous substances that, when inhaled, produce alcohol-like intoxication

injury epidemiology: the study of the occurrence, causes, and prevention of injury

insecticide: a pesticide that kills insects

insemination: introduction of semen into the uterus or oviduct

insoluble fiber: cannot be dissolved in water

insomnia: prolonged inability to obtain adequate sleep

intellectual wellness: having a mind open to new ideas and concepts

intrauterine device (IUD): a flexible, usually plastic device inserted into the uterus to prevent pregnancy

ionizing radiation: radiation such as X-rays that can damage cells and cause cancer; also used to treat cancer

ischemia: an insufficient supply of blood to the heart

isometric training: another term for strength training

isoprenoids: fat-soluble vitamins that may reduce the risk of some cancers

isopropyl alcohol: rubbing alcohol, sometimes used as an anesthetic

Kaposi's sarcoma: skin cancer that occurs with (and without) HIV infection

karyotype: visual display of all of a person's chromosomes that can detect chromosomal abnormalities characteristic of inherited diseases

kilocalorie: unit of energy. The amount of heat needed to raise one kilogram of water one degree centigrade. A kilocalorie is equivalent to 1,000 calories

labia majora: a pair of fleshy folds that cover the labia minora

labia minora: a pair of fleshy folds that cover the vagina

labor: the process of childbirth

lactase: enzyme secreted by glands in the small intestine that converts lactose (milk sugar) into simple sugars

lacto-ovo-vegetarian: one who excludes meats, poultry, and fish, but includes eggs and dairy products

lacto-vegetarian: one who excludes meat, poultry, fish, and eggs but includes dairy products

lactose: a molecule of glucose and galactose chemically bonded together; found primarily in milk

laminaria: a plug of sterile dried kelp (seaweed) which expands when in contact with water and can thus be placed in the cervical canal to dilate the cervix

laparoscopy: a surgical incision into the abdomen used to visualize internal organs

laryngospasm: spasm of the larynx

lean body mass: structural and functional elements in cells, such as body water, muscle, and bone

learned behavior tolerance: apparently "normal" behavior in someone with a high blood alcohol content

lecithin: an essential component of cell membranes

leukocytes: white blood cells that fight infections

life expectancy: average number of years a person can expect to live

lightening: the positioning of the fetus for birth by descent in the uterus

linoleic acid: an essential fat that must be obtained from food

lipids: fats such as cholesterol and triglycerides

lipoprotein lipase: an enzyme secreted in the digestive tract that catalyzes the breakdown of fats

literal message: a message that is conveyed by symbols

living will: a legal document that expresses your wishes regarding treatment should you become unable to make your own medical decisions

low-density lipoprotein (LDL): the carrier of "bad" cholesterol in blood

lowest observed failure rate: likelihood of becoming pregnant if using a birth control method consistently and as intended

LSD: one of the most common hallucinogens; alters brain systems and produces behavioral effects that vary among individuals

lupus erythematosus: an autoimmune disease that mostly affects women

lutenizing hormone: anterior pituitary hormone that causes a follicle to release a ripened ovum and become a corpus luteum; in the male it stimulates testosterone production and the production of sperm cells

Lyme disease: a serious, difficult to diagnose infectious disease caused by disease-carrying ticks

lymph nodes: nodules spaced along the lymphatic vessels that trap infectious organisms or foreign particles

lymphatic system: a system of vessels in the body that trap foreign organisms and particles; the immune system is part of the lymphatic system

macrophages: special cells of the immune system that engulf and destroy foreign cells and particles

magnetic resonance imaging scan: use of a strong magnetic field to produce images of internal parts of the body; especially useful for soft tissues

maintenance needs: human needs that include physical safety and survival requirements such as food and water

malaria: a disease of red blood cells that produces fever, anemia, and death

malignant tumor: a tumor whose cells spread throughout the body

mammogram: an X-ray of the breast

mandala: an artistic religious design used as an object of meditation

mantra: the sound or phrase that is repeated in the mind to help produce a meditative state

marijuana: the dried leaves, flowers, stems, and seeds of plants of the genus *Cannabis*; contains psychoactive chemicals

masturbation: self-induced sexual stimulation

maximum life span: the theoretical maximum number of years that individuals of a species can live

medical model: measure of health, inclusive of numerical data for the prevalence and incidence of diseases

medicine: drugs used to prevent, treat, or cure illness; medicines are drugs that are prescribed by a physician

meditation: relaxed state of mind produced by focusing the mind on internal images, sounds, or passing thoughts

megadoses: large doses of a substance; used in reference to excessive vitamin supplementation

melanoma: a particularly dangerous form of skin cancer

menopause: the cessation of menstruation in mid-life

menstruation: the regular sloughing of the uterine lining via the vagina

meridians: the channels along the body where energy flows and where acupuncture points are located

mesothelioma: a form of lung cancer caused by asbestos

metamessage: how the message is interpreted between sender and receiver

metastasis: the process by which cancer cells spread throughout the body

methyl alcohol: wood alcohol or methanol

mifepristone or RU 486: a drug that blocks the natural hormone progesterone; used to prevent or abort an early pregnancy

minerals: inorganic elements found in the body both in combination with organic compounds and alone

minilaparotomy: female sterilization procedure in which the fallopian tubes are ligated or cauterized through a small abdominal incision

moist snuff: a moist form of snuff made from air- and fire-cured tobacco leaves; most hazardous form of smokeless tobacco

mononucleosis: an infectious disease caused by the Epstein-Barr virus, common among college-age adults

monounsaturated fat: generally liquid at room temperature; common sources are olive oil and nuts

morbidity: ratio of persons who are diseased to those who are well in a given community

morning-after pill: a hormonal drug which, if taken within 72 hours after unprotected intercourse, temporarily disrupts the uterine environment to prevent implantation of the fertilized egg; morning-after pills also prevent ovulation

mortality: death rate: number of deaths per unit of population (e.g., per 100, 10,000, or 1,000,000) in a specific region, age range, or other group

multiple sclerosis (MS): an autoimmune disease that affects the central nervous system

mutation: a permanent change in the genetic information in a cell; only mutations in sperm and eggs are inherited

myelin: a substance that sheaths and insulates nerve fibers in the brain and spinal cord

myocardium: muscular wall of the heart that contracts and relaxes

myotonia: muscle tension

mysophobia: fear of dirt and germs

narcolepsy: extreme tendency to sleep during the day

naturopathy: an alternative medicine that uses nutrition, herbs, massage, and other techniques to promote healing

nicotine: an addicting chemical in tobacco that produces rapid pulse, increased alertness, and a variety of other physiological effects

nitrates: preservatives containing any salt or ester of nitric acid. Some individuals are sensitive to nitrates and may suffer from headache, diarrhea, or urticaria after ingesting them

nitrites: preservatives containing any salt or ester of nitrous oxide acid

nonessential amino acids: eleven amino acids required for protein synthesis that are synthesized by humans and are not specifically required in the diet

norepinephrine: a hormone and neurotransmitter that has many of the same functions as epinephrine

Norplant: hormone-containing capsule inserted under the skin

nosocomial diseases: an infectious disease contracted while in the hospital for an unrelated disease or problem

nutritional calorie: unit of energy; often used interchangeably with the term kilocalorie

obesity: increase in body weight beyond skeletal and physical requirements

occupational wellness: enjoyment of what you are doing to earn a living and/or contribute to society

open-heart surgery: surgery performed on the opened heart while the blood supply is diverted through a heart-lung machine

ophediophobia: fear of snakes

opiates: derived from the opium poppy, they are drugs that depress the central nervous system.

opportunistic infections: any infectious disease in a patient with a weakened immune system; often occurs in AIDS patients

orgasm: the climax of sexual responses and the release of physiological and sexual tensions

osteopathy: an alternative medicine that uses manipulation and medicines for healing; osteopaths receive training comparable to that of physicians and can prescribe drugs

osteoporosis: a condition in older people, particularly women, in which bones lose density and become porous and brittle

ova: a term for female eggs (singular: ovum)

ovaries: a pair of almond-shaped organs in the female abdomen that produces egg cells (ova) and female sex hormones

over-the-counter (OTC) drugs: drugs that do not require a prescription

overweight: excessive fat tissue, exceeding the "ideal" weight listed by gender, height, and frame size

ovulation: release of an egg (ovum) from the ovary

ozone hole: an ozone-deficient portion of the atmosphere above Antarctica that has been steadily growing since the problem was first reported in 1985

ozone layer: a layer of ozone molecules located in the stratosphere in a diffuse band extending from 10 to 30 miles above the earth's surface

pacemaker: an electrical device implanted in the chest to control the heartbeat

panic attacks: severe anxiety accompanied by physical symptoms

parasomnias: activities that interrupt restful sleep

parasympathetic nervous system: a division of the autonomic nervous system that tones down the excitatory effects of the sympathetic nervous system; slows metabolism and restores energy reserves

pathogens: disease-causing organisms

pathologist: a physician who specializes in the causes of diseases

pelvic inflammatory disease (PID): inflammation of the pelvic structures, especially the uterus and fallopian tubes; often caused by a sexually transmitted disease

penicillin: an antibiotic produced by mold and capable of curing many bacterial infections

penis: the male's organ of copulation and urination

pesticides: chemicals that kill insects and other unwanted organisms

phencyclidine (PCP): drug that, depending on the route of administration and dose, can be a stimulant, depressant, or hallucinogen; originally developed as an anesthetic

phenylpropanolamine (PPA): active ingredient in over-the-counter weight-control products

phobia: a powerful and irrational fear of something

physical dependence: a physiological state that depends on the continuous presence of a drug; absence of the drug may cause discomfort, nervousness, headaches, sweating (withdrawal symptoms) and sometimes death

physical wellness: maintenance of your body in good condition by eating right, exercising regularly, avoiding harmful habits, and making informed responsible decisions about your health

physician-assisted suicide: a form of active euthanasia in which a physician helps a patient who no longer desires to live because of pain or an incurable illness to commit suicide

phytochemicals: chemicals produced by plants

phytosterols: sterols of vegetable origin

placebo effect: healing that results from a person's belief in a treatment that has no medicinal value

placenta: the flat circular vascular structure within the pregnant uterus that provides nourishment to and eliminates wastes from the developing embryo and fetus and is passed as afterbirth after the baby is born

plague: a bacterial infectious disease that killed hundreds of millions of people in the past before antibiotics were discovered

plaque: deposit of fatty substances in the inner lining of arteries

platelets: cells in the blood that are essential for clotting

plumbism: disease caused by lead poisoning

poison: any chemical substance that causes illness, injury, or death

polychlorinated biphenyls (PCBs): a family of banned synthetic, organic chemicals that affect the human thyroid gland and reproductive systems of animals

polyunsaturated fat: generally liquid at room temperature; common sources are safflower, sunflower, soybean, and sesame oils

polyunsaturated fatty acid (PUFA): a saturated fat except for two or more parts that are unsaturated

post-traumatic stress disorder (PTSD): reactions following an event that is outside the range of usual human experience and would be distressing to almost anyone

prana: the life force in the body that is derived from cosmic consciousness

preferred provider organization (PPO): physicians who belong to the organization provide medical care at reduced costs that are negotiated by the organization

prevalence: predominance of particular diseases

progestin-only contraceptives: work by inhibiting ovulation and thickening of the cervical mucus; completely reversible

progressive relaxation: a specific technique that produces relaxation by tensing and relaxing muscles

prolactin: a hormone produced by the anterior lobe of the pituitary gland that stimulates milk secretion

proof: a number assigned to an alcoholic product that is twice the percentage of alcohol in that product

prostate gland: gland at the base of the bladder providing seminal fluid

proteins: the foundation of every body cell; biological molecules composed of chains of amino acids

psychoactive: a substance that primarily alters mood, perception, and other brain functions

psychological dependence: dependence that results because a drug produces pleasant mental effects

psychosomatic illnesses: physical illnesses brought on by negative mental states such as stress or emotional upset

pubic lice: small insects that live in hair in the genital-rectal region

puerperium: the six weeks after childbirth, also called postpartum period

radiation therapy: use of high-energy radiation such as X-rays to kill cancer cells and treat some forms of cancer

radon: a radioactive gas found in some homes that can increase the risk of cancer

rapid eye movement sleep (REM): stage of sleep in which dreams occur

reactive hypoglycemia: occurring after the ingestion of carbohydrate, with consequent excessive release of insulin

receptor: protein on the surface or inside a cell to which a drug or natural substance can bind and affect cell function

Recommended [Daily] Dietary Allowances (RDA): levels of nutrients recommended by the Food and Nutrition Board of the National Academy of Sciences for daily consumption by healthy individuals, scaled according to gender and age

relaxation response: the physiological changes in the body that result from mental relaxation techniques

releasing factors: hormones produced in the hypothalamus that control the release of hormones from the pituitary gland

retrovirus: a type of virus (such as the one that causes AIDS) that can invade cells and integrate its own genetic information into chromosomes

rheumatoid arthritis: an autoimmune disease that affects joints

risk factor: an element or condition involving certain hazard or danger

RNA: (ribonucleic acid): a chemical substance found in some viruses such as HIV that also carry genetic information; the RNA is converted to DNA when such viruses infect cells

rodenticide: a chemical that kills mice and rats

safety: an ever-changing condition in which one attempts to minimize the risk of injury, illness, or property damage from the hazards to which one may be exposed

saturated fat: generally solid at room temperature; comes from animal sources

scabies: infestation of the skin by microscopic mites (insects)

schizophrenia: a mental disorder that involves a disturbance in thinking, in perceiving reality, and in functioning

scrotum: the sac of skin that contains the testes

secondary hypertension: high blood pressure due to a recognizable disease or problem

secondary sex characteristics: anatomical features appearing at puberty that distinguish males from females

sedatives: CNS depressants used to relieve anxiety, fear, and apprehension

self-actualization: a state in which a person has achieved the highest level of growth in Maslow's hierarchy of needs

self-disclosure: sharing personal experiences and feelings with someone

self-efficacy: your belief that you are capable of handling the situation; self-esteem

semen: a whitish, creamy fluid containing sperm

seminal vesicles: sac-like structures that secrete a fluid that activates the sperm

seminiferous tubules: convoluted tubules in the testicles that produce sperm

senile dementia: loss of cognitive functions in elderly people

sex: has several definitions: 1) an individual's classification as male or female based on anatomical characteristics; 2) a set of behaviors; 3) the experience of erotic pleasure

sexual: characterized by or having sex; opposed to asexual

sexual assault: violent actions that include rape, incest, attempted rape, and unwanted sexual touching

sexual orientation: attraction toward and interest in members of one or both genders

sexual response cycle: the physiological response in both men and women as described in four phases

sexuality: a person's sense of self that is used to create sexual experiences

sexually transmitted disease (STDs): infections passed from person to person by sexual contact

sexually transmitted warts: hard growths caused by an infection with human papilloma virus, HPV, that appears on the skin of the genitals or anus

sick building syndrome: collection of symptoms reported by workers in some modern buildings

side effects: unintended and often harmful actions of a drug

sidestream smoke (passive smoking): smoke released into the environment directly from lighted tip of cigarettes

simple sugars: a class of carbohydrates called monosaccharides; all carbohydrates must be reduced to simple sugars to be digested

sinoatrial node: the region of the heart that produces an electrical signal that causes the heart to contract

sleep apnea: state of troubled or interrupted breathing while sleeping

smegma: a white, cheesy substance that accumulates under the foreskin of the penis

smog: air polluted by chemicals, smoke, particles, dust, and so on

snuff: a form of smokeless tobacco; made from powdered or finely cut leaves

social wellness: ability to perform the expectations of social roles effectively, comfortably, and without harming others

soluble fiber: can be dissolved in water

somatization: occurrence of physical symptoms without any bodily disease or injury being present

somnambulism: sleepwalking

specific metabolic rate: the amount of energy per gram of body weight consumed per day by mammals of different species

spectatoring: observing one's own sexual experience rather than fully taking part in it

spermicide: a chemical that kills sperm; particularly foams, creams, jellies, and suppositories used for contraception

spiritual wellness: state of balance and harmony with yourself and others

squamous cell carcinoma: a common form of skin cancer that is curable if detected early

starch: long chain of glucose molecules

sterility: not being able to be impregnated or impregnate

stimulants: drugs that produce nervous system excitement; including cocaine, caffeine, amphetamines

stomach ulcers: open sores that occur in the stomach or small intestine for reasons largely unknown

storage fat: also called depot fat; excess fat that is deposited in various parts of the body

strength training: the use of resistance to increase one's ability to exert or resist force for the purpose of improving performance

stress: the sum of physical and emotional reactions to any stimulus that disturbs the organism's homeostasis

stress response: the physiological changes associated with stress

stressor: any physical or psychological event or condition that produces stress

stroke: an insufficient supply of blood to the brain resulting in loss of muscle function, loss of speech, or other symptoms

subluxation: partial displacement of a vertebra from its correct position

sucrose: common refined "table" sugar; a molecule of glucose and a molecule of fructose chemically bonded together

sulfites: used as preservatives for salad, fresh fruit and vegetables, wine, beer, and dried fruit; in susceptible individuals, especially those with asthma, they can cause a severe reaction

suppositories: a medicine placed in a body orifice to dissolve and sometimes to be absorbed; birth control suppositories contain spermicidal chemicals

sympathetic nervous system: a division of the autonomic nervous system that reacts to danger or challenges by almost instantly putting the body processes in high gear

sympto-thermal method: using both the BBT and the mucus methods at the same time

syphilis: a sexually transmitted disease caused by spirochete bacteria (*Treponema pallidum*)

systole: the pressure in the arteries when the heart contracts

T-cells: cells of the immune system that attack foreign organisms that infect the body

tar: the yellowish brown residue of tobacco smoke

tartrazine: a yellow food dye, referred to by the FDA as "FD&C yellow No. 5"

teratogen: any environmental substance that affects the normal development of a fetus in people or other mammals; causes birth defects

testes: a pair of male reproductive organs that produce sperm cells and male sex hormones

theoretical effectiveness: how well a birth control method performs if it is used as intended and consistently

thyroxin: a hormone produced by the thyroid gland

tinnitis: a persistent ringing in the ears caused by repeated or sudden exposure to loud noises

tocotrienols: have some biological vitamin E activity

tolerance: a condition in which increased amounts of a drug or increased exposure to an addictive behavior are required to produce desired effects

toxemia: an infrequent complication of pregnancy characterized by high blood pressure, swelling, and possible convulsions

toxic shock syndrome: a severe bacterial illness characterized by a sudden high fever, vomiting, diarrhea, aches, and a sunburn-like rash; it usually occurs in menstruating females using superabsorbant tampons

trachea: upper part of respiratory tract

training effect: beneficial physiological changes as a result of exercise

tranquilizers: central nervous system depressants that relax the body and calm anxiety

tubal ligation: a surgical procedure in women in which the fallopian tubes are cut, tied, or cauterized to prevent pregnancy; a form of sterilization

tumor: a mass of abnormal cells

tumor viruses: viruses that infect cells, change their growth properties, and cause cancer

type A behavior: behaviors characterized by traits such as anger or hostility that contribute to the risk of heart disease

typical failure rate: likelihood of becoming pregnant considering all the potential problems associated with a birth control method

ultrasound scanning: use of sound waves to visualize the fetus in the womb

unconscious: whatever is in the mind but out of the awareness

undernutrition: restricting the daily caloric intake of an animal or person without causing malnutrition

unintentional injury: preferred term for accidental injury; result of an accident

universal donor: a person whose blood is accepted by everyone during transfusion

universal recipient: a person whose blood type is compatible with anyone else's blood

urethra: a tube that carries urine from the bladder to the outside

urethritis: an irritation or infection of the urethra caused by bacteria

uterus: the female organ in which a fetus develops

V

vacuum (suction) curettage: removal of fetal tissue by suctioning off the contents of the uterus

vagina: a woman's organ of copulation and the exit pathway for the fetus at birth

vaginitis: an infection of the vagina

varicose veins: swelling of veins (usually in the legs) due to defective valves

vasectomy: a surgical procedure in men in which segments of the vas deferens are removed and the ends tied to prevent the passage of sperm

vasocongestion: the engorgement of blood vessels in particular body parts in response to sexual arousal

vector: the carrier of infectious organisms from animals to people or from person to person

vegan: one who excludes all animal products from the diet including milk, cheese, eggs, and other dairy products

vegetarian: one who consumes no meat, poultry, or fish

veins: blood vessels that return blood from tissues to the heart

violence: use of force and power

vital statistics: numerical data relating to birth, death, disease, marriage, and health

vitamins: essential organic substances needed daily in small amounts to perform specific functions in the body

warm-up: low-intensity exercise done before full-effort physical activity in order to improve muscle and joint performance, prevent injury, reinforce motor skills, and maximize blood flow to the muscles and heart

water-soluble: soluble in water; there are nine water-soluble vitamins

weaned: to discontinue breast-feeding, using other means to provide nutrients

wellness: emphasizes individual responsibility for well-being through the practice of health-promoting life-style behaviors

Western blot test: a test to determine the presence of specific HIV proteins; very accurate

withdrawal symptoms: uncomfortable and sometimes dangerous reactions that occur after a person stops taking a physically addicting drug

xenoestrogens: environmental chemicals that mimic the effects of natural estrogen

yoga: a combination of physical movements and mental exercises that relax the mind and the body

you-statements: statements beginning with "You"; negative communication skill

yo-yo dieting: repeated cycles of weight loss and gain

zoophobia: fear of animals

zygote: the first cell of a new person, formed at fertilization

Index